Rapid Review
USMLE Step 3

David D. K. Rolston, MD
Staff Physician
Department of General Internal Medicine
Cleveland Clinic
Cleveland, Ohio

Craig Nielsen, MD
Staff Physician
Department of General Internal Medicine
Cleveland Clinic
Cleveland, Ohio

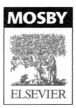
MOSBY

ELSEVIER

1600 John F. Kennedy Blvd.
Suite 1800
Philadelphia, PA 19103-2899

RAPID REVIEW: USMLE STEP 3

ISBN: 978-0-323-01981-1

Library of Congress Cataloging-in-Publication Data

Rolston, David.
  Rapid review for USMLE step 3 / David Rolston, Craig Nielson.—1st ed.
       p. ; cm.—(Rapid review series)
  ISBN 978-0-323-01981-1
  1. Medicine—Examinations, questions, etc. 2. Medicine—Outlines, syllabi, etc. I. Nielsen, Craig.
II. Title. III. Series.
  [DNLM: 1. Medicine—Examination Questions. WB 18.2 R755r 2008]
R834.5.R65 2008
610.76—dc22   2007022587

Publishing Director: Linda Belfus
Acquisitions Editor: James Merritt
Developmental Editor: Katie DeFrancesco
Design Direction: Steven Stave

Printed in the United States of America.

Last digit is the print number: 9 8 7 6 5 4 3 2 1

Rapid Review
USMLE Step 3

Rapid Review Series

Series Editor
Edward F. Goljan, MD

Behavioral Science, Second Edition
Vivian M. Stevens, PhD; Susan K. Redwood, PhD; Jackie L. Neel, DO;
Richard H. Bost, PhD; Nancy W. Van Winkle, PhD; Michael H. Pollak, PhD

Biochemistry, Second Edition
John W. Pelley, PhD; Edward F. Goljan, MD

Gross and Developmental Anatomy, Second Edition
N. Anthony Moore, PhD; William A. Roy, PhD, PT

Histology and Cell Biology, Second Edition
E. Robert Burns, PhD; M. Donald Cave, PhD

Laboratory Testing in Clinical Medicine
Edward F. Goljan, MD; Karlis I. Sloka, DO

Microbiology and Immunology, Second Edition
Ken S. Rosenthal, PhD; James S. Tan, MD

Neuroscience
James A. Weyhenmeyer, PhD; Eve A. Gallman, PhD

Pathology, Second Edition
Edward F. Goljan, MD

Pharmacology, Second Edition
Thomas L. Pazdernik, PhD; Laszlo Kerecsen, MD

Physiology
Thomas A. Brown, MD

USMLE Step 2
Michael W. Lawlor, MD

USMLE Step 3
David D. K. Rolston, MD; Craig Nielsen, MD

To my wife, Raj, for her immeasurable support, boundless encouragement in all that I have undertaken, and for being an unwavering source of inspiration. To my family for their support, and to my many students from whom I have learned much.

DR

To my lovely wife and children

CN

Contributors

Erica Anderson, DO
Former Senior Resident
Internal Medicine Residency Program
Cleveland Clinic
Cleveland, Ohio
Rheumatology

Iyad Azrak, MD
Former Senior Resident
Internal Medicine Residency Program
Cleveland Clinic
Cleveland, Ohio
Ophthalmology

Nadia Bajwa, MD
Former Chief Resident
Department of Pediatrics
Cleveland Clinic
Cleveland, Ohio
Pediatrics

Yvonne Braver, MD
Staff Physician
Department of General Internal Medicine
Cleveland Clinic
Cleveland, Ohio
Obstetrics and Gynecology

David Einstein, MD
Staff Physician
Department of Radiology
Cleveland Clinic
Cleveland, Ohio
Radiology

Tatiana Falcone, MD
Former Chief Resident
Department of Psychiatry
Cleveland Clinic
Cleveland, Ohio
Psychiatry

Natasha Frost, MD
Former Chief Resident
Department of Neurology
Cleveland Clinic
Cleveland, Ohio
Neurology

Paul Gubanich, MD
Sports Medicine Fellow
Department of Orthopedics
Cleveland Clinic
Cleveland, Ohio
Orthopedics

Thomas Helton, DO
Former Chief Medical Resident
Internal Medicine Residency Program
Cleveland Clinic
Cleveland, Ohio
Cardiology

Byron Hoogwerf, MD
Staff Physician
Department of Endocrinology
Cleveland Clinic
Cleveland, Ohio
Endocrinology

Jesse Jacob, MD
Former Chief Medical Resident
Internal Medicine Residency Program
Cleveland Clinic
Cleveland, Ohio
*Infectious Diseases; Preventive Medicine and
Miscellaneous Topics; Surgery*

Jacobo Kirsch, MD
Former Resident
Department of Radiology
Cleveland Clinic
Cleveland, Ohio
Radiology

Abigail Lara, MD
Former Senior Resident
Internal Medicine Residency Program
Cleveland Clinic
Cleveland, Ohio
Pulmonology

Martin Lascano, MD
Former Chief Medical Resident
Internal Medicine Residency Program
Cleveland Clinic
Cleveland, Ohio
*Nephrology and Urology; Preventive Medicine and
Miscellaneous Topics; Surgery*

Aruna Mani, MD
Former Senior Resident
Internal Medicine Residency Program
Cleveland Clinic
Cleveland, Ohio
Emergency Medicine

Frank Marrero, MD
Former Chief Medical Resident
Internal Medicine Residency Program
Cleveland Clinic
Cleveland, Ohio
Gastroenterology

Jonelle McDonald, MD
Staff Physician
Department of Dermatology
Cleveland Clinic
Cleveland, Ohio
Dermatology

Neil Mehta, MD
Staff Physician
Department of General Internal Medicine
Cleveland Clinic
Cleveland, Ohio
Ophthalmology

Tarek Mekhail, MD
Staff Physician
Department of Hematology and Medical Oncology
Cleveland Clinic
Cleveland, Ohio
Hematology and Oncology

Donald Moffa, MD
Staff Physician and Director of Medical Education
Department of Emergency Medicine
Cleveland Clinic
Cleveland, Ohio
Emergency Medicine

Marisha Newton, MD
Former Senior Resident
Internal Medicine Residency Program
Cleveland Clinic
Cleveland, Ohio
Endocrinology

Craig Nielsen, MD
Staff Physician
Department of General Internal Medicine
Cleveland Clinic
Cleveland, Ohio
Orthopedics

Alison Protain, DO
Former Chief Resident
Department of Pediatrics
Cleveland Clinic
Cleveland, Ohio
Pediatrics

David Rolston, MD
Staff Physician
Department of General Internal Medicine
Cleveland Clinic
Cleveland, Ohio
Gastroenterology

Andrew Russman, DO
Former Chief Resident
Department of Neurology
Cleveland Clinic
Cleveland, Ohio
Neurology

Dale Shepard, MD
Former Senior Resident
Internal Medicine Residency Program
Cleveland Clinic
Cleveland, Ohio
Otorhinolaryngology

Anita Shivadas, MD
Former Senior Resident
Internal Medicine Residency Program
Cleveland Clinic
Cleveland, Ohio
Obstetrics and Gynecology

Navneet Sidhu, MD
Former Chief Resident
Department of Psychiatry
Cleveland Clinic
Cleveland, Ohio
Psychiatry

Apra Sood, MD
Former Resident
Department of Dermatology
Cleveland Clinic
Cleveland, Ohio
Dermatology

Ramon Tiu, MD
Former Senior Resident
Internal Medicine Residency Program
Cleveland Clinic
Cleveland, Ohio
Hematology and Oncology

Series Preface

The *Rapid Review Series* has received high critical acclaim from students studying for the United States Medical Licensing Examination (USMLE) Step 1 and high ratings in *First Aid for the USMLE Step 1*. This volume provides a concise review for the USMLE Step 3 exam, summarizing most diseases' pathophysiology, presentation, diagnosis, and treatment in less than one page for efficient review.

SPECIAL FEATURES

Book

- **Outline format:** Concise, high-yield subject matter is presented in a study-friendly format.
- **Visual elements:** Abundant two-color schematics, black and white images, and summary tables enhance your study experience.
- **Two practice examinations:** Two sets of 50 USMLE Step 3–type multiple-choice questions (including images where necessary) and complete discussions (rationales) for all options are included.

New! Online Study and Testing Tool

- **More than 200 USMLE Step 3–type MCQs:** Multiple-choice questions that mimic the current board format are presented. These include complete rationales for all answer options. All of the questions from the book are included so you can study them in the most effective mode for you!
- **Test mode:** Select from randomized 50-question blocks or by subject topics for an exam-like review session. This mode features a 60-minute timer to simulate the actual exam, a detailed assessment report that can be printed or saved to your hard drive, and direct links to all or only incorrect questions. The links include your answer, the correct answer, and full rationales for all answer options, so you can fully analyze your test session and learn from your mistakes.
- **Study mode:** Like the test mode, in the study mode you can select from randomized 50-question sets or by subject topics to create a dynamic study session. This mode features unlimited attempts at each question, instant feedback (either on selection of the correct answer or when using the "Show Answer" feature), complete rationales for all answer options, and a detailed progress report that can be printed or saved to your hard drive.
- **Online access:** Online access allows you study from an Internet-enabled computer wherever and whenever it is convenient. This access is activated through registration on www.studentconsult.com with the pincode printed inside of the front cover.

Student Consult

- **Full online access:** You can access the complete text and illustrations of this book on www.studentconsult.com.
- **Save content to your PDA:** Through our unique Pocket Consult platform, you can clip selected text and illustrations and save them to your PDA for study on the fly!
- **Free content:** An interactive community center with a wealth of additional valuable resources is available.

Preface

Medical knowledge continues to increase by leaps and bounds and by all accounts will continue to do so. It is therefore a challenge to distill a large body of knowledge regarding a disease into a few short paragraphs. We believe that the essence of the core areas of knowledge that are tested in the USMLE Step 3 examination have been presented in this book. Each disease is discussed under the following headings: basic science; history and physical, laboratory, and diagnostic studies; formulating the diagnosis; evaluating the severity of the disease; and managing the patient. Unlike in traditional textbooks, the information is provided in "bullet format." We believe that this format, as well as the discussion under the various headings, will help the reader remember and understand the information more effectively. It is our hope that this book will be used not only as a study guide, but also as a handy reference for the diseases discussed.

The book is supplemented by USMLE Step 3–style questions with explanations as to why a particular answer is correct and the other choices are not. The questions and answers have been written to facilitate the reader's understanding of the subject.

We urge all readers to read standard textbooks as well to expand their knowledge in medicine, surgery, pediatrics, and obstetrics and gynecology so that they are better prepared for the Step 3 examination.

We gratefully acknowledge the help, guidance, and encouragement from all at Elsevier, particularly James Merritt, Katie DeFrancesco, and Nicole DiCicco.

David D. K. Rolston, MD, FACP
Craig Nielsen, MD, FACP

Contents

Neurology

I. Alzheimer's Disease
  A. Basic science
   - Alzheimer's disease is the most common form of dementia.
   - The etiology of Alzheimer's disease remains unclear, but genetics play a role. Mutations in chromosomes 1, 14, 19, and 21 have been associated with Alzheimer's disease.
   - There is a known association between Alzheimer's disease and Down syndrome (trisomy 21). Up to 90% of Down syndrome patients over age 30 have the pathologic changes of Alzheimer's disease.
   - In Alzheimer's disease there is a decrease in acetylcholine due to the loss of choline acetyltransferase.
   - The pathologic hallmarks of Alzheimer's disease are neuritic plaques (containing amyloid proteins) and neurofibrillary tangles (paired helical filaments containing tau proteins) in the cortex and hippocampus. There is often gross atrophy of the brain, mostly in the temporoparietal regions and frontal poles.
  B. History and physical examination
   - The most important risk factor for developing Alzheimer's disease is advanced age.
   - Patients present with a progressive decline in cognition and general functioning. A sudden change in cognitive function should prompt evaluation for another cause such as infection or intoxication. They have abnormalities in at least two of the following cognitive spheres: memory, language, spatial orientation, personality and social skills, abstract reasoning, and judgment. Impairment of memory is usually the first symptom.
   - An individual is said to have mild cognitive impairment (MCI) when cognitive impairment affects daily activities. MCI often progresses to Alzheimer's dementia.
   - Some patients have insight into their deficits, but others do not (anosognosia).
   - As the disease progresses, patients may become apathetic and may develop behavioral disturbances resulting in aggression, restlessness, and wandering. Patients eventually become totally unable to care for themselves. They are unable to speak or walk, and they lose basic biologic functions such as sphincter control. From 10% to 15% of patients also develop seizures.
   - On neurologic examination, mental status testing reveals cognitive impairment in two or more spheres. A mini-mental status examination may be normal early in the course of the disease, and more detailed neuropsychological testing

may be necessary to uncover a deficit. Disturbances of affect and behavior may also be noted. Except in advanced Alzheimer's, the remainder of the neurologic examination should be normal. Focal findings early in the course should alert one to other diagnoses, such as multi-infarct dementia or multiple system atrophy.

C. Laboratory and diagnostic studies

- Brain imaging can show atrophy, especially entorhinal and hyppocampal, although the presence of atrophy does not necessarily mean that someone has Alzheimer's disease. Diagnostic imaging and laboratory tests are generally performed to rule out reversible causes of dementia (discussed in Section I, D).

D. Formulating the diagnosis

- The diagnosis of Alzheimer's disease requires the clinical diagnosis of a dementia syndrome without another explanation and a postmortem confirmation of typical pathologic findings.
- The first step is to determine that the patient is actually demented. Demented patients have acquired fixed deficits in at least two cognitive spheres. Treatable and possibly reversible causes of dementia should be ruled out. These causes include pseudodementia secondary to depression, hypothyroidism, vitamin B_{12} and thiamine deficiencies, normal pressure hydrocephalus, chronic infections such as syphilis, subdural hematoma, brain tumors, and metabolic abnormalities including intoxications.
- Laboratory tests should include complete blood count and full chemistry profile, plus assessment of vitamin B_{12}, thyroid-stimulating hormone (TSH), and rapid plasma reagin (RPR). Human immunodeficiency virus (HIV) testing should also be considered.
- A computed tomography (CT) scan of the brain should be considered to rule out a mass lesion, normal pressure hydrocephalus, and subdural hematoma.
- Formal neuropsychological testing can help distinguish Alzheimer's disease from other nonreversible dementias such as frontal temporal dementia, vascular dementia (Binswanger's dementia), dementia associated with the parkinsonian syndromes, and the "reversible dementias."

E. Evaluating the severity of problems

- Alzheimer's disease is a progressive debilitating disease that ultimately leads to a loss of ability to care for oneself and a loss of control or performance of many basic biologic functions. Patients need increasing observation and supervision because poor judgment predisposes them to accidents. They may eventually be unable to eat and they are at risk for aspiration pneumonia.

F. Managing the patient

- There is no cure for Alzheimer's disease.
- Agents available for treating cognitive deficits in Alzheimer's disease include the cholinesterase inhibitors donezepil, rivastigmine, and galantamine. These agents enhance cholinergic function.
- Memantine, a NMDA (*N*-methyl-D-aspartate) receptor antagonist, can be used alone or to augment treatment with the cholinesterase inhibitors.
- Other treatments are directed at target symptoms and may include psychotropic medications for psychiatric and behavioral disturbances.

Medications that can worsen mental status should be avoided, and infections should be treated promptly.
- Patients need extensive supportive care and assistance with activities of daily living.

II. Brain Death
  A. Basic science
   - Death is defined as the total cessation of life. Death is determined by fulfilling certain defined criteria.
   - The first criterion that can be used to establish death is the irreversible cessation of circulatory and respiratory function.
   - The second criterion that can be used to determine death is the irreversible cessation of all brain function, including the brainstem (brain death).
   - Brain death is usually caused by hypoxic-ischemic brain injury, severe head trauma, or subarachnoid hemorrhage. Less frequently, severe metabolic disease or intoxication will cause irreversible loss of brain function.
   - This discussion pertains to adults and children older than 5 years of age. A prolonged observation period and a very individualized evaluation are necessary in children under age 5 before making the diagnosis of brain death.
  B. History and physical examination
   - Establishing brain death mandates that the physician identify a cause of coma that is sufficient to account for the loss of brain function (e.g., trauma).
   - If such history is not available, then reversible causes of severe coma must be considered and ruled out. Hypothermia, drug intoxication, neuromuscular blockade, circulatory failure (shock), and major metabolic derangements may all produce reversible coma.
   - In order for a person to be declared brain dead the physical diagnosis must demonstrate coma, absence of brainstem reflexes, and apnea.
   - The systolic blood pressure must be greater than 90 mm Hg, and a core body temperature must be 35°C or higher.
   - There can be no evidence of any drug intoxication that may result in coma (barbiturates).
   - These exclusion criteria were established to prevent misdiagnosis of patients with potentially reversible causes of coma or apnea. Furthermore, the physical examination should demonstrate no cerebral motor responses such as decorticate or decerebrate posturing. Spinal reflexes, however, may be preserved.
   - All brainstem reflexes (i.e., pupillary light response, oculocephalic reflex, oculovestibular reflex, cold caloric test, corneal reflex, gag reflex, and cough reflex) must be absent. There is no response to noxious stimulation. There is no spontaneous respiratory effort during formal apnea testing.
   - A repeat clinical evaluation, usually between 6 and 24 hours, is recommended.
  C. Laboratory and diagnostic studies
   - An apnea test should show no evidence of spontaneous respirations. The apnea test is performed by providing 100% oxygen through the ventilator (spontaneous respiration is absent and patients are connected to a respirator).

The ventilator is disconnected and oxygen provided through a tracheal cannula. The patient is said to be completely apneic if there is no respiratory effort when arterial P_{CO_2} is greater than 50 to 60 mm Hg.

- Blood work is obtained to rule out metabolic derangements (such as severe electrolyte disturbance), hepatic failure, and uremic disease. Screening for drug intoxication should be done.
- Other supportive tests may include EEG (electroencephalogram) demonstrating electrocerebral silence and vascular studies demonstrating circulatory cessation (angiogram or transcranial doppler).

D. Formulating the diagnosis
- Reversible causes of coma should always be considered. However, if reversible coma is ruled out and the three criteria of brain death (coma, absence of brain stem reflexes, apnea) are met, the patient may be pronounced dead.

E. Evaluating the severity of problems
- Disorders that may mimic brain death are generally life-threatening as well and mandate immediate treatment.

F. Managing the patient
- Until the diagnosis of death is made, the treatment is supportive.
- Patients being evaluated for brain death should be considered for organ donation.
- Once the patient is declared dead by brain death criteria the family should be notified of the death.

III. Brain Tumors
A. Basic science
- Brain tumors can be primary central nervous system tumors or metastatic tumors from systemic neoplasms.
- Primary brain tumors can be divided into several histologic classes (common examples of classes are in parenthesis): astryocytomas (glioblastoma multiforme), oligodendrogliomas, ependymomas, neuroectodermal tumors (medulloblastoma), meningeal tumors (meningioma), nerve sheath tumors (schwannoma), germ cell tumors (teratoma), tumors of blood vessel origin (hemangioblastoma), choroid plexus tumors, neuronal tumors (ganglioneuroma), and primary central nervous system (CNS) lymphomas.
- Glioblastoma multiforme is the most common primary brain tumor in adults. It is frequently associated with edema, necrosis, and a median survival period of less than 6 months.
- The most common metastatic brain tumors include lung carcinoma, melanoma, breast malignancies, gastrointestinal cancer, and renal cell carcinoma. Lung cancer is the most common cancer that metastatizes to the brain.
- Over half of metastatic brain lesions are multiple.
- Metastatic cancers that are commonly hemorrhagic include renal cancer, thyroid cancer, melanoma, and choriocarcinoma.

B. History and physical examination
- Clinical symptoms of brain tumors may be attributed either to local destructive effects of the tumor or to a mass effect in the brain. Mass effect produces increased intracranial pressure.
- Depending on the location of the tumor, the patient may present with hemiparesis (muscular weakness on one side of the body), aphasia (defective language function), personality change, seizure, visual disturbance, or ataxia (an impaired ability to coordinate movement).
- Increased intracranial pressure can cause papilledema, headache, nausea, vomiting, and cranial nerve palsies. More severe increases in pressure may lead to a Cushing response, characterized by bradycardia and hypertension. Cushing response is more commonly seen in children.

C. Laboratory and diagnostic studies
- CT or magnetic resonance imaging (MRI) with intravenous contrast material will show a mass. This may be ring enhancing with central necrosis or hemorrhage. There may also be extensive surrounding edema.
- Lumbar puncture should be avoided in patients with signs of mass effect, because this may precipitate herniation. Imaging should be done before lumbar puncture, especially if there are focal neurologic signs. Cerebrospinal fluid (CSF) is usually sterile but should be sent for routine studies and cytologic examination to look for malignant cells. CSF can help differentiate a tumor from other infectious and inflammatory processes.
- Biopsy is often necessary to determine the type of tumor before treatment can be initiated. In the presence of brain metastases, biopsy of the extracranial neoplasm is generally safer. A thorough investigation for the site of a primary cancer is therefore usually undertaken.

D. Formulating the diagnosis
- The diagnosis of a brain tumor is made primarily through imaging studies and biopsy.

E. Evaluating the severity of problems
- Signs of increased intracranial pressure, demonstrated either by physical examination or by CT scan, are alarming because brain herniation may follow and rapidly cause death.
- Seizures are also a serious complication and should be treated as they arise (see Section XI, Seizures). Prophylactic treatment may also be given.

F. Managing the patient
- Developing a treatment plan depends on the type of tumor identified.
- Prognosis is variable and is based on age, functional status (e.g., Karnofsky performance scale in which a score of 100 is normal, with no complaints and no evidence of disease; if the score <70 and the disease not treatable, the prognosis is poor), and type of tumor.
- Treatment almost always includes steroids (dexamethasone) to decrease edema. It can also include a combination of surgical resection, chemotherapy, and radiation.
- Response to treatment should be monitored with repeated imaging studies.

- An anticonvulsant (e.g., phenytoin) can be used if seizures occur.
- When there are signs of increasing cerebral edema and impending herniation, temporizing measures such as mannitol and hyperventilation can be used while preparing for surgical decompression.

IV. Cerebrovascular Disease
   A. Basic science
- The brain receives blood from two different vascular systems; the carotid and the vertebral.
- Stroke is defined as the acute onset of neurologic dysfunction secondary to cerebral ischemia, occurring in a vascular territory, lasting longer than 24 hours.
- A transient ischemic attack (TIA) is defined as acute neurologic dysfunction secondary to cerebral ischemia lasting less than 24 hours. In reality, most TIAs last less than 20 minutes. TIAs and ischemic strokes are caused by the same underlying pathology.
- The overall risk of stroke in a patient with a TIA is approximately 5% in the first month, 15% in 1 year, and 25% in 5 years. Patients with greater than 70% ipsilateral carotid stenosis are at greater risk of stroke and should be treated more aggressively.
- Stroke is the number one cause of morbidity and the third most common cause of death in the United States, following heart disease and cancer.
- The two major categories of stroke are hemorrhagic and ischemic.
- Hemorrhages can be intraparenchymal, subarachnoid, subdural, or epidural. Intraparenchymal hemorrhagic stroke will be discussed here.
   1. Intraparenchymal hemorrhage
- Intraparenchymal hemorrhage generally occurs in two patient populations: hypertensive patients and the elderly.
- Hypertensive stroke is related to lipohyalinosis of small intraparenchymal arteries. The most common locations for hypertensive stroke are in the basal ganglia, thalamus, cerebellum, and pons.
- In the elderly, intraparenchymal hemorrhage is often caused by amyloid protein deposits in the microvasculature leading to local areas of increased pressure and decreased vessel wall stability.
- Hemorrhages due to amyloid angiopathy are usually lobar, and there may be evidence of prior bleeding on imaging studies. Location can help differentiate amyloid angiopathy hemorrhages from the classic hypertensive hemorrhages.
- Less common causes of intraparenchymal hemorrhages are vascular malformations, trauma, coagulopathies, tumors, vasculitis, and cocaine, amphetamine, or ethanol abuse.
   2. Ischemic strokes
- Ischemic strokes are most commonly the result of thrombosis, emboli, or lacunar infarcts.
- Atherosclerotic disease is the principal pathologic entity in the formation of thrombus and emboli. Atherosclerotic plaques may rupture, causing

platelet adherence to vessel walls. This process leads to the formation of a thrombus. A thrombus may grow so large that it occludes the lumen of an artery, denying blood supply to distal brain tissue. The thrombus may also fracture, sending emboli distally occluding small vessels.

- Patients at greatest risk for embolic events are those with atrial fibrillation, cardiac thrombus, (secondary to myocardial infarction or cardiomyopathy), or bacterial endocarditis.
- Ischemic infarcts, especially embolic or large vessel events, can undergo hemorrhagic transformation.
- Lacunar strokes result from progressive thickening of small vessels that result in occlusion of penetrating arteries (lipohyalinosis and fibrinoid angiopathy).
- Hypertension, diabetes mellitus, and cigarette smoking are the most important modifiable risk factors for lacunes.
- Lacunar strokes occur primarily in the basal ganglia, pons, and subcortical white matter.

B. History and physical examination

- The major risk factors for stroke include hypertension, diabetes mellitus, hyperlipidemia, smoking, atrial fibrillation, previous stroke or TIA, carotid artery stenosis, valvular heart disease, coronary artery disease, coagulopathy, endocarditis, dilated cardiomyopathy, and antiphospholipid antibodies.
- Stroke usually presents as acute unilateral neurologic dysfunction that is maximal at onset. Cerebral edema may develop, leading to clouding of consciousness or a potentially fatal herniation of brain tissue.
- The severity of stroke can be assessed with the standardized NIH Stroke Scale (NIHSS). The lower the score, the better the prognosis. Patients seen within 24 hours of the stroke with a score greater than 15 have a poor prognosis if no treatment is given.
- Specific neurologic symptoms are attributable to the area of brain infarcted. The following is a partial list of these symptoms by the vasculature affected:
  1. Middle cerebral artery (MCA) occlusion
     - Occlusion of this artery, particularly the proximal MCA, is more often due to an embolus and results in contralateral paralysis, contralateral loss of sensation, and homonymous hemianopia.
     - When the dominant hemisphere is involved, aphasia may occur. When the nondominant hemisphere is involved, sensory neglect, spatial disorientation, and apraxia (loss of purposeful movement in the absence of paralysis) may occur.
  2. Posterior cerebral artery occlusion
     - Occlusion results in contralateral homonymous hemianopia, contralateral sensory loss, and rarely thalamic pain.
  3. Vertebrobasilar system occlusion
     - Occlusion results in cranial nerve abnormalities and sensory, motor, and cerebellar symptoms. Ophthalmoplegia and pupillary abnormalities may occur.

- Brainstem strokes can cause crossed syndromes with ipsilateral cranial nerve and contralateral extremity involvement.
- Large pontine strokes can result in "locked in syndrome" with preserved consciousness and only the ability to blink and have minimal eye movement.
- The physical examination should focus on the following:
  - Establish evidence of atherosclerosis or cardiac conditions (e.g., detecting an irregular cardiac rhythm, a third heart sound, murmur, or carotid artery bruit).
  - Perform mental status testing. Decreased level of consciousness is a common finding on physical examination in patients whose area of infarct is large or involves the brainstem.
  - Localize the area of brain affected. The constellation of deficits on neurologic testing identifies the involved region.

C. Laboratory and diagnostic studies
- Laboratory evaluation distinguishes hemorrhagic from ischemic stroke and helps to determine etiology and severity.
- A noncontrast head CT scan can identify a hemorrhage almost immediately. The CT scan of an ischemic stroke is usually negative for 24 hours except in very large infarcts.
- Complete blood count and blood chemistries and coagulation studies (when indicated) should identify evidence of infection, metabolic abnormalities, or coagulopathies.
- Cerebral angiography is the gold standard for evaluation of the cerebral vasculature. Angiography may be useful in detecting an area of vessel narrowing or occlusion.
- Carotid ultrasound is done for presumed carotid atherosclerotic disease of the neck.
- Transcranial doppler examination can provide an estimate of intracranial vascular disease including the posterior circulation.
- MRI with angiography may be used to localize the areas of ischemic lesions and provide noninvasive vascular evaluation.
- Echocardiography is helpful in the determination of potential cardiac or aortic sources of emboli.
- Holter monitoring or telemetry can identify arrhythmias.

D. Formulating the diagnosis
- The etiology and location of the stroke are determined by the history, physical examination, and laboratory evaluation.
- In patients with a gradual onset of neurologic symptoms (weeks, months) intracranial mass lesions should be ruled out with a contrast-enhanced CT scan or MRI.
- In cases with a relapsing and remitting course, demylinating diseases such as multiple sclerosis should be considered.

E. Evaluating the severity of problems
- Patients with hemorrhages, brainstem infarcts, or large hemispheric infarcts require close observation and supportive care.

- Decline in mental status, autonomic instability, and evidence of herniation all require emergent attention.
- Intubation may be necessary if respiratory function is threatened.
- The extent of recovery is dependent on the size of infarct, location of infarct, the patient's age, treatment, rehabilitation, and health status.

F. Managing the patient
- The patient's respiratory and circulatory function must first be stabilized. Intravenous normal saline should be used if necessary. Hypotonic solutions may increase cerebral edema. Hyperglycemia may cause ischemic tissue to infarct secondary to lactic acidosis. Elevated blood glucose should therefore be aggressively managed with insulin.
- Unless the patient has a hemorrhage, the mean arterial pressure should be maintained at 120 to 130 mm Hg. High blood pressure ensures cerebral perfusion to threatened but not yet infarcted tissue.
- Cerebral edema is usually at maximum levels by 72 to 96 hours. During this period the patient may require intubation and hyperventilation to reduce elevated intracranial pressure (ICP).
- Hyperventilation and mannitol are temporizing measures, and at this time surgical decompression should be considered.
- Seizures are a common sequela of embolic strokes. Acute seizures should be treated with benzodiazepines. Chronic seizures should be treated with anticonvulsants.
- Precautions against aspiration and deep venous thrombosis are indicated.
- Frequent neurologic evaluations should be done.
- Specific therapy depends on the etiology of the stroke.
- The only FDA-approved medical treatment for acute ischemic stroke is intravenous tissue plasminogen activator (IV tPA). IV tPA must be given within 3 hours of the onset of symptoms.
- There are several contraindications to tPA, including coagulopathy, gastrointestinal bleed, recent surgical procedure or noncompressible arterial puncture, recent stroke or intracranial hemorrhage, brain lesion at high risk for hemorrhage (such as tumor), pregnancy, systolic blood pressure greater than 185 mm Hg and diastolic greater than 110 mm of Hg that cannot be controlled with medication, early signs of large infarct on CT, and rapidly improving or minimal deficits. Seizures and severe hyper- or hypoglycemia are also relative contraindications. These relative contraindications are intended to prevent the thrombolysis of patients with stroke-like syndromes such as Todd's paralysis and focal neurologic deficits of hypoglycemia.
- When given to a patient without any contraindications there is a 6% rate of symptomatic intracranial hemorrhage.
- Patients who receive tPA should be closely monitored in an ICU or step-down setting.
- Antiplatlet agents or anticoagulants should not be given for 24 hours following the tPA infusion.
- Anticoagulation (heparin) is frequently used in patients with cardiac embolic disease, venous thrombosis, critical carotid stenosis, and vascular dissection. In

these patients IV heparin is given by continuous drip. The activated partial thromboplastin time (aPTT) is kept at approximately two times control levels.

- Long-term anticoagulation with warfarin may be necessary, and the prothrombin time (PT) international normalized ratio (INR) is usually kept between 2 and 3.
- Secondary stroke prophylaxis includes a reduction of risk factors as well as medical therapy, such as aspirin, clopidogrel, aspirin, and extended release dipyridamole combination or warfarin, depending on the etiology of the event. Warfarin reduces the risk of stroke in patients with atrial fibrillation.
- Patients with greater than 70% stenosis of the ipsilateral carotid artery should be considered for carotid endarterectomy or endovascular carotid stenting.
- Infectious etiologies of stroke, such as endocarditis or syphilis require the appropriate antibiotic therapy; bacterial endocarditis may require surgical intervention.
- Early rehabilitation may maximize recovery.

V. Guillain-Barré Syndrome
  A. Basic science
   - Acute inflammatory demyelinating polyradiculoneuropathy, Guillain-Barré syndrome (GBS), is the most common acute paralytic disease in Western countries.
   - Pathologically, GBS is usually characterized by an immunologically mediated multifocal attack upon myelinated spinal roots and peripheral nerves. Disruption of the normal conduction of nerve impulses results in a clinical syndrome of motor weakness, areflexia, and distal paresthesias.
   - The classic pathology of GBS is an endoneurial perivascular mononuclear cell infiltration with multifocal demyelination. The main immunologic targets are the ventral roots, proximal spinal nerves, and lower cranial nerves. However, GBS can also affect the full extent of a peripheral nerve.
   - A preceding infection may trigger an autoimmune response through molecular mimicry. During mimicry an immune response is directed against an epitope shared by both the organism and peripheral nerves.
   - Variant presentations of GBS include an acute motor or motor and sensory axonal neuropathy. These axonal variants produce a similar initial clinical presentation but are associated with a more severe course and poor recovery.
  B. History and physical examination
   - GBS affects people of all ages and shows limited geographic or seasonal variation.
   - A comprehensive evaluation of GBS begins with a detailed history of antecedent events, which can be seen in up to 70% of cases. These antecedent events include respiratory illness, gastrointestinal illness, vaccination, and surgery. These events typically occur 1 to 4 weeks before the onset of neurologic symptoms.
   - The etiologic agent responsible for the prodrome remains undetected in a majority of cases, but serologic evidence may show specific infectious agents, including *Campylobacter jejuni* (26%), *Cytomegalovirus* (15%), and *Mycoplasma pneumoniae* (10%).

- Characteristically, GBS begins with paresthesias of the extremities and then symmetrically ascending weakness. Severe cases include respiratory muscle weakness. Areflexia and/or hyporeflexia are always seen.
- By definition, GBS ceases to progress between 1 and 4 weeks after the onset of neurologic symptoms.
- Cranial nerve involvement occurs in about half of all patients and can be the predominant presentation.
- The Miller-Fisher variant of GBS, seen in 5% of cases, is characterized by ophthalmoplegia, ataxia, and areflexia. Motor strength in preserved. Between 10% and 20% of patients will require assisted ventilation, either for airway protection or diaphragmatic weakness during the course of their illness. Neuropathic pain occurs in a majority of patients.
- Dysautonomia may be seen in patients with GBS. Significant blood pressure variations and sinus arrhythmia are the hallmarks of GBS-associated autonomic dysfunction. Patients with these symptoms need their cardiac activity and hemodynamics closely monitored. Patients should have respiratory mechanics (e.g., negative inspired force and vital capacity) followed serially. This is especially important early in the disease because patients can rapidly decompensate.

C. Laboratory and diagnostic studies
- Patients with suspected GBS should have serologic, respiratory, and urinary studies to exclude a concomitant infectious etiology.
- Lumbar puncture and CSF analysis should be done in all patients without a contraindication. A hallmark of GBS is a low CSF white blood cell count and an elevated protein level (albumin-cytologic dissociation). Antibodies to the ganglioside GQ1b are found in most patients with the Miller-Fisher variant of GBS.
- During the first 3 weeks following the onset of motor weakness, nerve conduction studies may detect evidence of conduction block. These findings can help confirm the diagnosis of GBS.
- Following 3 weeks of motor weakness, needle electrode examination (electromyography [EMG]) may be helpful in differentiating the presence or degree of axonal injury. This provides prognostic information.
- Radiologic studies are usually normal; however, lumbosacral MRI scans with gadolinium may show enhancement of lumbar spinal roots. MRI imaging of the spine is useful to exclude other diagnoses, such as spinal cord compression or transverse myelitis.

D. Formulating the diagnosis
- GBS must be distinguished from other disorders with similar presentations. An extensive transverse myelitis may produce similar symptoms. Toxic exposure to arsenic, thallium, *N*-hexane, and organophosphates can produce an acute onset peripheral neuropathy. Critical illness neuropathy, tic paralysis, and botulism poisoning should be excluded in the proper clinical context. Careful attention needs to be given to clinical features that distinguish GBS from these other conditions.

E. Evaluating the severity of problems
- Close monitoring of respiratory and cardiac function during the early course of the disease are important.
- Serial neurologic examinations assessing for progression of disease are invaluable.
- Nerve conduction studies and tests of respiratory mechanics are helpful.

F. Managing the patient
- Treatment is individualized to each patient. Some patients have a mild presentation requiring limited hospital monitoring. Patient with rapidly ascending weakness and respiratory dysfunction need close monitoring and treatment should be started when the diagnosis is secured.
- Treatment with either intravenous immunoglobulin (IVIg) or plasmapheresis is of greatest benefit when begun within 2 weeks of symptoms onset. Serious complications of IVIg rarely include anaphylaxis when non-IgA depleted IVIg is given to IgA-deficient patients. Plasmapheresis has been shown to be efficacious in the treatment of GBS. Clinician preference dictates the use of these treatments.
- Corticosteroids have failed to show benefit in randomized controlled trials for the treatment of GBS.
- EMG may be useful in determining the degree of axonal injury after GBS which dictates the prognosis for recovery.
- Patients with weakness are at risk for deep venous thrombosis and should receive appropriate prophylaxis to prevent pulmonary embolism.
- Patients with GBS frequently benefit from physical and occupational therapy. Early initiation of rehabilitation plays an important role in recovery.

VI. Headache
A. Basic science
- The pathophysiology of headache remains debatable; however, a combination of vascular, trigeminal, and neurogenic inflammatory components all play a role.
- There are two types of headache syndromes: primary and secondary.
- Primary headache syndromes include migraine (vascular headache), tension-type (muscle contraction headache), and cluster. Other less common primary headache disorders exist.
- Secondary headache syndromes are caused by pathologic entities such as masses, subarachnoid bleeds, and giant cell arteritis.

B. History and physical examination
- A complete and accurate history is the key to the correct diagnosis of the etiology of headache.
- The physical examination should include complete neurologic, funduscopic, and neck examinations.
  1. Primary headache syndromes
     - The neurologic examination is normal in primary headache syndromes.
     a. Tension-type headaches
        - This is the commonest form of headache.

- Tension-type headaches are usually bilateral and pressure or "bandlike."
- They may be related to neck pain.
- Tension headaches can last hours or days and are not associated with autonomic symptoms (tachycardia, diaphoresis).
- Physical activity does not worsen the headache.

  b. Migraine headaches
  - Migraine headaches are commonly familial and are sometimes associated with a history of motion sickness.
  - Migraine without aura and migraine with aura are the most frequently encountered types.
  - The headache lasts 4 to 72 hours.
  - The pain is often unilateral and throbbing and is worsened by activity; however, a headache that always occurs on the same side should raise suspicion for a secondary cause.
  - Migraine may be triggered by specific foods or smells.
  - The aura typically consists of scintillating scotoma (flashes of light) that precede the headache by minutes and remit before the headache does.
  - The headaches usually last hours.
  - Headaches are associated with photophobia, phonophobia, nausea, and vomiting. The patient generally curtails all activity.
  - Episodes are relieved by sleep.
  - No other disease that can explain the headache should be present.

  c. Cluster headaches
  - Cluster headaches are typically found in young adult males.
  - They are excruciatingly severe, painful, unilateral headaches.
  - The orbital, supraorbital, and temporal regions are the usual sites of pain.
  - Patients with cluster headaches often present with ipsilateral autonomic signs including rhinorrhea, lacramation, miosis, ptosis, and impaired sweating.
  - The pain usually peaks in 10 minutes and lasts up to 3 hours. These headaches occur several times a day in "clusters" and then the patient will have a period of remission.
  - Unlike migraine, patients with cluster headaches often pace back and forth, and are sometimes driven to desperate measures owing to the severity of the pain.
  - These headaches may be triggered by alcohol consumption.

2. Secondary headache syndromes
   - Pathologic entities cause secondary headaches. Masses, subarachnoid bleeds, and giant cell arteritis may all cause secondary headaches.

   a. Mass lesions
   - Mass lesions typically cause headaches that are worse on awakening. Morning vomiting is a characteristic sign.
   - The location of the pain does not always correlate with the location of the mass.

- The headaches may at first be intermittent but eventually become more constant.
- Associated physical findings include papilledema; focal motor, sensory, or reflex abnormalities; and upper motor neuron signs (spasticity, hyperreflexia, Babinski sign).

  b. Subarachnoid hemorrhage
  - Subarachnoid, or intracranial parenchymal, hemorrhage may cause a sudden, severe "thunderclap" headache with vomiting, instantaneous loss of consciousness, or seizure.
  - Signs include focal neurologic abnormalities, fundus hemorrhage, and meningismus (signs of meningeal irritation, such as neck stiffness).

  c. Temporal arteritis or giant cell arteritis (see also Rheumatology section, Chapter 8, Section D)
  - Temporal arteritis occurs primarily in patients over 60 years old and is associated with headache (throbbing, continuous), vision loss, ocular motility abnormalities, jaw claudication, weight loss, and general malaise.
  - The temporal artery may be tender and firm.

C. Laboratory and diagnostic studies
  - There are no laboratory or diagnostic studies to support or refute the existence of primary headache syndromes.
  - The laboratory workup of secondary headache syndromes is discussed in the following sections.

D. Formulating the diagnosis
  1. Primary headache syndromes
     - Migraine and tension headaches demonstrate no associated focal neurologic abnormalities.
     - Migraine and tension headaches may be diagnosed based on their historical characteristics.

  2. Secondary headache syndromes
     - Mass lesions (such as tumor, abscess, and intracranial hemorrhage) can present with headache, focal neurologic signs, new onset seizures, or an increase in seizures in a patient with an underlying seizure disorder.
     - Head CT scan or MRI is abnormal in these patients. CT scan or MRI should be obtained in any patient with headaches and an abnormal neurologic examination. Imaging should also be considered in a patient with any features that are atypical for a primary headache syndrome (e.g., always unilateral headache or onset in the elderly).
     - Subarachnoid hemorrhage has a characteristic onset and should be considered in any patient who complains of a sudden severe headache. Noncontrast head CT scan should be performed, followed by lumbar puncture if the CT scan is negative.
     - Arteriovenous malformations should be considered in patients who have consistently unilateral headaches and seizures. A bruit may be heard over the malformation. Head CT scan or MRI with contrast is diagnostic.

- New onset headaches in elderly patients suggest a secondary headache syndrome. Ruptured aneurysms, tumors, and giant cell arteritis all become increasingly prevalent with increasing age.
- In giant cell arteritis, the sedimentation rate is elevated in approximately 90% of patients. Diagnosis is confirmed by the presence of multinucleated giant cells on temporal artery biopsy.
- Headaches are a common complaint of patients with depression. Other causes of headache include subdural or epidural hematoma, meningitis, sinusitis, glaucoma, systemic hypertension, carbon monoxide intoxication, hypothyroidism, analgesic overuse, and caffeine withdrawal.

E. Evaluating the severity of problems
  - Headache can be a sign of intracerebral mass lesion. The major complications of mass lesions are herniation and death.
  - Aneurysmal subarachnoid hemorrhage often causes death before medical care arrives, making the identification of prior "sentinel" bleeding imperative.
  - Giant cell arteritis can produce blindness by restricting blood flow in the ophthalmic and posterior ciliary arteries. It can also cause strokes, particularly in the posterior circulation.

F. Managing the patient
  1. Primary headache syndromes
     - Tension headaches are treated with aspirin, acetaminophen, or other analgesic therapy. Chronic tension headaches can be treated with a combination of medications (analgesics and tricyclic antidepressants) along with physical therapy and psychotherapy, such as cervical support, muscle relaxation training, and management of underlying stressors.
     a. Treatment of migraine headaches
        - Prophylaxis should be considered in patients with more than two headache days per week, when acute therapies are ineffective, or if the patient has a migraine variant such as basilar migraine or migraine with infarction that predisposes the patient to complications.
        - β-Blockers such as propranolol are useful in prophylaxis against migraine headaches in about 50% of patients. A calcium channel blocker (such as verapamil), tricyclic antidepressants (such as amitriptyline), and antiepileptics (such as divalproex and topiramate) may also prove effective.
        - Mild attacks may be treated with nonsteroidal anti-inflammatory drugs. The serotonin agonists (triptans), such as sumatriptan, have proved highly successful in ablating migraine headaches (70% relief of symptoms) and are now considered the therapy of choice for migraine headache. If serotonin agonists prove ineffective, ergotamines may be tried.
     b. Treatment of cluster headache
        - Prophylaxis: Cluster headache prophylaxis is similar to that of migraine. First-line prophylaxis for cluster headache is the calcium channel blocker verapamil. This can be combined with other agents such as lithium or valproic acid if needed.

- Acute treatment: First-line treatment is 100% oxygen at 8 to 10 L per minute by nonrebreather face mask for 15 to 20 minutes. This will often abort the attack. The serotonin agonists and ergotamines can also be used acutely.

2. Secondary headache syndromes
   - Patients with suspected mass lesions or subarachnoid hemorrhage should be immediately referred to neurosurgery for evaluation.
   - Hyperventilation and corticosteroids may prove acutely effective in reducing edema and mass effect due to tumors or abscesses.
   - Treat temporal arteritis immediately with high-dose corticosteroids (for example, prednisone 60 mg per day) to prevent blindness.

VII. Multiple Sclerosis
   A. Basic science
   - Multiple sclerosis (MS) is a chronic disease characterized by scattered areas of demyelination in the white matter tracts of the central nervous system.
   - Evidence suggests that multiple sclerosis is an autoimmune disease, with myelin as the predominant protein under attack. Environmental factors, genetics, and infectious agents are also thought to play a role.
   - The myelin sheath of peripheral nerves is antigenically different from myelin in central tracts and thus is not affected.
   - Deficits in multiple sclerosis are related to impaired neuronal transmission of signals through the demyelinated axons.
   B. History and physical examination
   - The incidence of multiple sclerosis in the United States general population is 0.1% and is more common in the northern latitudes.
   - Patients with a close relative have a higher risk of contracting multiple sclerosis, with an overall risk of approximately 5%.
   - Multiple sclerosis most often affects young adults. Most people become symptomatic between the ages of 15 and 50 years old.
   - Whites have a much higher incidence of multiple sclerosis than blacks or Asians. Females are affected twice as often as males.
   - Neurologic symptoms may present acutely or may be relapsing or progressive.
   - Although any area in the central nervous system may be affected, involvement of certain areas leads to particularly common manifestations of multiple sclerosis. These include the following:
     - Painful acute decrease in visual acuity in one eye (optic neuritis) from optic nerve lesions.
     - Diplopia and internuclear ophthalmoplegia (INO) from brainstem lesions.
     - Ataxia from cerebellar lesions.
     - Spasticity and weakness from motor neuron lesions in the brain or spinal cord which result in hyperreflexia and Babinski sign.
     - Urinary frequency and urgency from spinal cord lesions.
     - Sensory disturbances from lesions in the sensory tracts of the brain or spinal cord.

- Lhermitte's phenomenon, a transient electric shock-like sensation radiating down the spine with neck flexion, from cervical spine involvement
- Later in the course of multiple sclerosis persistent neurologic deficits result from accumulation of white matter damage in the spinal cord and brain.
- Common deficits include hemiparesis, spasticity, incontinence, and dementia. Seizures occur in up to 5% of multiple sclerosis patients, usually coinciding with active lesions near the cerebral cortex. Fatigue and depression are common throughout the disease course but do not clearly relate to nervous system lesions.
- The course of the disease is quite variable but can be grossly divided into relapsing versus progressive presentations.
- The most common presentation is the relapsing-remitting pattern of multiple sclerosis, which consists of clear attacks of MS symptoms interspersed with symptom-free periods. This frequently transforms into secondary progressive MS after several years and causes permanent deficits between attacks.
- Multiple sclerosis can also present as a primary progressive disease, in which symptoms steadily worsen without disease-free periods. Primary progressive MS is more likely to occur in slightly older individuals than the young women who classically present with relapsing-remitting MS.

C. Laboratory and diagnostic studies

- MRIs of the brain and spinal cord can confirm the existence of white-matter lesions in multiple areas. The classic MRI lesions are known as "Dawson's fingers," which are areas of demyelination extending perpendicularly from the ventricles.
- Evoked potentials of the visual, auditory, and somatosensory systems are also useful in establishing multiple lesions. Evoked potentials can remain positive even after resolution of symptoms.
- Cerebrospinal fluid gamma globulin elevation or oligoclonal banding can confirm the presence of immune-mediated process with the central nervous system.

D. Formulating the diagnosis

- The diagnosis of multiple sclerosis is based on history, physical examination, laboratory testing, and results of imaging.
- A diagnosis is based on recurrent attacks of deficits related to more than one area of the central nervous system. Attacks are separated in "time and space."

E. Evaluating the severity of problems

- At the onset of symptoms there is no way to accurately predict the frequency of attacks or subsequent disability that will occur.
- Life span is reduced only in those with the most extreme deficits, such as dysphagia, respiratory compromise, or urinary retention, because of the increased risk of overwhelming infections.

F. Managing the patient

- Acute attacks of symptoms can be treated with high-dose intravenous steroids (e.g., methylprednisolone 1000 mg per day for 3 to 5 days) to reduce symptoms more rapidly.

- FDA-approved medications to reduce the risk of developing attacks and long-term disability in relapsing-remitting MS include the beta interferons 1a and 1b, glatiramer acetate, and natalizumab.
- In aggressive disease, unresponsive to these medications, other chemotherapeutic agents are available such as mitoxantrone.
- Spasticity is treated with physical therapy, the centrally acting muscle relaxants baclofen and tizanidine, and benzodiazepines.
- Urinary frequency and urgency are reduced by anticholinergics (such as oxybutynin or tolterodine). Intermittent catheterization may be necessary if the bladder does not empty completely. Chronic catheterization should be avoided because of the risk of infection.
- Fatigue usually responds to brief naps, modafinil, methylphenidate, or amantadine.
- Depression is treated with standard antidepressants.
- Seizures are best treated with anticonvulsants such as phenytoin or carbamazepine.

VIII. Muscular Dystrophy
  A. Basic science
   - Muscular dystrophy (MD) is a group of genetically transmitted diseases characterized by progressive symmetric atrophy of groups of skeletal muscles without evidence of involvement or degeneration of neural tissue. In all forms of MD there is gradual loss of strength with increasing disability and deformity.
   - Each type differs in the group of muscles affected, the age of onset, rate of progression, and mode of genetic inheritance.
   - Five major muscular dystrophies are Duchenne's muscular dystrophy, Becker's muscular dystrophy, myotonic dystrophy, fascioscapulohumeral muscular dystrophy, and limb-girdle muscular dystrophy.
   - Duchenne's muscular dystrophy and Becker's muscular dystrophy are X-linked disorders localized to a gene producing the protein dystrophin.
  B. History and physical examination
   - The muscular dystrophies are characterized by progressive weakness and wasting of skeletal muscles.
   - Their age of onset varies among the specific disorders but as a group can present at any age.
   - In the evaluation for muscular dystrophy it is important to identify a family history, the rate of progression (typically very slow), and if systems other than skeletal muscle are involved.
  C. Laboratory and diagnostic studies
   - Electromyography, muscle biopsy, and immunoblotting are important diagnostic tests for establishing the diagnosis of a specific muscular dystrophy.
  D. Formulating the diagnosis
   - The key features needed to identify the presence of a specific dystrophy hinge on clinical presentation (age of onset), serum creatine kinase, neurophysiologic studies, and muscle biopsy.

E. Evaluating the severity of problems
  - The major concern in all of these diseases includes respiratory insufficiency, cardiac rhythm disturbances, and orthopedic complications.
F. Managing the patient
  - Treatment of these diseases is mostly symptomatic with the goal of improving ambulation with assistive devices.
  - Other therapy includes placement of a cardiac pacemaker and providing respiratory assistive devices (from simple nasal BiPAP to tracheostomy and mechanical ventilation) as necessary.
  - Myotonia (a condition in which a muscle or a group of muscles will not relax) has been treated with anticonvulsants (such as phenytoin or carbamazepine).

IX. Myasthenia Gravis
A. Basic science
  - Myasthenia gravis (MG) is the most common primary disorder of neuromuscular junction transmission. It is usually an acquired autoimmune disorder, but there are rare genetic causes.
  - The symptoms of MG are caused by antibodies that block the postsynaptic acetylcholine receptor. These antibodies prevent the binding of acetylcholine and signal transmission at the muscle end plate.
  - Women are affected more often than men, and patients with MG have a higher incidence of other autoimmune disorders (e.g., thyroid disease and diabetes).
  - The disease is characterized by remissions and exacerbations, especially early in the course of disease.
B. History and physical examination
  - Patients present with complaints of weakness, ptosis, diplopia, dysarthria, dyspnea, and dysphagia.
  - Symptoms fluctuate throughout the day and are worse with exertion and repeated muscle use (e.g., stairs or chewing).
  - Limb weakness is proximal and is asymmetric.
  - The disease can also be exacerbated by systemic illness, infections, thyroid disease, increases in body temperature, and pregnancy. MG is also exacerbated by several medications. The most common of these include D-penicillamine, succinylcholine and other neuromuscular blockers, acute high-dose steroids, quinine, procainamide, amnioglycoside antibiotics, β-blockers, calcium channel blockers, and magnesium-containing medications.
  - On physical examination there is decreased strength with repetitive muscle testing. Most patients will have ocular weakness and ptosis.
  - If there is any concern for respiratory weakness a vital capacity and negative inspiratory force should be followed. Dysphagia and dyspnea can result in respiratory compromise, aspiration, and death if unrecognized.
  - In the case of acute exacerbations the patient can quickly deteriorate; the physician should have a low threshold for admission and close monitoring.

C. Laboratory and diagnosis
- Several tests can assist in the diagnosis. A quick bedside test is the administration of IV edrophonium (Tensilon test). To perform this test there must be a fatigable muscle group in which improvement can be observed following injection (e.g., ptosis on upgaze). This must be done with blood pressure and pulse monitoring because of the cholinergic effects of edrophonium. A positive test is not specific for MG.
- Blood can be sent for acetylcholine receptor antibodies. These antibodies are binding, blocking, and modulating.
- Electromyography (EMG) with incremental decrements on repetitive stimulation also supports a diagnosis of MG.
- CT of the chest is performed to exclude tumor or enlargement of the thymus. Thymus removal in these cases correlates with improved disease control.
- MG should be differentiated from Lambert-Eaton myasthenic syndrome (a presynapic disorder that improves with exercise), botulism poisoning, myopathies, and acute neuropathies such as Guillain-Barré syndrome.

D. Evaluating the severity of problems
- The course of newly diagnosed MG and acute exacerbations is highly variable and should be approached cautiously. These patients are at risk for aspiration, respiratory compromise, and intubation. Respiratory parameters and arterial blood gases should be followed on hospitalized patients.

E. Managing the patient
- The first step is determining the severity of the disease and the need for hospitalization and respiratory support. Airway and circulatory support is the first priority.
- Symptoms can be managed with cholinesterase inhibitors (Mestinon), but disease control requires immunosuppression. Immunomodulating therapy can include steroids, chemotherepeutics, plasma exchange, and IVIg.
- In patients with an enlarged thymus on CT, thymectomy should be considered. Removing this source of antibodies improves long-term disease control.

X. Parkinson's Disease
A. Basic science
- Parkinson's disease (PD) is a common neurologic movement disorder caused by abnormalities in the basal ganglia. There is a loss of dopamine-containing neurons in the substantia nigra. Other neurotransmitter systems are involved as well, especially GABAergic neurons (neurons that produce gamma-aminobutyric acid), but to a lesser extent.
- Neuronal loss is progressive but its cause has not yet been clearly established. A minority of cases have been associated with various gene mutations; the best described is the *parkin1* gene.
- The pathologic hallmark of PD is the Lewy body, an intraneuronal cytoplasmic inclusion found mostly in the dopaminergic cells of the substantia nigra.

B. History and physical examination
- Parkinson's disease usually affects older adults, with a peak age of onset in the 60s.
- The four cardinal features of PD are resting tremor, bradykinesia (slowness of movement), rigidity, and postural instability.
- The most characteristic initial symptom is a resting tremor that is usually unilateral at onset. The tremor can involve the upper extremities, lower extremities, lower face, and jaw. Tremor of the face and jaw should be differentiated from head titubation seen in essential tremor.
- Patients may have difficulty initiating movements and may notice slowed voluntary movements. They have difficulty walking, and their gait is stooped and shuffling.
- Patients may exhibit a form of stooped posture known as camptocormia, which is distinct from a kyphotic stooped posture. They may also experience freezing (a sudden arrest in movement particularly when walking through a doorway).
- As the disease progresses, postural instability may result in frequent falls. In addition, handwriting becomes very small (micrographia).
- On neurologic examination, mental status testing is usual normal, or mild cognitive delay may be present.
- Symptoms of dementia, which precede the onset of parkinsonian symptoms by 1 year or more, may be present in a process known as diffuse Lewy body disease, which exhibits a distinctly different course and progression from PD.
- Cranial nerve deficits may include decreased upgaze (more characteristically seen in progressive supranuclear palsy), infrequent blinking, decreased facial expression (known as masked facies), soft voice (hypophonia), excessive drooling, and perhaps a tremor of the lower face or chin.
- Motor examination usually reveals a resting tremor that is often described as "pill-rolling" and has an average frequency of 4 Hz. Some patients may exhibit a postural tremor that, unlike essential tremor, has a delayed latency of onset after initiation of postural tone while outstretching the arms.
- Patients may exhibit a slowness of movement (bradykinesia). Passive manipulation of the extremities reveals rigidity, often with a "cogwheeling" quality (a ratchet-like movement).
- There is no weakness. Sensory, cerebellar, and reflex examinations are generally unremarkable.
- Gait, as described earlier, is remarkable for stooped posture, shuffling of the feet, and decreased arm swing.
- Patients often have difficulty initiating movement, but then steps become increasingly rapid and they find it hard to stop (festination).
- Patients have postural instability and may fall if not caught when pulled at the shoulders from behind (e.g., the pull test). The pull test may be performed with the examiner behind the patient, giving a warning to the patients, and allowing one step for normal balance adjustment after a brief, rapid pull upon the patient's shoulders.
- Seborrheic dermatitis is associated with PD.

C. Laboratory and diagnostic studies
- Although MRI may show decreased signal in the substantia nigra, imaging studies and blood tests are used mainly to rule out other diagnoses. The diagnosis of PD remains a clinical one.

D. Formulating the diagnosis
- The diagnosis of Parkinson's disease is not difficult when an accurate history and physical examination reveal the cardinal features.
- Many other causes of secondary parkinsonism should be considered whenever there are atypical features or when there is a young age at onset. These causes include effects of medications (such as antipsychotic agents, antidepressants, and metoclopramide), exposure to toxins (such as carbon monoxide, methanol, and manganese), metabolic disturbances (such as Wilson's disease, a treatable disorder of copper metabolism, or neurodegeneration with brain iron accumulation), other neurodegenerative diseases (Huntington's disease, an inherited neuropsychiatric disorder), and multiple cerebral infarcts.

E. Evaluating the severity of problems
- The course of PD is variable but is generally progressive. Patients can become quite debilitated as the disease progresses.
- Patients may develop swallowing problems, and alternative methods of feeding may need to be considered.
- Patients are at risk for aspiration pneumonia.
- Because of gait difficulties, patients are at risk for falls. They may become entirely unable to walk or perform the activities of daily living and need extensive supportive care to prevent other complications of immobility, such as decubitus ulcers.

F. Managing the patient
- Fortunately, many medications are available to provide symptomatic treatment of PD. The mainstay of treatment is the dopamine precursor levodopa, which, unlike dopamine, can cross the blood-brain barrier. It is given with carbidopa, a decarboxylase inhibitor, which prevents breakdown to dopamine in the periphery. The use of carbidopa results in fewer side effects (such as nausea) and allows for smaller doses of levodopa to be given.
- Patients who have been on levodopa for long periods may develop fluctuations between a rigid state and a nonrigid state (the "on-off" phenomenon) and can develop dyskinesias (involuntary movements) during the "on" phase. This medication can also cause psychosis in some patients, especially when given in high doses.
- Other medications used to treat PD include dopamine agonists (such as pergolide, pramipexole, and ropinorole).
- Catechol-*O*-methyltransferase (COMT) inhibitors are often used as adjuvant therapy in combination to prolong the effect of levodopa/carbidopa.
- Selegiline and rasagiline are specific monoamine oxidase B (MAO-B) inhibitors used for symptom control and to theoretically prevent disease progression.
- Anticholinergic medications and amantadine are sometimes used to help with tremor and bradykinesia.

- Patients with advanced PD who have rapid "off" periods between levodopa/carbidopa doses may benefit from the use of injectable apomorphine.
- Patients who have failed some form of medical therapy may be candidates for implantation of electrodes to stimulate targets in the basal ganglia. The subthalamic nucleus is currently the most common target for placement of these "deep brain stimulators." The use of this technology has expanded exponentially in recent years.
- Transplantation of adrenal medullary or fetal midbrain tissue remains experimental.

XI. Seizures
  A. Basic science
  - A seizure is an episode of neurologic dysfunction caused by abnormal electrical activity of neurons.
  - Epilepsy is a clinical syndrome characterized by recurrent, unprovoked seizure activity.
  - The etiology for seizures is classified as either primary (that is, idiopathic or unknown) or secondary.
  - Some causes of secondary seizures include trauma, infection, tumors, vascular lesions, anoxia, electrolyte disorders, toxins, and drugs (such as lidocaine).
  - The etiology of most seizures is idiopathic.
  - Various classification schemes currently are in use for describing seizures. The most commonly used system seeks to broadly classify seizures by their electroclinical characteristics into either generalized or partial (focal).
  - Generalized seizures involve loss of consciousness due to abnormal activation of the entire cerebral cortex.
  - The nomenclature depends on the type of movement noted, such as tonic, clonic, tonic-clonic, atonic, akinetic, or myoclonic.
  - Apnea, urine or stool incontinence, forced deviation (version) of the eyes, and postictal confusion are some of the associated manifestations.
  - Absence seizures are seen in children and are usually characterized by a brief episode of staring and behavioral arrest without associated postictal confusion.
  - Partial seizures stem from activation of localized regions of the cerebral cortex. Complex partial seizures display a loss of awareness, whereas simple partial seizures have retention of consciousness.
  - Partial seizures may be motor (unilateral tonic, clonic, or both), sensory (paresthesias or numbness), or autonomic. They may also be associated with psychic, affective, or cognitive symptoms preceding the seizures (auras). Focal seizures may secondarily generalize. The classic complex partial seizure presents with altered consciousness and automatisms such as lip smacking and is followed by a transient postictal state.
  - Febrile seizures are seen in children under the age of 5 with temperatures greater than 38°C, although the seizure may also occur soon after the patient has defervesced. They are sometime familial and are not associated with intracranial lesions. Children with a history of febrile seizures are at small

increased risk of developing epilepsy, especially temporal lobe epilepsy, as adults.

- Status epilepticus is a medical emergency in which seizures occur continuously for 30 minutes or longer, or recur without a fully lucid interval during this period. Mortality rate may be as high as 25%, and the patient may die of prolonged anoxia, trauma, or cardiovascular collapse. Specific measures to support the patient and initiate anticonvulsant treatment must be undertaken.
- Alcoholics may experience nonfocal motor seizures during periods of withdrawal. If untreated, these seizures may progress to delirium tremens.

B. History and physical examination

- A comprehensive evaluation of seizures begins with a detailed history surrounding the event. Both the patient and witnesses should be questioned regarding the onset and length of seizure activity, loss of consciousness, lateralizing features (such as versive eye movements, aphasia, unilateral motor activity, and features of an aura), and postictal confusion.
- The presence or absence of aura, localized or generalized motor activity, trauma, precipitating events, or illnesses should all be addressed.
- In patients with a known seizure disorder, questions regarding compliance with medical regimen, associated alcohol or drug use, sleep deprivation, and intercurrent illness need to be discussed.
- The most common reason for breakthrough seizures in known epileptics is missed medication.
- The neurologic examination should be thorough, looking for both changes in mentation and focal deficits.

C. Laboratory and diagnostic studies

- Laboratory studies should be done on an individual basis. Patients with an initial seizure require a more extensive workup including serum electrolytes, glucose, blood uras nitrogen (BUN), creatinine, calcium, magnesium, toxicology screens, urine hCG (human chorionic gonadotropin), and a complete blood count. Anticonvulsant levels may be helpful in detecting compliance with treatment.
- Radiology studies include a CT scan with or without contrast to rule out structural causes. In the search for structural lesions, MRI is more sensitive than CT, though it may not be available emergently.
- Electroencephalograms (EEGs) may help distinguish generalized from focal seizures. EEG is also useful in differentiating epileptic from nonepileptic seizures (also known as psychogenic or pseudoseizures).

D. Formulating the diagnosis

- Seizure disorders must be distinguished from other disorders that present similarly. The differential diagnosis includes syncope, narcolepsy/cataplexy, transient ischemic attacks (TIAs), movement disorders, psychogenic seizures, and malingering. Careful attention needs to be given to clinical features that distinguish seizures from other ailments.

E. Evaluating the severity of problems

- Seizures may be the manifestation of treatable disease, such as brain tumors, infections, stroke, arteriovenous malformations (AVMs), and metabolic derangements. As such, it is important to aim treatment at the cause when it is identifiable.

- Patients who are evaluated in the postictal state are not able to give a coherent history and may have transient focal deficits (Todd's paralysis).
- During the seizure patients may also have suffered an occult injury requiring emergent treatment (such as subdural hematoma or fractures).

F. Managing the patient

- Treatment is individualized to each patient. Certain seizures require more intense management than others (such as status epilepticus).
- General measures are taken to protect the patient against injury (such as padded bedrails), to stabilize the airway (oral/nasal airway or intubation), and to ensure adequate ventilation and circulation (such as large bore intravenous lines).
- Definitive control of seizures is geared toward treating the underlying cause (for example, correction of metabolic abnormalities such as hyponatremia).
- The choice of anticonvulsant depends on the type, frequency, and intensity of the seizure (Table 1-1). Maintenance anticonvulsants should be chosen depending on the most likely etiology. Phenytoin, valproic acid, and carbamazipine are some of the more frequently used anticonvulsants for outpatient maintenance therapy.
- Management of status epilepticus begins with the establishment of the airway and administration of thiamine and dextrose.
- Initial therapy of active seizures begins with benzodiazepines (i.e., lorazepam). Once the acute seizure has abated, phenytoin should be administered followed by valproic acid or phenobarbital, if necessary. If these measures are not effective, more drastic therapies such as barbiturate, midazolam, or propofol coma are used.

XII. Subarachnoid Hemorrhage

A. Basic science

- Subarachnoid hemorrhage usually results from trauma, a ruptured intracranial aneurysm, or an arteriovenous malformation.
- Traumatic subarachnoid hemorrhage usually occurs as result of major trauma and is often neurologically devastating.
- Subarachnoid hemorrhage from aneurysm rupture is associated with a death rate of 35% with the first bleed; an additional 15% of patients die in the ensuing weeks from a second rupture of the aneurysm.
- Peak incidence of aneurysm rupture is between the ages of 25 and 50 and is rare in children.
- Aneurysms are most commonly found at bifurcations in the circle of Willis, where the muscular layers of the cerebral arteries are less well developed.

B. History and physical examination

1. Traumatic hemorrhage
   - Patients with traumatic subarachnoid hemorrhage must be screened for other life-threatening injuries.
2. Aneurysmal hemorrhage

TABLE 1-1:

Drugs for the Treatment of Epilepsy in Adults

Drug	TREATMENT		Side Effects
	GTC	Focal Seizures	
Carbamazepine	Monotherapy	Monotherapy	Hyponatremia, drowsiness, dizziness, blood dyscrasia, hypertransaminasemia, rash
Phenytoin	Monotherapy	Monotherapy	Drowsiness, gingival hyperplasia, rash, blood dyscrasia, ataxia, folate deficiency, SJS
Primidone	Monotherapy	Monotherapy	Sedation, dizziness, rash, megaloblastic anemia, ataxia, diplopia, nystagmus
Phenobarbital	Monotherapy	Monotherapy	Drowsiness, rash, ataxia, behavioral and cognitive problems
Valproic acid	Monotherapy	Monotherapy	Hepatitis, weight gain, alopecia, drowsiness, ataxia, pancreatitis, thrombocytopenia, hyperammonemia, SJS
Lamotrigine	Adjunctive	Adjunctive	Rash, dizziness, diplopia, fatigue, somnolence, SJS
Gabapentin	Adjunctive	Adjunctive	Dizziness, somnolence, weight gain
Levetiracetam	Adjunctive	Adjunctive	Somnolence, dizziness, asthenia
Topiramate	Adjunctive	Adjunctive	Dizziness, diplopia, fatigue, nervousness, psychomotor slowing, weight loss, nephrolithiasis
Zonisamide	Not used	Adjunctive	Dizziness, somnolence, agitation, psychomotor slowing, weight loss, nephrolithiasis, oligohydrosis
Oxcarbazepine	Not used	Monotherapy	Hyponatremia, nausea, dizziness, fatigue, somnolence, headache

GTC, generalized tonic seizures; SJS, Stevens-Johnson syndrome.

- Aneurysms are usually asymptomatic until they rupture.
- There is often a history of exertion at the moment symptoms begin.
- After rupture has occurred, headaches are often described as the "worst headache" in the patient's life, or a "thunderclap" headache. The patient may develop syncope or appear obtunded and confused. Twenty-five percent of patients manifest focal neurologic deficits. Alterations in pulse and respiratory effort may occur. Nausea, vomiting, and meningismus may also be present as blood entering the CSF irritates the meninges. The patient's level of consciousness may rapidly progress to stupor or coma.
- Early attention to airway management is of critical importance.

C. Laboratory and diagnostic studies
- A noncontrast CT is the initial imaging modality of choice.
- Blood seen on noncontrast CT scan usually establishes the diagnosis of subarachnoid hemorrhage.
- CT fails to detect occult subarachnoid hemorrhage in about 5% of cases.

- If the CT scan is negative and subarachnoid hemorrhage is strongly suspected, a lumbar puncture is performed. The presence of xanthochromia (a characteristic heme-protein-mediated yellow color) to the CSF supernatant establishes the diagnosis of subarachnoid hemorrhage.
- CT angiography or conventional cerebral angiography is used to identify the cause of the hemorrhage (aneurysm, AVM) as well as asymptomatic vascular abnormalities (unruptured aneurysms).

D. Formulating the diagnosis
- The history, physical examination, CT scan, and lumbar puncture usually establish the diagnosis of subarachnoid hemorrhage.
- CT angiography or cerebral angiography can differentiate aneurysmal subarachnoid bleed from tumor, AVM, or subdural hemorrhage.
- Occasionally subarachnoid hemorrhage will mimic the symptoms of a myocardial infarction (i.e., ECG changes) through a sympathetically mediated process.

E. Evaluating the severity of problems
- Subarachnoid hemorrhage is an extremely serious disorder, with over 50% mortality rate within the first 2 weeks of presentation. If subarachnoid bleed is suspected, neurosurgical consultation should be sought immediately.

F. Managing the patient
- Once hemorrhagic cerebral aneurysm has been diagnosed, the patient's activities should be restricted to bed rest. The patient should be placed on agents such as docusate that prevent constipation and straining while defecating (straining causes increased intracranial pressure). Narcotics may be necessary for headache control.
- The major serious complications after subarachnoid hemorrhage (SAH) include rebleed, vasospasm, and hydrocephalus.
- The risk of rebleed is greatest in the first 24 hours after the ictus; early surgery is preventive.
- Serial transcranial doppler ultrasonography is frequently used to monitor the intracranial vessels for the presence of vasospasm. Vasospasm is usually maximum at 4 to 10 days after ictus and is treated with oral nimodipine, hypertensive/hypervolemic therapy, and possible angioplasty of vessels with critical stenoses to prevent ischemic infarction.
- Acute or delayed hydrocephalus can also occur after SAH and is managed with ventriculostomy or chronic CSF diversion (e.g., ventriculoperitoneal shunt) as needed.
- Other complications include hyponatremia and seizure.

Ophthalmology

I. Anatomy of the Globe and Orbit

- The orbital walls are composed of seven bones: ethmoid, frontal, lacrimal, maxillary, palatine, sphenoid, and zygomatic. The orbit is surrounded on three sides by sinuses: the frontal sinus above, the ethmoid and sphenoid sinuses medially, and the maxillary sinus below.
- Orbital fractures are most likely to involve the floor, medial wall, and roof. The lateral wall of the orbit is the thickest and strongest of the orbital walls. The medial orbital wall is paper-thin, as reflected in its name, lamina papyracea; it and the inferior wall are most prone to fracture.
- Following an ethmoid fracture, air may enter the orbit when the patient blows his or her nose, causing crepitus on palpating the orbit.
- In children, infections of the ethmoid sinuses may extend through the lamina papyracea to cause orbital cellulitis and exophthalmos.
- Orbital floor fractures are commonly known as "blowout" fractures. Clinical features of blowout fractures may include diplopia, enophthalmos, hypesthesia in the distribution of the infraorbital nerve, entrapment of orbital tissues or extraocular muscles with restricted upgaze, and radiographic evidence of fluid level or cloudiness of the maxillary sinus. Orbital roof fractures may be especially serious. Because of the potential involvement of the dura, brain, and frontal sinus, one should look for presence of cerebrospinal fluid rhinorrhea or pneumocephalus (i.e., air in the intracranial cavity). Usually, orbital computed tomography (CT) scanning, including coronal images, is most appropriate.
- The optic foramen, located at the apex of the orbit, transmits the optic nerve, the ophthalmic artery (which gives rise to the central retinal artery), and sympathetic fibers from the carotid plexus (Fig. 2-1).
- The superior orbital fissure lies adjacent to the optic foramen and transmits the sympathetic nerve plexus, all other orbital nerves (cranial nerve [CN] III, IV, VI, and the ophthalmic branch of CN V), and the superior ophthalmic vein. A lesion at the apex of the orbit can affect any or all of these structures.
- The transparent cornea occupies the center of the anterior pole of the globe and performs most of the refraction of light entering the eye. Abnormalities of the cornea may compromise its transparency, involve loss of corneal tissue, result in neovascularization of the normally avascular cornea, or result in corneal swelling.
- In contrast to the transparent cornea, the sclera is opaque and white. It is thicker than most of the cornea and provides insertions to the extraocular muscles. Inflammation of the sclera (or scleritis) may affect individuals with rheumatoid arthritis or other connective tissue diseases.

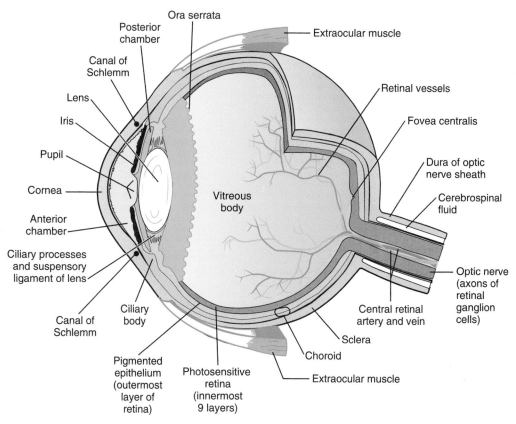

2-1: *General anatomy of the eyeball, including its tunics and chambers. (Adapted from Burns ER, Cave MD: Rapid Review Histology and Cell Biology, 2nd ed. St. Louis, Mosby, 2007, p 227.)*

- The limbus, which is the transition zone located between the peripheral cornea and the anterior sclera, is gray and translucent. This is an important area anatomically because many surgical procedures, including cataract extraction, involve entering the eye at this location.
- The inside of the lids and sclerae are covered by the normally clear conjunctiva. The conjunctiva may become erythematous or edematous or show inflammatory changes in a variety of conditions.
- The interior of the eye consists of three chambers. The anterior chamber is the space between the clear cornea and colored iris. This region is filled with aqueous humor produced by the eye. Blood in the anterior chamber is called a hyphema and may occur following ocular trauma or surgery. Ocular infections or inflammation may result in pus in the anterior chamber, known as a hypopyon.
- The posterior chamber is a small space between the iris and the lens immediately behind the dark pupillary space. Aqueous fluid is produced here, and it usually flows forward through the pupil, into the anterior chamber, and out the chamber angle, a space in the eye just interior to the limbus. In glaucoma, the intraocular

pressure in this space is elevated, usually owing to poor outflow of this fluid from the angle.
- The third space is the vitreous cavity, which is behind the lens and occupies the main volume of the eye. This chamber contains vitreous humor, a thick gel-like substance. Bleeding, infection, and inflammation may affect the vitreous. Surgical removal of the vitreous may become necessary in such conditions as vitreous hemorrhage (e.g., due to severe diabetic retinopathy or infections such as endophthalmitis) or for retinal detachment repair.
- Eye movements are controlled by six extraocular muscles: four rectus muscles and two oblique muscles. These muscles insert at varying distances posterior to the limbus and move the eyes in the various directions of gaze.
- Except for the lateral rectus, which is innervated by the abducens nerve (CN VI), and the superior oblique, which is innervated by the trochlear nerve (CN IV), the remaining extraocular muscles are innervated by the oculomotor nerve (CN III). Complete CN III paralysis results in an inability to move the eye up or in; ptosis (lid droop due to lid elevator paralysis); and a dilated pupil. A CN III palsy secondary to diabetes mellitus tends not to affect the pupil.
- Palsies of any of the muscles may result in diplopia or double vision. Common causes include strabismus as a child, diabetes, and intracranial lesions such as aneurysms and strokes. Imaging may be warranted if an intracranial or intraorbital lesion is suspected or the cause cannot be readily determined, or if it is long-standing. Figure 2-1 shows basic eye anatomy.

II. Cataracts
  A. Basic science
    - A cataract is an opacity of the lens of the eye that interferes with vision. Cataracts are most common in the elderly but are also seen in younger individuals. There are three main types of cataracts:
      - Congenital or juvenile onset
      - Secondary
      - Age related
    - Congenital cataracts are generally associated with systemic or ocular diseases, inherited traits, or exposure, but may be of undetermined cause. Associated conditions include galactosemia, hypoglycemia, and intrauterine infections.
    - Secondary cataracts are directly related to acquired systemic disorders, acquired ocular disease, physical trauma, medications, or local chemical agents. Examples include hypocalcemia, intraocular neoplasms, radiation, and steroids.
    - Age-related cataracts are the most common form and are caused by lens opacification as its chemical composition changes. Water content decreases, soluble protein becomes more insoluble, and calcium content increases. The lens becomes progressively harder as it opacifies. About 90% of all cataracts are age-related and begin development after 40 years of age.
  B. History and physical examination
    - The etiology of congenital and infantile cataracts may often be determined by seeking a prenatal history of maternal infections such as rubella or syphilis, a

family history of chromosomal abnormalities (e.g., trisomy 21 or 13), or a family history of cataracts.

- In older patients, it is important to determine any secondary causes of cataracts. These include trauma, drug exposure such as chronic steroid administration, dermatologic diseases (e.g., atopic dermatitis), metabolic disorders (e.g., diabetes mellitus or hypothyroidism), and other systemic syndromes or associated ocular abnormalities.
- Examination of a patient suspected of having a cataract generally includes visual acuity testing at distance and near, both in lighted conditions and dark. With the use of a slit lamp biomicroscope, one may determine the location and density of most opacities within the lens. A simple way to examine the lens is with a direct ophthalmoscope. Any opacities in the ocular media will appear as dark spots in the normal red reflex. Fundus evaluation by indirect and direct ophthalmoscopy is necessary to evaluate the macula, optic nerve, and retinal vessels.
- Posterior segment pathology may limit visual rehabilitation after an otherwise uneventful cataract extraction.

C. Laboratory and diagnostic studies
- Special tests estimating potential visual acuity are often helpful in assessing the contribution of the cataract to the patient's visual loss.
- Laboratory evaluation assists in determining inborn errors of metabolism and metabolic diseases that may result in cataracts.

D. Formulating the diagnosis
- The occurrence of an intralenticular opacity associated with a decrease in visual acuity in an eye suggests the diagnosis of cataract. It is confirmed with visual acuity testing, slit lamp examination, funduscopic examination, and potential acuity testing.
- Cataract may be confused with corneal opacity, anterior chamber opacity, and intraocular masses, including retinoblastoma.

E. Evaluating the severity of problems
- A cataract is clinically important if it causes a significant decline in visual function.
- Patients often complain of decreased visual acuity but may also experience increased glare, double vision, and decreased contrast sensitivity.
- Symptoms may worsen in either especially bright or dim light. Often patients will complain of difficulty driving at night because of increased glare with oncoming headlights.
- Patients often have severe compromise of their activities of daily living such as reading, driving, and working.

F. Managing the patient
- No medical treatment has been proved to prevent or reverse cataract development, although many are under investigation.
- Pupillary dilation may improve vision by allowing light to pass peripheral to the lens opacity. Spectacle correction may correct refractive errors induced by the cataract. Light absorption filters are useful for blocking those frequencies of light that create glare. These measures are useful for

patients when operative management is neither needed nor desired by the patient.

- Low vision aids including handheld monoculars and magnifying lenses may be useful for patients in whom surgery is contraindicated.
- The decision for surgical management is based primarily on whether reduced vision significantly interferes with the patient's activities. Other factors that must be assessed are the health of both eyes, the potential for vision, and the general health of the patient.
- For congenital cataracts, removal should be considered as soon as possible after birth, preferably before 3 months of age. A clear optical pathway is important during the early stages of visual pathway development to prevent amblyopia or "lazy eye" and to help development of binocular vision and stereopsis.
- Cataract surgery is usually performed using ultrasound power (phacoemulsification) to break up the nucleus of the lens prior to removal.
- An implant is almost always placed within the eye at the time of surgery for optical rehabilitation; that is, the power of the normal crystalline lens needs to be replaced at the time of surgery to avoid the need for thick "cataract" glasses. The implant is a plastic, acrylic, or silicone lens that acts to refract light once it enters the eye.
- Visual rehabilitation is usually rapid. Many patients gain their best corrected vision within the first few weeks after surgery.

III. Conjunctivitis
  A. Basic science
  - Conjunctivitis refers to any disorder causing inflammation of the conjunctiva, usually manifested as a "red eye."
  - There are many primary causes of conjunctivitis, including infections and allergy. Secondary causes of conjunctival inflammation include lid disease, corneal disease, orbital disease, and intraocular inflammation such as iritis. It is important to differentiate primary conjunctivitis from that due to adjacent ocular disease.
  - The conjunctiva may be primarily infected with viral entities (e.g., adenovirus) or with bacteria (e.g., staphylococci and streptococci). Most cases of bacterial conjunctivitis are confined to the conjunctiva, although there may be extension to other ocular structures. Ocular immune responses to infection, especially to viral antigens, may worsen ocular damage.
  - Certain bacteria are considered normal flora on the conjunctiva. These have been implicated as the etiology of infections in some patients due to compromised local immune function. In others, exposure to contagious individuals or fomites may spread bacteria or virus particles. Adenoviruses can live on dry surfaces for many hours and thus are highly contagious.
  B. History and physical examination
  - It is imperative to establish a history of the present illness. One should explore the course of development, the presence of a discharge (bacterial infections

produce more than viral), pain, recent upper respiratory infection (suggesting viral conjunctivitis), photophobia (suggesting iritis), foreign body sensation, itching (suggesting allergic conjunctivitis), burning, associated fever or rash, or decreased visual acuity.

- Elements of the past ocular history may be relevant, including glaucoma and contact lens wear. A history of atopic disease may be important in the diagnosis of allergic conjunctivitis. A history of herpes simplex virus labialis may be significant.

- Conjunctivitis usually does not decrease visual acuity. The pupils should be equal, round, and reactive to the light. Glaucoma or iritis may cause abnormal pupils. The periorbital skin should be inspected for lesions such as herpes simplex or zoster and for atopic or allergic changes. The conjunctiva should be grossly inspected for injection (redness) and chemosis (swelling). Gross purulence is usually present with bacterial conjunctivitis and sometimes with viral. Gonococcal conjunctivitis usually produces copious purulence. Adenovirus usually causes a watery discharge and swollen preauricular lymph nodes.

- The corneal surface and its light reflex should be inspected for whitish opacities (infectious infiltrates), foreign bodies, and decreased sheen and luster. Fluorescein dye may be instilled and observed with a cobalt blue light filter. Any dye uptake by the cornea indicates loss of corneal epithelium and thus suggests corneal disease. Any conjunctivitis in a contact lens patient should raise immediate suspicion for corneal disease, as corneal infections are increased in frequency in this population.

- Allergic conjunctivitis is often associated with conjunctival swelling and redness, lid swelling and erythema, and significant itching.

- Another less common cause of conjunctivitis is *Chlamydia* infection. In third world countries, trachoma is a common chronic conjunctivitis caused by *Chlamydia trachomatis* and is not sexually transmitted.

- To rule out other ocular diseases such as immune reactions, iritis, scleral or episcleral inflammation (scleritis, episcleritis), keratitis, or other conditions, an examination at a slit lamp is usually needed.

- **Red flags:** Warning signs of a more serious problem that should prompt evaluation by an ophthalmologist:
  1. Reduction of visual acuity
  2. Ciliary flush: A pattern of injection in which the redness is most pronounced in a ring at the limbus (the limbus is the transition zone between the cornea and the sclera)
  3. Photophobia
  4. Severe foreign body sensation that prevents the patient from keeping the eye open
  5. Corneal opacity or edema
  6. Irregular, asymmetric, or nonreacting pupil
  7. Severe headache with nausea
  8. Positive fluorescin test
  9. Contact lens use

C. Laboratory and diagnostic studies
  - Bacterial cultures are helpful if the patient does not respond to initial treatment.
D. Formulating the diagnosis
  - In the primary care setting, the history and physical examination usually suffice to make the diagnosis. Any suspicious history concerning ocular signs should prompt an ophthalmologic referral.
E. Managing the patient
  - If bacterial conjunctivitis is highly suspected, topical antibiotics can be started. Seven to 10 days of treatment is usually sufficient. Never use an antibiotic-steroid combination, or steroids alone, as this may lead to significant complications, including the potentiation of herpes simplex virus as well as worsened bacterial and viral infections.
  - Viral conjunctivitis usually runs its course but may lead to serious sequelae. Treatment usually consists of keeping the eye clear of accumulating discharge, cool compresses, and contagious precautions. Topical antibiotics may be added for possible bacterial infection if the diagnosis is in doubt.
  - Viral conjunctivitis can be contagious for approximately 2 weeks from the onset of symptoms. Patients should be advised to use prudent handwashing and to avoid sharing of towels or pillows. Due to the extremely infectious, often epidemic nature of viral adenovirus conjunctivitis, health care providers and others, including day care workers, must often be secluded if they cannot observe precaution.
  - Gonococcal conjunctivitis requires systemic antibiotics. Topical antibiotics are often helpful as well. Treatment for *Chlamydia* infection is also prudent given the significant rate of dual infection in this group. *Chlamydia* infection is often treated with oral doxycycline for 2 to 3 weeks. It is important to treat the sexual partners of these patients.
  - Allergic conjunctivitis can be treated with cool compresses and systemic antihistamines. Several topical products exist (e.g., antihistamines, mast cell stabilizers, and nonsteroidal anti-inflamatory drugs) and may provide symptomatic relief.

IV. Diabetic Retinopathy
  A. Basic science
  - Diabetic retinopathy is a significant cause of blindness in the United States. Its prevalence within the diabetic population increases with the duration of the disease and in patients with poorly controlled diabetes.
  - Within 7 years of diagnosis, more than half of the patients have some degree of retinopathy. This increases to over 90% for those with diabetes of many years' duration.
  - Diabetic retinopathy in the vast majority of cases precedes diabetic nephropathy.
  - Diabetic retinopathy is a microvascular disease of the retina. Sustained levels of hyperglycemia cause ongoing vessel damage with basement membrane thickening, endothelial cell loss, and, finally, capillary nonperfusion.

Intraretinal capillary closure leads to retinal ischemia and the release of a vasoproliferative factor. Neovascularization may occur on the optic nerve, retina, or iris. Leakage from capillaries leads to retinal edema which on resorption leaves behind "hard exudates" or lipoid deposits.

B. History and physical examination
- Examination of the retina with a direct ophthalmoscope shows changes that may be categorized in four stages.
  1. Background diabetic retinopathy (BDR)
     - Impaired autoregulation of the retinal vasculature and alterations in the retinal blood flow lead to microaneurysms, hemorrhages, and hard exudates. In severe cases flame hemorrages and cotton wool spots can be seen.
     - Patients without retinopathy should be seen by their ophthalmologist at least yearly. Once background retinopathy is detected, patients should be followed at least every 6 to 12 months, or even more often, depending on disease severity.
  2. Maculopathy/preproliferative stage
     - The central retina area is called the macula and is responsible for our precise central vision. Edema within the macula may lead to central visual loss. This is the commonest cause of visual loss in diabetic retinopathy.
     - Retinal thickening shows characteristic signs including the accumulation of a yellow lipid called hard exudate. This may take the form of a circinate ring in the macula.
     - Focal areas of edema may be treated with laser therapy. Diffuse edema has a poorer visual prognosis. Retinal ischemia may also be prominent resulting in significant visual loss. These patients need close ophthalmologic follow-up.
  3. Proliferative stage
     - Extensive ischemia leads to production of a vasoproliferative factor, which stimulates neovascularization. These abnormal vessels usually grow from the venous circulation. They are friable and tend to bleed easily. This may lead to hemorrhage within the retina or vitreous cavity, resulting in profound visual loss.
     - This stage generally occurs in diabetics who already manifest other end organ damage. These patients need urgent panretinal laser treatment to destroy hypoxic retina. Laser therapy will stop the production of the angiogenic factor, thus causing regression of neovascularization.
  4. Cicatricial stage
     - In this end stage, fibrous traction bands form between the retina and the vitreous face. These bands may eventually contract and may cause tractional retinal detachments. Surgery is often indicated to remove scar tissue and reattach the retina if needed. The visual potential of these patients is often low.
C. Laboratory and diagnostic studies
- Fluorescein angiography is often essential to define areas of leakage, aneurysm formation, ischemia, and neovascularization.

- Serum glucose monitoring and hemoglobin A_{1C} measurements are important in defining blood sugar control.

D. Formulating the diagnosis
- Characteristic retina changes in the setting of diabetes mellitus are diagnostic.

E. Evaluating the severity of problems
- Blindness is the end result of untreated diabetic retinopathy.

F. Managing the patient
   1. Metabolic control
      - It is generally agreed that tight serum glucose control may retard the onset or progression of retinopathy. Although some controversy exists, most ophthalmologists advocate maintaining as normal a serum glucose as possible.
   2. Laser photocoagulation
      - Laser therapy may significantly improve vision in some patients and prevent significant visual loss in others. There are two main groups of patients who benefit. The first group includes those with macular edema. The second group includes those with neovascularization.
      - Appropriate retinal examinations and adequate follow-up are extremely important.

V. Eyelid and Lacrimal System Pathology
- Anatomically, the lids consist of an outer thin layer of skin, a central collagenous plate (tarsus), and the inner conjunctiva. The skin is very thin and lacks subcutaneous fat. Fluid can easily accumulate beneath it. The tarsal plate is firm and rubbery and houses sebaceous glands that secrete lipid into the tear film. The conjunctival layer is in contact with the ocular surface and spreads tears over the eye with each blink. Muscular layers within the lid are responsible for opening and closing the lids.
- A wide spectrum of pathologic processes occur on or within the eyelids and can be categorized as infectious (bacterial and viral), degenerative, or neoplastic.

A. Eyelid inflammation and infections
   1. Blepharitis
      - The lipid glands within the lid may become plugged. This results in a deficiency of lipid in the tear film that normally lubricates and protects the ocular surface. This condition is known as blepharitis.
      - Patients may complain of eye and lid discomfort, including burning and itching, as well as a "gritty" sensation. Signs include eyelid erythema and edema, crusting or scaling of the eyelid margins, and a red eye.
      - The glands may become secondarily infected, usually with staphylococci, leading to bacterial toxin production with associated ocular inflammation.
      - Blepharitis may commonly accompany rosacea or acne vulgaris.
      - Treatment requires patient education as to the chronicity of the problem and eyelid hygiene (warm washcloth compresses followed by gentle scrubbing). An application of an antibiotic-corticosteroid ointment may reduce the infectious and inflammatory components of the disorder, but

this requires closer monitoring. If these measures are unsuccessful, oral doxycycline may be useful.

2. Chalazion
   - This very common, focal inflammation of the lids results from an obstruction of the meibomian glands. The lipid secretions break out of the glands into the surrounding tarsus, muscle, and soft tissues. An acute inflammatory response ensues, along with pain and erythema of the skin and lid.
   - In the acute inflammatory phase, the treatment consists of warm compresses, which soften the sebum and facilitate its passage out of the gland. This may be combined with a topical antibiotic and appropriate lid hygiene.
   - Frequently the lesions become chronic cysts that require incision and curettage to debulk the granulomatous mass. Spontaneous resorption may occur over weeks to months.
   - One should suspect a sebaceous carcinoma whenever a chalazion is unusually persistent or recurrent.

3. Hordeolum (stye)
   - Hordeola are acute bacterial infections involving the lid sweat glands or the lash (cilia) follicle. The onset can be rapid, and an inflammatory mass forms. These vary in size but may be so big as to distort the vision due to pressure on the globe due to astigmatism. Staphylococci are the usual offending bacteria.
   - A hordeolum points toward the lid margin and usually drains spontaneously, although its resolution can be hastened by the application of warm compresses, antibiotic ointment, and occasionally oral antibiotics.

4. Herpes simplex
   - Similar in appearance to herpes zoster, simplex lesions are confined to the epidermis. In comparison to zoster, simplex lesions usually do not scar, but recurrences are relatively common.
   - For the lid skin, local treatment is rarely needed. If vesicles are present on the eyelid margin, the eye may become involved, and thus topical treatment of the eye and lid with an antiviral may be warranted. Oral acyclovir may also be used. Timely ophthalmic referral should be made for any ocular signs or symptoms.

5. Preseptal/orbital cellulitis
   - Cellulitis of the eyelid may occur after seemingly minor trauma or because of a "pimple." The most common offending microbe is *Staphylococcus aureus.*
   - The orbital septum acts as a relative barrier to the spread of the infection posteriorly into the orbit. Preseptal cellulitis involves only anterior structures, does not extend into the orbit, and has no associated ocular motility or vision abnormalities.
   - Appropriate oral antibiotics, outpatient treatment, and close follow up are needed. Orbital cellulitis with proptosis and motility disturbances requires

urgent IV antibiotics and orbital imaging to rule out abscess formation. *Haemophilus influenzae* is a particular culprit when preseptal cellulitis occurs in a young child with coexistent upper respiratory infection. The eyelid frequently has a violaceous hue.

6. Dacryocystitis
   - Tears drain from the eye through a small opening in the medial upper and lower lid. This drains through the lacrimal sac (medial to the eye) and the nasolacrimal duct to the inner nose. Dacryocystitis, or infection of the lacrimal sac, is a common acute or chronic disease that typically occurs in infants or in persons over the age of 40.
   - In acute dacryocystitis the usual infectious organism is *Staphylococcus aureus* or, less frequently, beta-hemolytic streptococcus. In chronic dacryocystitis, *Streptococcus pneumoniae* is the predominant agent.
   - In cases of fungal infection, obstruction of the nasolacrimal duct by a dacryolith sometimes occurs.
   - In the acute form, inflammation, pain, swelling, and tenderness are present in the tear sac region. A mucopurulent discharge may be expressed from the puncta by applying pressure to the lacrimal sac.
   - Infantile dacryocystitis may result when the nasolacrimal duct fails to open spontaneously before birth or during the first month of life. Usually, there is a membranous blockage of the one of the valves of the nasolacrimal drainage system near the distal portion of the lacrimal sac beneath the inferior turbinate of the nose. Most obstructions open spontaneously within 4 to 6 weeks after birth. Massage of the lacrimal sac and application of topical antibiotics may be performed. If this conservative management fails, a nasal lacrimal duct probing should be performed.

B. Degenerative changes
   1. Entropion
      - Entropion is characterized as a tendency for the eyelid margin to rotate inward, with the lashes rubbing against the globe. The lower lid is most frequently involved.
      - This seldom occurs in patients under 40 years of age.
      - Senile entropion is a degenerative change resulting from tissue atrophy and detachment of fascial attachments to the lid.
      - Cicatricial entropion results from scarring of the lid conjunctiva with resultant inversion of the lid margin.
      - Entropion should be distinguished from trichiasis in which the eyelid margin is properly positioned, but eye irritation occurs from the misdirection of the eyelashes rubbing against the cornea.
   2. Ectropion
      - Ectropion is a tendency for the eyelid margin to rotate anteriorly, away from the globe. Like entropion, it is a degenerative change and is associated with horizontal lid laxity.
      - Exposure of the eye due to inadequate coverage may cause ocular complications.

- Paralytic ectropion is a common disorder in patients suffering from facial nerve disease such as Bell's palsy. These patients often cannot close the eye fully (lagophthalmos).
3. Dermatochalasis/blepharochalasis
    - Dermatochalasis refers to the redundant, baggy eyelid skin that occurs with age.
    - Blepharochalasis refers to a condition of thinned, stretched eyelid skin that results from repeated bouts of eyelid edema of no apparent cause.
4. Ptosis
    - Ptosis is a drooping of the upper lid, occurring in two distinct forms.
    - Congenital ptosis is characterized by a mild to severe degree of drooping, poor lid elevation function, and a poorly developed eyelid crease. It will be present at birth.
    - Acquired ptosis is characterized by gradual onset and may be due to previous eye surgery, trauma, or aging.
    - Other conditions associated with ptosis include Horner's syndrome, third cranial nerve palsy, and myasthenia gravis.

C. Neoplastic growths
- The most common malignant tumor of the lid is basal cell carcinoma, accounting for 90% of malignant eyelid neoplasms. Basal cell carcinomas are more commonly located on the lower eyelid or in the medial canthal region.
- Epithelial tumors such as seborrheic keratoses and squamous papillomas, as well as sudoriferous cysts, inclusion cysts, and cutaneous horns, are also quite common.
- Xanthelasmas are frequently seen lesions that characteristically localize to the nasal portion of both the upper and lower lids. They may occur spontaneously but are often associated with elevated serum cholesterol. These lesions are composed of lipid-filled histiocytes and are typically plaquelike, yellow, and soft.
- Sebaceous carcinomas usually arise from the meibomian glands and are the second most common eyelid malignancy. The upper lid is the usual site of origin. The tumor has a potential for local invasion and metastasis. Frequently they appear as a chalazion or as blepharoconjunctivitis. The diagnosis may be difficult or missed entirely for many months after onset.

VI. Glaucoma
  A. Basic science
- Glaucoma is an ocular disease characterized by elevated intraocular pressure (IOP). IOP is related to the aqueous humor of the eye. Aqueous humor is produced by the ciliary body in the posterior chamber, flows through the pupils into the anterior chamber, and then goes through the trabecular network in the angle and into Schlemm's canal. The greater the resistance to this flow in the trabecular network and Schelmm's canal, the greater is the intraocular pressure.

- Physiologically, IOP is determined by the rate of aqueous humor fluid production and outflow. The most common cause of increased IOP is secondary to outflow obstruction.
- Normal IOP is between 11 and 21 mm Hg. People with increased IOP are more likely to suffer from glaucomatous optic nerve damage, but increased IOP is not the sole factor. Some people with increased IOP do not develop optic nerve damage and therefore do not have glaucoma, whereas others develop optic nerve damage despite normal to low IOP and therefore do have glaucoma.
- The effect of glaucoma on the optic nerve is manifested as "cupping" or notching—an atrophy of the optic nerve head that leads to characteristic visual field loss. In glaucoma, the cup-to-disk ratio is increased; that is, the diameter of the cup takes up a disproportionate amount of the cross section of the optic disk. This finding suggests significant optic nerve damage. The damage may be due to a direct effect of elevated pressure on the nerve, disruption of axoplasmic flow, or vascular occlusion due to hemodynamic effects.

B. History and physical examination
- Clinically, glaucoma may present as acute or chronic varieties. Acute glaucoma usually involves closure of the anterior chamber angle. Closure occurs when the iris is pushed forward against the cornea, blocking the normal fluid outflow path. The most common causes of angle closure glaucoma are primary angle closure (an anatomic variant that is prone to closure), iris neovascularization, and others.
- Patients suffering an acute angle closure attack present with the sudden onset of pain, blurred vision, and photophobia. They may also complain of seeing halos around light sources that result from cornea swelling or edema. Upon examination, the eye may appear red, the cornea appears gray or hazy, and the anterior chamber will be shallow. IOP is usually very high (e.g., 40–80 mm Hg). One or both eyes may be involved. The patient may have experienced similar but perhaps milder episodes previously, especially while in a darkened area such as a movie theater. Iris dilation in this situation is a contributing factor. Pharmacologic dilation (e.g., during a routine examination) in predisposed individuals may also cause an attack of angle closure glaucoma. Predisposed individuals tend to be farsighted.
- Chronic glaucoma is far more common and usually is of the open angle variety. The gross anatomy appears normal, but there is resistance to fluid outflow of the eye at a microscopic level. Patients are usually asymptomatic, but a minority may experience a mild, nonspecific discomfort. Patients with this condition usually, but not always, have increased IOP, increased cupping or notching, and visual field defects. Risk factors for chronic open angle glaucoma include a positive family history of glaucoma or diabetes mellitus and a history of severe ocular trauma. Because early signs of this type of glaucoma (increased IOP and cup-to-disk ratio) are nonspecific, the initial diagnosis may be difficult, and these patients may require serial observations and visual field examination to obtain a definitive diagnosis.

C. Laboratory and diagnostic studies
- The IOP must be measured.
- Optic nerve damage is evaluated by observing changes in optic disk or nerve fiber layer. Currently, the most sensitive test of functional damage from glaucoma is visual field testing.

D. Formulating the diagnosis
- The differential diagnosis of a red, painful eye includes glaucoma, conjunctivitis, foreign body, corneal abrasion, keratitis, and intraocular inflammation (uveitis).
- The differential diagnosis of optic nerve damage includes glaucoma; optic neuropathy; optic neuritis; and compressive lesions of the optic nerve such as gliomas, meningiomas, aneurysms, and metastatic tumors.

E. Evaluating the severity of problem
- Acute angle closure glaucoma is a medical emergency. Prompt relief of increased IOP and correction of the underlying cause must be accomplished. Permanent loss of vision can result in as little as an hour to several days.

F. Managing the patient
- IOP can be lowered by giving topical β-blockers, oral or topical carbonic anhydrase inhibitors, and oral or IV osmotic agents such as mannitol. Topical pilocarpine (which constricts the pupil) can often be used to break the attack as it pulls the iris away from the chamber angle.
- In a primary angle closure attack, the definitive treatment is peripheral iridotomy in which a laser is used to make an opening in the iris, relieving the obstruction to flow.
- In chronic glaucoma, medical treatment is usually the first line of therapy. Treatments include topical β-blockers, apraclonidine, carbonic anhydrase inhibitors, and indirect or direct parasympathomimetics (e.g., pilocarpine, phospholine iodide).
- If patients fail or are intolerant of medical treatment, laser treatment of the trabecular meshwork (part of the outflow channel) may be helpful (argon laser trabeculoplasty). Some patients may be helped by glaucoma filtering surgery. This involves creation of a connection from the anterior chamber of the eye to a space further back on the eye, effectively shunting fluid from the anterior eye.
- All patients above age 50 should have eye examinations every 2 years to check for glaucoma; patients over age 65 should have annual examinations.

VII. Macular Degeneration
- Age-related macular degeneration is the leading cause of irreversible acquired legal blindness in developed countries. There are two types: atrophic ("dry") and neovascular ("wet"). Atrophic is by far the most common.
- Background: the fovea is responsible for fine visual acuity. The fovea and the surrounding retina form the macular area. Although the macula composes only 2% of the visual field, 25% of the cone photoreceptors are here and it correlates with half of the primary visual area of the brain.

- Atrophic age-related macular degeneration causes a gradual loss of central acuity down to 20/400 (peripheral vision is spared).
- Neovascular age-related macular degeneration (AMD) is somewhat amenable to treatment with laser photocoagulation and photodynamic therapy.
- Risk factors for both types include smoking and low levels of zinc and antioxidants in the diet. It has been found that taking high doses of antioxidants and zinc can reduce the risk of AMD by about 25%.

VIII. Hypertensive Retinopathy
  A. Basic science
  - Systemic hypertension may cause localized or generalized arteriolar constriction. This may affect vessels in either the retina (observable with an ophthalmoscope) or choroid. The choroid is an intricate network of smaller vessels between the retina and sclera.
  - Acutely and significantly elevated blood pressure may lead to vascular nonperfusion of the choroidal layer. This may affect the overlying retina with fluid leakage (retinal edema), ischemia, and eventual retinal photoreceptor loss. The optic nerve head may also become swollen on an ischemic or mechanical basis.
  - Chronically elevated systemic blood pressure leads to retinal vessel constriction secondary to autoregulation. This leads to vessel leakage of fluid into the retina, thickening of the vessel walls, and formation of aneurysms of retinal vessels.
  B. History and physical examination
  - The fundus should be examined with a direct ophthalmoscope. Dilation may be needed for an adequate examination. The following signs may be noted:
    1. Microaneurysms/macroaneurysms
       - Microaneurysms and macroaneurysms are small, red, dotlike vascular outpouchings in the retina. They are well defined and round and need not be adjacent to observable arterioles.
    2. Cotton wool spots
       - Nerve fiber infarction may cause cotton wool spots, which are white nebulous areas in the retina.
    3. Optic nerve swelling
       - The nerve head may be swollen; this is demonstrated by the loss of the normally sharp outer rim and the optic cup. The nerve bulges toward the vitreous cavity instead of being flush against the ocular wall.
    4. Retinal vessel changes
       - Narrowing of retinal arterioles
       - Decreased absolute diameter of the vessels
       - Thickening of retinal arteriole walls
       - Broader and brighter light reflex off the vessel wall

5. Arteriovenous crossing changes
   • Thickened arterioles may cause compression of veins at points where they cross; this is called nicking.
6. Hemorrhages
   • In hypertension retinal hemorrhages are usually flame-shaped but can be dot- or blot-shaped.
7. Hard exudates
   • Hard exudates are well-defined yellow accumulations of lipid within the retina that are due to chronic edema; these are seen more in patients with diabetes rather than in those with hypertension.

C. Laboratory and diagnostic studies
   • Fluorescein angiography may be performed by an ophthalmologist. Dye is injected into a peripheral vein, and specialized pictures are taken of the retinal vasculature as the fluorescent dye travels within it. Vessel wall anatomy, patency, and leakage can be well visualized.

D. Formulating the diagnosis
   • Characteristic retinal vascular changes in the setting of either acute or chronic systemic hypertension may be diagnostic.

E. Evaluating the severity of problems
   • Hypertensive retinopathy suggests that hypertensive changes have occurred elsewhere within the cardiovascular system, predisposing the patient to an increased risk of stroke and heart disease.

F. Managing the patient
   • Control of chronic hypertension may slow or halt disease progression. Argon laser photocoagulation may be performed to treat some retinal changes including fluid leakage, ischemia, and aneurysm formation.
   • If the retina shows signs of acute malignant hypertension (optic nerve head swelling, ischemic/necrotic changes), blood pressure should be brought down urgently but gradually to prevent optic nerve infarction.

IX. Retinal Vascular Occlusion
   A. Retinal artery occlusion
      • Occlusion of the central retinal artery (usually embolic) causes sudden, painless, unilateral blindness. This is a true ocular emergency and every minute counts. Retinal edema (sparing the relatively thin fovea, which is perfused by the choroid) creates pallor and the appearance of a "cherry red spot" in the macula.
      • Treatment is directed toward dislodging the embolus and includes ocular massage, paracentesis of the anterior chamber (to lower the pressure), and carbogen (95% O_2, 5% CO_2) inhalation to dialate retinal vessels. While waiting for the ophthalmologist, have the patient get into the Trendelenburg position and breath into a paper sack. You may massage the affected globe with the your index finger (5 seconds pressure, 5 seconds no pressure, repeat). Unfortunately, all these temporary measures are only rarely effective. Patients subsequently require a thorough systemic evaluation for the source of emboli.

B. Retinal vein occlusion
- Retinal vein occlusion causes sudden, painless, near-total loss of vision. Causes include hypertension, polycythemia vera, and Waldenström macroglobulinemia. Retinal edema is accompanied by hemorrhage, not a cherry red spot.
- Diagnosis is made with an ophthalmoloscopic examination showing a "blood and thunder" fundus with multiple hemorrhages.
- Unlike retinal artery occlusion, there is no effective acute treatment and it's not considered and emergency.

3

Otorhinolaryngology

I. Allergic Rhinitis
   A. Basic science
      - Allergic rhinitis is the nasal manifestation of the body's allergic response to environmental antigens. Binding of IgE to mast cells and basophils in the peripheral blood triggers the release of histamine, leukotrienes, and cytokines within the nose, causing swelling of the nasal lining and increased production of mucus.
   B. History and physical examination
      - A focused history should include symptoms, triggers, and personal or family history of atopy (eczema, urticaria, asthma).
      - Symptoms are commonly seasonal, but may be perennial if the allergens are food, dust, or animal dander. Symptoms include sneezing, nasal congestion, watery rhinorrhea, itchy, watery eyes, postnasal drip, and a scratchy or sore throat. Facial pain may be intermittently present as a result of edematous blockage of the sinus ostia. Decreased hearing may result from concurrent serous otitis media.
      - Physical examination will reveal pale, boggy, bluish nasal mucosa and swollen inferior turbinates. Nasal secretions will be clear or white. Conjunctival injection and prominent pharyngeal lymphoid follicles and a clear postnasal drip may be present.
   C. Laboratory and diagnostic studies
      - Skin testing may be used to determine the causative allergen to guide immunotherapy. Radioallergosorbent (RAST) testing, measurement of mucus eosinophils, and measurement of serum IgE are not usually necessary.
   D. Formulating the diagnosis
      - The diagnosis of allergic rhinitis is made clinically based on the history of the constellation of symptoms. Symptomatically, an upper respiratory infection or sinusitis may mimic some of those of allergic rhinitis. Chronicity of symptoms and the history will help differentiate allergic rhinitis from viral upper respiratory infection. Vasomotor rhinitis, a runny nose triggered by nonspecific triggers, such as cold weather, may present similarly to allergic rhinitis, but without the itching and sneezing.
      - In contrast to vasomotor rhinitis, allergic rhinitis is usually seasonal. Sinusitis will present with facial pain or pressure and purulent rhinorrhea.
   E. Evaluating the severity of problems
      - Allergic rhinitis, although potentially quite annoying, is not a life-threatening condition. Edema due to allergy may predispose a patient to bacterial sinusitis.

F. Managing the patient
- The first line of treatment is avoidance, if possible, of the offending allergen. Rugs, bed sheets, and heavy draperies are reservoirs for dust mites and should be removed or cleaned frequently. Patients with allergies to pollen should keep their windows closed and rely on air conditioning during the pollen season.
- Oral antihistamines, either the sedating over-the-counter forms or the newer prescription, nonsedating agents, are useful in treating both nasal and ocular symptoms. The physician must be aware of the anticholinergic side effects of the sedating over-the-counter antihistamines, which include dryness of the mouth, increased risk of urinary retention in patients with prostatic hypertrophy, acute angle closure in patients with narrow angle glaucoma, psychomotor impairment, and hypertension.
- Decongestants, such as pseudoephedrine or phenylpropanolamine, are useful for decreasing nasal congestion. They should be avoided, however, in patients with hypertension or cardiac disease because they may cause elevation of blood pressure.
- Increasingly, nasal glucocorticoid sprays are becoming the mainstay of therapy for allergic rhinitis. These drugs have no appreciable systemic side effects and minor nasal side effects (i.e., stinging). Candidal infection of the nose is a rare complication of intranasal steroid use. Nasal steroids may take 3 to 10 days to reach a therapeutic level in the nasal tissues, so they must be used continuously during the allergy season.
- Cromolyn sodium nasal spray may be used as an adjunct to intranasal steroids, but unfortunately must be used four times a day compared with the once or twice a day administration of nasal steroids. Allergen desensitization should be considered in patients whose symptoms are not relieved by medications.
- Patients with nasal polyps or turbinate hypertrophy unresponsive to medications may require surgery to relieve nasal obstruction.

II. Acute Upper Respiratory Infections
   A. Basic science
   - The common cold is a viral illness, usually associated with rhinoviruses, coronaviruses, respiratory syncytial virus, parainfluenza virus, or adenovirus. Parainfluenza and respiratory syncytial viruses are more common etiologic agents in children. Parainfluenza and adenovirus infections are likely to also cause lower respiratory infections. The viruses responsible for the common cold are transmitted both by direct contact and by aerosol particles.
   B. History and physical examination
   - The most frequent symptoms of the common cold are rhinorrhea (which may be clear or purulent) and nasal congestion. Typically, symptoms begin with a scratchy throat, followed by nasal congestion, then cough. Fever, malaise, and myalgias may also be present. Patients may report sick contacts within the past 3 days.
   C. Laboratory and diagnostic studies
   - No laboratory studies are necessary for diagnosing a common cold

D. Formulating a diagnosis
- A common cold is diagnosed based on the history and symptoms. A common cold should be distinguished from acute sinusitis and allergic rhinitis. If secondary bacterial infection occurs, the illness will be prolonged.

E. Managing the patient
- The common cold is self-limiting and is primarily treated by symptomatic therapies.
- Although many therapeutic agents, such as zinc, vitamin C, vitamin E, and *Echinacea,* have been reported to decrease the duration or severity of symptoms, clinical trials do not support their use.
- Over-the-counter decongestants and antihistamines may be useful for decreasing nasal symptoms. There is currently no antiviral therapy available and there is no role for antibacterial therapy in treating the viral infection.

III. Disorders of the Mouth
A. Basic science
- Structures in the mouth that may develop painful disorders include the teeth, gums, jaw, and oral mucosa.

B. History and physical examination
- The history in patients presenting with mouth pain should include characteristics of the pain, associated symptoms, history of trauma, and other comorbidities. The mouth should be examined, using a good light source and two tongue depressors to adequately visualize the entire mucosa. The examination should focus on the condition of the teeth; erythema of gums; evidence of vesicles, ulcerations, or plaques on the mucous membranes or palate; and pain upon palpation of the bones of the jaw or the temporomandibular joint.

C. Laboratory and diagnostic studies
- There are no specific laboratory studies. X-rays should be obtained if there is suspicion of dental caries or a dental abscess. Computed tomographic (CT) scans or magnetic resonance imaging (MRI) of the temporomandibular joint may be indicated in patients with temporomandibular joint syndrome who fail conservative treatment.

D. Formulating the diagnosis
- Proper diagnosis is guided by the history and physical examination. Dental caries is a common cause for pain and will be evident by examination and x-rays. Periodontal inflammation is usually painless, but may lead to abscess formation that may be seen by x-rays. Children, particularly infants, will have pain associated with eruption of new teeth, and may also present with drooling, low-grade fever, and irritability.
- Painful ulcers in the mouth are generally benign and can be recurrent, as in aphthous ulcers or herpes simplex virus ulcers. Ulcers due to herpes simplex are commonly on the buccal mucosa and are associated with a burning or tingling sensation. Chronic ulcers should be biopsied to rule out squamous cell carcinoma.

E. Evaluating the severity of problems
  - The severity of conditions leading to mouth pain is variable. Aphthous ulcers and ulcers from herpes simplex are relatively benign, but dental caries and abscesses should be treated promptly to avoid dissemination of infection.
F. Management of the patient
  - The key to management of patients with mouth pain is symptomatic relief and treatment of the underlying disorder.
  - Children who are teething often benefit from topical analgesics or cool compresses. Patients with a dental abscess or caries should be referred to a dentist.
  - Patients with mucosal lesions from primary herpes simplex virus infection may require oral acyclovir. Treatment is most effective if begun within 48 hours of symptoms.
  - The majority of patients with aphthous ulcers will benefit symptomatically from topical application of analgesics such as lidocaine. In more severe cases topical or systemic glucocorticoids may be indicated.

IV. Epistaxis
  A. Basic science
    - The most common site of epistaxis is the anterior, inferior portion of the nasal septum. This area, known as Kiesselbach's plexus, is the site of the confluence of branches of the anterior ethmoidal, sphenopalatine, and facial arteries. Because this area is near the nares, it is subject to trauma and desiccation with damage to superficial blood vessels. Posterior epistaxis is uncommon and may be secondary to vascular disease, although it is usually spontaneous.
  B. History and physical examination
    - Epistaxis occurs more commonly during the winter due to the effects of artificial heat and low humidity. Patients with underlying bleeding disorders and those on anticoagulants are at increased risk for epistaxis. The history should include the frequency, severity, duration, and side of the nosebleed.
    - The site of bleeding should be localized by physical examination. The anterior nasal cavity and pharynx should be observed with a good light source for evidence of bleeding. A nasal speculum and suction device may be required to properly localize bleeding. If the patient is not currently bleeding, it is best not to disturb any clots.
  C. Laboratory and diagnostic studies
    - A prothrombin time (PT) or partial thromboplastin time (PTT) should be obtained in patients on anticoagulation. A hematocrit should be obtained in patients with significant blood loss, and a platelet count is obtained if hypersplenism is suspected.
  D. Formulating the diagnosis
    - When there is blood dripping from the nose, the diagnosis is obvious. However, if a patient spits up blood, one might confuse epistaxis with hemoptysis or hematemesis. To accurately diagnose epistaxis, blood must be observed coming from a site in the nose.

E. Evaluating the severity of problems
- Most cases of epistaxis can be controlled with 10 minutes of continuous, direct pressure on the nares below the nasal bones. If bleeding persists in spite of conservative measures, further intervention is indicated.

F. Managing the patient
- Once localized, anterior bleeding may be controlled with topically applied vasoconstrictors (e.g., phenylephrine), oxidized cellulose, electric cautery, or chemical cautery with silver nitrate with the patient leaning forward to prevent aspiration or swallowing of blood. If these measures are unsuccessful, anterior nasal packing should be placed.
- For posterior bleeding, an otolaryngologist should be consulted for placement of a posterior packing or balloon tamponade, often followed by bilateral anterior packing. These patients may need hospital admission for observation and monitoring of oxygenation while the packing is in place. Bleeding that continues despite adequate packing may require surgical or angiographic intervention.
- All patients with a history of epistaxis will benefit from humidification of the nasal mucosa. This can be accomplished with saline nasal sprays and room humidifiers.

V. Head and Neck Cancer
A. Basic science
- Head and neck cancers can involve the oral cavity, pharynx, larynx, nasal cavity, paranasal sinuses, and salivary glands. The upper digestive and respiratory systems are lined by squamous epithelium, so the most common form of head and neck cancer is squamous cell carcinoma.
- Risk factors for head and neck cancer include smoking and drinking alcohol. The presence of both factors increases the risk of cancer geometrically.
- Like many cancers, squamous cell carcinomas often do not manifest their presence until they invade surrounding structures. Referred pain to the ear along cranial nerves IX and X may be the first manifestation of an oropharyngeal or hypopharyngeal tumor.
- The most common site for a head and neck cancer is the larynx.

B. History and physical examination
- The history in a patient with head and neck cancer may reveal sores in the oral cavity that do not heal, persistant hoarseness or sore throat, dysphagia, odynophagia, and hemoptysis. Even though these symptoms may be benign, they may all be signs of an occult malignancy. For example, ear pain with a normal ear examination should prompt examination of the base of the tongue and hypopharynx for evidence of malignancy. Many of these symptoms are caused by benign processes, but should not be ignored because occasionally they offer an opportunity to find an early stage cancer.
- A thorough examination of the tongue, buccal mucosa, floor of the mouth, and palate can be performed with two tongue depressors. The base of the tongue, hypopharynx, and larynx can be examined with a dental mirror, although flexible endoscopy may be required for better visualization.

C. Laboratory and diagnostic studies
- Fiberoptic laryngoscopy is an office procedure performed under topical anesthesia that can visualize those areas of the mouth and throat that are not visible perorally. Suspicious lesions should be biopsied. Nonpulsatile neck masses should be aspirated with a fine needle and sent for cytologic examination. A CT scan with intravenous contrast material or MRI can delineate the size and location of tumors and lymphadenopathy.
- There are no laboratory studies specific for head and neck cancer.

D. Formulating the diagnosis
- In a patient who smokes or drinks, a malignancy should be assumed to be present until proved otherwise if symptoms discussed above are persistent or if the patient has a nontender neck mass.
- Benign conditions with symptoms that may mimic head and neck cancers include gastroesophageal reflux, vocal cord polyps or nodules, and temporomandibular joint dysfunction.
- Diagnosis usually depends on appropriate imaging to determine the presence and extent of a mass and biopsies. Imaging will also help determine clinical staging.

E. Evaluating the severity of problem
- Severity of the disease, treatment, and prognosis depend on the site, histologic type of tumor, and stage of the disease.

F. Managing the patient
- Early stage primary cancers can be managed by radiation or surgical resection. Late stage cancers are best treated by surgical resection and radiation. Chemotherapy can be utilized for advanced disease, particularly for unresectable or metastatic disease. All patients should be encouraged to stop smoking and drinking alcohol.

VI. Otitis Externa
A. Basic science
- The external auditory canal is protected by hair, cerumen, and epithelial cells. The bacteria that normally colonize the ear canal include *Pseudomonas aeruginosa* and *Staphylococcus* species. Trauma to the skin in the ear canal and disruption of the cerumen barrier allow these bacteria to overgrow, resulting in otitis externa.

B. History and physical examination
- Otitis diffuse externa (swimmer's ear) is usually the result of trauma to the ear canal. The two most common causes are the excessive use of cotton swabs and maceration from water. The patient will complain of severe, worsening pain in the ear (otalgia), associated with purulent, foul-smelling drainage. As the drainage accumulates, hearing loss occurs. Patients may also report pruritus. If left untreated, the pinna, periauricular tissues, and temporal bone may be involved.
- Physical examination will reveal tenderness induced by pulling on the pinna or pushing on the tragus. The ear canal will be swollen and red. Drainage may

obstruct visualization of the tympanic membrane, which should be mobile with insufflation.

C. Laboratory and diagnostic studies
  - No laboratory or diagnostic studies are necessary to make the diagnosis of acute otitis externa. *Pseudomonas* and *Staphylococcus* are the most common infectious agents.

D. Formulating the diagnosis
  - The diagnosis is made clinically, based on the history and physical examination.
  - Potential causes of ear pain include dental infections, teething, temporomandibular joint disease, otitis media, and head and neck cancers.

E. Evaluating the severity of problems
  - Most outer ear infections are easily treated on an outpatient basis. Occasionally, patients with otitis externa will develop a chondritis or, rarely, osteomyelitis of the temporal bone (necrotizing otitis externa) and require intravenous antibiotics. Immunocompromised or diabetic patients who have ear pain out of proportion to physical findings have a high likelihood of having malignant otitis externa.

F. Managing the patient
  - Acute otitis externa is treated by removal of debris and pus from the canal. If the disease is mild, drying and acidifying agents such as acetic acid and alcohol or boric acid and acetic acid otic solutions can be used. Topical antibiotics are indicated in moderately severe cases. If the canal is too swollen, owing to severe disease, to allow the entry of drops, a wick should be inserted by an otolaryngologist. Severe disease may require oral antibiotics. Topical steroids may be used to decrease inflammation and promote healing. Cultures are only required for severe or resistant infections.
  - Patients should be advised to avoid inserting cotton swabs into their ears and to thoroughly dry the ear canal after swimming and showering to prevent recurrence.

VII. Otitis Media
  A. Basic science
  - The middle ear is lined by respiratory-type mucosa. The respiratory mucosa, including the eustachian tubes, becomes congested following an upper respiratory infection, allowing accumulation of a sterile transudate in the middle ear and mastoid air cells. Contamination of this fluid by viruses or bacteria from the respiratory tract leads to otitis media. Although most otitis media is due to viruses, the most common bacteria causing otitis media are *Streptococcus pneumoniae, Haemophilus influenzae, Moraxella catarrhalis,* and group A streptococcus.

  B. History and physical examination
  - Otitis media often follows a viral upper respiratory infection. Children with a history of cleft palate or Down syndrome are at increased risk for otitis media. Infants and young children may present with fever, irritability, and tugging at their ear. Older children and adults may report pain, hearing loss, fever,

tinnitus, and vertigo. Purulent drainage is uncommon and suggests perforation of the tympanic membrane.

- Physical examination with an otoscope will reveal a red, bulging, immobile tympanic membrane as determined by pneumatic insufflation. The tympanic membrane may also be cloudy or opaque. The presence or absence of a light reflex is not a reliable sign of infection. If the tympanic membrane is perforated, there may be pus in the ear canal. Movement of the pinna and tragus does not cause pain as it does in otitis externa.

C. Laboratory and diagnostic studies
- No laboratory or diagnostic studies are routinely necessary to make the diagnosis of acute media.
- Aspiration and culture of fluid from the middle ear may be useful in patients who repeatedly fail treatment with empiric antibiotics.

D. Formulating the diagnosis
- Otitis media is diagnosed based on a history of acute symptoms, signs and symptoms of middle ear inflammation, and a middle ear effusion. A crying child will have pink and injected ear drums even in the absence of infection.

E. Evaluating the severity of problems
- Most cases of otitis media respond to a course of empiric antibiotics such as amoxicillin with or without clavulanate or cefdinir. Serious complications of otitis media may be heralded by sudden hearing loss, vertigo, fever, and chills. Acute mastoiditis, facial nerve paralysis, meningitis, and brain abscess may occur in patients with serious untreated infections or patients who fail to respond to therapy.

F. Managing the patient
- Patients with otitis media should be given pain medications as needed. The 2004 guidelines of the American Academy of Pediatrics (AAP) and American Academy of Family Physicians (AAFP) recommend antibiotics for treating all infants younger than 6 months and all children 6 months to 2 years old with definitive otitis media or severe illness. Children over 2 years old can be observed for 48 to 72 hours if they don't have severe otitis media or if the diagnosis is uncertain. Acute otitis media should be treated initially with a 10-day course of amoxicillin. If fever or pain persists beyond 48 to 72 hours, the patient should be given a broader-spectrum antibiotic to cover penicillin-resistant *Streptococcus pneumoniae.*
- Patients with recurrent otitis media should be given a trial of low-dose prophylactic antibiotics. Chronic otitis media with conductive hearing loss and failure of prophylactic antibiotics are indications for the placement of tympanostomy tubes.

VIII. Sensorineural Hearing Loss
A. Basic science
- The inner ear is divided into two components, the cochlear and the vestibular apparatus.
- The cochlea converts mechanical energy from sound into neural signals. This occurs when the endolymph stimulates the movement of specialized hair cells.

The hair cells are topographically organized so that sounds of different pitch are recognized by hair cells at different locations within the cochlea. Malfunction or damage to the cochlea can result in sensorineural hearing loss or tinnitus (noise in the ear).

B. History and physical examination
- Sensorineural hearing loss may be congenital or acquired, but is most commonly associated with aging. People with sensorineural hearing loss will often report hearing people speak but being unable to discriminate distinct words. They often have difficulty hearing in the presence of background noise. History should include onset and progression of hearing loss, history of trauma, and previous noise exposure. Risk factors for sensorineural hearing loss include autoimmune diseases, collagen vascular disorders, tertiary syphilis, and exposure to ototoxic drugs, such as aminoglycosides, erythromycin, loop diuretics, and cis-platinum.
- Physical examination of the outer and middle ear by otoscopy is normal in patients with inner ear disorders. The Rinne or Weber test can help distinguish conduction from sensorineural hearing loss. Sound (from a 512-Hz tuning fork) localizes toward the ear with the conductive loss. Deficits may be mixed.

C. Laboratory and diagnostic studies
- All patients with hearing loss should have an audiogram performed in a soundproof booth by an audiologist. Patients with unexplained asymmetric or unilateral sensorineural hearing loss should have a further evaluation for the cause of their hearing loss.
- Serum studies are dictated by clinical suspicion and include sedimentation rate, antinuclear antibody, rheumatoid factor, complete blood count (CBC), thyroid-stimulating hormone (TSH), and Lyme titer.
- A CT scan of the head or MRI of the brain should be done if loss is asymmetric.

D. Formulating the diagnosis
- The most common cause of gradual sensorineural hearing loss is aging. The diagnosis of sensorineural hearing loss can be made by audiogram. Causes of sudden hearing loss include trauma, viral infections, autoimmune diseases, and stroke.

E. Evaluating the severity of problems
- Sudden hearing loss requires urgent intervention if hearing is to be salvaged. Audiography can be used to guide characterization of conductive versus sensorneural and symmetric versus asymmetric hearing loss. Results from this testing will determine the extent of the deficit and the need for further evaluation.

F. Managing the patient
- Age-associated sensorineural hearing loss or presbycusis can be managed with a hearing aid.
- Sudden sensorineural hearing loss should be evaluated to determine the etiology, and treated with a short course of high-dose steroids for a presumed viral infection while investigations are under way.

- Viral cochleitis is most often due to a herpes infection, is abrupt in onset, and results in asymmetric hearing loss. It is the commonest viral cause for sudden hearing loss. Besides urgent audiometry, a brain MRI scan should be ordered to exclude an ischemic event or multiple sclerosis. Acyclovir is indicated in treating acute herpes viral cochleitis.
- Other causes of hearing loss include otitis media, cerumen impaction, cholesteatoma, and otosclerosis, all of which cause conductive hearing loss.

IX. Sinusitis
   A. Basic science
   - There are four pairs of paranasal sinuses, which are lined with ciliated, pseudostratified, columnar epithelium. Most of the sinuses drain into the nasopharynx through the osteomeatal complex. Obstruction of drainage of the sinuses by viral-induced edema, inflammatory polyps, severe nasal septal deviation, or tumors can trigger bacterial sinusitis.
   - Acute sinusitis is usually due to a viral infection, and a small percentage of these infections lead to a secondary bacterial sinusitis. The duration of the illness is less than 4 weeks. Community-acquired bacterial sinusitis in adults is most commonly due to *Streptococcus pneumoniae* or *Haemophilus influenzae*. *Moraxella catarrhalis* is a common cause of acute sinusitis in children.
   - Chronic sinusitis is inflammation of the mucous membranes of the paranasal sinuses for longer than 12 weeks. Chronic sinusitis is due to persistent blockage of the osteomeatal complex or impaired mucociliary transport. Infections in chronic sinusitis are generally polymicrobial and include anaerobes.
   B. History and physical examination
   - Symptoms of acute and chronic sinusitis include nasal congestion, facial pain and headache, purulent nasal discharge, postnasal drip, and cough. Tooth pain and halitosis may also be present. For acute bacterial sinusitis, there is usually a history of an antecedent viral upper respiratory infection. Patients with acute bacterial sinusitis will have symptoms which have persisted or worsened over 7 to 10 days.
   - On physical examination, patients with acute sinusitis may have a low-grade fever. A purulent nasal discharge or postnasal drip does not necessarily indicate a bacterial infection. Generally there is tenderness to palpation over the infected sinuses. The nasal turbinates often have erythematous, inflamed mucosa with yellow or green mucopurulent discharge. Patients with chronic sinusitis often have postnasal drainage with secondary sore throat and cough.
   C. Laboratory and diagnostic studies
   - Most patients with acute sinusitis are treated empirically and imaging studies or nasal sinus cultures are usually not required. CT scans are the test of choice and may be useful for patients who fail medical treatment for acute sinusitis or to define the extent and location of chronic sinusitis. No laboratory studies are necessary for patients with chronic sinusitis, unless they fail to respond to antibiotics and an underlying systemic disease is suspected.

D. Formulating the diagnosis
- Acute sinusitis may be confused with a viral upper respiratory infection or allergic rhinitis. The diagnosis of acute bacterial sinusitis should be considered when symptoms last longer than 7 to 10 days, symptoms worsen, or facial pressure or pain, not normally present in a viral illness, develops.
- Chronic sinusitis is diagnosed by the presence of facial pain, pressure, or congestion and nasal discharge or postnasal drip that lasts longer than 12 weeks. If symptoms do not respond to treatment, other causes, such as fungal infection or systemic diseases, such as Wegener's granulomatosis or sarcoidosis, should be considered

E. Evaluating the severity of problems
- Because the sinuses are adjacent to the orbits and the brain, it is possible for infection to spread to these structures. Patients who develop sinusitis, high fever, severe headache or facial pain, eyelid swelling, impaired vision, periorbital edema, conjunctival edema, proptosis, or lethargy demand immediate evaluation and treatment. These patients may need a CT scan to rule out intracranial or orbital involvement.

F. Managing the patient
- Patients with acute sinusitis of less than 7 days' duration should be treated symptomatically with decongestants, nasal saline lavage, and nasal glucocorticoids. Antibiotics that can be used include amoxicillin, doxycycline, and trimethoprim-sulfamethoxazole. Patients with continued symptoms may require amoxicillin-clavulanate or cefuroxime to cover resistant *Streptococcus pneumoniae*. Patients with chronic sinusitis should be treated with antibiotics for 3 to 6 weeks, often with amoxicillin-clavulanate or cefuroxime. Patients with recurrent symptoms may benefit from surgery to open the osteomeatal complex.

X. Tonsil and Adenoid Disorders
  A. Basic science
  - The adenoids and tonsils are lymphatic structures that function as the first line of defense against oral and respiratory infections. These structures may become a site of repeated infection or they may hypertrophy to the extent that they obstruct the oral or nasal airways.
  - The tonsils are separated from the pharyngeal musculature by a fibrous capsule. If the infection spreads from the tonsil into this potential space, a peritonsillar abscess forms.
  - The adenoids may contribute to otitis media by acting as a reservoir for bacteria to spread to the middle ear via the eustachian tubes.

  B. History and physical examination
  - Adenotonsillitis may be of viral or bacterial etiology. Patients with infection of the adenoids or tonsils complain of a sore throat, fever, nasal congestion, and difficulty swallowing. Symptoms of infection due to a group A streptococcus usually begin abruptly.
  - On physical examination, the tonsils will be enlarged and red and may be covered with an exudate. Some viral infections, such as coxsackievirus, cause

vesicles to form on the tonsils. There may be a fine, papular, generalized rash in patients with a *Streptococcus* infection.

- Trismus (inability to open the mouth) and a muffled voice are signs of a peritonsillar abscess. The tonsil on the side of the abscess is often obscured.

C. Laboratory and diagnostic studies

- A throat culture or rapid "strep" test may be used to diagnose infection with group A β-hemolytic organisms.
- A Monospot test may be indicated to test for infection with Epstein-Barr virus in young patients with tonsillitis and generalized adenopathy, or in patients who do not respond to initial antibiotics. A white blood cell count with differential may suggest infectious mononucleosis within the first 3 days of infection when the Monospot test is negative.

D. Formulating the diagnosis

- The diagnosis of adenotonsillitis or peritonsillar abscess is made clinically, although usually a CT scan is necessary to determine the extent and location of a peritonsillar abscess.

E. Evaluating the severity of problems

- Most patients with tonsillitis can be treated as outpatients; patients with a peritonsillar abscess need drainage and intravenous antibiotics.
- If a patient cannot drink because of the pain, he or she should be admitted for intravenous antibiotics and hydration.
- Occasionally, acute adenotonsillar enlargement can impinge on the airway, necessitating placement of a nasopharyngeal airway to relieve the obstruction.

F. Managing the patient

- The decision to treat adenotonsillitis is usually based on the severity of symptoms. The antibiotic of choice for bacterial tonsillitis is penicillin because of its narrow spectrum, good efficacy, and low cost. Erythromycin is an alternative drug for patients allergic to penicillin.
- Peritonsillar abscesses should be drained by needle aspiration or by incision and drainage. The carotid artery lies in close proximity to the tonsils; therefore, abscess drainage is usually performed by an otolaryngologist.
- Patients with recurrent tonsillitis or upper airway obstruction from adenotonsillar hypertrophy will benefit from adenoidectomy or tonsillectomy, or both.

XI. Upper Airway Obstruction

A. Basic science

- The upper airway consists of the nose, nasopharynx, oral cavity, oropharynx, laryngopharynx, and trachea. Obstruction at any level may impede respiration. Upper airway obstruction can be secondary to foreign body aspiration, epiglottitis, allergic reactions, tumors, trauma, subglottic stenosis, choanal atresia, or laryngeal cancer.
- The primary function of the larynx is protection of the lung from aspiration. A reflex arc is mediated through the sensory and motor branches of the vagus nerve to adduct the vocal cords during swallowing.

B. History and physical examination
- Signs of upper airway obstruction may include shortness of breath, pain or difficulty swallowing, change in voice, and stridor.
- Physical findings may include visible swelling of upper airway structures or drooling, depending on the cause. Stridor can be differentiated from wheezing, a lower respiratory sign by its inspiratory nature. Stridor is loudest in the neck in contrast to wheezing, which is louder in the chest.

C. Laboratory and diagnostic studies
- Anteroposterior and lateral neck x-rays should be ordered to evaluate the upper airway. Fiberoptic laryngoscopy may also be necessary, but should not be attempted in children suspected of having epiglottitis. Because of potential airway instability, all examinations should be done in the emergency room under close physician supervision or in the operating room.
- An arterial blood gas measurement is not a helpful diagnostic or prognostic test in upper airway obstruction, as it may be normal until respiratory arrest occurs.

D. Evaluating the severity of problems
- Upper airway obstruction is a medical emergency.

E. Managing the patient
- The location and degree of obstruction and the severity of respiratory distress should be assessed quickly. If the patient's airway is severely compromised, an endotracheal tube must be placed. When an endotracheal tube cannot be placed, a surgical airway, such as a cricothyroidotomy, must be established.
- Further management is dependent on the cause of the obstruction. Foreign objects should be visualized, if possible, with indirect laryngoscopy and removed with forceps. If this is impossible, a flexible laryngoscopy and bronchoscopy should be performed.
- Patients with severe epiglottitis should be treated with immediate endotracheal intubation because of airway instability. Patients should preferably be intubated in the operating room by an anesthesiologist with an otolaryngologist in attendance. Once stabilized, intravenous antibiotics should be given to treat the underlying infection.
- Patients with allergic reactions presenting with edema of the lips, tongue, and uvula are at risk for progressive airway compromise. These patients should immediately be given subcutaneous epinephrine followed by nebulized epinephrine, intravenous antihistamines, and intravenous steroids, as necessary. Patients may require intubation for airway protection or a surgical airway if intubation is not possible.

XII. Vertigo
A. Basic science
- The inner ear vestibular apparatus is one part of the body's vestibular system. It is responsible for alerting the brain to changes in head position. Malfunction or damage to the vestibular apparatus can result in peripheral vertigo.
- Damage to the eighth cranial nerve or the vestibular nuclei and pathways (which travel through the cerebellum and brain stem) can cause central vertigo.

B. History and physical examination
- Peripheral vertigo may last minutes, hours, or days. Patients report the sensation that they (or their environment) are spinning. Patients with peripheral vertigo may be nauseated, vomit, or fall, but they will never have syncope or vision or speech difficulties.
- Patients with benign paroxysmal positional vertigo (BPPV) report symptoms provoked by particular movements. The history should include the time course of the vertigo, aggravating factors, exposure to ototoxic drugs such as aminoglycosides or loop diuretics, history of head trauma, and history of stroke.
- Physical examination of the outer and middle ear (otoscopy) will be normal. Peripheral vertigo may be initiated with a change in head position. Nystagmus with peripheral lesions is usually horizontal, and gait abnormalities are minimal. In central vertigo, nystagmus may be of any variety, but vertical nystagmus is associated only with central vestibular dysfunction.
- Evaluation of vertigo should include checking the pulse for an irregular heart rhythm and a complete neurologic examination.

C. Laboratory and diagnostic studies
- Many tests have been recommended to evaluate inner ear disorders. All patients should have a behavioral audiogram performed by an audiologist in a soundproof booth. A magnetic resonance image will help rule out a brain stem tumor, hemorrhage, or infarct.

D. Formulating the diagnosis
- The most common cause of peripheral vertigo is vestibular neuronitis, a viral infection of the vestibular nerve. Patients report the sudden onset of unremitting vertigo that lasts for several days before symptoms begin to spontaneously relent. The initial step should be to distinguish central from peripheral causes of vertigo.
- Ménière's disease is a clinical diagnosis. Patients with Ménière's disease have episodic bouts of vertigo, hearing loss, and a sensation of clogged ear that last from 1 to 24 hours. Tinnitus may be constant or intermittent. Ménière's disease usually affects only one ear at a time. As the vertigo is recurrent, the diagnosis of Ménière's cannot be made on first presentation.
- Basilar artery insufficiency, orthostatic hypotension, and cardiac arrythmias can also cause the sensation of vertigo or lightheadedness. Diabetic peripheral neuropathy may give a patient the feeling of unsteadiness.

E. Evaluating the severity of problems
- Peripheral vertigo must be differentiated from central vertigo. Untreated peripheral vertigo will not result in permanent injury; however, central vertigo may be life-threatening and needs to be identified immediately.

F. Managing the patient
- Symptoms of peripheral vertigo may be relieved with the following:
  1. Benzodiazepines for vestibular sedation constitute the fastest, most effective treatment for acute vertigo.
  2. Antihistamines (e.g., meclizine or diphenhydramine) are given for vestibular system sedation.

3. Anticholinergics (e.g., scopolamine or atropine) are used for control of nausea.

- BPPV can often be treated successfully with maneuvers that remove debris from the posterior semicircular canal. Reduction of sodium intake and administration of a diuretic (to decrease the production of endolymph) may control the vertigo of Ménière's disease.

- Some patients with unrelenting vertigo may require vestibular nerve section or other ablative procedures directed toward the malfunctioning vestibular apparatus.

Pulmonology

I. Acute Respiratory Failure
  A. Basic science
   - Acute respiratory failure occurs when the lungs are unable to maintain normal levels of either oxygen or carbon dioxide or both in the systemic arterial blood. Respiratory failure can lead to death if not reversed.
   - Respiratory failure can be hypoxemic ($PO_2 < 60$ mm Hg), hypercarbic ($PCO_2 > 45$ mm Hg), or a combination. Hypoxemic respiratory failure occurs when arterial oxygen tension falls below 60 mm Hg while breathing room air; arterial CO_2 tension is normal or reduced. Hypercapnic respiratory failure occurs when arterial CO_2 tension rises above 45 mm Hg, associated with a respiratory acidosis (pH < 7.35); arterial oxygen tension is secondarily reduced.
   - The prototypic example of acute hypoxemic respiratory failure is the adult respiratory distress syndrome (ARDS). Many clinical disorders lead to ARDS, but the most common are sepsis, major trauma, and aspiration of gastric contents. The mechanisms of injury are poorly understood but probably involve both cellular and humoral proinflammatory mediators, which cause loss of integrity of the capillary and alveolar epithelium, leading to protein rich alveolar edema. Despite appropriate support, the mortality rate remains at 35% to 40%. One third of the deaths occur within 72 hours as a direct result of the underlying illness. Most of the remaining deaths occur within 2 weeks from infection and multiple organ failure. The prognosis for survivors appears good. Quality of life is typically decreased for up to 1 year following ARDS. As many as 80% of survivors of ARDS may have mild abnormalities in their pulmonary function tests indefinitely. The abnormalities include a decrease in diffusion capacity of carbon monoxide and mild obstructive and restrictive patterns of lung disease.
   - Hypercapnic respiratory failure is caused by disorders that impair ventilation and affect the respiratory muscles. In disorders of impaired ventilation, there is a diminished removal of CO_2 by alveolar ventilation. This may often occur secondary to obstructive lung diseases (e.g., chronic obstructive pulmonary disease [COPD], asthma), upper respiratory obstruction (e.g., foreign body aspiration, bacterial epiglottitis, and inhalation injury), and chest wall diseases that increase the stiffness of the chest (e.g., kyphoscoliosis).
   - Hypercapnic respiratory failure frequently complicates disorders that interfere with the nervous system, both central and peripheral. Disorders that affect the central nervous system effectively decrease the drive to breathe by causing respiratory center suppression (i.e., overdose of CNS depressant drugs, diseases

BOX 4-1

NERVOUS SYSTEM DISORDERS ASSOCIATED WITH HYPERCAPNIC RESPIRATORY FAILURE

Central respiratory center depression
   Sleep apnea
   Overdoses of CNS depressant medications
   Hypothyroidism
   Metabolic acidosis
   Rabies
Motor neuron dysfunction
   Spinal cord Injury (C3–C5)
   Tetanus
   Anterior horn cell diseases (amyotrophic lateral sclerosis, poliomyelitis)
Peripheral Neuropathy
   Guillain-Barré syndrome
   Critical illness polyneuropathy
   Diphtheria
   Porphyria
   Tick paralysis
   Ingestion of the neurotoxin found in puffer fish
Diseases of the neuromuscular junction
   Myasthenia gravis
   Eaton-Lambert syndrome
   Toxins that inhibit cholinesterase (e.g., organophosphates)
   Botulism
   Prolonged exposure to no depolarizing neuromuscular blocking agents

of the medulla, hypothyroidism, rabies). Motor neuron disease causes an interruption of the transmission of impulses from the respiratory centers to the respiratory muscles, spinal cord injury to the third through the fifth cervical nerve roots, and tetanus. Disorders of the peripheral nervous system and the neuromuscular junction typically cause a generalized paralysis or weakness of all muscles involved with respiration (Box 4-1). Weakness in the inspiratory muscles as well as hyperinflation of the chest decrease the amount of force the muscles are able to generate, thus decreasing the alveolar ventilation and increasing arterial CO_2. A variety of disorders are associated with respiratory muscle weakness (Box 4-2). Weakness of expiratory muscles causes an impaired cough reflex, which predisposes patients to retention of secretions and leads to the development of pneumonia.

BOX 4-2

CAUSES OF RESPIRATORY MUSCLE WEAKNESS

Aging
Malnutrition
Denervation
Myopathies
Muscular dystrophy
Poliomyelitis
Drug-induced (corticosteroids, neuromuscular blocking agents)
Endocrinopathies (hyperthyroidism, Cushing's syndrome)
Metabolic derangements
Electrolyte disorders (particularly low levels of K^+, PO_4^-, Mg^-)
Hyperinflation

B. History and physical examination
   • Typically, patients with ARDS rapidly develop respiratory distress within the first 72 hours of the inciting event with evidence of pulmonary edema, manifested by pink, frothy sputum, and diffuse crackles upon examination of the chest and concomitant increasing FIO_2 requirements. History should be directed at discovering the underlying event.
   • The clinical features of patients with acute hypercapnic respiratory failure depends, in part, on the underlying cause. Acute hypercapnia can produce dramatic changes in central nervous system function, including obtundation and coma. However, patients with hypercapnic respiratory failure due to central nervous system disorders or neuromuscular disease may not develop respiratory distress. Patients with intrinsic lung, airway, or chest wall disorders will generally complain of dyspnea and exhibit tachypnea and use accessory respiratory muscles. Patients with severe exacerbations of COPD or asthma typically present with a recent history of worsening dyspnea, confusion, and agitation. They are tachypneic with diffuse wheezing and decreased expiratory flow rates. Patients with acute upper airway obstruction present with severe dyspnea and tachypnea. If the airway obstruction is extrathoracic (above the vocal cords), stridorous breath sounds are heard on inspiration, whereas obstruction in the lower trachea generates wheezing. Patients with respiratory muscle weakness present with variable complaints of dyspnea and difficulty in coughing. Worrisome signs include ineffective cough, difficulty in handling secretions and swallowing, increasing respiratory rate, and use of accessory muscles of respiration.

C. Laboratory and diagnostic studies
- All patients with acute respiratory failure should have arterial blood gas (ABG) measurements with comparison of the results with previous ABGs, if available. The amount of oxygen the patient is on at the time the ABG is obtained is an important factor in the clinical decision-making tree. Additionally, a chest x-ray should be obtained. An electrocardiogram (ECG) should be reviewed to look for a cardiac cause.

D. Formulating the diagnosis
- The differential diagnosis of acute respiratory failure includes disorders that affect the parenchyma of the lung, such as pulmonary edema or obstructive airway disease, or problems that decrease ventilation in a normal lung, such as upper airway obstruction or diminished respiratory drive or muscle strength (see Boxes 4-1 and 4-2).
- *ARDS* is defined by the combination of severe dyspnea of acute onset, diffuse alveolar infiltration manifested by bilateral opacities on chest radiograph, pulmonary artery occlusion pressure at or below 18 mm Hg or absence of left atrial hypertension (i.e., the absence of left ventricular failure), and marked hypoxemia defined as a $PaO_2:FIO_2$ ratio below 200. Patients with $PaO_2:FIO_2$ below 300 are said to have acute lung injury.
- Pulmonary edema must be ruled out. The history, physical examination, ECG, and echocardiography can help accomplish this. When the distinction between ARDS and left ventricular failure is not clear, pulmonary artery catheterization will be required.
- In considering the differential diagnosis of hypercapnic respiratory failure, it is useful to categorize disorders according to the component of the respiratory system affected. Obstructive lung diseases such as COPD and asthma cause hypercapnic respiratory failure primarily by increasing pulmonary dead space (hyperinflation) and precipitating respiratory muscle fatigue, which decreases the elastic recoil of the lung. In patients with COPD, acute respiratory failure may be precipitated by respiratory tract infections, congestive heart failure, pulmonary emboli, or pneumothorax, which accentuate the loss of the elastic recoil of the lung. Upper airway obstruction causes hypercapnia by decreasing total ventilation.

E. Evaluating the severity of problems
- In hypercapnic respiratory failure, the severity of disease is reflected by the degree of hypercapnia detected by the ABG measurement and its concomitant effect of pH on the blood. Similarly, the severity of hypoxemic failure is gauged by the magnitude of hypoxemia detected on the ABG test and indirectly through pulse oximetry. The need for urgent/emergent intubation for mechanical ventilation in all types of acute respiratory failure is dictated by the ability of the lungs to maintain adequate oxygenation and ventilation and a clinical evaluation of the degree of the patient's respiratory distress.

F. Managing the patient
- The physician should consider the possibility of upper airway obstruction in every patient with acute respiratory failure. To manage acute respiratory failure successfully, the physician must accomplish three goals: (1) establish an airway,

(2) administer an appropriate amount of oxygen, and (3) maintain adequate alveolar ventilation. Furthermore, the underlying cause of respiratory failure should be identified and treated.

- Most patients with severe respiratory failure of either type will require mechanical ventilation. With regard to ventilator settings, the degree of hypoxemia may be largely controlled with increasing concentrations of oxygen and positive end-expiratory pressure. Hypercapnia is treated by increasing alveolar ventilation by adjusting the respiratory rate and tidal volume.

II. Asthma
  A. Basic science
    - Asthma is a disease characterized by chronic inflammation of the airway passage and bronchial airway hyperresponsiveness when exposed to irritants, causing *reversible* bronchoconstriction.
    - Pathologic changes include the following: airway smooth muscle contraction; microvascular leakage causing airway edema; stimulation of mucus-secreting cells; interruption of the ciliated epithelium of the airways by inflammatory cell mediators, such as leukotrienes and histamine; thickening of the basement membrane by increasing deposits of collagen; and infiltration of inflammatory cells such as eosinophils, mast cells, activated T-lymphocytes, and neutrophils. Chronic changes of asthma include the foregoing changes as well as hypertrophy and hyperplasia of airway smooth muscle.
    - Because of these changes, alveoli develop impaired gas exchange, which is most pronounced during an acute attack. The alveolar oxygen content becomes depleted. Thus, venous blood returns to the left ventricle with much less oxygen than normal (decrease in PO_2) due to ventilation/perfusion (V/Q) mismatches.
    - In the United States, more than 20 million people have asthma. Asthma may present at any age. About 50% develop asthma by the age of 10 years, with a 2:1 male-female ratio. This ratio equalizes by the third decade of life.
    - Asthma is loosely classified as either allergic or nonallergic. Allergic asthma (or extrinsic asthma) typically develops in childhood. Many asthmatic patients have associated allergic conditions such as hay fever or eczema. Common allergens include pollen, house dust, drugs, feathers, and animal dander. The airways of allergic asthmatics contain mast cells with IgE directed against specific antigens. Contact with these antigens results in release of histamine, bradykinin, and leukotrienes (early inflammatory response). Continued exposure to the antigen leads to an influx of eosinophils and lymphocytes (late inflammatory response), which can lead to irreversible damage to the airway epithelium.
    - Nonallergic (intrinsic) asthma occurs in older individuals with normal IgE levels. Precipitants include exercise, drugs (e.g., aspirin, β-blockers), chemicals, gastroesophageal reflux, atmospheric pollution, chronic sinusitis, and viral infection. Although asthma may improve during adolescence and with age, the condition may recur.

B. History and physical examination
- Most attacks develop unexpectedly and are marked by shortness of breath, wheezing; and a hacking, nonproductive cough. The patient may give a history of a preceding upper respiratory infection.
- Patients should be asked about the severity of their asthma, known precipitants, previous hospitalizations (ICU admissions and intubations), and medication compliance.
- In an acute attack the patient appears apprehensive and may be unable to complete a full sentence. The patient may bend over to ease breathing. Wheezing, tachycardia, or the use of accessory respiratory muscles may be found. During a severe asthmatic attack, airflow may be so severely limited, that wheezing is not heard on physical examination and pulsus paradoxsus may be detected.
- Patients with severe, chronic asthma develop attenuated sensitivity to the severity of the airflow limitation; thus, the typical signs and symptoms that signify an asthma attack may be absent.

C. Laboratory and diagnostic studies
- During an acute asthma attack, an arterial blood gas should be obtained. A rising (or "normal") PCO_2 with dyspnea represents a severe exacerbation and impending respiratory failure. The patient should be placed on a continuous pulse oximeter to monitor changes in arterial oxygenation.
- A chest x-ray should be ordered for patients. Hyperinflation is typically seen secondary to air trapping.
- Pulmonary function tests should be obtained during the workup of a chronic asthmatic patient, preferably not during an acute attack. Spirometry will reveal a reversible, obstructive pattern, with an FEV_1/FVC ratio less than 70%. Bronchial airway reversibility is defined as a change in FEV_1 of 15% or more after administration of two puffs of a β-agonist. In chronic asthma, restriction may occasionally be seen, reflecting smooth muscle hypertrophy of the airways. In certain individuals, allergy skin tests should be done, as this may help identify a precipitant. Bronchoprovocation challenge tests should be performed only in patients in whom the diagnosis of asthma is in question.

D. Formulating the diagnosis
- The diagnosis is based on the prior history, the typical symptoms of asthma (cough, dyspnea, and wheezing), and reversal of symptoms and airflow limitations after the administration of a β-agonist.

E. Evaluating the severity of problems
- Asthmatic episodes vary greatly in frequency, duration, and the severity of symptoms. The symptoms may range from episodic wheezing, mild bouts of coughing, and slight dyspnea to severe attacks that can lead to total airway obstruction and respiratory failure (Table 4-1 provides a classification of asthma.)
- Features of a severe attack include a heart rate above 120 beats/minute, tachypnea (>30 beats/minute), pulsus paradoxus (>20 mm Hg fall in systolic blood pressure during inspiration), cyanosis, reduced or absent air entry on chest examination, and a peak expiratory flow rate less than 120 mL/second.

TABLE 4-1:
Classification of Asthma

Severity	Symptoms	Nighttime Symptoms	PFTs (FEV₁ or PEFR)
Mild intermittent	≤2/week	≤2/month	≥80% predicted of normal between exacerbations
Mild persistent	>2/week but <1/day	>2/month	≥80% predicted
Moderate persistent	Daily symptoms Daily β-agonist use Exacerbations ≥2/week	1/week	60–80% predicted
Severe persistent	Continual symptoms Frequent exacerbations	Frequent	≤60% predicted

FEV₁, forced expiratory volume at 1 second; PEFR, peak expiratory flow rate; PFTs, pulmonary function tests. Data from National Asthma Education and Prevention Program, Expert Panel Report 2, 1997.

Patients with these signs should be hospitalized in a carefully monitored setting.

- Intubation and mechanical ventilation may be necessary if the patient develops increasing hypercapnia indicating respiratory muscle fatigue, or severe hypoxia indicating impending respiratory failure.

F. Managing the patient

- The management of an acute asthma attack includes oxygen and nebulized albuterol. Nebulized albuterol may be administered continuously if necessary. In a severe asthma attack, intravenous corticosteroids (e.g., methylprednisolone) should be given. Subcutaneous epinephrine and aminophylline can be given during severe exacerbations if there are no contraindications, but these are second-line agents.

- The treatment of chronic asthma involves drug therapy and identification and avoidance of asthma triggers. Effective outpatient management includes frequent monitoring of airflow measurements using a peak flowmeter so that a baseline can be obtained and adjustments to medications made based on the changes in peak flow. Three main types of agents are used in the long-term treatment of asthma: bronchodilators, corticosteroids, and other anti-inflammatory agents. Refer to Table 4-2 for indications for treatment of asthma.

1. Bronchodilators

   a. Albuterol (β₂-agonist)

      - Albuterol acts on airway smooth muscle, causing bronchodilation. It is given as a metered dose inhaler (MDI) or nebulizer. Albuterol often provides rapid relief of symptoms and thus referred to as a "rescue" medication. Side effects include tremor, tachycardia, and irritability. β-Agonists with a longer half-life (9 to 12 hours) such as salmeterol and formoterol are used for maintenance therapy and never during an acute attack.

TABLE 4-2:
Medical Treatment of Asthma Based on Asthma Classification

Severity	Treatment
Mild intermittent	Inhaled short-acting β_2-agonist as needed
Mild persistent	Anti-inflammatory agents: inhaled corticosteroids, consider leukotriene pathway modifier or cromolyn
Moderate persistent	Add long-acting β_2-agonist, increasing doses of inhaled corticosteroids, add leukotriene pathway modifier or consider theophylline; continue short-acting β_2-agonist
Severe persistent	Inhaled corticosteroids; long-acting β_2-agonist; theophylline; oral corticosteroids

    b. Ipratropium
- Ipratropium is an inhaled anticholinergic medication that causes bronchodilation by decreasing vagal tone. Its use in asthma is limited to severe acute exacerbation of asthma in combination with β_2-agonists. However, it may be approximately 60 minutes before maximal bronchodilatation is achieved. This drug is not a potent bronchodilator.

2. Methylxanthines
- The methylxanthines include theophylline (given by mouth) and aminophylline (given intravenously). They are used as second-line agents and are not as effective as β-agonists in causing bronchodilation; additionally, methylxanthines have many side effects, including nausea, vomiting, and cardiac arrhythmias. These drugs also have pharmacokinetic interactions with many drugs such as warfarin and anticonvulsants; the chronic use of theophylline requires therapeutic (i.e., drug level) monitoring.

3. Anti-inflammatory agents
    a. Corticosteroids
- Glucocorticoids are given as MDIs, IV, or orally. They decrease the activation and stimulation of proinflammatory cells and are not bronchodilators. Corticosteroid MDIs should be used initially. Oral candidiasis is usually the only side effect and can be prevented by rinsing the mouth with water after each use. Oral or parenteral corticosteroids are usually reserved for acute exacerbations or for those individuals not controlled by MDIs. Side effects of chronic use of corticosteroids includes weight gain, elevated blood glucose levels, hypertension, adrenal suppression, and osteoporosis especially with long-term use of higher doses.

    b. Cromolyn sodium and nedocromil sodium
- Cromolyn sodium and nedocromil sodium are mast cell stabilizers administered via an MDI; this combination is a particularly useful anti-inflammatory agent in younger patients and patients with allergen-induced bronchospasm.

    c. Leukotriene-modifying agents
- Leukotriene-modifying agents (montelukast, zafirlukast, and zileuton) include 5-lipoxygenase inhibitors, which inhibit the cysteinyl leukotrienes and leukotriene B_4 and D_4 receptor antagonists of the cysteinyl leukotrienes C_4, B_4, and D_4. These agents are effective in treating aspirin-induced asthma, allergen-induced asthma, and exercise-induced asthma.

    d. Omalizumab
- Omalizumab is an intravenous medication that works by blocking IgE. Omalizumab is reserved for select patients with allergic severe persistent asthma associated with elevated IgE levels despite optimal medical treatment.

III. Chronic Obstructive Pulmonary Disease
  A. Basic science
- Chronic obstructive pulmonary disease (COPD) refers to a spectrum of chronic respiratory diseases (emphysema, chronic bronchitis, and small airway disease) characterized by cough, sputum production, dyspnea, irreversible airflow obstruction, and impaired gas exchange.
- Chronic bronchitis is defined as presence of a productive cough for at least 3 months of the year for 2 successive years in a patient in whom other causes of chronic cough, such as infection and carcinoma, have been excluded.
- Emphysema is defined by such pathologic criteria as an abnormal enlargement of airspaces distal to the terminal bronchioles accompanied by the destruction of alveolar walls with or without fibrosis.
- Risk factors for the development of COPD include both external factors (i.e., cigarette smoking, occupational exposure, and environmental exposures) and internal factors (i.e., genetic problemss such as α_1-antitrypsin disease, atopy, and asthma). Chronic bronchitis and emphysema are most often associated with cigarette smoking.

  B. History and physical examination
- The symptoms associated with COPD do not usually manifest until after the patient has been smoking at least a pack of cigarettes a day for more than 20 years. Patients typically present in the fifth decade of life with a chronic productive cough which worsens after a viral respiratory infection. This is followed by slowly progressive dyspnea in the sixth or seventh decade of life and tends to be most severe with activities involving the upper extremities. Hemoptysis may occur in chronic bronchitis but should always raise the possibility of lung cancer in a person with a smoking history.
- Physical examination may reveal little abnormality except wheezing. In moderate to severe obstructive lung disease, the expiratory phase of respiration is prolonged and there is evidence of hyperinflation ("barrel chest," decreased diaphragmatic motion due to hyperinflation), or use of accessory muscles. Signs of pulmonary hypertension (parasternal heave, loud P_2, tricuspid regurgitation), right ventricular hypertrophy, or right-sided heart failure (*cor pulmonale*) may be present in end-stage COPD.

TABLE 4-3:
GOLD Classification for COPD Severity

Stage	Characteristics
0: At risk	→Normal spirometry →Chronic symptoms (cough, sputum production)
I: Mild COPD	→FEV_1/FVC < 70% →FEV_1 ≥ 80% predicted →With or without chronic symptoms (cough, sputum production)
II: Moderate COPD	→FEV_1/FVC < 70% →30% ≤ FEV_1 < 80% predicted (IIA: 50% ≤ FEV_1 < 80%, IIB: 30% ≤ FEV_1 < 50% predicted) →With or without chronic symptoms (cough, sputum production, dyspnea)
III: Severe COPD	→FEV_1/FVC < 70% →FEV_1/FVC < 30% predicted or FEV_1 < 50% predicted plus respiratory failure or clinical signs of right-sided heart failure)

COPD, chronic obstructive pulmonary disease; FEV, forced expiratory volume; FVC, forced virtal capacity.

C. Laboratory and diagnostic studies
  • The presence of COPD is often evident from the history and physical findings. However, the severity of the disease and evaluation of its response to therapy are based on pulmonary function tests, chest radiography, and arterial blood gases.
  • Chest radiographs often show low, flattened diaphragms. In severe emphysema, the lung fields may be hyperlucent, with diminished vascular markings and evidence of bullae. CT scan of the chest will define the presence or absence of emphysema.
  • Pulmonary function testing will reveal that the FEV_1 and the FEV_1/FVC ratio fall progressively as the severity of COPD increases and may show some evidence of reversibility; however, this is generally not complete reversibility as in asthma. Total lung capacity (TLC), functional residual capacity (FRC), and residual volume (RV) may be normal or increased. The diffusing capacity of the lung for carbon monoxide (D_{LCO}) is reduced in patients with moderate to severe emphysema because of parenchymal damage. (Table 4-3 gives the Global Initiative for Chronic Obstructive Lung Disease [GOLD] classification of the severity of COPD.) Arterial blood gases reveal worsening hypoxemia and hypercarbia with increasing severity of the disease.
  • An acute exacerbation of COPD is defined as worsening of dyspnea, an increase in sputum production from baseline, and the development of purulent sputum. The most frequent causes of acute exacerbations of COPD are respiratory infections. Bacterial pathogens cultured during an acute exacerbation are a mixture of organisms, including *Streptococcus pneumoniae*, *Haemophilus influenzae*, *Moraxella catarrhalis*, and *Pseudomonas aeruginosa*. Viral infection may be the related to nearly 40% of acute exacerbation. Bacterial cultures are rarely necessary before beginning antimicrobial therapy in outpatients. In hospitalized patients, Gram stain and culture may reveal a

gram-negative or, rarely, a staphylococcal infection. Other causes of exacerbations include continued smoking, noncompliance with medical therapy, and natural progression of the disease.

D. Formulating the diagnosis
- Although the history and physical examination suggest the possibility of COPD, a chest radiograph excludes other diagnoses (e.g., tuberculosis, lung cancer) and may reveal the findings of emphysema or a complicating pneumonia.
- Forced expiratory spirometry and arterial blood gas measurements quantify the degree of airway obstruction and the presence and severity of hypoxia and hypercapnia. The response of FEV_1 to a bronchodilator may help to differentiate COPD from asthma and may suggest that airflow obstruction will respond to corticosteroids.
- The prognosis of patients with mild airway obstruction is favorable; it is poor in those with severe obstruction, especially if accompanied by hypercapnia. In patients presenting with values of FEV_1 less than 0.75 L, the mortality rate at 1 year is approximately 30%.

E. Evaluating the severity of problems
- Although infection is a common cause of COPD exacerbation, pulmonary emboli, pulmonary edema, pneumothorax, and other causes of dyspnea should be excluded. Acute respiratory failure in COPD is defined as an arterial PCO_2 greater than 50 mm Hg, or an arterial PO_2 less than 50 mm Hg, in association with recent clinical worsening.
- The goal of treatment is (1) to improve hypoxemia by administering oxygen to raise the PO_2 to 60 mm Hg and (2) to reverse airway obstruction with inhaled β_2-agonists, anticholinergics, or methylxanthines (see Section II, Asthma). Adequate hydration should be maintained, and empiric antibiotics may be started. A course of steroids is usually given and then tapered quickly as the clinical status permits.
- Most patients can be managed conservatively; however, worsening hypoxemia and hypercapnia in association with clinical deterioration mandates mechanical ventilation.

F. Managing the patient
- Cigarette smoking is the most important risk factor, and patients should be urged to quit smoking. Occupational and environmental irritants should be eliminated, if possible. Preventive strategies aimed at decreasing the risk of respiratory infections should be administered; influenza vaccine should be given annually; the 23-strain pneumococcal vaccine should be given.
- Ambulatory therapy consists of symptomatic treatment directed against the reversible elements of airways obstruction (e.g., secretions, bronchospasm, and inflammation) and long-term oxygen therapy in patients with hypoxemia, which improves functioning of the patient without affecting lung physiology.
- The mainstays of symptomatic therapy are β_2-agonists (both short- and long-acting), anticholinergic agents, and methylxanthines, oxygen therapy, and corticosteroids.

1. Bronchodilators
   - Sympathomimetic β_2-adrenergic agonists such as metaproterenol, albuterol, and terbutaline are effective bronchodilators. They relieve smooth muscle spasm and enhance mucociliary clearance.
2. Anticholinergics
   - Unlike atropine, inhaled ipratroprium bromide is not systemically absorbed and is free of anticholinergic side effects. In many studies, ipratroprium has had a greater bronchodilating effect in COPD than the β_2-aerosols.
3. Methylxanthines
   - The mode of action of theophylline is poorly understood. Small changes in FEV_1 as well as improvement in symptoms and exercise capacity occur with chronic use. Toxicity is poorly related to its blood level. More serious toxicities, such as arrhythmias and seizures, occur at blood levels greater than 20 mg/mL.
4. Glucocorticoids
   - In hospitalized patients, glucocorticoids decrease length of stay. The currently recommended dose of prednisolone is 30 to 40 mg per day for 2 weeks. Long-term use with inhaled corticosteroids show improvements in 6-minute walk and lung function.
5. Antibiotics
   - An upper respiratory infection is the most common identifiable cause of a COPD exacerbation. Antibiotic-treated exacerbations are shorter in duration and less likely to have serious consequences. Routine cultures are not indicated before instituting therapy. Prophylactic use of antibiotics has not been shown to decrease the frequency of exacerbations.
6. Home oxygen
   - Long-term oxygen therapy prolongs life in hypoxemic COPD patients as well as improves the quality of life. Indications include a resting room-air arterial PO_2 of 55 mm Hg or less, oxygen saturation of less than 89%, or a PO_2 between 56 and 59 mm Hg in the presence of erythrocytosis or cor pulmonale.
7. Pulmonary rehabilitation
   - Pulmonary rehabilitation is a multidisciplinary program, which has been shown to improve exercise tolerance, reduce dyspnea, improve quality of life, and decrease number of hospitalizations.
8. Surgery for COPD
   - Lung volume reduction surgery (LVRS) has been shown to be potentially therapeutic for advanced COPD due to emphysema. LVRS involves resection of the severely emphysematous and nonfunctional areas of the lung in order to improve the elastic recoil of the lung and decrease chest wall hyperinflation.
   - Lung transplantation is reserved for end-stage COPD to improve the quality of life. Lung transplantation has not been shown to improve survival at 2 years after transplant.

IV. Interstitial Lung Diseases
  A. Basic science
  - Interstitial lung diseases (ILDs) have a variety of causes (known and unknown) and result either in inflammation and fibrosis or a granulomatous reaction in the interstitum. The initiating event is an injury to the interalveolar septum. Excessive repair leads to progressive deposition of extracellular matrix proteins and distortion of normal alveolar architecture. The hallmark of active ILD is "alveolitis," that is, infiltration of the alveolar space with inflammatory cells and ultimately fibrosis.
  - The known causes of ILDs includes a list of more than 100 causes. Some of the most common causes are infections and exposures (to dusts, fumes, radiation, and drugs); however, the cause of ILDs in most patients is unknown. Patients in whom the cause of ILD is unknown most often receive the diagnosis of idiopathic pulmonary fibrosis (IPF).
  - *Sarcoidosis* is an ILD that requires special attention. It is a poorly defined granulomatous disease that is characterized by the presence of noncaseating granulomas that involve the lung parenchyma and intrathoracic lymph nodes in greater than 90% of patients. The skin, bone, and eyes can be involved. Cardiac and nervous system involvement is uncommon. It is commonly diagnosed as an incidental finding of bilateral hilar lymphadenopathy on chest x-ray. If there is no involvement of the parenchyma, this form is type I sarcoid. If in addition to the hilar lymphadenopathy there is parenchymal involvement, the radiologic type is type II. Type III is diffuse parenchymal involvement without hilar lymphadenopathy.
  - Spontaneous remission occurs in nearly 2 of every 3 patients, and a history of a waxing and waning course is typical. Factors associated with a poor prognosis include African-American descent, disfiguring cutaneous facial involvement, chronic hypercalcemia that doesn't respond to therapy, and chronic pulmonary involvement.
  B. History and physical examination
  - The typical patient with ILD is middle-aged and presents with the insidious onset of dyspnea on exertion and a dry, nonproductive cough. A careful history may elicit clues to an environmental or occupational exposure that may be the cause of the ILD. A period of latency often occurs between the development of the ILD and exposure to the inciting exposure. A smoking history is important as it may have played a role in causing the ILD as well as influencing the course of the disease.
  - Physical examination usually reveals bibasilar end inspiratory crackles (i.e., "velcro rales"). Bibasilar crackles in a middle-aged individual without signs of congestive heart failure (e.g., elevated jugular venous pressure, S_3 gallop) should raise the suspicion of ILD. Wheezing is uncommon. Clubbing of the fingers is common in patients with IPF but rare in other causes of ILD (e.g., sarcoidosis) and is an indication of advanced fibrosis. In advanced disease, evidence of pulmonary hypertension and cor pulmonale appear. Weight loss is common when the disease is advanced.

C. Laboratory and diagnostic studies
- There are no laboratory abnormalities diagnostic of ILD; however, an elevated erythrocyte sedimentation rate (ESR), lactic dehydrogenase (LDH), and hypergammaglobulinemia are common. Laboratory assessment is generally directed at generating support for diagnosis of a specific ILD (e.g., angiotensin-converting enzyme levels and blood calcium levels for sarcoidosis).
- Patients commonly come to medical attention because of an abnormal chest x-ray. Radiographic abnormalities commonly seen in ILD are of an alveolar filling pattern (i.e., diffuse or patchy infiltrates, nodules, air bronchograms, and obliteration or silhouetting of normal thoracic structures) or of the interstitial changes (i.e., reticular or reticulonodular pattern). A high-resolution thoracic CT scan also is an important test in evaluating early airspace or interstitial changes of ILD.
- Pulmonary function testing in patients with ILD typically reveals a restrictive pattern (i.e., vital capacity, functional residual capacity, and total lung capacity are reduced). Pressure-volume measurements will reveal reduced lung compliance. The DLCO is reduced as a result of a destruction of alveolar capillary units. The resting arterial blood gas measurement may reveal a normal or reduced PO_2 and a mild respiratory alkalosis. The arterial PO_2 usually falls with exertion.

D. Formulating the diagnosis
- A careful clinical history and physical examination with particular emphasis on possible occupational or environmental exposures and the determination of whether the ILD is occurring in the setting of a systemic illness will allow the majority of patients to be identified. It is important to exclude potentially treatable chronic infectious processes such as mycobacterial and fungal disease.
- Following this initial evaluation, the next important issue is to confirm the diagnosis and determine the level of impairment in order to obtain information on the prognosis and decide on therapeutic options. Fiberoptic bronchoscopy with bronchoalveolar lavage and transbronchial biopsies should be the first step in the majority of cases. If adequate lung tissue is not obtained by the transbronchial approach, traditional open lung biopsy or video-assisted thoracoscopic biopsy is required in order to obtain adequate lung tissue.

E. Evaluating the severity of problems
- Cardiopulmonary exercise testing can be done and quantifies the amount of work the patient can perform and the need for supplemental oxygen during periods of exertion. Signs of pulmonary hypertension and overt right ventricular failure (cor pulmonale) indicate advanced disease.

F. Managing the patient
- Management of the patient with ILD is determined by the cause. The patient with an occupational or environmental exposure should be removed from the offending agent. Smokers should be encouraged to quit.
- Corticosteroids are the mainstay of therapy for IPF, collagen vascular disease–associated ILD, inorganic dust exposure, acute radiation pneumonitis, and drug-induced disease.

- The goals of therapy are to suppress the ongoing inflammatory response and prevent further fibrosis. Objective response commonly takes 6 to 12 weeks in most forms of ILD and occurs in only 20% to 30% of patients; however, many forms of ILD are not responsive to therapy. Many patients will relapse and require lifelong therapy.
- Patients with IPF who demonstrate progression of disease on corticosteroids may be candidates for cytotoxic therapy with cyclophosphamide or azathioprine. Other immunosuppressive agents that have been used include cyclosporine, methotrexate, D-penicillamine, and colchicine. The treatment of choice for patients who do not respond to therapy is lung transplantation. All patients should be encouraged to maintain an exercise routine to improve oxygen utilization.

V. Obstructive Sleep Apnea Syndrome
   A. Basic science
   - Obstructive sleep apnea syndrome (OSA) is characterized by repetitive episodes of complete or partial obstruction of the upper airway during sleep resulting in apneas (complete cessation of airflow for at least 10 seconds) or hypopneas (50% reduction in airflow for more than 10 seconds). The underlying mechanism for these obstructive episodes is a combination of abnormal upper airway anatomy and normal sleep-induced reduction in pharyngeal muscle tone.
   - These apneas and hypopneas may lead to hypoxemia and hypercapnia, which can cause nocturnal arrhythmias, particularly bradyarrhythmias. The respiratory events also cause transient (3 to 5 seconds) arousals, sometimes several hundred times at night, resulting in sleep fragmentation, with symptoms of chronic sleep deprivation such as excessive daytime sleepiness and personality changes.
   - The prevalence of obstructive sleep apnea syndrome is approximately 4% for males and 2% for females 30 to 60 years of age. The prevalence increases with increasing age. Approximately 75% of patients with OSA are obese (weight > 120% of predicted). There is an association between obstructive sleep apnea syndrome and hypertension, some of which is due to shared risk factors (obesity, male sex), but OSA also appears to be an independent risk factor for systemic hypertension. Pulmonary hypertension occurs in 15% to 20% of patients with OSA.
   - A subset (10% to 15%) of OSA patients suffers from the obesity hypoventilation syndrome (pickwickian syndrome). This syndrome is characterized by waking hypoventilation ($PaCO_2 > 45$ mm Hg) manifested by both daytime hypercapnia and hypoxemia, and the subsequent development of pulmonary hypertension, right-sided heart failure, and polycythemia if left untreated.
   B. History and physical examination
   - Symptoms of OSA arise either as a direct manifestation of the obstructive episode or as a sequela of chronic sleep disruption. Clinical presentations include frequent awakenings during the night, sometimes with choking. Often

the patient is unaware of the choking and frequent arousals. Morning headaches secondary to hypercapnia occur in 10% to 15%. Impotence can occur in males. Almost all patients with OSA snore, though most snorers do not have OSA. In addition to snoring, bed partners may report apneic episodes, which often are terminated with a snort and a jerk. Also, patients typically suffer from excessive daytime sleepiness. Increased irritability and an impaired ability to concentrate may arise from chronic sleep fragmentation.

- Risk factors for OSA include male sex and obesity, anatomic abnormalities (e.g., nasal obstruction, mandibular or maxillary hypoplasia, macroglossia, and tonsillar or adenoid hypertrophy), neuromuscular diseases, hypothyroidism, acromegaly, and Down syndrome.
- Physical examination should be directed toward identifying predisposing anatomic abnormalities including a neck circumference greater than 17 inches in males as well as sequelae of OSA, such as systemic or pulmonary artery hypertension.

C. Laboratory and diagnostic studies
- Laboratory evaluation plays a limited role. Patients with severe OSA, especially those with obesity hypoventilation syndrome, may be polycythemic or have elevated serum bicarbonate. Thyroid-stimulating hormone level, if normal, will help exclude hypothyroidism. Arterial blood gases are typically indicated only for patients with severe OSA.
- Imaging studies such as cephalometrics, or CT/MRI imaging of the upper airway, sometimes may identify sites of collapse during sleep. Although these approaches have generated research interest, clinical applicability has yet to be defined.
- The diagnosis of OSA requires a nocturnal polysomnogram (sleep study), during which respiratory efforts, nasal and oral airflow, and oximetry is measured. Sleep staging is also frequently performed. Overnight oximetry is sometimes used as a screening test. An oximetry study showing oxyhemoglobin desaturation is very suggestive of OSA. The absence of desaturation below 90% does not, however, exclude the diagnosis, as many patients can be very symptomatic but do not desaturate.

D. Formulating the diagnosis
- The history is the determining factor in deciding whether to work up a patient for OSA. Current indications for a sleep study include excessive daytime sleepiness, frequent nocturnal awakenings, observed apneic episodes during sleep, cyclic nocturnal arrhythmias, waking hypoventilation, or pulmonary hypertension without an obvious cause. Snoring, obesity, or hypertension alone without other symptoms of OSA are not indications for a sleep study.

E. Managing the patient
- All patients with OSA should be advised to avoid alcohol and sedative drugs, especially at bedtime, as these can worsen disease severity. Some patients have obstructive episodes only while supine; sleep position training to keep them on their side can eliminate these obstructive episodes. In obese patients, weight loss is critical because weight loss alone can be curative. Underlying conditions, such as hypothyroidism or chronic nasal congestion, should be treated. Patients

with excessive daytime sleepiness should not engage in potentially dangerous activities (e.g., driving), in which falling asleep could be lethal, until they have been adequately treated.

- The first-line and most effective therapy for OSA is continuous positive airway pressure delivered by a nasal mask (nasal CPAP). Nasal CPAP works by creating a pneumatic splint, which holds the pharynx open during sleep, preventing obstructive respiratory events. The major drawback to nasal CPAP is poor acceptance of the device by patients, resulting in poor compliance.
- Several surgical procedures have been used to treat OSA. Currently the most popular procedure is uvulopalatopharyngoplasty (UPPP), which involves resecting the uvula, portions of the soft palate, tonsils and adenoids (if present), as well as the tonsillar pillars. Unfortunately, this procedure is effective in only 40% to 50% of cases. Some studies suggest that procedures combining UPPP with surgery to advance the base of the tongue forward may be more effective. Tracheostomy, by bypassing the site of obstruction, is generally curative, but this procedure is reserved only for those with severe OSA who fail other treatment modalities. In children, enlarged adenoids are the major cause of OSA, so tonsillectomy and adenoidectomy is indicated as a first-line treatment. Dental appliances that act to advance the mandible and tongue can be of some benefit, especially in milder cases.

VI. Pleural Effusion

 A. Basic science

- The pleural space normally contains less than 10 to 15 mL of fluid, which is formed continuously in small amounts. Excess fluid, known as a pleural effusion, results when the net fluid formation exceeds the clearance capacity of the pleural lymphatics (300–400 mL/day) or when a process (such as a parasite or neoplasm) diminishes or blocks lymphatic flow. The fluid of a pleural effusion can be a transudate or an exudate. This differentiation is based on laboratory analysis of the fluid.

 B. History and physical examination

- Although a pleural effusion can be asymptomatic, symptoms may be due to the underlying condition responsible for the effusion (e.g., abdominal pain in pancreatitis, fever and sputum production in pneumonia, or joint pain in systemic lupus erythematosus or rheumatoid arthritis) or due to the size of the effusion (shortness of breath). Irritation of the pleural surfaces or mediastinal shift can produce a dry, nonproductive cough. A process involving the visceral pleura can result in dull, aching pain, whereas parietal pleura involvement leads to sharp, knifelike pain worsened with deep inspiration.
- Physical examination findings depend on the size of the effusion and include impaired chest expansion, decreased resonance by percussion, and decreased tactile fremitus by palpation. If the effusion is large enough, the trachea can be shifted to the contralateral side. Breath sounds are diminished or absent over the effusion.

C. Laboratory and diagnostic studies
　1. Diagnostic imaging
　　• A posteroanterior and lateral chest radiograph is the first step in confirming a pleural effusion. A lateral decubitus film can detect as little as 100 mL and determine if the fluid is free flowing or loculated (trapped in pockets from adhesions).
　　• Ultrasound is useful for confirming the free-flowing nature of the fluid and selecting a site for thoracentesis when loculation is suspected.
　　• CT scanning can be useful in distinguishing small pleural effusions from atelectasis or masses and can be useful in detecting the presence and degree of loculation.
　2. Invasive procedures
　　a. Thoracentesis
　　　• A thoracentesis is needed in almost every case of a newly discovered pleural effusion to help with definitive diagnosis and management. Exceptions to the need for diagnostic thoracentesis include effusions secondary to congestive heart failure or pneumonia that is improving with therapy.
　　b. Pleural biopsy
　　　• Pleural biopsy is indicated if malignancy or granulomatous disease is suspected, or when several thoracenteses have revealed nondiagnostic exudative material.
D. Formulating the diagnosis
　• The first decision point depends on the characterization of the fluid as a transudate or exudate. Exudates have at least one of the following criteria, whereas transudates will have none: (1) ratio of pleural fluid protein to serum protein greater than 0.5, (2) ratio of pleural fluid LDH to serum LDH greater than 0.6, (3) pleural fluid LDH above two thirds of the upper limit of normal for a simultaneously taken serum LDH. Table 4-4 shows commonly found pleural effusions and their associated laboratory tests.
　• Congestive heart failure is the most common cause of a transudative effusion; exudative effusions are most commonly the result of malignancy, although in developing countries tuberculosis remains an important cause. If the fluid is a transudate, no further workup is needed, and efforts are focused on treating the underlying condition. Exudates, however, require further investigation. The diagnostic effort can be focused with data from the following tests on the pleural fluid:
　　1. LDH
　　　• Very high LDH, especially without elevated protein, suggests malignancy.
　　2. Protein
　　　• Level above 6.0 g/dL suggests tuberculosis (TB) or parapneumonic effusion.
　　3. Glucose
　　　• Level below 60 mg/dL suggests TB, rheumatoid arthritis, malignancy, or a parapneumonic process.

TABLE 4-4:
Characteristics of Pleural Effusions

Etiology	Appearance	WBCs/mm³	RBCs/mm³	pH	Glucose (mg/dL)	Comments
Transudates: Protein ≤ 3 g/100 mL,* LDH < 200 IU, LDH ratio < 0.6						
Congestive heart failed	Clear, straw-colored	<1,000 lymphs	<5,000	Normal	~Serum	Bilateral cardiomegaly
Cirrhosis	Serous to serosanguineous	<1,000	<5,000	Normal	~Serum	Right-sided
Nephrotic syndrome	Serous	<1,000 monos	<5,000	Normal	~Serum	Bilateral
Meigs' syndrome	Serous to serosanguineous	<1,000 lymphs	<10,000	Normal	~Serum	Right-sided, occasionally left or bilateral
Exudates: Protein ≥ 3 g/100 mL,* LDH > 200 IU, LDH ratio ≥ 0.6						
Uncomplicated parapneumonic	Turbid	5–40,000 PMNs	<5,000	Normal to ↓	~Serum	
Complicated parapneumonic	Turbid to purulent	5–40,000 PMNs	<5,000	↓↓	↓↓	
Empyema	Purulent	25–100,000 PMNs	<5,000	↓↓↓	↓↓	
Tuberculosis	Serosanguineous	5–10,000 lymphs	<10,000	Normal to ↓	Normal to ↓	+ AFB + ADA
Malignancy	Turbid to bloody	1–100,000 lymphs	1–100,000	Normal to ↓	Normal to ↓	+ cytology
Pulmonary embolism	Bloody	1–50,000 PMNs	1–100,000	Normal	~Serum	No infarct→ Transudate
Rheumatoid arthritis	Turbid	1–20,000 PMNs, lymphs, eos	<1,000	↓	↓↓↓	↑ RF, ↓CH50
Pancreatitis	Serosanguineous to turbid	1–50,000 PMNs	1–10,000	Normal	~Serum	Left-sided ↑ Amylase
Esophageal rupture	Turbid to purulent	<5,000–>50,000	1–10,000	↓↓↓	↓↓	Left-sided ↑ Amylase
Hypoalbuminemia	Serous	<1,000 monos	<5,000	Normal	~Serum	Small, bilateral

*With normal serum protein concentration.
ADA, adenosine deaminase; AFB, acid fast bacilli; CH50, total complement; eos, eosinophils; LDH, lactic dehydiagenaze; lymphs, lymphocytes; monos, monocytes; PMNs, polymarphonuclear cells; RBCs, red blood cells; RF, rheumatoid factor; WBCs, white blood cells.

4. White blood cell count
   - This is rather nonspecific; counts greater than 10,000/mm³ are seen with TB, malignancy, infection, collagen vascular disease, and pulmonary infarction.
5. Differential white blood cell count
   - Lymphocyte predominance suggests TB, sarcoidosis, and malignancy. Neutrophil predominance suggests bacterial infection, pulmonary embolism, or pancreatitis. Although it is nonspecific, eosinophilia is seen with bleeding and pneumothorax.

6. Red blood cell count
   - Generally, counts greater than 100,000 cells/mm^3 are required to define an effusion as grossly bloody. Grossly bloody effusions are seen in trauma, malignancy, TB, and pulmonary embolism.
7. Amylase
   - This is elevated in pancreatitis, esophageal perforation, and adenocarcinoma.
8. Triglycerides
   - An elevated triglyceride level (>150 mg/dL) is diagnostic of chylothorax.
9. pH
   - A parapneumonic effusion with a pH below 7.20 suggests a complicated effusion with risk of empyema. In malignancy, a pH below 7.30 connotes a poor prognosis.
10. Gram stain and culture
    - Empyema is defined if either is positive in a parapneumonic effusion. If TB is suspected, acid fast bacilli (AFB) stain should be performed.
11. Cytologic examination
    - The diagnostic yield for metastatic malignancy is 60% on a single specimen. Three separate specimens will improve the yield to 90%.

E. Evaluating the severity of problems
   - Respiratory compromise from large effusions requires therapeutic thoracentesis until diagnosis permits definitive management.

F. Managing the patient
   - In most cases of effusions, a definitive diagnosis is possible, and therapy is directed at the underlying disorder. Parapneumonic and malignant pleural effusions, however, merit further attention.
   1. Parapneumonic effusions
      - Parapneumonic effusions are effusions associated with pneumonia, pulmonary abscesses, or bronchiectasis. The crucial management decision, besides selection of appropriate antibiotics, centers on whether tube thoracostomy is needed to drain the effusion. Indications for chest tube drainage are pleural fluid that shows gross pus, positive Gram stain, positive pleural fluid culture, glucose less than 60 mg/dL, or pH below 7.20.
      - Complicated parapneumonic effusion is defined as an effusion that requires a chest tube for drainage or that is grossly infected (an empyema).
   2. Malignant effusion
      - Proper therapy for a malignant effusion depends upon the mechanism responsible for it. Endobronchial lesions causing obstructions should be treated with a stent or a laser therapy. Radiation therapy should be instituted if the effusion is due to mediastinal lymphatic blocking. Pleurodesis (the production of adhesions to obliterate the pleural space) may be performed when pleural metastases exist. Before considering pleurodesis, one needs to ascertain whether the patient has symptoms attributable to the effusion and, if so, demonstrate symptomatic improvement after therapeutic thoracentesis. If these conditions are met, pleurodesis is done (via tube thoracostomy or video-assisted thoracic

surgery) with chemical irritants such as doxycycline or talc, or a chemotherapeutic agent such as bleomycin.

VII. Pneumothorax
   A. Basic science
   - A pneumothorax is defined as gas present in the pleural space. Pneumothoraces are characterized as traumatic, spontaneous, or iatrogenic. Spontaneous pneumothoraces are further subdivided into primary, if there is no known underlying lung pathology, or secondary, if related to a known cause of spontaneous pneumothorax such as COPD, cystic fibrosis, or menses (Box 4-3).
   - Normally the pressure in the pleural space is negative relative to alveolar pressure and atmospheric pressure. A pneumothorax develops if a communication is established between either the alveoli or the chest wall, in which case air will enter the pleural space until the intrapleural pressure equals the atmospheric pressure. This increased pressure results in compression of the underlying lung and outward expansion of the hemithorax. If a ball-valve effect is present, air will move into the pleural space during inspiration but will be trapped during expiration, creating a life-threatening situation known as a tension pneumothorax.
   B. History and physical examination
   - The symptoms of pneumothorax are usually sudden in onset and include dyspnea and sharp chest pain. The symptoms are typically more severe and less well tolerated in those with secondary rather than primary pneumothorax because of the underlying lung disease. A history of antecedent penetrating or blunt trauma is usually obvious in cases of traumatic pneumothorax.
   - Physical findings in pneumothorax can include tachypnea, with decreased tactile fremitus and decreased to absent breath sounds on the ipsilateral side. Percussion resonance is increased on the side with the pneumothorax. The trachea may be shifted to the opposite side. Additional signs that may be present when a tension pneumothorax is present include tachycardia, hypotension, elevated jugular venous pressure, distended external jugular veins, weak peripheral pulses, and cyanosis.
   C. Laboratory and diagnostic studies
   - A plain chest radiograph is usually adequate to confirm the diagnosis of pneumothorax, in which case a visceral-pleural line can be seen. Occasionally, a pneumothorax will be loculated and better visualized on a lateral radiograph or CT scan.
   D. Evaluating the severity of problems
   - Imaging has no role in confirming the presence of tension pneumothorax, as the condition is life-threatening, and a delay in diagnosis can be fatal. In the case of suspected tension pneumothorax, the clinician should proceed immediately to needle or tube thoracostomy.
   E. Managing the patient
   - In a case of suspected tension pneumothorax, a large-gauge needle should be inserted immediately into the ipsilateral second intercostal space in the

BOX 4-3

CAUSES OF SECONDARY SPONTANEOUS PNEUMOTHORAX

Disease of the airways
    Chronic obstructive pulmonary disease
    Cystic fibrosis
    Status asthmaticus
Interstitial lung diseases
    Langerhans cell granulomatosis
    Sarcoidosis
    Lymphangioleiomyomatosis
    Tuberous sclerosis
    Rheumatoid disease
    Idiopathic pulmonary fibrosis
    Radiation fibrosis
Infectious diseases
    Necrotizing gram-negative pneumonia
    Anaerobic pneumonia
    Staphylococcal pneumonia
    AIDS with *Pneumocystis* pneumonia
    Mycobacterium tuberculosis infection
Malignancy
    Sarcoma
    Lung cancer (all types)
Others
    Catamenial
    Pulmonary infarction
    Wegener's granulomatosis
    Marfan syndrome
    Ehlers-Danlos syndrome
    Berylliosis
    Idiopathic pulmonary hemosiderosis

midclavicular line. An alternative is the insertion of a chest tube if equipment and skilled personnel are immediately available. In either case, an immediate rush of air through the needle or chest tube upon insertion confirms the diagnosis.

- In cases of traumatic or iatrogenic pneumothorax, where there is greater than 30% to 40% pneumothorax, tube thoracostomy will be required to reexpand the lung. If the size of the pneumothorax is smaller than 30%, observation, with supplemental oxygen, is standard therapy.

- In primary pneumothorax, initial management can include aspiration of the air with a 16-gauge needle. Recurrence rates are high (>50% in 2 years), and recurrences should be managed with tube thoracostomy and sometimes with open thoracotomy and instillation of a pleural sclerosing agent.
- Most cases of secondary pneumothorax should be managed with tube thoracostomy, as simple aspiration is frequently ineffective; chemical pleurodesis should be considered to prevent recurrence.

VIII. Pulmonary Embolism
   A. Basic science
- Pulmonary emboli are blood clots originating in the venous system that dislodge, traverse the right side of the heart, and occlude portions of the pulmonary vasculature. Rarely, thrombotic material from upper extremity or right cardiac sources or nonthrombotic material such as tumor, intravascular foreign bodies, or bone marrow can manifest as pulmonary emboli. However, the vast majority of pulmonary emboli come from venous thrombosis in the proximal veins of the lower extremities.
- Approximately one third of deaths from acute pulmonary emboli occur within 1 hour of the onset of symptoms. Thrombi confined to the calf veins are unlikely to embolize. Patients with large emboli may present with right ventricular failure and shock. Patients who have recurrent asymptomatic or minimally symptomatic embolization will develop pulmonary hypertension, which leads to progressive right-sided heart failure and ultimately death.

   B. History and physical examination
- The predisposing factors leading to pulmonary emboli are those that predispose to deep venous thrombosis: stasis, vascular injury, and enhanced clotting (Virchow's triad). Clinical settings include sedentary or bedridden patients, patients with trauma, postoperative patients, patients with cancer (especially adenocarcinoma), patients who are pregnant or woman older than 35 years of age using oral contraceptives, patients with a previous history of pulmonary embolism or deep venous thrombosis, those having long duration of air travel, and persons with obesity. The common genetic mutations that contribute to thrombosis are factor V_{Leiden} and prothrombin gene mutations.
- Patients with acute pulmonary embolism complain of sudden onset of dyspnea or syncope. Pleuritic chest pain suggests a peripheral embolus. Nonproductive cough or hemoptysis occurs in about half of patients. On physical examination, the patient is anxious, tachypneic, and tachycardic and may have low-grade fever. If the emboli are large, the patient may be hypotensive and cyanotic. There may be jugular venous distention and a loud second heart sound. Breath sounds are generally normal. Wheezing from the release of bronchoconstrictive mediators may occur.

   C. Laboratory and diagnostic studies
- Elevated D-dimer levels (<500 ng/mL) are present in the majority of patients. However, D-dimer has a low specificity. The chest x-ray may be normal or may show a variety of abnormalities, including unilateral pleural effusion, an

elevated diaphragm or atelectasis from splinting, focal oligemia, or a localized pleural-based infiltrate indicating pulmonary infarction. The ECG usually shows sinus tachycardia but may also show right ventricular strain, right bundle branch block, right axis deviation, or a supraventricular arrhythmia; the "classic" $S_1Q_3T_3$ pattern is rare. Arterial blood gases may show hypoxia and a respiratory alkalosis. The alveolar–arterial oxygen gradient is probably not as helpful as previously thought.

- The finding of multiple segmental perfusion defects without corresponding ventilation defects in a ventilation-perfusion lung scan is highly suggestive of pulmonary embolism and is virtually diagnostic when combined with a typical clinical history. Conversely, the absence of any perfusion defects as large as a single segment makes emboli very unlikely. However, many scans lie between these two extremes and are read as "indeterminate," that is, requiring further study.
- Further tests may include noninvasive studies of the veins of the legs such as venous plethysmography or duplex scanning. These tests are highly sensitive and specific for proximal deep venous thrombosis. A positive finding both increases the specificity of the indeterminate lung scan and necessitates anticoagulant therapy that treats pulmonary embolism as well as the venous thrombosis. CT of the chest with intravenous contrast material easily detects large central pulmonary emboli. The newer scanners are effective in detecting emboli in peripheral bronchi as well. Pulmonary angiography remains the gold standard.

D. Formulating the diagnosis
- Patients presenting with the signs and symptoms of pulmonary embolism, hypoxia, and a "high probability" lung scan have a greater than 95% probability of having emboli and should be treated as such. Patients whose history and physical examination are less suggestive of emboli (i.e., low pretest probability who have normal or low probability scans) should not be treated. Other patients presenting with dyspnea, pleuritic chest pain, and hypoxia may have alternative diagnoses such as pneumothorax, pneumonia, or empyema, which become obvious with evaluation. However, many patients with equivocal clinical presentation and hypoxia require further study, including pulmonary angiogram.
- Untreated, pulmonary emboli have a 30% mortality rate, which decreases to less than 5% with therapy. Some patients survive multiple unrecognized episodes and present with irreversible pulmonary hypertension and right ventricular failure.

E. Evaluating the severity of problems
- Patients in shock and patients who require intubation and mechanical ventilation obviously require management in an intensive care unit. Patients with underlying cardiac or pulmonary disease, those requiring high (>50%) concentrations of inspired oxygen, and those with three or more segmental defects on perfusion scanning are also at increased risk of dying from additional emboli and may benefit from intensive monitoring.

F. Managing the patient
- Hypoxia must be relieved immediately with supplemental oxygen. Shock must also be treated rapidly, first with intravenous isotonic crystalloid and then, if necessary, with the vasopressors. Patients with suspected pulmonary emboli should also begin treatment with intravenous heparin (bolus and continuous infusion) immediately while diagnostic studies are obtained. Unless the patient has a major contraindication to anticoagulation, the risk of additional emboli far exceeds the risk of hemorrhage while awaiting definitive tests.
- Anticoagulation with heparin is the mainstay of acute therapy for pulmonary emboli. Heparin activates antithrombin III, allowing endogenous thrombolysis and preventing clot propagation, but does not directly dissolve existing clot. Heparin should be administered by continuous infusion to elevate the activated partial prothrombin time (PTT) to two to three times its control value. Low-molecular-weight heparin has now been shown to have equivalent treatment efficacy to unfractioned heparin and has less variable bioavailability than heparin.
- Patients in shock or with refractory hypoxia should be considered for thrombolytic therapy or embolectomy. Thrombolytics more rapidly reverse the hemodynamic abnormalities, although the ultimate degree of pulmonary clot resolution is similar to that in patients receiving heparin alone. Contraindications to thrombolysis include active bleeding from a noncompressible site, pregnancy, recent surgery, and central nervous system trauma and surgery, bleeding, or infarct in the preceding 2 months. After thrombolytic therapy, patients are continued on heparin. During this time, patients are converted to oral warfarin. Oral anticoagulation should be continued for 3 to 6 months and requires close monitoring of the prothrombin time. Anticoagulation may be continued indefinitely in patients who have had recurrent emboli or have risk factors that cannot be corrected such as a hypercoaguable state. If there is a contraindication to warfarin, such as pregnancy, patients may self-inject subcutaneous heparin.
- Patients who hemorrhage on anticoagulants, who develop recurrent emboli despite appropriate anticoagulation, or in whom any additional embolization would be fatal should be considered for vena caval filters. This is performed via transvenous placement of a wire filter in the inferior vena cava, which intercepts clots embolizing from the lower extremities.
- The prevention of pulmonary emboli is achieved through the prevention of deep venous thrombosis. Patients with venous insufficiency should avoid sitting for long, continuous periods. Hospitalized bedridden patients, particularly those with fractures, surgery, or venous insufficiency, should receive 5000 units of subcutaneous low-molecular-weight heparin three times daily or wear sequential compression stockings.

IX. Sarcoidosis
A. Basic science
- Sarcoidosis is a systemic disease characterized by the presence of noncaseating granulomatous inflammation in involved organs. Although

much research has been undertaken to find the cause of sarcoidosis, its etiology remains unknown. The CD_4 T-helper lymphocyte (T_H1) and a panel of cytokines, including interleukin 2 and interferon, are thought to contribute to the pathogeneisis of the disease. This inflammatory response may be self-limiting and spontaneously regress, or it may progress to fibrosis.

B. History and physical examination
- The onset of sarcoidosis usually occurs between the ages of 20 and 40 years. It can, however, occur in children and adults. In the United States, it is approximately 14 times more common in blacks than in the white population. The sex distribution is equal.
- The clinical presentation of patients with sarcoidosis falls into three broad categories: (1) the asymptomatic patient with an abnormal chest x-ray, (2) the patient with pulmonary symptoms, and (3) the patient with extrapulmonary manifestations.
- Over 90% of patients with sarcoidosis have lung involvement, with dominant symptoms being nonproductive cough and dyspnea on exertion. The patients may have very little symptomatology despite extensive radiographic abnormalities. The chest examination is often unremarkable. Any organ system can be involved.
- The most common skin manifestations are erythema nodosum (which often heralds acute sarcoidosis and generally has a better prognosis) and chronic plaques. Granulomatous anterior uveitis detected by slit-lamp examination is the most common eye finding.
- Other disorders seen on physical examination may include lupus pernio (nodular skin lesions around the nares and cheeks), hepatosplenomegaly, lymphadenopathy, intrathoracic (hilar, paratracheal, mediastinal) as well as peripheral nodes such as cervical and axillary nodes, arthritis, cranial (most commonly the facial nerve) and peripheral nerve deficits, and lacrimal and parotid gland enlargement.

C. Laboratory and diagnostic studies
- Fiberoptic bronchoscopy provides the most common source of biopsy tissue. However, in appropriate patients, biopsies may be obtained from other affected tissues (e.g., the skin).
- Pulmonary function tests typically show restrictive lung disease on spirometry and lung volume studies; however, an obstructive pattern can be seen with endobronchial sarcoidosis.
- The use of angiotensin-converting enzyme (ACE) levels in the diagnosis and management of sarcoidosis is controversial. It is elevated in 60% of patients with sarcoidosis but has a low specificity and little predictive value. Similarly, the clinical usefulness of gallium scans is limited.
- Laboratory abnormalities common to sarcoidosis include leukopenia, eosinophilia, hypercalcemia, hypercalciuria, and an elevated erythrocyte sedimentation rate. The rheumatoid factor and antinuclear antibody can be falsely elevated.

D. Formulating the diagnosis
- The diagnosis of sarcoidosis requires compatible clinical, radiographic, and laboratory findings with supporting histopathologic features demonstrating noncaseating granulomas. Care must be taken to rule out infectious diseases such as tuberculosis and, in the presence of hilar or peripheral adenopathy, lymphoma. Given sarcoid's systemic involvement, it may mimic many other disease processes.

E. Evaluating the severity of problems
- Clinical symptoms such as progressively worsening dyspnea on exertion, besides abnormal pulmonary function testing and chest x-ray findings, serve as monitors for the severity and progression of pulmonary sarcoidosis. Transaminases and alkaline phosphatase can be used to monitor liver involvement. Other laboratory tests such as blood urea nitrogen (BUN), creatinine, calcium, complete blood cell count, and cerebrospinal fluid analysis can be used to define the other organ involvement in sarcoidosis.

F. Managing the patient
- Many patients with sarcoidosis do not require therapy because spontaneous remission occurs.
- Patients with symptomatic pulmonary disease and extrapulmonary sarcoidosis, especially those with ocular, central nervous system, hepatic, and myocardial involvement should be considered for therapy. The mainstay of therapy is glucocorticoids, which are usually taken systemically but can be used as a topical application in sarcoid confined to the skin or eyes. Other medications that may be useful include methotrexate, hydroxychloroquine, and azathioprine.

5 CHAPTER

Cardiology

I. Angina Pectoris
  A. Basic science
     • Angina pectoris is divided into three broad categories: stable angina, unstable angina, and variant (or Prinzmetal's) angina.
     • Stable angina is characterized by episodic chest pain, lasting 2 to 5 minutes, exacerbated by exertion or stress, and relieved by rest usually in less than 5 minutes or by nitroglycerin.
     • Unstable angina is also divided into three general categories: (1) new onset exertional angina; (2) angina with increasing severity, duration, or requiring more nitroglycerin (crescendo angina); and (3) angina at rest (or angina decubitus).
     • Finally, variant angina usually occurs at rest, without provocation, and is thought to be secondary to spasm of epicardial coronary arteries.
  B. History and physical examination
     • History is the most useful tool in arriving at a diagnosis of angina. Typically, the patient is a male over 50 years of age or female over 60 years. Anginal pain is frequently retrosternal, and is described as a pressure or squeezing sensation. There may be radiation to the neck, jaw, shoulders, and at times down the left arm. Patients may also complain of nausea, vomiting, lightheadedness, diaphoresis, and shortness of breath. Angina can manifest without chest pain and can present as fatigue, lightheadedness, and dyspnea, all referred to as anginal equivalents.
     • Risk factors for angina are the same as those for coronary artery disease and include hypertension, hyperlipidemia, male gender, postmenopausal females, age greater than 55, family history of heart disease before age 45 in males and age 55 in females, diabetes mellitus, cigarette smoking, and obesity.
     • Physical examination is often normal, but may reveal an anxious patient with rales, cardiomegaly, left ventricular akinesia or dyskinesia, an S_3, S_4, or an apical systolic murmur indicative of mitral regurgitation due to papillary muscle ischemia.
  C. Laboratory and diagnostic studies
     • An electrocardiogram (ECG) taken during an anginal attack will show changes 50% of the time, usually ST depression; ST elevation may be seen during episodes of variant angina but cardiac enzymes are not typically elevated.
     • Chest x-ray may reveal other causes of chest pain and indirect evidence of cardiac disease such as cardiomegaly.
     • Other laboratory work is not helpful in making the diagnosis of angina.

D. Formulating the diagnosis
- A prior history of angina is critical when diagnosing stable angina. All new onset angina is unstable angina until proved otherwise.
- A diagnosis of unstable angina should be entertained if the chest pain is new, different, progressive, or not responding to nitroglycerin, or if pain occurs at rest.
- Prinzmetal's variant angina tends to occur in younger patients with fewer risk factors, recurs at the same time of day, and frequently is associated with transient ST segment elevation; coronary angiography demonstrates transient coronary spasm, which can be induced with a vasoconstrictor such as ergonovine.

E. Evaluating the severity of problem
- If any of the features of unstable angina are present, there is a 40% incidence of acute infarction and a 17% incidence of death in the next 3 months; thus, it is imperative to make the diagnosis. In unstable angina, medical therapy can reduce the risk of acute myocardial infarction to 8% and the risk of early death to 3%.

F. Managing the patient
- The most critical part of managing the patient with angina is to recognize and admit those patients with an acute myocardial infarction or unstable angina.
- With respect to stable angina, modifiable risk factors should be identified and corrected (e.g., smoking cessation). Diseases such as hypertension, diabetes, and hyperlipidemia should be treated with diet and medications. Aggravating factors such as hyperthyroidism and aortic valve disease should be identified and treated appropriately.
- The cornerstone of acute therapy is sublingual nitroglycerin (tablet or spray). Long-acting preparations can be used, but with caution to prevent the development of tolerance. β-Blocking agents have also been shown to be useful in the management of stable angina; additionally, they reduce infarct size and lower the risk of death in acute myocardial infarction. β-Blockers are contraindicated in patients with acute decompensated congestive heart failure (CHF), bradycardia, second- and third-degree atrioventricular (AV) block, severe chronic obstructive lung disease, or severe asthma. Long-acting calcium channel blockers are probably as effective as β-blockers in the management of stable angina and are the primary therapy for variant angina. Calcium channel blockers are particularly useful in patients with side effects to β-blockers such as depression and fatigue and significant AV conduction defects. Unless contraindicated, all patients with angina or any coronary artery disease should be on aspirin (ASA) 75 to 325 mg daily.
- Unstable angina is treated in a similar fashion with antianginal drugs (IV nitroglycerin), ASA, β-blockers, and IV unfractionated heparin or low-molecular-weight heparin. Glycoprotein IIb/IIIa inhibitors are additional therapy for patients with elevated troponins or in patients undergoing percutaneous coronary intervention. Otherwise, management is tailored to modify risk factors (i.e., statins for hyperlipidemia and angiotensin-converting

enzyme [ACE] inhibitors for low ejection fractions). Serial cardiac enzymes should also be performed to rule a myocardial infarction.

II. Aortic Aneurysm
- Aortic aneurysm is defined as a pathologic dilatation of all three layers of the aorta and is most commonly found in the infrarenal abdominal aorta. Most aortic aneurysms are asymptomatic.
- The current screening recommendation is a one-time abdominal aorta ultrasound in men aged 65 to 75 years who are hypertensive and have ever smoked.
- When thoracic aortic aneurysms present symptomatically they are usually associated with abdominal or back pain. Other symptoms include cough and hoarseness of voice.
- Computerized tomography (CT) scan is the best noninvasive diagnostic test for thoracic aneurysms and ultrasonography is used for abdominal aneurysms.
- Surgical repair is indicated if the aneurysm is the cause of symptoms, is larger than 5 to 6 cm (thoracic) or larger than 5.5 cm (abdominal) or if it has enlarged more than 1 cm in a year. Treatment with β-blockers reduce the rate of expansion.

III. Aortic Dissection
- Aortic dissection is the extravastion of blood into and along the aortic media. The most common risk factor is hypertension. Patients with inflammatory aortitis (e.g., syphilis), Marfan syndrome, and Ehlers-Danlos syndrome are predisposed to aortic dissection.
- Thoracic aortic dissection typically presents with the acute onset of "tearing" chest pain in the sixth and seventh decades of life. Syncope and shortness of breath may be associated symptoms. Physical findings depend on the site of the dissection and include a disparity in the upper limb pulses and blood pressure in type A dissection, acute aortic regurgitation, pulmonary edema, hemiplegia, paraplegia, and signs of pericardial tamponade.
- Rapid diagnosis is best made with CT scan. Surgery is generally indicated for type A (ascending dissection), and conservative medical therapy is indicated for uncomplicated, stable type B (descending dissection). β-Blockers should be given intravenously to reduce the heart rate to about 60 beats/minute and systolic blood pressure to 120 mm Hg.

IV. Arrhythmias and Conduction Disorders
  A. Basic science
    - A basic understanding of electrocardiography is assumed.
  B. History and physical examination
    - It is important to know if the patient is symptomatic because of the arrhythmia or conduction disturbance. An arrhythmia without symptoms may be well tolerated and may not require intervention. Symptoms such as syncope, presyncope, lightheadedness, weakness, shortness of breath, nausea, and chest pain should be sought. Signs such as diaphoresis, tachypnea, hemodynamic instability, and altered mental status demand urgent evaluation.

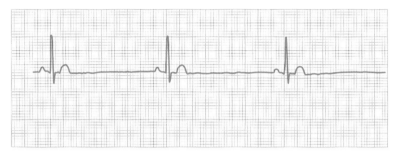

5-1: *Sinus bradycardia. (Redrawn from Cerra FB: Manual of Critical Care. St. Louis, Mosby, 1987.)*

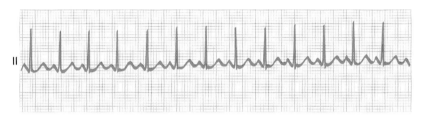

5-2: *Sinus tachycardia. (Redrawn from Goldberger AL, Goldberger E: Clinical Electrocardiography, 5th ed. St. Louis, Mosby, 1994.)*

C. Laboratory and diagnostic studies
- The basic evaluation of a patient with an arrhythmia is a thorough analysis of the 12-lead ECG. Single-lead rhythm strips (e.g., lead II) are helpful in determining the regularity of the rhythm. Holter monitors allow continuous recording of a patient's rhythm, and event monitors allow recordings when the patient develops symptoms and activates the device manually. Electrophysiologic studies are evaluations of the conduction system performed during a cardiac catheterization; they allow attempts at inducing and ablating the arrhythmia in a controlled setting.
- Laboratory studies should be limited to cardiac enzymes, thyroid-stimulating hormone (TSH; also thyrotropin), serum electrolytes (particularly potassium, calcium, and magnesium), and drug levels of therapeutic agent(s) that the patient is taking.

D. Formulating the diagnosis
1. Sinus bradycardia (Fig. 5-1)
   - P waves are normal. Heart rate is less than 60 beats/minute. Some athletic patients have normal resting rates between 40 and 60 beats/minute.
2. Sinus tachycardia (Fig. 5-2; see also Fig. 5-5A)
   - P waves are normal. Heart rate is between 100 and 150 beats/minute.
3. Premature atrial contractions (PACs) (Fig. 5-3A)
   - P waves are abnormal in contour and axis. QRS complexes occur early with a short RR interval but are otherwise normal.

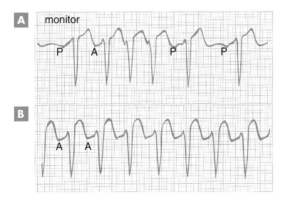

5-3: A, Sinus beat (P) followed by three premature atrial contractions (A). **B,** Atrial tachycardia has developed. Tracings in parts A and B were taken a few seconds apart. (Redrawn from Goldberger E: Treatment of Cardiac Emergencies, 5th ed. St. Louis, Mosby, 1990.)

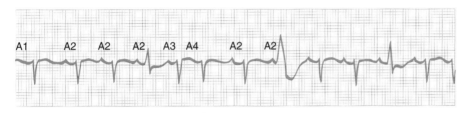

5-4: Multifocal atrial tachycardia. A1, A2, A3, and A4 show premature atrial beats from varying foci. Notice that fourth, eighth, and eleventh QRS complexes are aberrant. (Redrawn from Goldberger E: Treatment of Cardiac Emergencies, 5th ed. St. Louis, Mosby, 1990.)

4. Atrial tachycardia (Fig. 5-3B)
   - P wave axis and contour are abnormal. Look for associated block (may be variable block) as this is pathognomonic of digitalis toxicity.
5. Multifocal atrial tachycardia (MAT) (Fig. 5-4)
   - Abnormal P waves are present with at least three different contours or axes and the rhythm is irregular. MAT is commonly associated with chronic lung disease.
6. Supraventricular tachycardia (SVT) (Fig. 5-5C)
   - P wave is buried in or following the QRS complex (retrograde P wave). QRS is normal (unless conduction occurs aberrantly because of partial refractoriness or an aberrant pathway). SVT is frequently caused by a re-entrant circuit that can produce a fast, regular ventricular response rate (150 to 250 beats/minute).
7. Atrial flutter (Fig. 5-5D)
   - Atrial flutter features sawtoothed "P waves." Often a 2:1 block is present, giving a ventricular rate of 150. Rhythm is typically regular unless a variable block is present.

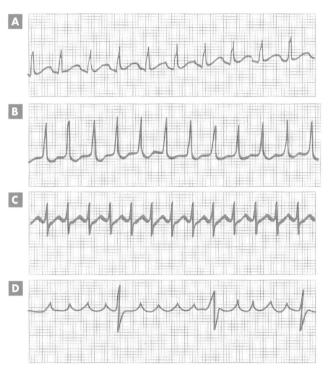

5-5: *Four look-alike narrow-complex tachycardias.* **A,** *Sinus tachycardia.* **B,** *Atrial fibrillation.* **C,** *Paroxysmal supraventricular tachycardia (PSVT) due to atrioventricular (AV) nodal reentrant tachycardia.* **D,** *Atrial flutter with 2:1 block. When the ventricular rate is 150 beats/minute, these four arrhythmias may be difficult, if not impossible, to tell apart with the standard ECG. In this example of sinus tachycardia* **(A)** *the P waves can barely be seen. Notice that the irregularity of the atrial fibrillation* **(B)** *is very subtle. In PSVT* **(C)** *the rate is quite regular without evident P waves here. In atrial flutter* **(D)** *the F waves cannot be seen clearly in this lead. (Redrawn from Goldberger AL, Goldberger E: Clinical Electrocardiography, 5th ed. St. Louis, Mosby, 1994.)*

8. Atrial fibrillation (AFib) (Fig. 5-5B)
   - Atrial fibrillation shows an irregular baseline without discernible P waves with an irregular ventricular response and is classically referred to as a irregularly irregular rhythm. The ventricular response may be quite fast (120 to 180 beats/minute), requiring prompt intervention.
9. Atrioventricular block (AVB)
   a. First degree (Fig. 5-6)
      - Prolonged PR is greater than 0.20 second. This may be normal but is also associated with digitalis toxicity, β-blockers, and calcium channel blockers (diltiazem and verapamil).
   b. Second degree, Mobitz type I (Fig. 5-7)
      - PR progressively lengthens until a QRS is dropped (Wenckebach phenomenon).

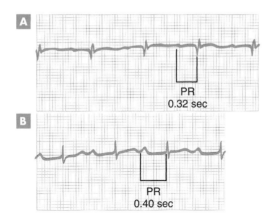

5-6: With first-degree atrioventricular (AV) block the PR interval is uniformly prolonged above 0.2 second with each beat. Parts A and B are from different patients. (Redrawn from Goldberger AL, Goldberger E: Clinical Electrocardiography, 5th ed. St. Louis, Mosby, 1994.)

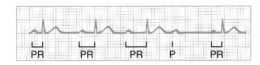

5-7: In second-degree atrioventricular (AV) block (Mobitz type I) the PR interval lengthens progressively with successive beats until one P wave is not conducted at all; then the cycle repeats. (Redrawn from Goldberger AL, Goldberger E: Clinical Electrocardiography, 5th ed. St. Louis, Mosby, 1994.)

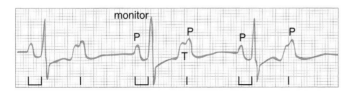

5-8: Mobitz type II atrioventricular (AV) block. Notice that every alternate P wave is blocked. (Redrawn from Goldberger E: Treatment of Cardiac Emergencies, 5th ed. St. Louis, Mosby, 1990.)

   c. Second degree, Mobitz type II (Fig. 5-8)
   - A QRS is unexpectedly dropped after a normal P wave and the PR interval remains constant. This may occur with a regular or irregular block pattern. The ratio of conducted to blocked beats may be irregular, or may be fixed (2:1, 3:1, etc.). This pattern implies a block below the atrioventricular node (high-grade second-degree block) and has a propensity to progress to third-degree heart block. High-grade second-degree AV block and third-degree AV block require urgent intervention.
   d. Third degree (AV dissociation) (Fig. 5-9)
   - P waves are normal and regular but are independent of the QRS complexes (which are also regular but may be wide).

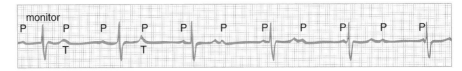

5-9: *Complete atrioventricular (AV) block. (Redrawn from Goldberger E: Treatment of Cardiac Emergencies, 5th ed. St. Louis, Mosby, 1990.)*

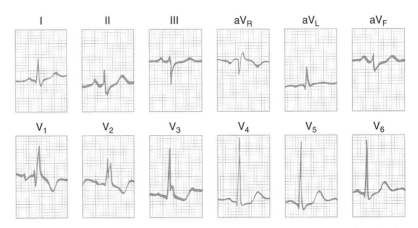

5-10: *Right bundle branch block. Note the wide rSR′ complex in lead V₁ and the QRS complex in lead V₆. (Redrawn from Goldberger AL, Goldberger E: Clinical Electrocardiography, 5th ed. St. Louis, Mosby, 1994.)*

10. Right bundle branch block (RBBB) (Fig. 5-10)
    - Wide QRS (>0.120 msec) is present with a broad S wave in leads I and V$_6$. An rSR′ ("rabbit ear") pattern is in V$_1$.
11. Left bundle branch block (LBBB) (Fig. 5-11)
    - Wide QRS (>0.120 msec) is present with a QS wave in leads V$_1$ and III, and notched R wave in leads I and V$_6$ ("haystack appearance").
12. Premature ventricular contractions (PVCs) (Fig. 5-12)
    - There is no P wave prior to a wide QRS complex, which appears early (short RR interval). A compensatory pause follows this complex.
13. Ventricular tachycardia (VT) (Fig. 5-13)
    - P waves may or may not be present, but there is AV dissociation with a wide QRS and a rate of greater than 100 beats/minute with a regular rhythm. The patient will not necessarily be unstable, as occasionally VT at a slow rate is well tolerated. Unstable VT requires emergent unsynchronized cardioversion/defibrillation.
14. Ventricular fibrillation (VFib) (Fig. 5-14)
    - There is an undulating baseline without discernible QRS complexes. This rhythm (as opposed to VT) is not compatible with a pulse or consciousness. This rhythm, like unstable VT, always requires emergent unsynchronized cardioversion/defibrillation.

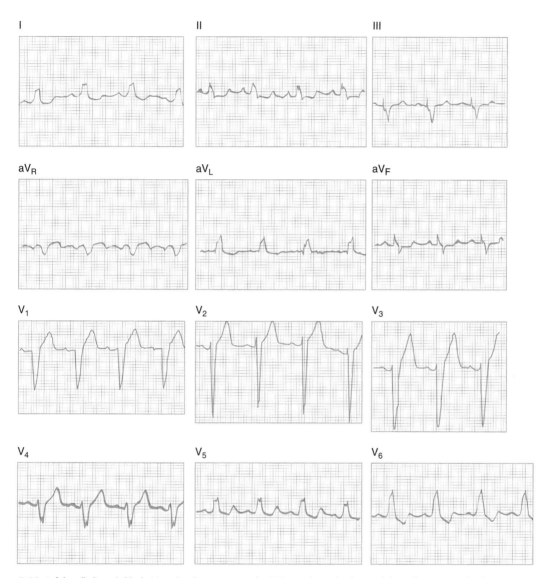

I	II	III
aV_R	aV_L	aV_F
V_1	V_2	V_3
V_4	V_5	V_6

5-11: *Left bundle branch block. Note the characteristic wide QRS complex in lead V_1 and the wide R wave in lead V_6 with slight notching at the peak. (Redrawn from Goldberger AL, Goldberger E: Clinical Electrocardiography, 5th ed. St. Louis, Mosby, 1994.)*

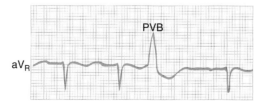

5-12: *Premature ventricular beat (PVB). (Redrawn from Goldberger AL, Goldberger E: Clinical Electrocardiography, 5th ed. St. Louis, Mosby, 1994.)*

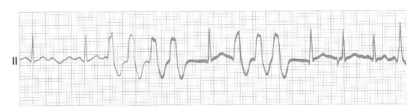

5-13: *Nonsustained ventricular tachycardia. (Redrawn from Goldberger AL, Goldberger E: Clinical Electrocardiography, 5th ed. St. Louis, Mosby, 1994.)*

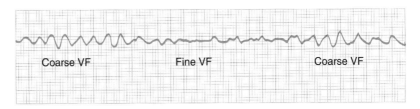

5-14: *Ventricular fibrillation (VF). (Redrawn from Goldberger AL, Goldberger E: Clinical Electrocardiography, 5th ed. St. Louis, Mosby, 1994.)*

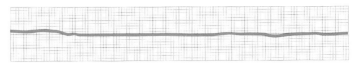

5-15: *Complete ventricular standstill produces a straight-line pattern (asystole) during cardiac arrest. (Redrawn from Goldberger AL, Goldberger E: Clinical Electrocardiography, 5th ed. St. Louis, Mosby, 1994.)*

15. Asystole (Fig. 5-15)
   - There are no QRS complexes and the patient is pulseless.
16. Pulseless electrical activity (PEA)
   - The PEA classification recognizes any electrical activity without an obtainable pulse or blood pressure.
   E. Evaluating the severity of problems
   - As with any potentially life-threatening condition, attention must first be directed toward the ABCs. If the airway is not patent or maintainable, the patient should be intubated. If circulation is inadequate as evidenced by a low blood pressure or mental status changes, then rapid intervention including pharmacologic agents or immediate cardiac pacing or cardioversion should be employed, depending on the identified rhythm.
   F. Managing the patient
   - Asymptomatic arrhythmias require evaluation, but may not require therapy unless the potential for adverse or life-threatening events is present. Patients with a history of syncope and a normal 12-lead ECG require an evaluation for a potential arrhythmogenic source; with careful follow-up many of these

patients can be evaluated during a short inpatient stay with monitoring, or with an outpatient Holter monitor or event monitor.

- Atrial fibrillation is the most common sustained atrial arrythmia. It may be paroxysmal or sustained. Atrial fibrillation may occur in individuals with no cardiac disease (e.g., after surgery, severe emotional stress, or acute alcoholic intoxication). Hypertension, cardiovascular disease, rheumatic heart disease, atrial septal defects, and chronic lung disease may cause persistent atrial fibrillation. If the onset of atrial fibrillation is acute, pulmonary embolus, pneumonia, CHF or thyrotoxicosis should be considered. The first goal is to control the rapid ventricular rate that sometimes accompanies it and restore hemodynamic stability. β-Blockers, calcium channel blockers, and digoxin are used for rate control. In the absence of an intracardiac thrombus, electrical cardioversion may be attempted. If the patient is hemodynamically unstable, then immediate cardioversion is required irrespective of the presence of an intracardiac thrombus. If the atrial fibrillation is new onset (<48 hours) then cardioversion may be attempted and no evaluation for an intracardiac thrombus is necessary. If the onset is longer than 48 hours or unknown then a transesophageal echogram (TEE) cardiogram needs to be performed to exclude an intracardiac thrombus. Patients who are not successfully cardioverted should be anticoagulated and the heart rate controlled with the above-mentioned agents. The utility of antiarrhythmics in this setting is debated.

- Symptomatic bradyarrhythmias should be treated initially with external or internal pacing, withdrawal of drugs with bradycardic side effects, and evaluation for other potential sources, including myocardial infarction. Atropine is the initial drug of choice but is often only a temporizing measure. Permanent pacemakers are implanted in patients with documented symptomatic brachycardia secondary to sinus note dysfunction, following catheter ablation of the atrioventricular node or following cardiac surgery when an atrioventricular block persists.

- Tachyarrhythmias may be atrial or ventricular. Atrial fibrillation is a common symptomatic arrhythmia. Atrial premature complexes are generally aymptomatic. Ventricular tachyarrythimias are treated according to the width of the QRS complex and hemodynamic stability. Wide complex tachycardias are assumed to be ventricular tachycardia. Initial therapy should be with amiodarone if the patient is hemodynamically stable. Synchronized cardioversion should be performed on any patient with unstable vital signs. If the patient is in extremis, unsynchronized cardioversion should be performed.

- Narrow complex tachyarrhythmias can be treated (and diagnosed) with adenosine, which causes transient AV block. If the arrhythmia is supraventricular in origin, it may be slowed enough to allow P waves or other diagnostic clues to appear. In patients with Wolff-Parkinson-White (WPW) syndrome or other reentry arrhythmias, adenosine will often terminate the arrhythmia. When adenosine is unsuccessful, intravenous amiodarone, diltiazem, or β-blockers can be used. For patients with supraventricular tachycardia (SVT) and unstable vital signs, synchronized cardioversion should be performed.

TABLE 5-1:

Laboratory Evaluation of the Cardiomyopathies

	Chest X-Ray Examination	Electrocardiogram	Echocardiogram
Dilated cardiomyopathy	Moderate to severe cardiomegaly with pulmonary congestion	Sinus tachycardia, arrhythmia, bundle branch block	Dilated cavities with normal wall thickness, MR, TR, and decreased ejection fraction
Hypertrophic cardiomyopathy	Often unremarkable	LVH, exaggerated septal Q waves, arrhythmias	Normal or small LV cavity with asymmetric hypertrophy, possible outflow obstruction
Restrictive cardiomyopathy	Mild to moderate cardiomegaly	Low voltage, AV conduction abnormalities	Normal to mild dilatation of ventricle, reduced systolic function, pericardial effusion

AV, atrioventricular; LVH, left ventricular hypertrophy; LV, left ventricular; MR, mitral regurgitation; TR, tricuspid regurgitation.

G. Indications for emergent pacemaker placement
- Certain rhythms may require placement of a transvenous or external pacemaker until a permanent pacemaker is placed. These rhythms are symptomatic sinus bradycardia or sinus arrest, and second-degree (especially Mobitz II) and third-degree heart block.

V. Cardiomyopathy
   A. Basic science
   - Cardiomyopathy describes a primary disorder of the myocardium. Before the diagnosis of cardiomyopathy is made, secondary causes of heart dysfunction, such as infection, (e.g., Chagas' disease, adenovirus, HIV), ischemia, systemic disorders (e.g., sarcoid, amyloidosis, hemochromatosis), connective tissue diseases (e.g., systemic lupus eythematosus, Wegener's granulomatosis), and endocrine causes (e.g., thyrotoxicosis, hypothyroidism, pheochromyocytoma) must be identified or ruled out.
   - The cardiomyopathies are classified pathophysiologically as dilated, hypertrophic, or restrictive (Table 5-1). Dilated cardiomyopathy is characterized primarily by systolic dysfunction and accounts for about one third of all patients with congestive heart failure. Hypertrophic cardiomyopathy (previously known as idiopathic hypertrophic subaortic stenosis) is characterized by diastolic dysfunction. Restrictive cardiomyopathy has elements of both systolic and diastolic dysfunction. The most common cause type of cardiomyopathy is ischemic cardiomyopathy secondary to underlying coronary artery disease.
   B. History and physical examination
   - Patients with dilated cardiomyopathy develop signs and symptoms due to the associated biventricular failure. Complaints include exertional dyspnea, fatigue,

weight gain, orthopnea, and cough. Physical findings may consist of jugular venous distention, cardiomegaly, S_3 and S_4 gallop, peripheral edema, hepatosplenomegaly, ascites, and a mitral or tricuspid regurgitation murmurs.

- Common symptoms in patients with hypertrophic cardiomyopathy are related to pulmonary congestion (e.g., exertional dyspnea and paroxysmal nocturnal dyspnea). Angina, palpitations, and syncope are other typical complaints. Sudden death secondary to a ventricular arrhythmia may be the first manifestation.
- The physical examination is notable for brisk carotid upstrokes, a prominent sustained apical impulse, and an S_4. A diamond-shaped systolic murmur is heard in patients who have developed outflow obstruction as a consequence of hypertropic cardiomyopathy. This murmur typically increases during a Valsalva maneuver.
- Patients with restrictive cardiomyopathy present with signs and symptoms much like those in patients with dilated cardiomyopathy, although clinical evidence of cardiomegaly is less dramatic.

C. Laboratory and diagnostic studies

- All patients suspected of having cardiomyopathy should have a chest x-ray, ECG, and echocardiogram. Table 5-1 lists common findings of these tests.
- Endomyocardial tissue biopsy is becoming more common, although not routine, in the evaluation of these patients because it often identifies diseases that cause cardiomyopathy (e.g., amyloidosis, sarcoidosis, hemochromatosis, myocarditis, and unusual infections).
- Cardiac catheterization may be useful in measuring pressure/volume relationships and in identifying individuals suspected of having coronary artery disease.

D. Formulating the diagnosis

- The diagnosis of cardiomyopathy is made by the history and physical examination and confirmed by laboratory studies as outlined earlier. The primary cause of the cardiomyopathies is idiopathic.
- Conditions frequently associated with dilated cardiomyopathy include alcoholism, doxorubicin and high-dose cyclophosphamide, endocrinopathies, and pregnancy. Peripartum cardiomyopathy typically occurs in the last trimester of pregnancy or within 6 months of delivery. Those who recover should be advised against further pregnancies.
- Hypertrophic cardiomyopathy may be seen in families; a genetic defect has been identified as a risk factor. Chronic hypertension may be seen in association with this disease.
- Restrictive cardiomyopathy is commonly confused with constrictive pericarditis; it may be seen in association with amyloidosis, post–radiation therapy, or endomyocardial fibrosis (a progressive idiopathic disease typically seen in children and young adults in tropical and nontropical Africa).

E. Managing the patient

- Because the cause of the cardiomyopathies is often unknown, therapy is directed at symptomatic relief. In patients with dilated cardiomyopathy, this includes eliminating aggravating factors such as alcohol and treating endocrinopathies when present. Further management consists of therapy for congestive heart failure, such as ACE inhibitors, angiotensin-receptor blockers, digitalis, diuretics including spirinolactone, and vasodilators (see Section VI for details). When systolic function is severely impaired, chronic anticoagulation should be considered to limit thromboembolic events.

- Symptomatic patients with hypertrophic cardiomyopathy are often responsive to negative inotropes, including β-blockers and calcium channel blockers. Antiarrhythmics should not be used in the absence of arrhythmias. Surgical removal or ablation of part of the myocardial septum may benefit some patients with outflow obstruction.
- The basic tenets of treatment for restrictive cardiomyopathy are similar to those for dilated cardiomyopathy.

VI. Congestive Heart Failure
   A. Basic science
   - Congestive heart failure (CHF) is the inability of the heart to supply sufficient output to meet metabolic demands. Manifestations of CHF derive from tissue hypoperfusion (forward failure) as well as pulmonary and systemic venous congestion (backward failure). In addition, several compensatory processes occur that augment cardiac output. The most important are (1) cardiac dilatation and hypertrophy, (2) elevated systemic vascular resistance and myocardial contractility (due to increases in sympathetic tone and circulating catecholamines), and (3) increased plasma volume due to activation of the renin-angiotensin-vasopressin and aldosterone systems. Beyond a certain point, each of the compensatory mechanisms will no longer improve cardiac output and instead will exacerbate the underlying cardiac insufficiency. The interplay between the primary pump failure and the secondary compensatory mechanisms determines the course of CHF in a given individual.
   B. History and physical examination
   - The classic symptoms and signs of CHF are due to venous congestion. A failing left ventricle causes pressures in the pulmonary circuit to rise. Eventually the right ventricle begins to fail, and pressures in the systemic venous system rise.
   - Interstitial edema typically leads to a dry, hacking cough. The patient perceives decreased pulmonary compliance and impaired oxygenation as dyspnea. At first, shortness of breath will occur with exertion, but as pump failure worsens, dyspnea will appear with less and less activity. The patient will complain of fatigue and eventually will note dyspnea at rest.
   - With a failing heart, the patient may experience dyspnea when recumbent (orthopnea). During sleep, fluid that had seeped into the interstitium will shift back into the vasculature. The subsequent volume overload will precipitate sudden shortness of breath or paroxysmal nocturnal dyspnea (PND). The kidneys will attempt to reduce the apparent volume expansion, resulting in nocturia.
   - Pump failure will reduce renal perfusion, activating the renin-angiotensin system and promoting sodium and water retention. The patient will complain

of weight gain and edema. Other symptoms of heart failure including fatigue, anorexia, and in the older patient with diffuse cerebral arteriosclerosis, confusion.

- Obesity, smoking, hypertension, diabetes, coronary artery disease, and a family history of coronary artery disease are commonly associated with CHF.
- Physical examination of the chest often reveals wheezing in mild CHF, but the cardinal sign is the presence of crackles. An effusion, typically right-sided or bilateral, may be present. The heart, when percussed, will be enlarged with the PMI displaced laterally, and a heave will often be present. S_3 or S_4 heart sounds may be present. A S_3 is more frequently heard in heart failure. Inspection of the neck will reveal jugular venous distention. Palpation of the liver will reveal hepatomegaly, and frequently hepatojugular reflux can be elicited. Dependent edema is common, usually noted first at the ankles, but in advanced cases will also be evident more proximally. In the bedridden, presacral edema may be noted.

C. Laboratory and diagnostic studies

- The B type natriuretic peptide (BNP) is helpful in distinguishing cardiac from noncardiac causes of dyspnea. A BNP of less than 100 pg/mL makes the diagnosis of acute heart failure unlikely. Other laboratory tests may be warranted based on the history and physical findings to help establish or exclude diagnoses (glucose in diabetes, ferritin in hemochromatosis, ACE level in sarcoid, protein electrophoresis in amyloid, and TSH in thyroid dysfunction).
- The chest x-ray may show cardiomegaly, characteristic patterns of vascular redistribution and engorgement, and interstitial edema. The ECG can be helpful in diagnosing underlying disease or rhythm disturbances, but there are no diagnostic changes that are specific to CHF. An echocardiogram should be performed in all patients with heart failure to identify a cause and to assess systolic and diastolic ventricular function and valvular dysfunction.

D. Formulating the diagnosis

- When the history and physical examination indicate the presence of dyspnea, pulmonary congestion, and edema, the diagnosis of CHF is obvious. When the clinical picture is incomplete, other diagnoses must be considered. Common noncardiac causes of dyspnea include chronic obstructive pulmonary disease (COPD), asthma, and pneumonia. The differentiation between CHF, COPD, and pneumonia on physical examination alone can be difficult (BNP may help), and these diseases commonly coexist. Peripheral edema may be due to venous incompetence and thrombosis, trauma, renal disease, malignancy, and cirrhosis. Careful attention to details of the history and physical examination coupled with the chest x-ray and appropriate laboratory studies will enable a correct diagnosis.

E. Evaluating the severity of problems

1. The New York Heart Association criteria are as follows:
   - Class I: symptoms of heart failure only at levels that would limit normal individuals
   - Class II: symptoms of heart failure with ordinary exertion

- Class III: symptoms of heart failure on less than ordinary exertion
- Class IV: symptoms of heart failure at rest

2. The Amercican College of Cardiology and the American Heart Association have suggested the following stages of heart failure (HF):
   - Stage A: high risk for HF, without structural heart disease or symptoms
   - Stage B: heart disease with asymptomatic left ventricular dysfunction
   - Stage C: prior or current symptoms of HF
   - Stage D: advanced heart disease and severely symptomatic or refractory HF
   - Acute pulmonary edema is characterized by the abrupt onset of life-threatening congestive symptoms (e.g., severe shortness of breath, hypoxia, pink frothy sputum), often in association with significant forward failure. Treatment includes vigorous diuresis, supplemental oxygen, and management of hypertension when present. In severe cases, respiratory support via endotracheal intubation and mechanical ventilation will be required. Additionally, intra-aortic balloon counterpulsation may be employed to reduce afterload, and left ventricular assist devices (LVADs) can help support a failing heart refractory to medical therapy.

F. Managing the patient
   - Dietary salt restriction is important. The medical management of chronic CHF is directed toward reducing preload and afterload and improving contractility. The mainstay of chronic therapy has traditionally been diuretics, which decrease fluid retention and lower preload. Various agents, used singly or in combination, include loop diuretics (furosemide and bumetanide), thiazides, and the aldosterone antagonists (spironolactone). Additionally, venodilators, primarily nitrates, reduce preload by increasing venous capacitance.
   - Afterload is reduced primarily by arterial vasodilatation. The agents used most commonly are nitrates (weak arterial vasodilator), ACE inhibitors (e.g., captopril, enalapril), angiotensin-receptor blockers (e.g., losartan), hydralazine, and nitrates. Inhibition of the renin-angiotensin-aldosterone pathway is the mainstay of CHF treatment.
   - Inotropic drugs improve contractility. Currently, digitalis preparations are the primary agents chronically used for this purpose and have been shown to decrease the number of hospitalizations but not the mortality rate. In acute situations dobutamine, milrinone, or amrinone can be used intravenously. Nesiritide, a recombitant brain natruretic peptide, is helpful in acutely decompensated CHF.
   - Finally, severe refractory CHF may be amenable to cardiac transplantation in selected cases.

VII. Hypertension
   A. Basic science
      - Hypertension occurs in 15% to 30% of adults and in more than 60% of patients over the age of 65 in the United States. It is usually asymptomatic and found on routine screening. The presence of hypertension increases a patient's risk for vascular and renal diseases. If left untreated, hypertension reduces life expectancy by 10 to 20 years.

- Approximately 90% of patients with hypertension have no known cause and are said to have primary, or essential, hypertension. Family history, obesity, and a high-sodium diet also contribute to the development of hypertension.
- About 10% of hypertension is due to renal disease (renal vascular insufficiency; parenchymal renal disease); other causes include pheochromocytoma, primary hyperaldosteronism, Cushing's syndrome, coarctation of the aorta, and medications such as oral contraceptives and steroids.

B. History and physical examination
- Attention should be directed toward identifying any family history of hypertension and cardiovascular disease. The patient's history of medication use, diet, exercise, and other cardiovascular risk factors should be explored.
- Physical examination should focus on (1) stigmata of the causes of secondary hypertension such as a round face, truncal obesity, and abdominal striae (Cushing's syndrome), disproportionately better muscular development in the upper extremities and differences in pulse volume in the upper compared to the lower extremities (coarctation of aorta), and renal bruits on abdominal examination; and (2) evidence of target organ damage due to hypertension. The five primary target organs affected by hypertension are as follows:
  1. Brain (hemorrhagic and lacunar strokes, encephalopathy)
  2. Eye (fundal hemorrhages, exudates, papilledema)
  3. Heart (left ventricular hypertrophy, CHF, acute coronary syndrome)
  4. Kidney (nephrosclerosis, microscopic hematuria and proteinuria)
  5. Vessels (aortic dissection, peripheral vascular disease)

C. Laboratory and diagnostic studies
- Initial studies of a newly diagnosed hypertensive patient should include hematocrit, electrolytes, glucose, serum creatinine and blood urea nitrogen, lipid profile, urinalysis for proteinuria and hematuria, and an ECG. Some physicians would also request a TSH, serum calcium, phosphorus, chest x-ray, and echocardiogram.
- Additional diagnostic studies may be appropriate if the history and physical examination provide clues to secondary hypertension. Historical clues that are suggestive of secondary hypertension include age of onset younger than 35 or older than 55, abrupt onset of severe hypertension, hypertension resistant to medical management, and target organ damage at the time of diagnosis.

D. Formulating the diagnosis
- The diagnosis of hypertension should be based on at least two blood pressure measurements over time. Transient mild to moderate hypertension in response to stress or medication is not pathologic. If persistent hypertension is documented without evidence of secondary hypertension on history, physical examination, and laboratory evaluation, then essential hypertension may be presumed.

E. Evaluating the severity of problems
- See Table 5-2 for hypertension classification and treatment.
- Isolated systolic hypertension is a systolic blood pressure above 140 mm Hg and a diastolic pressure below 90 mm Hg. This is more common in the elderly in whom vascular compliance is lost.

TABLE 5-2:

Classification of Blood Pressure for Adults Aged 18 Years and Older*

Category	Systolic Pressure (mm Hg)	Diastolic Pressure (mm Hg)	Treatment
Normal	<120	<80	None
Prehypertensive	120–139	80–89	None unless diabetes or CKD[†]
Stage 1	140–159	90–99	Thiazide if no comorbidities
Stage 2	>160	>100	Thiazide + one additional agent

*These definitions apply to adults who are not taking antihypertensive drugs and who are not acutely ill. When systolic and diastolic blood pressures fall into different categories, the higher category should be selected to classify the individual's blood pressure status. Isolated systolic hypertension is defined as a systolic blood pressure of 140 mm Hg or more and a diastolic blood pressure of less than 90 mm Hg and staged appropriately. Diagnosis is based on the average of two or more readings taken at each of two or more visits after an initial screening.
[†]Diabetics and chronic kidney disease (CKD) patients should be treated to reach a goal blood pressure of <130/80 mm Hg.
Data from Joint National Committee: The Seventh Report of the Joint National Committee on Prevention, Detection, Evaluation, and Treatment of High Blood Pressure: The JNC VII Report. JAMA 2003;289(19):2560–2572.

- Patients presenting acutely with an exacerbation of hypertension may be classified as having a hypertensive emergency when acute target organ damage is evident, regardless of the numerical value of the blood pressure. This condition demands immediate treatment, often with parenteral agents. In contrast, patients with a hypertensive urgency have no target organ damage but display a dangerously high diastolic blood pressure (i.e., >120 mm Hg), which, if allowed to persist, may be expected to cause target organ damage within 24 to 48 hours. This condition requires prompt treatment and follow-up to ensure reduction of blood pressure within 24 to 48 hours.

F. Managing the patient
- The treatment of hypertension is usually a lifelong process. Nonpharmacologic interventions include weight reduction in obese patients, regular aerobic exercise, reduction in dietary sodium intake, and stress reduction. These interventions alone may control stage 1 hypertension. Attention to other cardiovascular risk factors such as diabetes is also important.
- If nonpharmacologic interventions are ineffective in controlling hypertension within months, many effective antihypertensive medications are available. Therapy must be tailored to the individual's needs and complete health profile. Severe (stage 2 hypertension) or refractory patients may require simultaneous administration of two or more classes of agents. Classes of antihypertensive agents include the following:
  1. Diuretics (e.g., thiazides, furosemide, bumetanide)
  2. β-Blockers (e.g., atenolol, metoprolol, labetalol, propranolol)
  3. Calcium channel blockers (e.g., nifedipine, verapamil, diltiazem)
  4. Angiotensin-converting enzyme (ACE) inhibitors (e.g., captopril, enalapril, lisinopril, ramipril)
  5. Angiotensin-receptor blockers (ARBs) (e.g., losartan, valsartan, irbesartan)

6. Adrenergic inhibitors (e.g., clonidine, prazosin)
7. Direct vasodilators (e.g., hydralazine, minoxidil, guanethidine)
8. Mineralocorticoid receptor antagonists (spironolactone, eplerenone)
- The patient presenting with a hypertensive emergency, showing evidence of acute target organ damage, must have immediate control of blood pressure. Intravenous vasodilators (e.g., nitroprusside, diazoxide) and intravenous β-blockers (e.g., labetalol, esmolol, or metoprolol) are used. Initial goal should be a 25% reduction in mean arterial pressure over 2 to 3 hours. If pheochromocytoma is suspected, β-blockers should not be given alone or unopposed α-adrenergic stimulation may result in paradoxic worsening of hypertension. Instead, phentolamine should be used in conjunction with a β-blocker. Intensive care unit treatment and monitoring are appropriate in all patients with hypertensive emergency.

VIII. Murmurs
  A. Basic science
- Blood flow through the heart is laminar, and therefore the normal cardiac examination reveals only the first and second heart sounds. Additional heart sounds include gallops, opening snaps, ejection and midsystolic clicks, rubs, and murmurs. Murmurs are the most common extra sound and represent turbulent flow.
- Murmurs are designated as functional or structural. Functional murmurs are not associated with any anatomic abnormality, whereas structural murmurs are.
  B. History and physical examination
- When a murmur is found, a directed history should be taken, including duration of the murmur, if known, and the results of any prior workup. If the patient has been advised regarding endocarditis prophylaxis, the presence of a murmur from a valve dysfunction is likely; similarly, a prior history of bacterial endocarditis or rheumatic fever implies a murmur of structural origin.
- The presence or absence of fatigue and dyspnea should be noted, as these imply advanced valvular dysfunction, as does historical evidence of CHF (e.g., peripheral edema, orthopnea, paroxysmal nocturnal dyspnea).
- The cardiac examination should include the basics of inspection, palpation, percussion, and auscultation. Percussion, however, rarely provides useful information. Auscultation allows the grading, quality, timing, and pattern of a murmur to be determined. Additionally, the radiation and loudest point of a murmur may be used to assess its source. Added sounds such as an opening snap, ejection click, and S_3 or S_4 can often be recognized only on auscultation.
  C. Laboratory and diagnostic studies
- The commonly used diagnostic aids include ECG, chest x-ray, echocardiography, and exercise tolerance test (ETT). Radionuclide imaging and cardiac catheterization are used less often to assess the effects of and need to intervene in specific murmurs.
- An ECG can reveal evidence of atrial or ventricular enlargement. It is an inexpensive and noninvasive way to assess the effects of a murmur. It is also

useful in following the effects of a known structural murmur on a given cardiac chamber. However, ECG has very low sensitivity and specificity when used for these purposes.

- The chest x-ray is a low-risk method of assessing cardiac chamber size. Additionally it provides evidence of pulmonary congestion and is useful in the initial evaluation of murmurs and the follow-up of known structural murmurs.
- Echocardiography can assess chamber size, wall thickness, valve orifice dimension, valve movement, presence of regurgitant flow, presence of valvular vegetation, and estimation of ventricular ejection fraction. It is the best noninvasive test for evaluating murmurs.
- The use of exercise testing is best reserved for patients with known structural abnormalities. It is useful to follow exercise tolerance in valvular heart disease as it may help in deciding when surgical intervention is required.

D. Formulating the diagnosis

1. Aortic murmurs
   - Aortic stenosis murmurs are characteristically high pitched, crescendo-decrescendo harsh systolic ejection murmurs that are best heard at the right upper sternal border (aortic area) and radiate into the carotids or the mitral area. A later peak and long duration of murmur are associated with a more severely stenotic valve. The presence of an aortic ejection click indicates the stenosis is valvular rather than supravalvular or subvalvular and a delayed or diminished carotid pulse (pulsus parvus et tardus) may be present in severe aortic stenosis.
   - Aortic insufficiency (AI) murmur is a high-pitched blowing decrescendo early diastolic murmur that may be heard along the left to sternal border. The murmur is best heard with the patient leaning forward and in full expiration. Handgrip exercise, which causes an acute elevation in blood pressure, causes the murmur to become louder, while a decrease in blood pressure as with amyl nitrate causes the murmur to become softer. Because of reversed flow across the aortic valve in diastole, the systolic stroke volume of the left ventricle is greatly increased, giving rise to an aortic ejection murmur which does not necessarily indicate aortic stenosis. Patients with severe AI may also have a water-hammer pulse (rapid upstroke and decline) and wide pulse pressures. There is also a myriad of other physical findings (Mueller's sign of pulsating uvula, deMusset's sign of head bobbing with each heart beat, Traube's sign of a pistol shot sound over the femoral arteries, Duroziez's sign of a to and fro femoral bruit, Becker's sign of retinal arterial pulsations) that may be appreciated in AI.

2. Mitral murmurs
   - The classic mitral stenosis murmur is a low-pitched, decrescendo, rumbling mid-diastolic murmur best heard at the apex in the left lateral decubitus position and accentuated by mild exercise. It is best heard with the bell of the stethoscope. The length of the murmur correlates with the severity of stenosis. A preceding opening snap indicates pliable and noncalcified mitral valves.

- Mitral regurgitation produces a high-pitched blowing, holosystolic murmur that typically begins with S_1. It is loudest at the apex and radiates to the ipsilateral axilla. The murmur is augmented with exercise. A late systolic murmur heard at the mitral area usually indicates mild mitral regurgitation as in mitral valve prolapse.

3. Pulmonary murmurs
   - Stenotic murmurs are systolic ejection murmurs best heard along the left sternal border. The intensity of P_2 is also decreased and there may be a right parasternal heave if severe right ventricular hypertrophy is present.
   - Pulmonary insufficiency murmur is a low-pitched, diamond-shaped diastolic murmur best heard at the left sternal border. The intensity of the murmur increases with inspiration and P_2 is accentuated. However, it tends not to radiate and may be associated with a right parasternal heave. There are no associated pulse character changes.

4. Tricuspid murmurs
   - Tricuspid stenosis shares the timing and quality (low-pitched, diastolic) of mitral stenosis but is usually well localized to the left lower sternal border. It does not to radiate but is strongly accentuated by inspiration.
   - Tricuspid regurgitation is a pansystolic murmur that shares the same timing and quality as mitral regurgitation but is localized to the left lower sternal border. It is characteristically accentuated by inspiration and is associated with neck vein engorgement that may be pulsatile. The liver may also demonstrate pulsatile enlargement due to hepatic congestion.

5. Innocent or flow murmurs
   - These murmurs do not indicate valvular disease. They are typically heard in children, young adults, and the elderly. Flow murmurs may also be heard in anemia, thyrotoxicosis, hypertension, and pregnancy. They are always ejection systolic murmurs, which occur early in systole, have a grunting or musical character, and may become louder with maneuvers that increase cardiac output.

E. Evaluating the severity of problems
   - New murmurs accompanied by symptoms deserve urgent medical attention.

F. Managing the patient
   - Management and prognosis of the patient with a murmur depends on the cause of the murmur and the clinical situation. A patient with mitral regurgitation found during a routine examination will be managed very differently from the patient who develops mitral regurgitation as a consequence of papillary muscle rupture complicating an acute myocardial infarction. Patients with murmurs due to a structural valve disease (e.g., aortic stenosis) should be followed such that a decision to intervene surgically can be made before the onset of cardiac decompensation. It is imperative that the patient is educated regarding the need for endocarditis prophylaxis before undergoing dental or surgical procedures. It is beyond the scope of this chapter to discuss the management of valve disorders.

IX. Myocardial Infarction
   A. Basic science
   - Myocardial infarction (MI) is necrosis of heart muscle caused by an inadequate blood supply. Factors implicated in the pathogenesis include progression of coronary artery arteriosclerosis to the point of total occlusion, subintimal hemorrhage or thrombosis at the site of an existing narrowing or plaque resulting in plaque rupture and subsequent platelet aggregation at the rupture site, and coronary artery embolism or spasm.
   - Infarction, like ischemia, results in alterations in myocardial cell contractility and depolarization secondary to hypoxemia. These cellular derangements are the cause of clinical complications. Impaired contractility can lead to left ventricular pump failure, resulting in CHF and ultimately cardiogenic shock. Electrical differences between adjacent areas of normal and ischemic myocardium can cause arrhythmias. The term "acute coronary syndrome" (ACS) encompasses the spectrum from unstable angina to non-ST segment elevation myocardial infarction to ST segment elevation myocardial infarction.
   B. History and physical examination
   - Pain is the most common presenting complaint in patients with acute myocardial infarction (AMI). Typically the pain is squeezing or crushing pain in character, lasts longer than 15 minutes, is located in the substernal or epigastric region, with 30% of patients complaining of radiating pain down the arms. Less common complaints include pain in the jaw, neck, back, or abdomen. The severity, quality, and location of pain vary considerably among individuals. Atypical presentations referred to as anginal equilavents are more common in the elderly, women, and diabetics. Between 20% and 25% of known MIs are clinically unrecognized or "silent" (most commonly in diabetic or hypertensive patients). As with angina pectoris, pain may be accompanied by other symptoms including dyspnea, diaphoresis, nausea, vomiting, hypertension, lightheadedness, or palpitations.
   - Risk factors for coronary artery disease include cigarette smoking, hyperlipidemia, hypertension, diabetes, and family history of cardiac disease. Males older than 50 years and females older than 60 years are also at increased risk.
   - The physical examination is most useful in evaluating the complications resulting from myocardial infarction. Although a patient's general appearance may be deceptively normal, most appear anxious and diaphoretic. Physical findings to note include neck vein distension, pulmonary crackles, and new or more pronounced heart murmurs or extra sounds.
   C. Laboratory and diagnostic studies
   - In the emergency setting, there is no single laboratory test that can be used for establishing a diagnosis of acute MI. Therefore, diagnosis is dependent on clinical suspicion in combination with ancillary tests.
   - The early workup of AMI includes ECGs and serial cardiac biomarkers, such as creatine kinase and troponins. A normal ECG does not exclude the diagnosis, because at least 15% of patients ultimately "rule in" for MI with

completely normal initial tracings. ECG in AMI can include ST segment elevation, Q waves, and loss of R wave progression.

D. Formulating the diagnosis

- With clinical suspicion or ECG findings, patients should be admitted to a monitored setting for definitive diagnostic testing and treatment. Serial cardiac enzyme measurements can then be used over a 24-hour period to establish the diagnosis of myocardial infarction. Cardiac troponin is the most sensitive, specific, and rapidly available biomarker for detecting myocardial damage because it is found almost exclusively in cardiac myocytes. However, false positive results have been reported in patients with renal insufficiency, so caution must be used when interpreting results in this setting. Thus, cardiac troponin is typically used in conjunction with serial creatine kinase (MB fraction) to assist in making the diagnosis of AMI.

E. Evaluating the severity of problems

- The major complications of myocardial infarctions are arrhythmias, congestive heart failure, and cardiogenic shock.
- Continuous cardiac monitoring is necessary in all patients with suspicion for AMI. Ventricular fibrillation is the most dangerous arrhythmia, although bradycardia, tachycardia, and heart block are also common.
- Pump failure is the primary cause of in-hospital deaths from AMI and is the pathophysiologic mechanism responsible for CHF and cardiogenic shock.

F. Managing the patient

- All patients with suspected MI should have continuous cardiac monitoring and receive supplemental oxygen. Intravenous access should be established immediately. Pain relief, rest, mild sedation, and a quiet atmosphere can reduce anxiety and thereby lower heart rate, a major determinant of oxygen consumption.
- Commonly employed agents in the treatment of AMI include the following:

  1. β-Blockers
     - β-Blockers reduce the size of infarction by reducing the oxygen consumption and demands on ischemic areas of myocardium. They may decrease in-hospital mortality rate. They are recommended in all patients unless they are contraindicated by acute CHF, bradycardia, severe bronchospasm, or hypotension.

  2. Aspirin
     - Aspirin decreases platelet aggregation and limits arterial constriction by blocking the formation of thromboxane A_2. Aspirin significantly reduces the risk of death and should be given as early as possible. Aspirin should be continued daily.

  3. Heparin
     - Heparin prevents recurrence of thrombosis after thrombolysis has occurred and is essential in maintaining vessel patency.

  4. Nitroglycerin
     - Nitroglycerin relaxes vascular smooth muscle of the venous system (decreasing preload), dilates coronary arteries, antagonizes vasospasm, and

increases coronary blood flow to ischemic myocardium. Because nitrates can also induce hypotension, blood pressure must be closely monitored.

5. Morphine
   - Morphine acts as both a sedating and analgesic agent, reducing oxygen demand. Morphine can cause nausea, vomiting, hypotension, and bradycardia. Caution must be advised when using morphine in this setting because it can mask ongoing ischemia.

6. Thrombolytics (tissue plasminogen activator [tPA], streptokinase, tenecteplase [TNC] and reteplase [rPA])
   - Thrombolytics are an important adjunct in the treatment of AMI. They act to dissolve clot, thus reopening blocked coronary arteries and preventing the further progression of myocardial injury. Greatest benefit is achieved under the following conditions: (1) patients with ST elevation greater than 1 mm in two contiguous leads, (2) cases in which pain was not responsive to nitroglycerin, and (3) when the thrombolytic is given within 3 hours of the infarction. Thrombolytics are contraindicated in the following situations: (1) active bleeding, (2) major surgery or trauma in the past 3 weeks, (3) recent head trauma or stroke in the past 3 months, (4) suspected aortic dissection, (5) known traumatic cardiopulmonary resuscitation, (6) pregnancy, (7) history of cerebrovascular hemorrhage, and (8) hemorrhagic diabetic retinopathy.
   - Percutaneous transluminal coronary intervention (PTCI) has largely replaced the use of thrombolytics in selected centers, as it provides a more reliable and safe method of reperfusion when rapidly available. Optimal reperfusion time is 90 minutes from hospital arrival to balloon-up (angioplasty).

X. Pericarditis
   A. Basic science
      - The pericardium is made up of two layers, the visceral pericardium and the parietal pericardium. The visceral pericardium is a serous membrane overlying the epicardium. The parietal pericardium consists of dense collagenous tissue that forms a sac surrounding the heart. The space between these two structures normally contains up to 50 mL of fluid.
      - Pericarditis, the most common pathologic process involving the pericardium, may result from local and systemic diseases. There are three etiologic categories:
         1. Infectious: viral (e.g., coxsackievirus, adenovirus, and echovirus), bacterial (e.g., staphylococcus, streptococcus, tuberculous), and mycotic (histoplasmosis)
         2. Noninfectious: idiopathic, neoplastic (lymphoma, leukemia, metastatic carcinoma of lung and breast), uremia, myxedema, sarcoidosis, and postirradiation
         3. Hypersensitivity or autoimmune-related: collagen vascular disease (lupus, rheumatoid arthritis, scleroderma), drug-induced (procainamide, hydralazine), postmyocardial infarction syndrome (Dressler's syndrome)
      - Pericarditis can be classified as an acute (<6 weeks), subacute (6 weeks to 6 months), or chronic (>6 months) process. Subacute and chronic pericarditis

can result in constrictive pericarditis and place the patient at high risk for congestive heart failure.

B. History and physical examination
   - In acute pericarditis the most common symptom is a burning or sharp substernal chest pain of sudden or gradual onset that may radiate to the neck, back (especially to the left trapezius), epigastrium, and left arm; it is often exacerbated by deep inspiration, coughing, and positional changes (worse when supine, relieved when leaning forward). The most common associated symptoms include dyspnea, odynophagia (i.e., pain on swallowing), and low-grade temperature, especially with infectious etiologies. Differentiating the chest pain of acute pericarditis from that of an acute myocardial infarction is difficult.
   - The hallmark of pericarditis is the pericardial friction rub. The pericardial rub is best heard at the left sternal border with the patient leaning forward or in the hands-and-knees position. The quality is similar to that of sandpaper and is often irregular or triphasic. This sign is frequently transient, necessitating serial examinations when the diagnosis is strongly suspected. When an effusion is present, heart tones may be muffled and the rub absent. Additionally, with an effusion the patient may develop pulsus paradoxus. Other less specific signs include tachycardia, tachypnea, and fever.
   - A diagnosis of pericarditis is likely if two of the following three criteria are present: (1) chest pain, (2) pericardial rub, (3) diffuse ST elevation.

C. Laboratory and diagnostic studies
   - Primary diagnostic studies include serial ECGs, posteroanterior (PA) and lateral chest radiographs, and echocardiography. The ECG will classically show diffuse ST elevations across most leads and PR segment depression in all leads except aVR. With a large effusion present, electrical alternans may be present. Chest radiography can help in ruling out other diagnoses such as pneumonia, pneumothorax, and pneumomediastinum. Its value in positively diagnosing pericarditis is limited, especially if no previous radiographs exist for comparison. Echocardiography is the best study for diagnosis of acute pericarditis with an effusion. It is the study of choice for serial follow-up of patients.
   - The remaining laboratory evaluation is aimed at discovering the cause for pericarditis: CBC with differential cell count for infectious etiologies; BUN/creatinine for uremia; serial viral titers; serologic studies such as ANA and RA latex fixation for immunologic disaeses; blood cultures for bacterial etiologies. Creatine kinase, CK-MB, and troponins may be elevated when associated myocarditis exists.

D. Formulating the diagnosis
   - The presence of a pericardial rub virtually confirms the diagnosis of pericarditis. Life-threatening conditions such as myocardial infarction, pulmonary thromboembolism, pneumothorax, and esophageal rupture (i.e., Boerhaave's syndrome) should be excluded.

E. Evaluating the severity of problems
   - The major acute complication of pericarditis is that of cardiac tamponade (rare). CHF can occur in patients with constrictive pericarditis, which is seen

primarily in subacute and chronic cases. Therefore, careful evaluation and ongoing monitoring of vital signs, cardiac rhythm, and respiratory status are mandatory in patients diagnosed with pericarditis.

F. Managing the patient
- There is no specific treatment for acute idiopathic pericarditis. Bed rest and in stable patients, high-dose nonsteroidal anti-inflammatory drugs (NSAIDs) (e.g., aspirin or indomethacin) are recommended both for pain relief and as anti-inflammatory agents. If an underlying cause is discovered, treatment should be modified accordingly. In patients who develop tamponade, pericardiocentesis and, if recurrent, pericardiectomy are indicated. Patients who develop constrictive pericarditis will require pericardial resection, with medical management (dietary sodium restriction and diuretics) serving only as an interim measure.

XI. Rheumatic Heart Disease
A. Basic science
- Rheumatic heart disease can be defined as the acute and chronic effects of rheumatic fever on the heart. Rheumatic fever is characterized by inflammatory lesions involving the joints, heart, skin, and nervous system. It occurs in 3% of individuals after an episode of untreated group A streptococcal pharyngitis. The latent period between antecedent pharyngitis and rheumatic fever ranges from 1 to 5 weeks. Rheumatic fever does not occur after nonpharyngeal streptococcal infections.
- Rheumatic fever most commonly occurs between ages 5 and 15 years. Because crowding promotes the spread of disease, it is the major environmental factor relating to the occurrence of rheumatic fever.
- Forty percent to 50% of individuals with rheumatic fever have a pancarditis. Rheumatic heart disease most commonly affects the mitral and aortic valves. Healing of the valvulitis may result in thickening of the leaflets, fusion at the commissures, and adhesions of the chordae tendineae, leading to various degrees of stenosis and regurgitation, the most common cardiac sequelae. Chronic rheumatic carditis presents as chronic heart failure, usually secondary to mitral regurgitation.
- Almost all patients with rheumatic fever recover within 12 weeks. Death can occur as a result of a fulminant acute course, or from permanent residual valvular damage. Chronic persistent carditis may assume a fatal course over months to years or resolve spontaneously with little residual cardiac pathologic change.

B. History and physical examination
- Rheumatic fever most commonly presents as an acute febrile illness associated with large joint polyarthritis, which is typically fleeting. A history of recent streptococcal pharyngitis is important in aiding diagnosis, although 30% of patients do not recall an antecedent infection. Only rarely are cardiac symptoms the presenting complaint. Far more commonly cardiac involvement

is an incidental finding. Therefore, a careful cardiac examination focusing on new murmurs (or a change in a preexisting murmur) is essential. Signs of congestive heart failure may be subtle. A pericardial friction rub may be present. Three characteristic murmurs may occur: an apical systolic, apical mid-diastolic, and basal diastolic murmur. Erythema marginatum is a nonpruritic, erythematous, centrally clearing, macular rash involving the trunk and proximal extremities, sparing the face and hands. Subcutaneous nodules (erythema nodosum) range in size from several millimeters to 2 cm and may be found over areas of bony prominence and along extensor tendons. Erythema margination, subcutaneous nodules, and Sydenham's chorea occur in less than 10% of patients.

C. Laboratory and diagnostic studies
   - No laboratory test is pathognomonic for rheumatic fever or rheumatic heart disease, but an elevated erythrocyte sedimentation rate (ESR), elevated C-reactive protein (CRP), and leukocytosis are helpful in establishing presence of an inflammatory process. Anemia secondary to suppression of erythropoiesis is common. Streptococcal antibodies such as antistreptolysin-O (ASO) and anti-DNAase B are elevated. The most common ECG finding is a prolonged PR interval and sinus tachycardia.
   - Doppler flow echocardiography is useful in identifying pericardial effusion and valvular lesions. It is also useful in establishing the significance of flow disturbances and following the long-term progression of valvular disease.

D. Formulating the diagnosis
   - The modified Jones criteria are useful in establishing a diagnosis. Two of the major criteria (carditis, polyarthritis, Sydenham's chorea, erythema marginatum, and subcutaneous nodules) or one major criterion and two minor criteria (fever, arthralgia, elevated ESR or CRP, prolonged PR interval, and evidence of a recent group A streptococcus infection) indicate a high probability of rheumatic fever.

E. Evaluating the severity of problems
   - The severity of the cardiac complications cannot be predicted at the onset of the disease. Prognosis is related to the severity of the carditis, the degree of valvular involvement, and the significance of hemodynamic flow abnormalities by doppler flow echocardiogram. Recurrent rheumatic fever portends a bad prognosis.

F. Managing the patient
   - Prevention of rheumatic fever by treatment of streptococcal pharyngitis is successful if instituted within 7 to 9 days of onset. Therapy should be continued for a minimum of 10 days.
   - There are no treatments that cure rheumatic fever or change the course of the acute attack. Aggressive supportive therapy may, however, alter the morbidity and risk of death from the disease. Upon diagnosis, rheumatic fever should be treated with a course of penicillin to ensure eradication of streptococcus from the pharynx. Parenteral therapy is preferred, and a single dose of 1.2 million units of benzathine penicillin IM is adequate.

- Aspirin is effective in treating the pain and inflammation due to join involvement. The dose can be increased until resolution of symptoms occurs, or systemic toxicity such as tinnitus, headache, dizziness, or blurred vision develops. Other nonsteroidal agents may also be effective but data on their efficacy are lacking. Prednisone may offer benefit to patients who lack significant response to NSAIDs. Either steroids or NSAIDs must be continued for several weeks following the return of the ESR to normal and then the dose tapered.
- Because rheumatic fever may recur, prophylaxis with penicillin, sulfonamides, or erythromycin is indicated. It must be continued for at least 5 years following an episode; prophylaxis must also be continued in patients under 25 years old, and in those at high risk for recurrent streptococcal infection (e.g., military recruits, parents of young children, and health care workers). Prophylactic antibiotics should also be given before an invasive procedure (e.g., tooth extraction) to prevent endocarditis.
- Surgical valve replacement and balloon or surgical valvuloplasty remain the only definitive treatment modalities when significant valvular disease is present.

XII. Superficial Thrombophlebitis
  A. Basic science
  - Superficial thrombophlebitis is a venous disorder characterized by inflammation and thrombosis of a superficial vein. It is generally caused by minor trauma or an indwelling catheter.
  B. History and physical examination
  - The vessel involved is tender to palpation and appears red and edematous. A cord may be felt. Characteristically, there is no swelling in other parts of the involved extremity.
  C. Laboratory and diagnostic studies
  - Doppler examination of the superficial vessel is not routinely performed but may be useful in revealing extension of thrombophlebitis to deeper vessels.
  D. Formulating the diagnosis
  - The differential diagnosis includes deep venous thrombosis, lymphangitis, and cellulitis. Migratory superficial thrombophlebitis is associated with Buerger's disease and malignancy, particularly of the pancreas.
  E. Evaluating the severity of problems
  - Although it is important to rule out deep vein thrombosis, superficial thrombophlebitis rarely progresses to deep venous thrombosis or pulmonary embolism.
  F. Managing the patient
  - The treatment for this condition is mainly directed at the control of the inflammation, with the application of warm compresses, elevation of the limb, and the use of nonsteroidal anti-inflammatory medications. Mobility is important, as deep venous thrombosis might actually follow forced bed rest. A follow-up examination should be scheduled in 2 days, and the patient should be asked to return immediately if the area of inflammation enlarges in spite of therapy.

XIII. Varicose Veins
  A. Basic science
    • Varicose veins are abnormally prominent, distended, tortuous veins that usually affect the lower extremities. Varicose veins are present in approximately one fifth of the population. They develop either on a familial basis, as a consequence of deep venous occlusion or increased intra-abdominal pressure (e.g., during pregnancy) or, in the majority of cases, idiopathically. Women are affected two to three times as often as men.
  B. History and physical examination
    • Varicose veins are initially asymptomatic. Patients may report to their physician for cosmetic reasons. Patients may seek help for a sense of heaviness in the lower extremities, accompanied by edema, especially after prolonged standing. These symptoms often disappear if the patient lies down and elevates the limbs. The symptoms may be more severe when the venous distention is caused by a deep occlusion.
    • As the condition becomes chronic, persistent edema, induration, and cutaneous hyperpigmentation (secondary to hemosiderin deposition) may occur. Eventually cutaneous atrophy, venous stasis dematitis, ulcers, and recurrent cellulitis may develop.
  C. Laboratory and diagnostic studies
    • The Trendelenburg test may be used to assess the competency of the communicating veins. The patient is placed in the supine position with the legs elevated. A tourniquet is applied around the thigh, close to the groin. The patient is then placed in the upright position. Filling of the veins within 30 seconds suggests incompetence.
    • Perthes' test assesses the competency of the deep vessels. A tourniquet is placed high in the calf to temporarily occlude the superficial vessels. Following this, the patient is asked to exercise for a short time. Pressure and discomfort in the calf suggest occluded deep vessels.
  D. Formulating the diagnosis
    • The diagnosis of varicose veins is made by the history and physical examination. Generally, inspection will suffice.
  E. Evaluating the severity of problems
    • If deep venous insufficiency is suspected, continuous-wave doppler plethysmography or descending venography may be used to confirm the diagnosis.
  F. Managing the patient
    • Young patients often need only reassurance. They should be advised to increase mobility and avoid long periods of standing if possible.
    • The therapy of varicose veins should be primarily directed to the control of edema and symptoms. These can usually be accomplished by the application of graduated compression stockings and elevating the lower extremities whenever possible. The stockings should be applied when the swelling is at a minimum (before getting out of bed) and worn during waking hours.
    • If stasis dermatitis is present, the application of low-dose steroid creams may improve symptoms. Antibiotics are indicated to treat cellulitis. If ulcers are

present, meticulous skin care is essential. This often accomplishes healing. If the ulcer is refractory, then surgical stripping of the superficial veins may be considered. However, the superficial veins must not be stripped if the varices are caused by a deep venous thrombosis, because they work as collaterals. In that event, excision of the ulcer followed by skin grafting should be considered.

- Finally, in the presence of arteriosclerotic disease, no therapy is often advised. The decreased flow through the arteries actually limits the degree of venous engorgement.

6

Gastroenterology

I. Acute Diarrhea

A. Basic science

- Diarrhea is the passage of loose stools usually associated with increased stool frequency. Diarrhea of duration less than 14 days is referred to as acute diarrhea. The annual incidence of acute diarrhea is approximately 5%.
- Acute diarrhea is most commonly infectious (caused by viruses, bacteria, and protozoa).
- Viral diarrhea is by far the most common cause of acute diarrhea. Bacterial diarrhea can cause the most severe forms of diarrhea.
- Infectious diarrhea is usually caused by one of the following mechanisms:
    1. Enterotoxins stimulate water and electrolyte secretion into the bowel lumen (e.g., *Staphylococcus aureus, Vibrio cholerae,* and enterotoxigenic *Escherichia coli*).
    2. Cytotoxins cause direct injury to bowel (e.g., *E. coli* O157:H7 and *Clostridium difficile*).
    3. Some bacteria invade the mucosa, causing edema and ulceration, e.g., *Salmonella, Shigella,* and enteroinvasive *E. coli* and the parasite *Entamoeba histolytica.*
    4. By adhering to the mucosa (e.g., enteroadherent *E. coli, Giardia,* and *Cryptosporidium*).
- Although acute diarrhea is most commonly infectious, other disease processes that should be considered include inflammatory bowel disease, ischemic bowel, irritable bowel syndrome, medications including laxatives or magnesium-containing antacids, diverticulitis, and rarely food allergies.

B. History

- Acute diarrhea can be categorized as bloody or nonbloody. The presence of blood and mucus in the stool indicates mucosal ulceration caused by invasive organisms. Watery diarrhea is usually due to toxins (which may be preformed and ingested as with *Clostridium perfringens* and *Bacillus cereus*) or due to viruses. If acute diarrhea occurs in hospitalized patients and other causes such as medications or enteral feeds have been excluded, then *Clostridium difficile* is the likely pathogen.
- The history should document the presence or absence of fever, recent antibiotic use, recent travel, sick contacts, history of inflammatory bowel disease, medication use (especially laxatives, antibiotics, and cholinergic agents), recent social events such as parties, and a history of immunodeficiency as in human immunodeficiency virus (HIV) infection or immunosuppression

with medications. Dizziness, lightheadedness, and increased thirst reflect intravascular volume depletion.

C. Physical examination
- Patients with diarrhea may be dehydrated. Dehydration is manifested by tachycardia, orthostatic hypotension, loss of skin turgor, and the absence of sweating most noticeable in the axillae. The presence of fever should be noted. The elderly can present with mental status change. Abdominal examination may reveal diffuse tenderness, but peritoneal signs are absent. It is important to remember that acute diarrhea may be the initial presentation of a more ominous condition such as sepsis or toxic shock syndrome or be an early manifestation of chronic diarrhea.

D. Laboratory and diagnostic studies
- Laboratory and radiologic studies and sigmoidoscopy are not indicated in the immunocompetent patient with mild diarrhea. If the patient appears toxic or dehydrated a white blood cell count and serum electrolytes will generally reveal a leukocytosis (if due to bacteria with the exception of *Salmonella*) and electrolyte abnormalities, which may reveal hypokalemia, hyponatremia, prerenal azotemia, and metabolic acidosis.
- Stool should be examined for the presence of blood and leukocytes and when appropriate sent for evaluation of *C. difficile* toxins and the presence of ova and parasites. Stool cultures are indicated when the stool contains leukocytes or blood, when there is a need to distinguish a flare of inflammatory bowel disease from an acute infectious diarrhea, and in immunocompromised patients and patients with severe comorbidities.
- Endoscopy is rarely indicated in acute diarrhea but should be considered if there is no improvement after 1 week of conservative therapy. Immunocompromised patients may need endoscopy to rule out opportunistic infections.

E. Formulating the diagnosis
- The history and physical examination may provide clues to the cause and to the severity of diarrhea.

F. Evaluating the severity of problems
- Physical appearance and signs of dehydration indicate the degree of severity.

G. Managing the patient
- Initial treatment should include assessment of fluid status and, if indicated, intravenous fluid and electrolyte resuscitation. Intravenous hydration should continue until the patient is able to take sufficient fluids and electrolytes by mouth to maintain hydration despite ongoing fluid losses. The oral fluid of choice is the glucose-electrolyte solution recommended by the World Health Organization (WHO).
- The use of antimicorbial agents is generally discouraged. However, it is reasonable to prescribe antimicrobials empirically to patients with traveler's diarrhea, when there are outbreaks of protozoal or bacterial diarrhea or when the patient appears toxic. EHEC should not be treated with antibiotics because of the increased risk for developing the hemolytic uremic syndrome. Paradoxically, antibiotics prolong the duration of diarrhea due to *Salmonella*

typhi. In diarrhea due to *Salmonella enteritidis,* antibiotics should be reserved only for patients who are very ill or are immunocompromised. Most diarrheas due to a parasite require treatment with the appropriate antimicrobial agent.

- Antidiarrheal agents such as opiates and loperamide, and intraluminal agents such as bismuth subsalicylate and adsorbants such as kaolin do reduce stool frequency and abdominal cramps. Concerns that these agents may prolong diarrhea duration, increase the severity of illness, or cause toxic megacolon have not been borne out when these medications were used judiciously.

II. Acute Pancreatitis
   A. Basic science
   - Acute pancreatitis is defined as abdominal pain associated with elevations in pancreatic enzymes (lipase, amylase). The process is related to inflammation within the gland. The major causes of pancreatitis in the United States are gallstones and alcohol consumption. Although the precise mechanisms leading to pancreatitis are unknown, dysfunction of the exocrine function is thought to be the contributing factor. Enzymatic activity in the local tissues leads to autodigestion and ischemia within the gland. This in turn leads to a spectrum of disease from mild interstitial inflammation to frank pancreatic necrosis. Interstitial pancreatitis is mild inflammation that is usually limited to the gland. Necrotizing pancreatitis is more severe inflammation, leading to the death (necrosis) of pancreatic tissue. This process not only affects peripancreatic tissues, but also affects more distant organs, leading to adult respiratory distress syndrome and acute renal failure, for example.
   - Other complications of acute pancreatitis include hypocalcemia, hyperglycemia, acidosis, acute fluid collections around the pancreas, pancreatic pseudocyst, sterile pancreatic necrosis, infection (pancreatic abscess, infected pancreatic necrosis), ascites, pleural effusion, and pancreatic ductal scarring/stricturing (leading to chronic pancreatitis).
   - Besides alcohol and gallstones, there are several other important causes of pancreatitis:
     1. Anatomic variation: pancreas divisum
     2. Mechanical factors: post-ERCP (endoscopic retrograde cholangiopancreatography), trauma
     3. Medications: azathioprine, thiazide diuretics, sulfonamides, protease inhibitors
     4. Infections: viral, bacterial, parasitic (in order of decreasing frequency)
     5. Metabolic: hypertriglyceridemia (>1000 mg/dL), hypercalcemia
     6. Genetic mutations: cystic fibrosis
     7. Miscellaneous: scorpion sting
   B. History and physical examination
   - Patients present with severe unrelenting colicky epigastric pain that often radiates to the back, nausea, and vomiting. Patients may also present with fever. Low-grade fever is common and does not necessarily mean that the patient has an infection. High fevers, especially with shaking chills, are indicative of infection. Other historical clues may include alcohol consumption

or a history of gallstones. Keep in mind that patients may not be forthcoming with their use of alcohol and that pancreatitis is sometimes the first manifestation of cholelithiasis. In the absence of a history of alcohol or gallstones, a careful history must be taken for other causes of pancreatitis, especially medications (azathioprine or thiazides) or recent abdominal trauma or ERCP. Other causes of acute pancreatitis will likely not be discovered in the initial history.

- Hypotension, tachycardia, and fever are often observed. Physical findings consistent with acute pancreatitis are abdominal (epigastric) tenderness with or without guarding. Periumbilical (Cullen's sign) and flank (Grey Turner's sign) ecchymoses are rare findings that represent retroperitoneal hemorrhage due to necrotizing pancreatitis. Bowel sounds may be diminished or absent owing to ileus. Findings consistent with biliary obstruction may be present (jaundice, RUQ [right upper quadrant] tenderness, palpable RUQ or epigastric mass). Rarely, clinical evidence of hypocalcemia (Chovstek's sign) may be present.

C. Laboratory and diagnostic studies

- Serum amylase and lipase elevations (more than three times the upper limit of normal) are suggestive of acute pancreatitis. Lipase is considered to be more specific for pancreatic processes. Be aware that amylase may be elevated in many other disease processes including vomiting, parotid disease, and various intra-abdominal pathologic states other than pancreatitis. AST (aspartate aminotransferase), ALT (alanine aminotransferase), alkaline phosphatase, CBC (complete blood count), BUN (blood urea nitrogen), serum creatinine, calcium, LDH (lactic dehydrogenase), and glucose should be checked to assess the severity of illness. Upon presentation, the WBC (white blood cell) count, glucose, AST, and LDH are important prognostic indicators. After 48 hours have passed, the PaO_2, calcium, BUN, HCT (hematocrit), and base deficit are important prognostic factors. These data from the initial assessment and at 48 hours compose the Ranson's score, which helps to predict overall mortality risk in acute pancreatitis.
- An ALT greater than three times the upper limit of normal is suggestive of gallstone pancreatitis.
- Radiologic tests for acute pancreatitis include plain abdominal x-ray, contrast-enhanced abdominal computed tomography (CT), and abdominal ultrasound.
- CT scan can confirm the diagnosis of pancreatitis with a standard severity grading scale. It is indicated in patients presenting with severe pancreatitis and in patients that have unresolving abdominal pain after 7 to 10 days. In addition, CT can help identify cholelithiasis (although this is not the optimal test: RUQ ultrasound is) and can identify alternative pathologic processes that may be causing the patient's symptoms.
- Plain x-rays of the abdomen can reveal pancreatic calcifications (significant in chronic pancreatitis) and the "sentinel loop"—a dilated loop of small bowel adjacent to the pancreas.
- Ultrasound of the abdomen is helpful to identify cholelithiasis, biliary sludge, and biliary dilatation.

D. Formulating the diagnosis
- Making the diagnosis of pancreatitis is generally straightforward in most patients.

E. Managing the patient
- All but the mildest cases of pancreatitis require hospitalization. Pain control with narcotics is generally necessary. Aggressive volume resuscitation is paramount due to the third-spacing of fluid in the abdomen and ongoing fluid losses due to vomiting. Bowel rest may be required in cases of severe abdominal pain and vomiting, but recent data suggest improved outcomes when patients that can tolerate it are fed. It has been shown that early feeding, when possible, preserves the gut's mucosal barrier and reduces the incidence of pancreatitis-associated infections. Adequate oxygenation and management of metabolic complications (hyperglycemia, hypocalecemia, and other electrolyte abnormalitites) are important as well.
- Assessment of the severity is important early in the course with reevaluation at 48 hours. This is done by using Ranson's score, based on Ranson's criteria:
  1. At diagnosis:
     - Age older than 55 years
     - WBC count above $16,000/mm^3$
     - Glucose level over 200 mg/dL
     - AST above 250 U/L
     - LDH above 350 U/L
  2. At 48 hours:
     - HCT ↓ more than 10%
     - BUN ↑ more than 5 mg/dL
     - Base deficit above 4 mEq/L
     - Ca less than 8 mEq/L
     - PaO_2 less than 60 mm Hg
     - Fluid sequestration greater than 6 L
  3. Prognosis is based on Ranson's score:
     - Up to 2 criteria: mortality rate less than 5%
     - 3 to 4 criteria: mortality rate 15% to 20%
     - 5 to 6 criteria: mortality rate 40%
     - 7 or more criteria: mortality rate approaches 99%
- Ranson's score reflects overall systemic complications related to the pancreatitis. Keep in mind that the presence of severe necrosis, abscess, or pseudocysts (even with a low Ranson's score) portends a poor prognosis. Any patient with a Ranson's score above 4 should be managed in an intensive care setting.
- Systemic antibiotics are indicated only when there is evidence of severe infection (high fever, chills, and leukocytosis) or positive Gram stain or culture from fluid collection or pseudocyst. The antibiotic of choice in treating pancreatitis-associated infection has classically been imipenem because of its penetration into inflamed pancreatic tissues and broad spectrum of coverage.

III. Cirrhosis
  A. Basic science
  - Cirrhosis is a result of progressive hepatic fibrosis, which leads to hepatic architecture distortion, followed by nodular regeneration. These changes due to cirrhosis are generally irreversible. Any chronic liver disease can lead to cirrhosis.
  - The most common causes of liver injury (cirrhosis):
    1. Alcoholic liver disease
       - Alcohol consumption can lead to the histopathologic changes of fatty liver, hepatitis, and cirrhosis. The histologic changes seen in alcoholic fatty liver and alcoholic hepatitis are reversible with alcohol abstinence. Even with established cirrhosis, fibrosis can improve and portal pressure decrease with abstinence. Cirrhosis tends to develop after consumption of 80 g of alcohol daily for 10 to 20 years.
    2. Chronic viral hepatitis
       - Hepatitis B and C (see Chapter 20, Infectious Disease). Chronic hepatitis B leads to cirrhosis in approximately 15% to 20% of patients. Chronic hepatitis C leads to cirrhosis in approximately 20% to 30% of patients.
    3. Primary sclerosing cholangitis (PSC)
       - PSC is a condition of idiopathic intra- and extrahepatic biliary obstruction caused by continual inflammation and stricture formation in medium and large biliary ducts. Cholangiography reveals significant multifocal stricture formation and dilation of bile ducts, which give rise to a beaded appearance. Biliary abnormalities may also be seen by ultrasound. There is a significant correlation with inflammatory bowel disease, particularly ulcerative colitis. Antinuclear antibodies, anti–smooth muscle antibodies, and p-ANCA (perinuclear antineutrophil cytoplasmic autoantibodies) are often positive but not diagnostic.
    4. Primary biliary cirrhosis (PBC)
       - PBC is an autoimmune disorder caused by inflammation and destruction of intrahepatic bile ducts. It is rarely found before the age of 30 years. Patients may also have evidence of other autoimmune disorders, especially the sicca syndrome. Symptoms include pruritus, hyperpigmentation of the skin, and joint pains secondary to an inflammatory arthropathy. Hepatomegaly and other signs of chronic liver injury occur years later. IgM antimitochondrial antibody is present in 95% of patients, and alkaline phosphatase levels are almost always elevated. Jaundice occurs late in the disease.
    5. Autoimmune hepatitis
       - Autoimmune hepatitis is a chronic hepatitis of unknown cause associated with hyperglobulinemia and the presence of circulating autoantibodies. Most patients respond to treatment with immunomodulating drugs such as prednisone.
    6. Nonalcoholic steatohepatitis (NASH)/nonalcoholic fatty liver disease (NAFLD)

- There is histopathologic fatty liver with features indistinguishable from alcoholic hepatitis in the absence of a concurrent history of viral hepatitis or excessive alcoholic consumption. The etiology is not entirely known, but these conditions are associated with the metabolic syndrome (obesity, type 2 diabetes, insulin resistance, and dyslipidemia), extensive bowel resection, and medications such as amiodarone and tamoxifen. Patients with this disorder can progress to advanced liver disease (i.e., cirrhosis), especially in the diabetic.

7. Hereditary hemochromatosis
   - Hereditary hemochromatosis is an autosomal recessive disorder in which mutations in the *HFE* gene cause increased intestinal iron absorption circumventing normal mechanisms that prevent absorption of iron when stores are normal (or elevated). This leads to excessive iron deposition in multiple tissues (liver, heart, pancreas, and pituitary). Look for the classic triad of cirrhosis, diabetes mellitus, and abnormal skin pigmentation in patients with elevated serum iron markers. Hereditary hemochromatosis is virtually never seen in African Americans.

8. Wilson's disease
   - Wilson's disease is a rare inherited autosomal recessive disorder of copper metabolism (cellular copper export). Males and females are equally affected. It is generally seen in individuals 5 to 40 years of age. The manifestations of the disease are due to failure to excrete unneeded and excessive copper in the bile for loss in the stool. This may be due to a failure to excrete copper packaged in ceruloplasmin into the bile. This leads to tissue copper deposition which causes hepatic disease (acute hepatitis, chronic active hepatitis, cirrhosis), neurologic impairment (movement disorders), hematologic abnormalities (hemolytic anemia), renal impairment, and psychiatric abnormalities (irritability, depression). Treatment is with penicillamine or zinc acetate.

9. Alpha$_1$-antitrypsin (AAT) deficiency
   - Liver disease is caused by polymerization of the dysfunctional AAT resulting in accumulation of AAT molecules in hepatocytes. AAT dysfunction also causes emphysema (typically pan-acinar) due to defective inhibition of elastase in the lungs. A variant of AAT deficiency in which AAT is absent leads to severe pulmonary manifestations but no liver manifestations (AAT cannot polymerize in the liver if it is absent).

10. Venous congestion
    - Passive venous congestion can lead to cirrhosis. Etiologies of venous congestion are right-sided heart failure, pericardial fibrosis, and Budd-Chiari syndrome. Budd-Chiari syndrome is defined as an occlusion of the hepatic veins or the inferior vena cava.

B. History and physical examination
  - The history should include a history of alcohol intake and evaluation for risk factors and for hepatitis B and C (prior blood transfusions, high-risk sexual behavior, occupational exposures, history of hepatitis, and family history of

liver disease). Gastrointestinal bleeding may be a consequence of variceal bleed, portal gastropathy, or ulcers.

- On presentation, patients may be asymptomatic or have increased susceptibility to infections or have evidence of malnutrition or pruritus.
- On examination, there may be signs of liver failure such as palmar erythema, spider angiomas, encephalopathy, gynecomastia, and testicular atrophy, and jaundice may be present. Also look for signs of portal hypertension such as caput medusae, ascites, and splenomegaly.
- The consequences of cirrhosis include portal hypertension which can cause varices, portal hypertensive gastropathy, and ascites. Upper gastrointestinal (GI) endoscopy should be obtained in all patients with gastrointestinal bleeding.
- Ascites is fluid in the peritoneal cavity. In cirrhosis it is a consequence of portal hypertension, hypoalbuminemia, and increased renal sodium reabsorption.
- Spontaneous bacterial peritonitis (SBP) is a complication associated with ascites. SBP presents with fever, diffuse abdominal discomfort, and leukocytosis. The classic signs of peritonitis are absent. Ascitic fluid analysis reveals a leukocyte count greater than 500 cells/dL or a polymorphonuclear count greater than 250 cells/dL. Gram stain may be positive for bacteria. All patients admitted to the hospital who have ascites should be evaluated for SBP.
- Hepatic encephalopathy refers to mental status changes due to multiple toxins that normally are removed by the liver. Increased ammonia levels may be detected.
- Coagulopathy results in increased prothrombin time (PT) and partial thromboplastin time (PTT). There is easy bleeding or bruising due to thrombocytopenia and abnormal and diminished production of the vitamin K–dependent clotting factors (V, VII, IX, and X).
- Hepatorenal syndrome is progressive azotemia, oliguria, and urine sodium level below 10 mEq/L.

C. Laboratory and diagnostic studies

- Screening laboratory studies include a complete blood count, serum electrolytes, and liver function studies (transaminases, alkaline phosphatase, prothrombin time, protein, and albumin).
- Thrombocytopenia and anemia are common findings in cirrhosis and are a consequence of hypersplenism.
- Liver function enzymes such as AST may not be elevated because little viable tissue exists to cause elevations. AST is commonly elevated in alcoholic cirrhosis and is usually greater than ALT by a 2:1 ratio.
- In a patient with newly diagnosed cirrhosis an attempt should be made to establish the etiology.
- The following investigations may be done depending on the clinical situation:
  1. Tests of hepatocellular damage: In alcoholic hepatitis and cirrhosis the AST is greater than ALT (ratio > 2:3).
  2. Alkaline phosphatase is usually elevated in primary biliary cirrhosis and primary sclerosing cholangitis.

3. Hepatitis serologic test may indicate the presence of past exposure to hepatitits B. Hepatitis C infection can be detected by ELISA (enzyme-linked immunosorbent assay) or PCR (polymerase chain reaction).

4. Elevated serum copper, decreased serum ceruloplasmin, and increased 24-hour urine copper levels are seen in Wilson's disease.

5. Protein electrophoresis may provide a clue to AAT deficiency. IgM level is increased in primary biliary cirrhosis.

6. Antinuclear antibodies and elevated serum globulins are detected in autoimmune hepatitis.

7. Ultrasonography and CT scan of the abdomen may provide evidence that cirrhosis is present but do not help in determining the cause of cirrhosis.

- Primary biliary cirrhosis is a disease of women between the ages of 30 and 65 years. The etiology is unknown. Pruritus and fatigue are usually the presenting complaints. Jaundice and inflammatory arthropathy may be present. Excoriations, hepatosplenomegaly, and signs of liver cell failure and portal hypertension may be present.

- Alkaline phosphatase is usually elevated. Elevated bilirubin is a poor prognostic sign. Abdominal ultrasound, endoscopic retrograde cholangiopancreatography (ERCP), or cholangiography is indicated only if the clinical picture and laboratory data do not support the diagnosis.

- Liver biopsy may be helpful in establishing the cause for the cirrhosis.

D. Formulating the diagnosis

- The diagnosis of cirrhosis should be entertained in any patient who presents with jaundice. Clinical findings such as palmar erythema, spider angiomata, varices, encephalopathy, and ascites may be present to variable degrees and help support the clinical suspicion of cirrhosis and portal hypertension. The cause of cirrhosis may be less obvious. Pruritis suggests biliary disease.

E. Evaluating the severity of problems

- Morbidity and death are most commonly due to complications of cirrhosis. Treatment should be directed at correcting these complications.

- Significant worsening liver function studies may suggest worsening cirrhosis, but improvement of these tests does not correlate with improvement of disease and may, in fact, signal end-stage disease.

- Hepatorenal syndrome involves worsening renal insufficiency in the presence of liver failure. The cause is not known. Renal biopsy is unremarkable.

F. Managing the patient

- Management is directed initially at removing the cause, for example, alcohol, and treating the complications of cirrhosis.

1. Variceal bleeding

- Variceal bleeding must be treated aggressively with volume and blood resuscitation, reversal of coagulopathy with vitamin K, and fresh frozen plasma. Bleeding should be stopped with octreotide or vasopressin. Balloon tamponade (Blakemore tube) may be used as a temporizing measure if the patient is too unstable to undergo endoscopy. Upper endoscopy to band or sclerose the varices should be done as soon as the patient is stable. Transjugular intrahepatic portosystemic shunt (TIPS) is an option to urgently reduce portal pressure in order to reduce variceal bleeding. Worsening encephalopathy is a complication of the procedure. Surgical portosystemic shunt is also an option if bleeding continues. If the bleeding persists liver transplantation should be considered.

- β-Blocking agents, elective sclerosis, portosystemic shunts, and liver transplantation are options to consider for preventing variceal bleed.

2. Hepatic encephalopathy
- Treatment of hepatic encephalopathy should include correcting any precipitating cause such as gastrointestinal bleed or an infection. Protein restriction and oral lactulose or neomycin are the mainstay of treatment.
- Other causes of mental status changes should be eliminated, including intracranial bleeding, drug ingestion, alcohol ingestion or withdrawal, and meningitis.

3. Spontaneous bacterial peritonitis
- Diagnosis of spontaneous bacterial peritonitis is confirmed by peritoneal fluid analysis. Treatment with antibiotics should be commenced promptly as this is potentially a life-threatening condition. SBP prophylaxis with norfloxacin or trimethoprim-sulfamethoxazole should be instituted in cirrhotics with a history of prior SBP.

4. Ascites
- Ascites due to liver disease and portal hypertension should be managed conservatively. In the presence of worsening ascites consider an increase in the salt intake or noncompliance with diuretics if the patient was previously on diretics. Salt restriction and bed rest may improve ascites. Diuretics (lasix 40 mg/day and spironolactone 100 mg/day) should be started. Periodic paracentesis, TIPS, and liver transplantation are treatments for ascites not responsive to bed rest, salt restriction, and diuretics.

5. Liver transplantation
- Liver transplantation should be considered for patients with the hepatorenal syndrome, refractory ascites, Child class B or C, or MELD (model for end-stage liver disease) score of 26 or higher. Contraindications to transplantation include advanced HIV, extrahepatic malignancy, continued substance abuse, uncontrolled sepsis, and end-stage cardiac or pulmonary disease.

IV. Colorectal Cancer/Familial Adenomatous Polyposis
   A. Basic science
   - Colorectal cancer is the second leading cause of cancer death in the United States, with 160,000 Americans newly diagnosed each year.
   - About 98% of all colon malignancies are adenocarcinomas.
   - Most colorectal cancer is sporadic, occurring from a variety of environmental causes. Genetic factors probably play a role as well. The peak incidence is between the ages of 60 and 80 years. Risk factors for developing colon cancer include a history of colon cancer in first-degree relatives, inflammatory bowel disease, colonic polyps (especially adenomatous, serrated, or villous polyps),

and several familial polyposis syndromes such as familial polyposis, Gardner's syndrome, and Turcot's syndrome.

B. Clinical presentation

- If the cancer is in the cecum or ascending colon and if the patient is symptomatic, the patient usually presents with symptoms of anemia, vague abdominal discomfort, or overt rectal bleeding. With cancers in the descending colon, change in bowel habits and rectal bleeding and signs and symptoms of colonic obstructive are the more common modes of presentation. Examination may be normal or may reveal a palpable mass, abdominal distention, and tenderness suggestive of colonic obstruction or a rectal mass on digital rectal examination.
- Screening is most effectively carried out by colonscopy, although fecal occult blood testing and flexible sigmoidoscopy are still recommended.
- Surgical resection with adjuvant chemotherapy and radiotherapy are the current treatment modalities depending on the staging of the cancer. Follow-up is with fecal occult blood testing, colonoscopy, and CEA levels.
- *Familial adenomatous polyposis (FAP)* is the most common adenomatous polyposis syndrome. FAP accounts for about 1% of all colorectal cancer cases. FAP is an autosomal dominant syndrome caused by a germline mutation.
- FAP patients develop hundreds to thousands of colorectal adenomas, usually in adolescence. Polyps occur diffusely throughout the colon and rectum. Polyps can occur in the stomach and the small intestines.

C. History and physical examination

- FAP patients are initially asymptomatic. Symptoms usually occur in later stages of this syndrome and include rectal bleeding, change in bowel habits, and abdominal pain.
- Patients can develop colonic obstruction. Colorectal cancer, primarily in the left colon, occurs in virtually all FAP patients if colectomy is not performed. The average age at diagnosis of colorectal cancer is 39 years.
- FAP can be associated with various extracolonic lesions. These include skin epidermoid cysts, osteomas noted particularly on the mandible, pigmented ocular fundus lesions (POFLs) found on ophthalmologic examination, and desmoid tumors found of the skin or in the abdomen. FAP patients are at increased risk for intestinal cancers, especially duodenal, periampullary carcinomas and rectal cancer in those with subtotal colectomy. Extraintestinal cancers reported in association with FAP include tumors of the thyroid gland, adrenal gland, biliary tree, brain, and pancreas.

D. Laboratory and diagnostic studies

- The diagnosis of FAP is confirmed by finding 100 or more adenomatous polyps on endoscopic examination of the colon and rectum. In an at-risk patient, the finding of greater than three POFLs on indirect ophthalmoloscopic examination has a 100% positive predictive value for the diagnosis of FAP. Detection of the *APC* gene mutation has virtually 99% sensitivity and specificity for FAP.
- Suspicion of hereditary colorectal cancer should be raised in individuals with multiple family members with colorectal cancer or adenomatous polyps,

members with colorectal cancer at young age (younger than 50 years of age), and family members with multiple adenomatous polyps.

- The diagnosis of FAP is made in patients with mutation of the *FAP* gene or those who have greater than 100 adenomatous polyps on endoscopic examination of the colorectum.

E. Evaluating the severity of problems

- Major complications in FAP consist of the extracolonic manifestations of FAP just described. After colorectal cancer, the most common cause of death is duodenal cancer.

F. Managing the patient

- Colectomy is the only effective therapy that eliminates the development of colorectal cancer in FAP patients. Surgery should be done at the time of diagnosis of FAP to minimize risk of colorectal cancer. Postoperative follow-up is important. Patients with subtotal colectomy require routine endoscopic surveillance of the remaining rectum for recurrent adenomas and carcinoma. Also, in patients with ileoanal pull-through, endoscopic biopsy surveillance of the pouch should be considered. Most authorities recommend upper endoscopic surveillance (with biopsy and brushing) of the stomach, duodenum, and periampullary region.
- Because FAP is a genetic disease, screening of at-risk first-degree relatives by endoscopy of the colorectum and genotyping is imperative.

V. Constipation

A. Basic science

- Constipation is defined as a decrease in defecation frequency coupled with an increase in stool hardness. The patient often has extreme difficulty with defecation and often has a feeling of incomplete evacuation.
- Constipation can be classified as acute or chronic.
- Acute constipation often indicates an organic disease state (e.g., mechanical bowel obstruction, adynamic ileus from trauma, or peritoneal irritation).
- Chronic constipation requires 12 weeks (which need not be consecutive) of infrequent stools or difficult defecation. Chronic constipation may indicate:
  1. A neurological problem (irritable bowel disease, Hirshsprung's disease)
  2. An electrolyte disorder (hyperglycemia, hypercalcemia)
  3. An endocrine disorder (hypothyroidism, diabetes mellitus, estrogen/progesterone changes in pregnancy)
  4. A musculoskeletal problem (pelvic floor dysfunction)
  5. A psychological disorder (depression, eating disorders)
  6. Medications (opiates, anticholinergics, 5-HT$_3$ antagonists)
- Chronic constipation is more common in females and the elderly.

B. History

- The physician should determine whether constipation is acute or chronic. Family history of constipation or GI problems should be obtained. A history of abdominal surgery (hysterectomy, bowel surgery), neurologic disease or injury, endocrine disorders, pregnancy, and psychological disorders should be documented. Note should be made of any changes in the patient's diet or exercise regimen and the use of new medications, particularly opiates, tranquilizers, and anticholinergics.

- Recent onset of constipation, bloody stools, pain, fever, anemia, or weight loss may indicate a tumor.

C. Physical examination
- Physical examination in acute constipation may show evidence of intestinal obstruction, or peritonitis, whereas in chronic constipation other than hemorrhoids and mucosal prolapse the examination is normal.

D. Laboratory and diagnostic studies
- Thyroid-stimulating hormone (TSH), thyroxine (T_4), and standard serum chemistries should be obtained to determine if other abnormalities exist that may cause constipation (e.g., hypothyroidism, diabetes mellitus, hypercalcemia, and hypokalemia).
- If the cause of constipation is unclear after a carefully taken history, a thorough physical examination, a colonscopy, or barium enema may be necessary. A colonic transit study or studies of pelvic floor function may be necessary as well because anorectal and pelvic floor dysfunction is an important cause of chronic constipation in some individuals.

E. Formulating the diagnosis
- History, physical examination, and the results of diagnostic studies will usually reveal the cause of the patient's constipation.

F. Evaluating the severity of problems
- Constipation may be a symptom of a life-threatening disease state (e.g., colonic malignancy). However, constipation may be idiopathic or a component of the irritable bowel syndrome.

G. Managing the patient
- If history and physical examination indicate a possible organic cause of constipation (weight loss, anemia, hematochezia, occult fecal blood), then diagnostic testing and treatment should be instituted.
- If a non-life-threatening cause is suspected based on initial history and physical examination (i.e., no abnormal laboratory values and no signs or symptoms of organic disease), then dietary, lifestyle, or pharmacologic therapy should be instituted.
- The patient should be advised to adhere to a high-fiber diet. Increasing dietary fiber (fruits and vegetables) increases stool bulk and makes stools softer, ensuring easier stool elimination. Adequate water intake must be ensured when patients increase their fiber intake. Agents that increase stool bulk, such as psyllium, may make defecation easier.
- If the patient improves on the high-fiber diet, the workup should end and the patient told to continue his or her present regimen. Unabsorbed polyethylene glycol-electrolyte solutions cause feces that are softer and have increased bulk. This facilitates evacuation of feces. Laxatives and cathartics should be used carefully. Patients often become dependent on these medications and develop an inability to defecate without their use.
- Laxatives and cathartics are classified as follows:

1. Detergent laxatives
   - These agents (docusate) act by allowing water to enter into the stool, increasing the stool size and thereby stimulating peristalsis.
2. Osmotic agents
   - These agents (sorbitol, laculose) are poorly absorbed large molecules and act by osmotically drawing water into the colon. The excess water in the colon softens the stool and stimulates peristalsis. These agents may contain large amounts of sodium, magnesium, or phosphate and must be used with care in patients with cardiac and renal disease. These agents may cause electrolyte abnormalities if abused.
3. Stimulant cathartics
   - These agents (bisacodyl, castor oil) act by irritating the bowel. Abuse leads to severe electrolyte abnormalities. Normal colonic neuromuscular function could be compromised with chronic use of these medications as well.
   - Enemas and suppositories stimulate colonic and rectal contraction and soften stools.

VI. Crohn's Disease
   A. Basic science
   - Crohn's disease is a chronic inflammatory bowel disease. The etiology is not known. The disorder results in ulcerations (apthous/serpiginous/stellate) in the gastrointestinal tract. The ulcers may occur anywhere in the GI tract but tend to cluster around the distal ileum and cecum. The ulcers are deep and often transmural (mucosa to serosa). The transmural inflammation can result in fibrosis (and therefore obstruction), sinus tracts, and fistula formation. Any part of the gastrointestinal tract can be involved, although the ileum is most frequently affected. Involvement can be limited to the small intestine or the colon.
   - Characteristically, Crohn's disease is distinguished from ulcerative colitis by the presence of perianal disease with or without rectal involvement, mucosal skip lesions, and the presence of fistulas. The disease is thought to be an immune-mediated inflammatory response to unknown environmental triggers. There appears to be a genetic predisposition to Crohn's disease.
   - The disease usually occurs in patients before the age of 30 years, but a second peak incidence can be seen around 60 years of age. Smoking has been associated with a near twofold increase in the incidence of Crohn's disease.
   B. History
   - Crohn's disease is characterized by frequent attacks of diarrhea, severe abdominal pain, weight loss, anorexia, fatigue, fever, and vomiting. Additionally, patients may have other "extraintestinal" symptoms and signs such as migratory nonerosive arthritis, ankylosing spondylitis, erythema nodosum, pyoderma gangrenosa, uveitis, and kidney stones.
   C. Physical examination
   - Patients may present with few symptoms or may manifest with fever, right lower quadrant pain, abdominal distention, abdominal mass, signs of obstruction or perforation.

D. Laboratory and diagnostic studies
- The diagnosis is established by endoscopy in a patient who has a clinical presentation consistent with Crohn's disease. Granulomas are seen in a third of all biopsies. Barium studies (enema or small bowel follow-through) may show a narrowed lumen and skip lesions. In severe cases a string sign may be present. Barium studies are helpful in determining the length of stricture formation and its location.
- CBC may demonstrate a leukocytosis. Serum chemistries may demonstrate a low albumin. The erythrocyte sedimentation rate (ESR) may be elevated. These changes reflect the severity of inflammation and disease duration.

E. Formulating the diagnosis
- History, physical examination, and endoscopic findings are helpful in establishing the diagnosis. Other diseases that produce an acute abdomen and may be confused with Crohn's disease include appendicitis, pelvic inflammatory disease, and infection with *Yersinia enteritis*.

F. Evaluating the severity of problems
- Fistulas, hemorrhage, and abscess formation are the major complications of Crohn's disease. Toxic megacolon is less commonly seen compared to ulcerative colitis.
- Life-threatening complications include perforation and electrolyte imbalance.

G. Managing the patient
- Specific treatment includes the following:
  1. Anticholinergics, loperamide (to relieve cramps and diarrhea)
  2. Sulfasalazine and 5-ASA drugs such as mesalamine
     - Sulfasalazine and 5-ASA drugs are useful in treating mild exacerbations and preventing relapse.
  3. Antibiotics such as ciprofloxacin or clarithromycin
     - Antibiotics may also be helpful in inducing remission.
  4. Steroids
     - In patients who do not go into remission prednisone 60 mg/day with a tapering dose after 4 weeks should be prescribed. However, steroids are contraindicated in patients with abscess or infection.
  5. Azathioprine, 6-mercaptopurine, and methotrexate
     - These drugs should be reserved for refractory patients.
     - Infliximab is a chimeric mouse/human monoclonal antibody directed against tumor necrosis factor-alpha. It is indicated in severe refractory Crohn's disease.
     - These agents take months to work.
  6. Elemental diets or hyperalimentation
     - These options are probably better than bowel rest in active disease.
  7. Surgery
     - Surgery should be avoided as far as possible. Surgery is not curative, and the disease will return in the vast majority of patients.

VII. Diverticular Disease

A. Basic science

- Diverticula are pouchlike herniations through the muscular layer that can occur in the small bowel or colon. Because diverticula in the colon become symptomatic more frequently than small bowel diverticula this discussion will focus on colonic diverticular disease. Diverticula form as a result of elevated intraluminal colonic pressure. They tend to occur in narrow regions of the colon (descending and sigmoid colon) where intraluminal pressure is elevated.

- Diverticula are common and usually asymptomatic. However, two disease states may occur as a result of diverticulosis:

  1. Diverticulitis

     - Diverticulitis is inflammation of the diverticula or a localized perforation of a diverticulum. The penetration of fecal matter (fecalith) through the thin-walled diverticula or high intraluminal pressure in the bowel causes perforation, which leads to inflammation and abscess formation or fistula formation into the tissues surrounding the colon. With repeated inflammation, the lumen of the colon may become strictured and cause obstruction.

  2. Diverticular bleeding

     - The diverticula erode through the vasa recta (vessels) on the outside of the colon, causing bleeding. Bleeding may be massive but is often self-limited.

B. History and physical examination

- The history and physical examination reveal no abnormality when diverticulosis (i.e, diverticula) alone is present. When evaluating a patient with a possible diverticulitis the patient should be asked about previous gastrointestinal disease, change in bowel habits, and previous colonic diagnostic studies.

  1. Diverticulitis

     - Typically, the patient is age 50 years or older. The pain is often present in the left lower quadrant and can be severe in intensity. Right-sided diverticulitis is uncommon but well documented. Fever, nausea, vomiting, constipation, or diarrhea may also be present.

  2. Diverticular bleed

     - Patient often describes painless rectal bleeding; blood is a maroon or deep red color. The patient may feel lightheaded or dizzy, indicating potential hemodynamic instability.

- Physical examination should include vital sign assessment and orthostatic measurements if bleeding is suspected. Abdominal, rectal, and pelvic (in females) examination must be performed. If bleeding and hypotension are present, upper GI bleed must be ruled out with a gastric lavage that is negative for blood and positive for bile. Tenderness and a mass on an abdominal examination is indicative of diverticulitis. Bleeding associated with diverticulitis is uncommon.

C. Laboratory and diagnostic studies
   1. Diverticulitis
      - A leukocytosis with a left shift is often found. X-ray of the abdomen may show evidence of a displaced colon, air in the peritoneum if a free perforation is present, and mucosal abnormalities. A CT scan of the abdomen may show a thickened colon, inflammatory changes and extraluminal gas. These findings are highly suggestive of diverticulitis.
   2. Diverticular bleed
      - Blood for CBC, blood type, and crossmatch should be drawn. Angiography is the best method for diagnosing and treating active bleeding. Colonoscopy is indicated if a mass is palpated or the cause of bleeding is not identified. Exploratory laparotomy may be necessary if bleeding continues and the cause remains in question after colonoscopy and angiography.
D. Formulating the diagnosis
   1. Diverticulitis
      - History and physical examination usually point to the diagnosis. Diseases that may be confused with diverticular diseases include Crohn's disease, irritable bowel syndrome, ischemic colitis, colon cancer, appendicitis, and bacterial colitis due to *Shigella, Campylobacter,* or *Salmonella.* A left lower quadrant mass, fever, leukocytosis, and a left shift suggest abscess or perforation.
   2. Diverticular bleed
      - Diverticular bleeding must be differentiated from upper GI bleeding and other causes of colonic bleed such as ateriovenous malformations.
E. Evaluating the severity of problems
   1. Diverticulitis
      - Diverticulitis may lead to sepsis, perforation, abscess, or intestinal obstruction.
   2. Diverticular bleed
      - Patients may exsanguinate. Vitals signs must be closely monitored.
F. Managing the patient
   1. Diverticulitis
      - Patients who do not appear ill may be treated with oral ciprofloxacin and metronidazole, liquid diet, and at follow-up double contrast barium enema or colonoscopy.
      - Patients who appear ill should be treated with IV antibiotics (metronidazole and a third-generation cephalosporin, e.g., ceftriaxone), kept NPO (nothing by mouth), and monitored closely. If the patient does not improve or worsens, a CT scan of the abdomen should be performed to rule out abscess or other abdominal disease. Severe persistent pain or signs of peritonitis should prompt surgical intervention.
   2. Diverticular bleed
      - Most diverticular bleeding will cease spontaneously. In patients in whom bleeding does not stop, infusion of intra-arterial vasopressin may be necessary. If vasopressin does not stop the bleeding, intravascular embolization or surgery with diverticular resection may be necessary.

VIII. Esophageal Cancer
    A. Basic science
- Esophageal cancer accounts for approximately 1% of cancer in the United States. About 50% are squamous cell carcinomas and 50% are adenocarcinomas. Elderly black males in urban areas account for the majority of cases.
- Several factors are implicated in the pathogenesis of esophageal cancer, including alcohol, tobacco; dietary carcinogens (i.e., nitrosamine, fungal toxins); and predisposing conditions such as Barrett's esophagus, which can lead to an adenocarcinoma, lye stricture, achalasia, celiac disease, and radiation-induced strictures.

    B. History and physical examination
- Patients with esophageal cancer typically present with progressive difficulty in swallowing. At first patients report difficulty swallowing solids, but as the disease progresses patients are unable to swallow liquids. Other symptoms can include weight loss, chest pain, odynophagia (painful sensation while swallowing), gastrointestinal bleeding, and aspiration of food and secretions.
- Extension of cancer into soft tissues surrounding the esophagus can result in laryngeal paralysis due to recurrent laryngeal nerve involvement, causing hoarseness of voice, superior vena cava obstruction, or Horner's syndrome. In addition, spread of cancer into the mediastinum may cause tracheoesophageal or aortoesophageal fistula.

    C. Laboratory and diagnostic studies
- Barium contrast studies of the esophagus provide information about the length of esophageal involvement by the cancer and also about the presence of any fistulas. Typically, marked narrowing of the esophageal lumen with an irregular and ragged pattern to the esophageal mucosa is noted. An achalia-like picture (pseudo-achalasia) can be seen if the tumor involves the cardia.
- Esophagoscopy should follow an abnormal barium esophagogram. Biopsy and cytologic brushing of the esophagus should be collected and strictures dilated when feasible.

    D. Formulating the diagnosis
- Diagnosis is suspected by the clinical presentation and confirmed by histologic or cytologic evaluation.

    E. Evaluating the severity of problems
- Additional information concerning the extent and spread of cancer can be obtained by CT of the thorax and abdomen. An esophagogram with a water-soluble contrast agent may be necessary to determine if a tracheoesophageal fistula is present.

    F. Managing the patient
- Patients with dysphagia should always undergo diagnostic testing with upper gastrointestinal endoscopy, contrast studies, manometry, or a combination of these modalities.
- Most patients are diagnosed with esophageal cancer only after experiencing symptoms. Because difficulty with swallowing does not occur until the development of significant narrowing of the esophageal lumen, most patients

have advanced and incurable disease. The prognosis for esophageal cancer is poor (5% survival rate 5 years after diagnosis).

- Surgical resection is the mainstay of attempts at curative treatment. Surgery is sometimes combined with chemotherapy and radiation. Over one third of patients have inoperable disease due to tumor involvement of mediastinal structures or distant metastases.
- Most patients will ultimately receive palliative care, and attention should focus on general supportive care with restoration of nutritional status. In order to allow the patient to eat and swallow saliva the esophageal lumen must be restored to an adequate size. This can be accomplished by per oral dilatation or radiotherapy. After dilation, esophageal stents can be placed endoscopically through the tumor in an attempt to maintain luminal patency. In addition, the stenotic lumen can be enlarged by using a laser or heater probe to ablate the tumor.

IX. Gastritis
  A. Basic science
  - Gastritis refers to inflammation of the gastric mucosa characterized by erosions and subepithelial hemorrhages and is usually due to infectious agents, most often *Helicobacter pylori,* or a hypersensitivity reaction. The term "gastropathy" refers to evidence of epithelial cell damage without mucosal inflammation and is often a result of medications such as nonsteroidal anti-inflammatory drugs (NSAIDs) or bile reflex.
  - Gastritis is classified as (1) nonatrophic most often due to *H. pylori,* (2) atrophic secondary to poorly defined autoimmune processes and possibly *H. pylori,* (3) chemical due to bile or NSAIDs, (4) radiation-induced injury, (5) noninfectious causes such as Crohn's disease and sarcoidosis, (6) eosinophilic, mainly as a result of food sensitivity, and (7) infectious cause, including *H. pylori* and cytomegalovirus.
  - Injury to the gastric mucosa can occur from a variety of sources, including the following:
    - Local injury resulting from trauma from suction through a nasogastric tube or therapeutic endoscopic techniques
    - Generalized injury due to the disruption of mucosal barrier:
      1. NSAIDs (inhibit prostaglandin synthesis)
      2. Ethanol
      3. Ischemia (decreased mucosal blood flow)
      4. Radiation
      5. Reflux of bile acids, pancreatic secretions, and duodenal contents, especially from a poorly functioning pyloroplasty or antrectomy
  - Other predisposing factors include sepsis, shock, burns, and organ system failure (heart, kidneys, lungs, liver). Acute gastritis is estimated to occur in 80% to 90% of critically ill hospitalized patients. It is very common in patients with severe burns, head injury, or severe hemorrhage.
  - Injury to the gastric mucosa allows hydrochloric acid access to unprotected gastric tissue. This results in tissue injury, which leads to mucosal friability, erosions, and extravasation of blood into the mucosa and stomach lumen.

- *Helicobacter pylori* is an important cause of gastritis characterized by superficial inflammation of the gastric mucosa. The antrum is consistently involved with variable involvement of the fundus. It is also an important cause of gastric and duodenal ulcer and is associated with primary gastric B cell lymphoma and adenocarcinoma.

B. History and physical examination
- Patients may give a history of alcohol abuse or NSAID use. Gastritis usually causes mild dyspepsia. Less common symptoms include nausea and midepigastric pain.
- Because hospitalized patients may be too ill to complain about dyspepsia or nausea, the first sign of gastritis in the hospitalized patient may be blood from the nasogastic aspirate, occult blood in stool, anemia, or abrupt GI hemorrhage with a fall in hematocrit.
- Physical examination may reveal evidence of blood loss such as pallor, tachycardia, hypotension, and dizziness. The abdominal examination is generally unremarkable.

C. Laboratory and diagnostic studies
- The diagnosis is best made by endoscopy, which allows inspection of the gastric mucosa, and permits taking of biopsies for the urease test for *H. pylori* as well as for histologic examination. Barium contrast studies are usually not helpful because the lesions are superficial.

D. Formulating the diagnosis
- Acute gastritis should be suspected based on clinical symptoms. Evidence of blood loss in a hospitalized individual should prompt evaluation for gastritis.

E. Managing the patient
- Treatment of gastritis is to remove the offending agent when possible. H_2 blockers, sucralfate, antacids, and proton pump inhibitors will facilitate healing. If gastritis is due to *H. pylori* one of several regimens that combine antimicrobials and a proton pump inhibitor should be used, such as a combination of a proton pump inhibitor, amoxicillin, and clarithromycin for 10 to 14 days. Another common strategy is to use a proton pump inhibitor combined with bismuth and two antibiotics (e.g., metronidazole and tetracycline) for 14 days.
- Patients with life-threatening gastritis may require vasopressin infusion. Endoscopic coagulation may be a temporizing measure.
- Surgery is performed for intractable hemorrhage (antrectomy with vagotomy or oversewing a regional lesion). Surgical morbidity and mortality rates can be high, depending on the severity of the associated illnesses.
- In the high-risk patient as in an ICU setting prophylactic use of intravenous H_2 blockers, proton pump inhibitors, or oral sucralfate is often used.

X. Irritable Bowel Syndrome
A. Basic science
- Irritable bowel syndrome (IBS) is caused by altered intestinal motility. This is thought to occur due to abnormalities in intestinal electrical rhythm. Intestinal

motility may decrease abnormally, leading to constipation, or increase abnormally, leading to diarrhea.

- Patients with IBS have visceral hypersensitivity and have a lower pain threshold. Stress plays a major role in the severity of symptoms. IBS is seen more frequently in females. The age of onset is typically between ages 30 and 50 years.

B. History and physical examination

- Abdominal pain is a common symptom of IBS. Bloating is common. IBS presents in one of three ways:
  1. Chronic abdominal pain with constipation
     - Patients may have a bloating sensation; heartburn and back pain are common. Pain is often relieved with flatus or passage of stool.
  2. Intermittent diarrhea
     - This is usually worse in the morning hours.
  3. Alternating constipation and diarrhea.
     - Physical examination is normal. If bleeding is present, the patient should undergo colonoscopy.

C. Laboratory and diagnostic studies

- Laboratory and diagnostic studies should eliminate other causes for the patient's symptoms. If diarrhea is present, stool studies, including examination for blood, fecal leukocytes, and cultures may be indicated. Consider testing for lactose intolerance and gluten sensitivity because these conditions can masquerade as IBS. The patient's TSH level should be checked to rule out hyperthyroidism or hypothyroidism.

D. Formulating the diagnosis

- Symptoms which are *not* typical of IBS includes abdominal pain that often awakens/interferes with sleep, weight loss, diarrhea that often awakens/interferes with sleep, blood in the stools, fever, and an abnormal physical examination.
- The Rome II diagnostic criteria of IBS always presume the absence of a structural or biochemical explanation for the symptoms.
- Irritable bowel syndrome can be diagnosed based on at least 12 weeks or more, which need not be consecutive, in the preceding 12 months, of abdominal discomfort or pain that has two out of three of these features:
  1. Relieved with defecation
  2. Onset associated with a change in frequency of stool
  3. Onset associated with a change in form (appearance) of stool
- Symptoms that cumulatively support the diagnosis of IBS:
  1. Abnormal stool frequency (may be defined as greater than three bowel movements per day and less than three bowel movements per week)
  2. Abnormal stool form (lumpy/hard or loose/watery stool)
  3. Abnormal stool passage (straining, urgency, or feeling of incomplete evacuation)
  4. Passage of mucus
  5. Bloating or feeling of abdominal distention

E. Evaluating the severity of problems
- Irritable bowel syndrome does not result in increased mortality rate. It may result in considerable morbidity.

F. Managing the patient
- Irritable bowel syndrome is a chronic condition. The patient should be reassured that the disease is not life-threatening. Changes in lifestyle and stress reduction may alleviate symptoms. Medications that may aggravate the patient's symptoms of constipation or diarrhea should be avoided.
- Management includes symptomatic treatment; loperamide, diphenoxylate, and the bile-sequestrating agent cholestyramine may be used for diarrhea, and fiber, polyethylene glycol solutions, stimulant laxatives such as phenophthalein and bisacodyl, and the prokinetic agents metoclopramide and tegaserod may be given for constipation. Bloating may respond to simethicone and abdominal pain to anticholinergics and antidepressants.

XI. Lactose Intolerance

A. Basic science
- Lactase is an enzyme located in the brush border of the small intestine. Lactase converts the disaccharide lactose into the monosaccharides glucose and galactose. Glucose and galactose are actively transported by the gut epithelium into the body. A deficiency of lactase results in the inability to digest lactose. Lactose is an osmotically active sugar and draws water into the gut lumen. Gut bacteria break down the undigested lactose producing gas and acid by-products. These cause bloating, flatus, and abdominal discomfort.
- Ninety percent of Asians, 45% of blacks, and a significant proportion of whites develop lactase deficiency after childhood.

B. History and physical examination
- A history of upset stomach, bloating, flatus and diarrhea after the consumption of milk products is classic for lactase deficiency. Patients often have a family history of lactose intolerance.
- Physical examination is normal.

C. Laboratory and diagnostic studies
- High hydrogen gas levels, measured by a gas breath analyzer, after a lactose test dose supports the diagnosis of lactase deficiency. Hydrogen is a byproduct of bacterial breakdown of lactose. In otherwise well patients, a trial of lactose avoidance that results in resolution of symptoms is sufficient to make the diagnosis without any further testing.

D. Formulating the diagnosis
- History, physical examination, and resolution of symptoms with lactose avoidance with or without the results of breath gas analysis are diagnostic for lactase deficiency. Lactase deficiency may be confused with irritable bowel syndrome.

E. Evaluating the severity of problems
- Lactase deficiency is a benign disorder that can cause significant morbidity and social embarrassment.

F. Managing the patient
- Patients should avoid milk products or other lactose-containing compounds.
- Patients may be able to tolerate lactose-containing products if they first add artificial lactase to those products.

XII. Lower Gastrointestinal Bleeding
A. Basic science
- Lower GI bleeding is the passage of blood (which may appear bright red or maroon) per rectum. It can originate from a number of sources:
  1. Brisk upper GI bleeding
  2. Diverticulosis: vessel erosion through thinned diverticular wall
  3. Ateriovenous malformation
  4. Ischemic colitis
  5. NSAIDs: secondary to colonic ulcerations
  6. Infection: *Shigella, Salmonella,* amebiasis, or *Campylobacter jejuni*
  7. Neoplasms: generally cause occult bleeding, which is not visible
  8. Inflammatory bowel disease: ulcerative colitis more often than Crohn's colitis
  9. Anal fissures, hemorrhoids and radiation colitis
B. History and physical examination
- The history should determine the amount, duration, and frequency of bleeding, color of stools, whether pain is present, past medical history of cirrhosis or other GI pathology and medications. In any patient with a bleed it is important to determine hemodynamic stability before additional physical examination is carried out and investigations done. Signs that may provide a clue to the cause of the bleed include jaundice, ecchymoses, telangiectasia or buccal pigmentation, caput medusa, ascites, abdominal distention, abdominal bruits, absent bowel sounds, and peritoneal signs. Digital rectal examination detects the presence and character of blood (gross versus occult).
- The stools are usually tarry black (melena) if the bleeding is from the upper GI tract (i.e., proximal to the ligament of Trietz). However, a brisk upper GI bleed can manifest with the passage of bright red blood per rectum and is indicative of a life-threatening bleed. If an upper GI bleed is suspected, a nasogastric tube should be passed into the stomach and the gastric contents sampled for bleeding.
- If the bleed is from diverticula, the stools are usually dark red or maroon. Pain is mild or absent. Diverticular bleeding frequently recurs.
- Infections cause abdominal pain and bloody diarrhea.
- Bleeding from a cancer is generally associated with weight loss, anemia, change in bowel habits, and bowel obstruction.
- Inflammatory bowel disease is generally associated with abdominal pain, tenesmus, and bloody diarrhea.
C. Laboratory and diagnostic studies
- A CBC, PT, and PTT serum chemistry should be done in all patients. If blood transfusion is anticipated, blood should be sent for typing and crossmatching.
- Depending on the degree and suspected site of bleeding, several different diagnostic modalities may be employed. These include anoscopy, flexible

sigmoidoscopy, and colonoscopy. Angiography is helpful if there is ongoing bleeding. Labeled red blood cells (^{99m}Tc) can be used for patients unable to undergo angiography, or if angiography is nondiagnostic.
- If upper GI bleeding is suspected or confirmed, nasogastric aspiration upper GI endoscopy should be performed.

D. Formulating the diagnosis
- Diagnosis is generally evident after history, physical examination, and diagnostic testing.

E. Evaluating the severity of problems
- Most lower GI bleeds are not life-threatening and thus do not require emergency treatment. However, if the patient appears to be hemodynamically unstable (i.e., tachycardic, hypotensive), volume resuscitation should be instituted immediately.
- Some patients may appear hemodynamically stable despite a relatively large amount of blood loss. Tachycardia is usually the first clue that they are unstable. These patients can then "crash" rather quickly. Therefore, the physician must have a high level of suspicion in each bleeding patient and be able to support them quickly with volume repletion. This requires adequate IV access (two large-bore antecubital catheters or a central venous introducer; a standard central line is inadequate), and blood products should be ready to be given at short notice.

F. Managing the patient
- The treatment of lower GI bleeding is dependent on the cause. Diverticulosis is the most common cause of massive lower GI bleeding. Arteriovenous malformations are a common cause of lower GI bleeding in the elderly. The lesions are usually located in the right colon. A hemicolectomy may be necessary in patients with persistent bleeding.
- Ischemic colitis is a GI manifestation of atherosclerotic vascular disease. The bleeding is generally mild and self-limited. However, if the ischema is left untreated, the consequence can be fatal.
- The management of other causes of lower GI bleeding (e.g., inflammatory bowel disease, hemorrhoids, cancer) is discussed elsewhere.

XIII. Peptic Ulcer Disease
A. Basic science
- Peptic ulcer disease (PUD) is defined as an ulceration of the stomach or duodenum mucosa. Pepsin and hydrochloric acid play a role in the formation of ulcerations and erosions in the gastrointestinal mucosa. Hydrochloric acid is secreted by parietal cells in the stomach. Hydrochloric acid production is regulated by both neurohumeral (vagus nerve) and hormonal influences (e.g., gastrin, histamine, and acetylcholine). Hydrochloric acid production lowers stomach pH, which activates the enzyme pepsin.
- The stomach and duodenum are covered by a thick coat of bicarbonate-laden mucus that protects the mucosa from enzymatic degradation. Prostaglandins, produced by the mucosa, enhance the stability of the mucous layer. Genetic

factors appear to play a role in peptic ulcer formation, as does susceptibility to *H. pylori* infection, which is an important cause of gastric and duodenal ulcers.

- Peptic ulcers arise when the mucosal defense mechanisms are overwhelmed. This may occur by either of two mechanisms:
  1. Ineffective defensive barrier
     - The most common causes:
       a. *H. pylori* infection causes ulceration by disrupting the mucosal barrier.
       b. NSAIDs (worse when combined with corticosteroids) lead to ulceration by inhibiting the prostaglandin-mediated mucosal barrier.
       c. Severe physiologic stress, such as seen in patients with major burns or septic shock, can lead to ulceration.
  2. Overproduction of hydrochloric acid
     a. Hypersecretion of gastrin (Zollinger-Ellison syndrome)
     b. Mastocytosis
- Duodenal ulcers occur in the first few centimeters of the duodenal bulb. Gastric ulcers are mostly located in the lesser curvature of the stomach.

B. History and physical examination
- Typically, the patient presents with epigastric pain approximately 2 to 3 hours after a meal. The pain is described as boring, burning, dull, aching, or nagging. Epigastric pain that awakens the patient from sleep is characteristic. Most patients have pain relief when they eat food. The pain may radiate to the back. Patients may also be completely asymptomatic, as can often be seen with NSAID-induced PUD.
- Physical examination may reveal some upper abdominal tenderness; however, the examination may be entirely normal. Weight loss occurs in 50% of those with benign ulcers, but cancer must be considered when weight loss is present.
- Patients with active bleeding ulcers may present with anemia, melena, or hematemesis. Perforation, a complication of duodenal ulcers, may present as abrupt, severe pain radiating to the back. On examination peritoneal signs are present.

C. Laboratory and diagnostic studies
- In patients taking NSAIDs or with other risk factors, endoscopy is the preferred initial study for the detection of peptic ulcer disease. If a gastric ulcer is found, a biopsy should be performed to rule out malignancy. Duodenal ulcers are rarely associated with malignancy. Gastric biopsies should also be taken to detect *H. pylori* infection.
- Initial laboratory studies include a complete blood count (to determine if anemia is present). If the clinical picture suggests posterior penetration of the ulcer into the pancreas, amylase and lipase levels should be measured. If a perforation is suspected, erect plain x-rays of the abdomen should be taken to rule out perforation. Analysis of gastric acid and gastrin levels are appropriate if there is concern for Zollinger-Ellison syndrome. However, gastrin is secreted in response to low pH levels. Therefore, the gastrin levels will be elevated if the patient is taking antacids, H_2-receptor blockers, or proton pump inhibitors.

D. Formulating the diagnosis
- Peptic ulcer disease should be considered in any patient with upper abdominal pain. An active GI bleed should be considered in the patient presenting with hematemesis, bloody stools, unexplained anemia, or orthostatic symptoms.
- The differential diagnosis in patients with symptoms suggestive of PUD includes nonulcer dyspepsia, gastritis, pancreatitis, aortic dissection, and gallbladder disease.

E. Evaluating the severity of problems
- Massive GI bleed is a medical emergency calling for rapid and aggressive fluid resuscitation, packed red blood cell transfusions, and therapeutic intervention. GI perforation is a medical emergency calling for immediate surgical consultation and surgery.

F. Managing the patient
- In the absence of symptoms such as weight loss or anemia or a history of NSAID use, empiric antisecretory therapy with or without *H. pylori* testing is a reasonable approach to treating patients with dyspeptic symptoms. If risk factors (i.e., NSAID use) are present, then endoscopy should be performed.
- Empirically treated patients should respond to therapy in 7 to 10 days. If symptoms persist, *H. pylori* should be ruled out by noninvasive means and eradicated if present. If noninvasive *H. pylori* testing is negative, endoscopy should be done.
  1. Medications
     - Antacids reduce the amount of acid in the stomach. Antacids should be given 1 hour after meals and at bedtime. Poor compliance due to taste, frequency of intake, and diarrhea limit the use of antacids as single therapy.
     - H_2 antagonists, such as cimetidine, ranitidine, nizatidine, and famotidine, work to block the action of histamine and subsequently acid secretion. Decreased hydrochloric acid production inhibits the activation of pepsin. Proton pump inhibitors such as omeprazole and lansoprazole work by preventing acid secretion by blocking H^+K^+-ATPase.
     - Eradication of *H. pylori* in affected individuals dramatically reduces ulcer recurrence. Currently used regimens to eradicate *H. pylori* use a combination of antimicrobial agents and a proton pump inhibitor.
- All patients with active GI bleeding on presentation must be monitored closely for signs of hypovolemia and exsanguination. Vital signs, orthostatic blood pressures, and hemoglobin or hematocrit must be monitored closely. Fluid resuscitation and use of packed red blood cells are indicated in unstable patients. Gastric aspiration via nasogastric tube should be attempted.
- Red blood indicates an active bleed. Samples that resemble coffee grounds suggest bleeding that has stopped. Active bleeding may require emergent endoscopy to treat any bleeding vessels by injection, heater probe coagulation, or endo-clipping. In the event that endoscopic maneuvers cannot stop the bleeding, emergent surgery is indicated.
- Patients with an acute abdomen should proceed to surgery rather than have endoscopic evaluation; these patients may have a perforated bowel or incarcerated paraesophageal hernia.

XIV. Ulcerative Colitis
   A. Basic science
- Ulcerative colitis (UC) is a chronic, episodic, inflammatory disease of the large intestine and rectum. It is characterized by blood and mucus diarrhea.
- Ulcerative colitis has a bimodal peak of onset occurring in the second and sixth decades. Smoking has been shown to have somewhat of a protective affect against UC.

   B. History and physical examination
- Attacks of blood and mucus diarrhea are accompanied by tenesmus, abdominal pain, fever, chills, anemia, and weight loss. Children with this disease may suffer retarded physical growth. The debilitating symptoms often prevent the patient from carrying on the normal activities of daily living.
- Additionally patients may have other non-GI symptoms such as arthritis, erythema nodosum, pyoderma gangrenosum, or uveitis.
- If extraintestinal manifestations are absent, the physical examination is often normal.

   C. Laboratory and diagnostic studies
- Serum chemistries may show a low albumin. Erythrocyte sedimentation rate (ESR) is elevated and there may be anemia.
- Barium x-rays will demonstrate loss of haustra in the colon and mucosal ulceration. Flexible sigmoidoscopy or colonoscopy will show continuous and circumferential erythema and ulceration; the rectum is invariably involved, and aphthous ulcers are rarely present.
- Stool cultures must be sent to rule out infectious diarrhea as the source of the patient's symptoms.

   D. Formulating the diagnosis
- Diagnosis of the disease is based on the history, physical examination, the results of barium x-ray films of the colon, and colonoscopy with biopsy. It may be difficult to differentiate ulcerative colitis from Crohn's disease.

   E. Evaluating the severity of problems
- Toxic megacolon is a life-threatening complication of ulcerative colitis. The colon dilates and loses tone causing an ileus. Toxic megacolon may lead to perforation, septicemia, and death. If treatment is not instituted immediately, 40% of patients will die.

   F. Managing the patient
- Patients need periodic colonoscopy to detect occult GI cancers. Colonoscopy should be performed 7 years after the first severe UC flare. Specific therapy for ulcerative colitis includes the use of anticholinergics and loperamide to relieve cramps and diarrhea and sulfasalazine to decrease chronic inflammation. Other aminosalicylates include mesalamine, olsalazine, and balasalazide. Corticosteriods are effective for acute exacerbations.
- Immunosuppressive agents azathioprine and 6-mercaptopurine are used in refractory patients. These agents take months to work.
- Neither elemental diet nor bowel rest have been shown to alter the course of the disease.

- Patients with severe disease of life-threatening complications (toxic megacolon, cancer) usually require surgery. Total proctocolectomy with ileostomy is a permanent cure for ulcerative colitis. Patients with toxic megacolon should be started on ampicillin and gentamicin, made NPO, placed on IV hydration and IV steroids, and watched closely for signs of peritonitis.

XV. Upper Gastrointestinal Bleeding
  A. Basic science
    - Upper GI bleeding may be due to any of the following:
      1. Capillary bleeding (e.g., due to gastritis from ethanol or nonsteroidal usage)
      2. Venous bleeding (e.g., due to esophageal varices and usually due to liver disease with associated portal hypertension)
      3. Coagulopathies and other serious medical problems
        - High mortality rate is associated with this type of bleeding.
      4. Arterial bleeding due to ulcer erosion into one of the gastric arteries
        - This may also result from fistula formation between aorta and duodenum. The mortality rate is high in these situations.
  B. History and physical examination
    - The following elements of the history are important:
      1. Duration of the bleeding
      2. Hematochezia (defecating blood): may indicate rapid upper GI bleed; more usually it is due to a lower GI bleed
      3. Hematemesis (vomiting blood): indicative of upper GI bleed
      4. Ethanol: chronic heavy drinking associated with gastritis, alcoholic cirrhosis, and esophageal varices
      5. NSAIDs: chronic nonsteroidal use is associated with gastritis and peptic ulcer disease
      6. Pain: raises the possibility that the lesion is inflammatory (e.g., gastritis, esophagitis, peptic ulcer disease)
      7. Painless GI bleeding: indicative of noninflammatory lesions such as varices or cancer
      8. History of severe vomiting and hematemesis: may indicate a Mallory-Weiss tear
      9. Past medical history of cirrhosis, varices, bleeding disorders, epistaxis, peptic ulcer disease, or cancer: may point to a particular pathologic state
    - Pallor, tachycardia (pulse above 100), decreased blood pressure (systolic BP below 100), or orthostatic blood pressure changes are signs of significant blood loss and hemodynamic instability. An abdominal mass may be felt if a cancer is present. Signs of cirrhosis or portal hypertension (splenomegaly, caput medusae, and ascites) may indicate esophageal varices.
  C. Laboratory and diagnostic studies
    - Endoscopy is the diagnostic study of choice for identifying the cause of upper GI bleeding. Angiography may be helpful if endoscopy does not detect the bleeding lesion and the patient continues to bleed.
    - All patients should have a CBC and serum chemistries including liver function tests, PT, and PTT.

- A nasogastric tube should be passed into the patient's stomach and gastric fluid aspirated to check for bright red blood (active bleeding) or a coffee ground appearance (intermittent bleeding). A negative aspirate does not exclude upper GI bleeding.

D. Formulating the diagnosis

- History, physical findings and endoscopic findings will establish the cause of the GI bleed in the majority of patients. Concurrently with the diagnosis of GI bleeding, the physician needs to assess the degree of GI bleeding and institute IV fluids and blood transfusions as needed.
- Bleeding may be classified as follows:
    1. Occult bleed: no hemodynamic instability.
    2. Overt bleed: acute bleeding with stable vital signs and hematocrit
    3. Massive bleed: acute bleeding with unstable vital signs

E. Evaluating the severity of problems

- Active GI bleeding is a medical emergency. Major complications of upper GI bleeding occur with aspiration of blood. Therefore, patients with no gag reflex or who are unconscious should be intubated.

F. Managing the patient

1. Occult bleeding

- Endoscopy or barium contrast studies, on a nonemergent basis, should be done to establish the diagnosis. Treatment depends on the pathologic entity.

2. Overt and massive GI bleeding

- The patient should be stabilized; this includes the following:
- Vital signs are frequently measured.
- IV fluids (two large-bore IVs) are given.
- Packed red blood cells are needed to keep hematocrit above 30.
- Perform continuous gastric aspiration (NG tube).
- Endoscopy should be performed to localize the bleeding site. Treatment depends on the pathologic entity.
- Gastritis is treated with proton pump inhibitors, H_2 blockers and antacids. *H. pylori* infection must be treated.
- Bleeding ulcer is treated by heat cautery, injection sclerosis, or, in cases of recalcitrant bleeding, partial gastrectomy.
- Esophageal varices are treated with vasopressin, endoscopic sclerotherapy, or a Sengstaken-Blakemore tube (esophageal tamponade tubes). In cases of recalcitrant bleeding, transjugular intrahepatic portasystemic shunt (TIPS) or portacaval shunt surgery should be considered.

7 CHAPTER

Psychiatry

I. Adjustment Disorders
   A. Basic science
   - An adjustment disorder is defined as the development of emotional or behavioral symptoms in response to an identifiable stressor occurring within 3 months of the stressor. The symptoms do not exceed 6 months, unless the stressor becomes chronic or has enduring consequences. There is marked distress in excess of what would be expected given the circumstances or it leads to marked social or occupational dysfunction.
   - Disturbed emotions occurring in the course of an adjustment disorder include depressed mood, anxious mood, or a combination of both. Disturbances of conduct also can develop (violence, truancy, reckless driving, and so on), especially in children. Other possible manifestations include physical complaints, social withdrawal, or a decline in work or academic performance. These patients do not meet the criteria for major depression or a full-blown anxiety disorder. If the disturbance lasts for more than 6 months in the absence of enduring stressors, other diagnoses should be considered.
   - The prevalence of adjustment disorders ranges from 2% to 8% of the general population. They are a common psychiatric diagnosis in patients hospitalized for medical or surgical problems.
   B. History and physical examination
   - A careful psychiatric history and mental status examination must be performed. A physical examination is also helpful to rule out potential medical causes for the presenting symptoms.
   C. Laboratory and diagnostic studies
   - As with all acute presentations, an organic cause must be excluded; however, there are no laboratory evaluations routinely used to make the diagnosis of adjustment disorder.
   D. Formulating the diagnosis
   - Adjustment disorders should be distinguished from normal bereavement and from the anticipated emotional and behavioral disturbances that patients with personality disorders exhibit when exposed to stress. Also, they differ from posttraumatic stress disorders.
   - Complications of adjustment disorders include the development of a major depressive episode, substantial psychosocial impairment, and suicidal ideation.
   E. Evaluating the severity of problems
   - Suicidal assessment should always be done. If suicidal ideation is present, patients require aggressive therapy, generally including hospitalization.

F. Managing the patient
- The treatment of adjustment disorders varies depending on the circumstances. Supportive individual psychotherapy, group therapy, and marital and family therapies can all be of substantial help. Social interventions (e.g., changing work or school environments or temporary disability) may aid in speeding resolution of the disorder.
- Pharmacologic interventions, mostly benzodiazepines, may assist in the management of severe anxiety or agitation. The use of antidepressants for "adjustment disorder with depressed mood" is frequently practiced but remains controversial. Psychiatric hospitalization is reserved for suicidal patients who require close supervision.

II. Anxiety Disorders
  A. Basic science
- Anxiety disorders, as a group, are the most common psychiatric disorders with a 12-month prevalence rate as high as 25%. Anxiety is characterized by a sense of foreboding or dread and can occur for no obvious reason (primary). It may also be a result of an illness or be a medication side effect (secondary).
- The primary anxiety disorders are panic disorder, social phobia, obsessive-compulsive disorder, posttraumatic stress disorder, and generalized anxiety disorder. Social phobia is the most common anxiety disorder. A blend of physical and environmental triggers combine to create anxiety disorders. First-degree relatives of individuals with panic disorder are four to eight times more likely to develop panic disorder.
  B. History and physical examination
    1. Panic disorder
- Panic disorder has a lifetime prevalence of 1.5% to 3.5%, and is more commonly diagnosed in females. The first attack typically occurs in late adolescence or early adulthood.
- Panic attacks are discrete periods in which there is a sudden unexplained intense apprehension, fearfulness, or terror, often associated with a sense of doom. Physical symptoms, such as shortness of breath, palpitations, chest pain, choking, or smothering sensations are present. Often the patient fears losing control or going crazy.
- Panic disorder is recurrent, unpredictable panic attacks followed by at least 1 month of persistent concern about having another panic attack. This may be associated with agoraphobia, which is anxiety about or avoidance of places and situations from which escape might be difficult. Agoraphobia can occur without panic attacks.
    2. Social phobia
- Social phobia is the resultant anxiety provoked by exposure to certain types of social or performance situations and often leads to avoidant behavior.
    3. Obsessive-compulsive disorders (OCD)
- The lifetime prevalence of OCD is 2% to 3% in the general population. Individuals with obsessive-compulsive disorder have pervasive obsessions, defined as persistent ideas, thoughts, impulses, or images that are intrusive,

or compulsive behaviors, defined as ritualistic or repetitive behaviors or mental acts that serve to neutralize anxiety and often disrupt the patient's life.

- The most common obsessions are repeated thoughts about contamination, repeated doubts, a need to have things in order, horrifying images, and sexual imagery. Common compulsions include handwashing, ordering, and checking. Mental acts typically are praying or counting or repeating words silently.
- Individuals usually recognize that the obsessions and compulsions are excessive and unreasonable. The severity of the illness fluctuates.

4. Posttraumatic stress disorder (PTSD)
- PTSD is characterized by the re-experiencing of an extremely traumatic event, usually as dreams and intrusions of traumatic events in one's thoughts, and accompanied by symptoms of increased arousal, such as hypervigilence, irritability, and an exaggerated startle response, and by avoidance of any stimuli associated with the trauma.
- The lifetime prevalence of PTSD in the general population is 8%.
- Individuals who suffer from PTSD are prone to developing problems with substance abuse, especially alcohol.

5. Generalized anxiety disorder (GAD)
- GAD is twice as commonly diagnosed in females. The prevalence in the general population is 5%.
- It is characterized by persistent and excessive anxiety and uncontrollable worry lasting at least 6 months. Somatic symptoms and symptoms of increased arousal are present and are similar to the experienced in a panic attack. GAD is often associated with major depression or dysthymia.

C. Laboratory and diagnostic studies
- Laboratory testing is usually done to rule out medical conditions or substance use leading to symptoms of anxiety and typically includes thyroid function tests, complete blood count (CBC), glucose, electrolytes, urine toxin screen and calcium. An electrocardiogram (ECG) should be considered during an attack. Panic attacks can be precipitated by carbon dioxide inhalation or sodium lactate infusion. Some studies suggest a higher incidence of mitral valve prolapse in those with panic disorder.

D. Formulating the diagnosis
- Medical illness, iatrogenic causes, and toxicologic effects may be the source of the patient's anxiety and should be excluded. Central nervous stimulants (such as cocaine, amphetamines, and caffeine), medications (such as high-dose steroids), central nervous system depressants (such as barbiturates and alcohol), endocrine diseases (such as hyperthyroidism, hyperparathyroidism, and pheochromocytoma), respiratory diseases (such as chronic obstructive pulmonary disease, pneumonia, hyperventilation, and pulmonary embolus) and cardiac disorders (such as arrhythmias) should be excluded.

E. Evaluating the severity of problems
- Coexistence of several anxiety disorders is common. Major depression and substance abuse often coexist in individuals with anxiety disorders. It is always

very important to assess for safety. The risk of suicide should be assessed in all patients with an anxiety disorder.

F. Managing the patient

- Antidepressants are the treatment of choice for the majority of the anxiety disorders. Selective serotonin reuptake inhibitors (SSRIs) are usually effective and are the first line of treatment. Other antidepressants such as tricyclic antidepressants and monoamine oxidase inhibitors (MAOIs) have also been used. MAOIs are particularly effective for social anxiety and refractory anxiety disorders. Obsessive-compulsive disorder can be successfully treated with clomipramine, fluoxetine, or fluvoxamine. Cloimipramine is often poorly tolerated because of its potent anticholinergic effects.

- Benzodiazepines such as diazepam, lorazepam, alprazolam, and clonazepam effectively treat anxiety-related symptoms of hyperarousal. However, there exists potential for abuse and development of tolerance with this type of medication and such drugs should be used on a short term basis.

- Psychotherapy and somatic treatments are known to be effective. Cognitive behavioral therapy has been shown to successfully treat anxiety disorders.

III. Attention Deficit Hyperactivity Disorder

A. Basic science

- Attention deficit hyperactivity disorder (ADHD) affects 3% to 7% of elementary school children. The prevalence of this disorder is four to five times higher in boys than in girls. ADHD is thought to be a childhood disorder; however, long-term prospective studies indicate that a significant subset of children with ADHD continue to manifest symptoms into adulthood and continue to require medication.

- ADHD is thought to be a disorder of the neurotransmitter systems in the brain that control sustained attention, impulsivity, and motor activity. The neurotransmitters dopamine and norepinephrine have been implicated as the primary modulators of attention and arousal in the central nervous system (CNS). The dopamine hypothesis of ADHD suggests that the depletion of dopamine, or the unavailability of dopamine to receptors, results in the alteration of sustained attention and arousal. Siblings of children with ADHD are twice as likely to develop ADHD. Parents have a higher incidence of alcohol abuse, sociopathy, hyperkinesis, and conversion disorder.

B. History and physical examination

- Most children presenting for evaluation of possible ADHD symptoms do so between the ages of 6 and 12 years. Typically symptoms of motor hyperactivity and impulsivity result in problematic behavior in the classroom setting and at home.

- Core symptoms of ADHD are the following: excessive or inappropriate motor activity, difficulty with tasks requiring sustained attention, and difficulties with impulse control. Some children have predominantly hyperactive symptoms, and others may have predominantly inattentive symptoms.

- Evaluation may consist primarily of obtaining clinical history, observing the patient, and obtaining collaborative data from other sources such as school.

C. Laboratory and diagnostic studies
- There are no medical tests specifically designed for the evaluation of ADHD. The diagnosis must always be made by combining the clinical presentation and history of the patient with supportive data obtained from other resources such as the classroom teacher or psychometric tests.

D. Formulating the diagnosis
- The diagnosis of ADHD is based on the presence of core clinical symptoms. The existence of an underlying learning disability needs to be considered in every child presenting with ADHD symptoms. This may be assessed by careful consultation with the classroom teacher or may require more extensive psychological testing such as an IQ or achievement test. Children also will need assessment for underlying medical conditions, which may include lead toxicity, fetal alcohol syndrome, thyroid dysfunction, other endocrine abnormalities, and brain injury. Children with mental retardation, pervasive developmental disorder, and other developmental disorders are also frequently distracted and inattentive.

E. Evaluating the severity of problems
- Consultation with a pediatric neurologist is indicated for those children who may have complex symptoms such as absence seizures or tic disorders. Child psychiatrists are frequently consulted when there are complex underlying psychosocial issues or other psychiatric diagnoses present.

F. Managing the patient
- The treatment of ADHD requires an approach that coordinates school-based services, parents, physicians, and therapists. Prognosis is optimized by improving the child's social functioning, diminishing aggression, improving family environment, and treating co-morbid depression or anxiety.
- Nonpharmacologic treatments include classroom changes such as smaller teacher-to-student ratios, social skills training, and remedial services for any learning disabilities. Therapies that teach the child to think of alternative behaviors before acting on impulse have proven successful. Parent education and training focused on parenting skills can be extremely useful and are always a necessary part of any treatment program.
- For children requiring pharmacologic interventions, medications can be highly effective in alleviating symptoms. Stimulant medications are the first line of therapy and include methylphenidate and dextroamphetamine. The most common side effects of stimulant treatment may include insomnia, decreased appetite, tics, irritability, and decreased growth rate. Nonstimulant medications used in the treatment of ADHD include bupropion, atamoxetine, and α-adrenergic agonists such as clonidine and guanfacine.

IV. Delirium and Dementia
A. Basic science
- Delirium is a syndrome that is a direct consequence of a general medical condition. The hallmark of delirium is impairment in consciousness, occurring with global impairment of cognitive function. Agitation, hallucinations, and tremors may also be present.

- Causes of delirium include substance intoxication or withdrawal, medications, postoperative states, hypoxia, metabolic abnormalities resulting from renal, hepatic, or pulmonary disease, infections, and frequently a combination of these factors. Patients with CNS disease (e.g., dementia or cerebrovascular accidents), elderly patients, and patients with hearing or visual impairment are more susceptible to a delirium.
- Dementia is characterized by chronic, global, nonreversible intellectual impairment with memory deficits and at least one of the following: aphasia, apraxia, agnosia, or a disturbance in executive function. The deficits represent a decline from a previous level of functioning and cause significant impairment in social or occupational functioning.
- Alzheimer's disease is the most common cause of dementia, representing 50% to 60% of those diagnosed with dementia.
- Vascular dementia, which is secondary to cerebrovascular diseases, represents approximately 20% of cases.
- Other causes of dementia include alcoholic dementia, metabolic abnormalities (hypothyroidism, vitamin B_{12} deficiency), human immunodeficiency virus (HIV) infection, hydrocephalus, neoplasms, Huntington's disease, head trauma, infections, Parkinson's disease, postanoxia, and combinations of these. Dementias can also be categorized as cortical (Alzheimer's, frontal lobe, degeneration), subcortical (Parkinson's disease, Huntington's disease, HIV, multiple sclerosis, Wilson's disease), or mixed (vascular).

B. History and physical examination
- A complete history and thorough physical examination is imperative in evaluating any change in mental status. Onset, clinical course, and baseline function must be established. The history often differentiates delirium from dementia.
- Delirium usually has an acute onset with a fluctuating course, sleep-awake alteration, and impairment of attention, disorientation, and rapid improvement when the causative factor is identified and corrected. Hallucinations, delusions, and psychomotor agitation or retardation may also be present. Alcohol withdrawal delirium (i.e., delirium tremens) occurs 2 to 7 days after cessation of alcohol intake and is characterized by confusion, visual or tactile hallucinations, tremor, agitation, and autonomic hyperactivity.
- Dementia commonly has an insidious onset and is chronically progressive with deficits predominantly in memory. Judgment, calculation, language, and problem-solving are affected. Hallucinations, psychomotor agitation, disorientation, and attention difficulties occur less frequently. Delirium superimposed on dementia is not uncommon.
- A careful physical examination must be performed, including complete neurologic and mental status examinations, with emphasis on cognitive functioning. Mini-mental status examinations may be helpful as a screening tool and gauge of severity of impairment. Formal neuropsychological testing may also be of value. Bilateral asterixis (a flapping tremor) of the hands is typically seen in delirium due to hepatic, renal, or pulmonary induced metabolic states.

C. Laboratory and diagnostic studies
- Laboratory data are useful in determining possible causes of mental status changes. The underlying cause of a delirium must be established to render appropriate treatment. The workup may include CBC with differential count, sedimentation rate, complete blood chemistries including liver and renal function tests, arterial blood gas, urinalysis, urine drug screen, drug levels, appropriate cultures (e.g., urine, blood), an ECG, a chest x-ray, a computed tomographic (CT) scan of the head, and, if indicated, a lumbar puncture.
- In evaluating dementia, potentially reversible causes must be identified. Laboratory evaluation includes the workup just described with the addition of vitamin B_{12} and folate levels, thyroid function tests, HIV tests, heavy metals, rapid plasma reagin (RPR), and electroencephalogram (EEG) as clinically appropriate.

D. Formulating the diagnosis
- The differential diagnosis of an acute change in mental status includes delirium, dementia, and primary psychiatric disorders such as depression, schizophrenia, mania, and dissociative disorders. Previous psychiatric history, course of illness, and impairment in level of consciousness and cognition will differentiate delirium from other psychiatric conditions.
- Dementia must be differentiated from benign senescent forgetfulness, which lacks the impairment in social or occupational functions of dementia; delirium that has an acute onset, and fluctuating level of consciousness; and depression, or "pseudo-dementia." Depressed patients must be distinguished from those with dementia by history of previous depression, complaints about cognitive deficits, lack of effort in responses, and inconsistent results in cognitive testing. Patients with dementia may also develop depressive disorders.

E. Evaluating the severity of problems
- Medical illness often complicates delirium and dementia; the magnitude of organic disease should be aggressively sought as symptoms may be masked by the patient's mental state.

F. Managing the patient
- The primary treatment of delirium is the identification and correction of the underlying cause. The patient should be placed in a safe environment with close monitoring. Restraints may be necessary to ensure safety. Vital signs, fluid input and output, and appropriate laboratory tests should be monitored. All nonessential medications should be discontinued.
- High-potency neuroleptics such as haloperidol or atypical antipsychotics are used to treat target symptoms, including hallucinations, delusions, paranoia, anxiety, and agitation. The initial dose of haloperidol may be from 0.5 mg to 10 mg IM depending on the patient's age, weight, and medical condition. The total dose in a 24-hour period necessary to calm the patient is then given in divided doses on a routine basis. Short- or intermediate-acting benzodiazepines such as lorazepam are preferred for insomnia or agitation. Once the delirium has cleared, the neuroleptic should be tapered over the next week to a month.
- Alcohol withdrawal delirium is treated using adequate doses of benzodiazepines (higher doses than those used for uncomplicated alcohol withdrawal).

Multivitamins, folate, and thiamine should also be given. Antipsychotics are sometimes needed to control severe agitation, delusions, or hallucinations.

- Reversible causes of dementia must be treated. Other causes are managed through supportive interventions. Treat any concurrent medical conditions.
- Behavioral difficulties may be successfully treated through nonpharmacologic interventions such as frequent reorientation and the provision of a consistent, safe, familiar environment.
- Associated depression should be treated with antidepressants. SSRIs are preferred over tricyclic antidepressants, which have anticholinergic side effects that can induce a confusional state, particularly in the elderly.
- Low-potency neuroleptics and benzodiazepines and should be avoided. Educational and supportive interventions are helpful to the family and caregivers.
- Treatment of Alzheimer's disease includes acetylcholinesterase inhibitors such as donepezil, rivastigmine, galantamine, and memantamine. These cognitive enhancing agents do not stop the cognitive decline but may slow the rate of decline by 6 months to a year. The cholinesterase inhibitors have cholinergic effects, such as nausea, vomiting, diarrhea, and bradycardia; the dosage must be tapered very slowly.

V. Eating Disorders: Anorexia, Bulimia, and Obesity
   A. Basic science
      - Eating disorders include anorexia nervosa and bulimia nervosa and are characterized by a pattern of disturbed or unconventional feeding habits. These conditions share some features but are distinct entities. They frequently begin in childhood and adolescent years, potentially lasting into adulthood.
      - Anorexia is defined by preoccupation with body image, refusal to maintain ideal body weight, intense fear of gaining weight, purposeful behavior directed at losing weight, and amenorrhea.
      - Bulimia is more prevalent than anorexia and includes recurrent binge eating and recurrent inappropriate behaviors to compensate for binge eating, such as self-induced vomiting.
      - Obesity is classified in the DSM-IV as a physical condition that is affected by psychological factors and which may result from overeating to reduce anxiety or a failure to perceive appetite, hunger, and satiety.
      - A combination of genetic, biologic, and environmental factors may predispose one to eating disorders.
   B. History and physical examination
      1. Anorexia nervosa
         - Anorexia typically begins in early adolescence and rarely occurs after age 40; it is characterized by a body weight 15% below expected normal for age and height. It is 10 to 20 times more common in females. Anorexia nervosa is potentially fatal in nearly one fifth of cases. It is more common in Western culture where there is an abundance of food and where attractiveness is linked to being thin.

- Resulting amenorrhea is usually secondary to weight loss, and in prepubescent females menarche may be delayed by this illness.
- It is rare for the victim of anorexia to complain of weight loss; most individuals are brought to professionals by friends or family after a substantial weight loss has occurred. Patients with anorexia nervosa maintain considerable denial and are prone to a lack of insight. Therefore, it is necessary to obtain further history from the family or other outside sources to assess the degree of weight loss.
- Anorexia is commonly associated with comorbid depression, social phobia, and obsessive-compulsive disorder.
- Serious cognitive distortions exist, including descriptions of intense fear of gaining weight or becoming fat, even though one is underweight. A disturbance of perception of one's body weight, shape, or size leads to claims of "feeling fat" even when emaciated.
- In females, amenorrhea, or evidence of three consecutive missed menstrual cycles, is included diagnostically. Examination will reveal a thin individual who may have bradycardia and hypotension. Hypercaroteinemia may be present in those who eat large amounts of vegetables.

2. Bulimia nervosa
- Bulimia combines the morbid fear of obesity with an equally compelling passion for eating. It is manifested by recurrent episodes of binge eating, lack of control, overeating, and routine self-induced vomiting or purging. To prevent weight gain, bulimic patients follow strict diets, abuse laxatives and diuretics, and exercise excessively. Along with marked overconcern with body shape and weight, these individuals ingest sweet, high-calorie food such as ice cream and cake.
- Individuals with bulimia nervosa typically are female, are within normal weight range, and have a higher rate of mood and anxiety disorders than average. Substance abuse involving alcohol and stimulants occurs in about one third of cases.
- Self-induced vomiting can lead to finger lacerations and calluses, dental caries, and characteristic "moth-eaten" teeth. Further common findings include salivary gland swelling, and repeated vomiting can lead to metabolic alkalosis, esophageal tears, and cardiac arrhythmias. Cardiomyopathy may occur with the abuse of syrup of ipecac.

3. Obesity
- Obesity is defined as a body mass index of greater than 30 kg/m². Obesity may contribute to various medical ailments, including orthopedic abnormalities, hypertension, diabetes, hyperlipidemia and reduced respiratory capacity, which may progress to pickwickian syndrome.

C. Laboratory and diagnostic studies
- Laboratory abnormalities found in anorexia nervosa include subtle hematologic (anemia) and chemical profile changes. Elevated blood urea nitrogen due to dehydration, metabolic alkalosis, and sinus bradycardia on ECG may also be present.

- Purging behavior in bulimia nervosa can lead to electrolyte abnormalities including lowered serum sodium, potassium, and chloride. Loss of stomach acid via emesis produces a metabolic alkalosis; and elevated serum amylase (salivary isoenzymes) may be found because of excessive vomiting.
- Diagnostic studies (including skeletal imaging, pulmonary function tests, and a cardiovascular workup) may be necessary to evaluate the potential consequences of obesity. Thyroid function studies should be done to ensure that hypothyroidism is not contributing to obesity.

D. Formulating the diagnosis
- Anorexia nervosa must be differentiated from bulimia as well as other causes of weight loss. Organic causes include hypothalamic-pituitary axis tumors, Addison's disease, hyperthyroidism, and various GI disorders. In addition, psychiatric conditions such as depression, drug dependence, somatization disorders, and psychotic disorders, with delusions regarding food, may result in significant weight loss.
- Bulimia must be distinguished from anorexia and psychiatric disorders including depression and dysthymia.
- Organic causes of obesity include hypothalamic lesions and hypothyroidism.

E. Evaluating the severity of problems
- Patients with anorexia nervosa can become so malnourished that hospitalization is necessary for parenteral hyperalimentation.
- Serious electrolyte derangements may occur in bulimics secondary to laxative abuse and vomiting; these should be sought and corrected.

F. Managing the patient
- Depending on the degree of weight loss in anorexia, admission to an inpatient psychiatric or medical unit may be required. The mainstay of treatment focuses on weight gain and monitoring and correction of metabolic complications. Treatment includes setting goals of desired weight with supervision of meals. In severe cases nutritional supplements and nasogastric feedings may be in order. Pharmacotherapy has limited efficacy; except when depression coexists. Psychotherapy is aimed at changing attitudes and distorted body images.
- In bulimia nervosa, hospitalization to correct life-threatening electrolyte and metabolic abnormalities may be required. Psychotherapy is aimed at normalizing eating habits and attitudes about food and the individual's pursuit of ideal body weight. Antidepressants have been shown to reduce bingeing and purging behaviors in bulimia independent of depression.
- In the treatment of obesity, low-calorie diets offer immediate, accessible weight loss methods. Unfortunately, these results are often temporary. Such diets lower the body's resting metabolic rate to an energy-conserving level that thwarts further desirable weight loss. One way to avoid this problem is regular exercise to return the resting metabolic rate to normal levels. A combination of social supports, group therapy, self-help programs (such as Weight Watchers), and behavioral therapies have shown to be more effective than pharmacologic treatment.
- Studies reveal that it is easy to take off weight but very difficult to keep it off. The short- and long-term effects of therapies for obesity vary greatly. Appetite

suppressants are moderately successful, though only while being taken. In the long term, behavior therapies and cognitive treatments tend to be more efficacious than medication, but all three treatments generate similar and modest outcomes. Surgical techniques such as vertical banded gastroplasty, adjustable gastric banding, and Roux-en-Y gastric bypass are being increasingly carried out in morbidly obese persons (BMI > 40 kg/m^2) or in those individuals with a BMI of 35 to 40 kg/m^2 if they have comorbidities such as diabetes.

VI. Mood Disorders
   A. Basic science
   - Mood disorders are characterized by a disturbance in mood along with changes in activity level, cognitive abilities, and socio-occupational functioning.
   - There are primarily two types of mood disorders: major depressive disorder (unipolar depression) and bipolar disorder (manic-depressive illness). Whereas patients suffering from major depressive disorder experience single or recurrent episodes of depression, those suffering from bipolar disorder experience episodes of mania (bipolar I) or hypomania (bipolar II) with or without episodes of depression.
   - The lifetime prevalence for major depressive disorder ranges from 10% to 25% for females and 5% to 12% for males. The onset is frequently between the ages of 20 and 50. The lifetime prevalence for bipolar disorder is equal for men and women and ranges from 0.5% to 1.6%. The onset of bipolar disorder is usually earlier than major depression and occurs in the second or third decade of life.
   - Hypomania consists of manic symptoms that do not meet the full criteria for a manic episode. Cyclothymia is distinguished from bipolar type 2 by less severe episodes of depression and hypomania.
   - Dysthymia comprises chronic symptoms of depression lasting at least 2 years without meeting criteria for a major depressive episode.
   - Other disorders included in this spectrum are mood disorder secondary to substance abuse, mood disorder secondary to medical conditions, and postpartum depression.
   - The precise causes of mood disorders are unknown. Both biologic and psychosocial factors have been implicated. Biologic theories focus on brain norepinephrine and serotonin abnormalities. The dopaminergic system has also been theorized to play a role. Mood disorders tend to run in families. The evidence of heritability of bipolar disorder is stronger than that for major depressive disorder. However, the mode of genetic transmission remains uncertain.
   B. History and physical examination
   - The central feature of a major depressive disorder is either depressed mood or loss of interest or pleasure in nearly all activities for at least 2 weeks. Other symptoms associated with depression include anxiety or agitation, changes (increase or decrease) in appetite, changes in weight, (>5% in a month), insomnia or hypersomnia, and psychomotor agitation or retardation.

Decreased energy; feelings of worthlessness or guilt; difficulty in thinking, concentrating, or making decisions; and recurrent thoughts of death or suicide may be present. Occasionally depression may be associated with psychotic symptoms in the form of delusions and hallucinations.

- The most serious consequence of a major depressive episode is attempted or completed suicide. Suicide risk is especially high for individuals with psychotic features, a history of previous suicide attempts, a family history of suicide, or a history of substance abuse. Between 10% and 15% of patients with mood disorders commit suicide.

- Additional signs and symptoms associated with depression include decreased libido, inability to experience pleasure (anhedonia), and poor concentration. These symptoms frequently result in neglect of work, family, and friends and lead to social withdrawal and isolation.

- Patients with bipolar disorder may suffer from depression as well as manic episodes. The hallmark of a manic episode is elevated, expansive, or irritable mood. During the period of elevated mood, patients may also experience inflated self-esteem or grandiosity, decreased need for sleep, excessive and pressured speech, flight of ideas, distractibility, and psychomotor agitation. Expansiveness, unwarranted optimism, grandiosity, and poor judgment often lead to an imprudent involvement in pleasurable activities such as buying sprees, reckless driving, poor business investments, and indiscriminate sexual behavior. Such symptoms should last for a period of 1 week to make the diagnosis of a manic episode. Impairment is usually severe enough to cause marked impairment in functioning or to require hospitalization to protect the individual from the negative consequences of actions that result from poor judgment. Patients may also have associated psychotic symptoms such as delusions and hallucinations. Occasionally patients may develop catatonic symptoms in the form of stupor, mutism, negativism, and posturing.

- Acquiring a history of past psychiatric illnesses, including response to medications or treatment, is essential. A family history regarding psychiatric disorders is important. Information about alcohol and drug abuse must also be included. The presence of medical problems or recently prescribed (or nonprescribed) medications may suggest a nonpsychiatric cause for the mood disorder. Childhood events including physical or sexual abuse, as well as current life stressors, might play an important role in the current mood disorder. Screening for manic and hypomanic symptoms should be done for any patient presenting with depression.

- Careful attention must be paid to the vital signs and neurologic examination. A detailed mental status examination must search for any signs of altered sensorium or prominent cognitive deficits. The clinician must address the issues of suicide, homicide, insight, and judgment.

C. Laboratory and diagnostic studies
   - The clinician's first task is to separate primary mood disorders from those due to physical diseases and drug ingestion. Laboratory studies including CBC, electrolytes, liver function tests, urinalysis, urine drug screen, and thyroid-stimulating hormone (TSH) levels may be obtained. An ECG is useful,

especially prior to starting medications that can affect the QT interval. Radiologic studies, such as CT or magnetic resonance imaging (MRI) of the head, are useful in patients with abnormal neurologic findings and when electroconvulsive treatment (ECT) will be given.

- Psychological testing can be useful in the diagnosis of mood disorders. These tests can help clinicians detect the presence of suicidal ideation and psychotic thought processes and give a profile of the patient's personality style. They can also be helpful in differentiating depression from dementia.

D. Formulating the diagnosis

- The clinician must always consider possible organic causes for mood disorders. A variety of medical and neurologic conditions and pharmacologic agents cause symptoms of both depression and mania. The following is a list of diseases that can be associated with symptoms suggestive of a mood disorder.
- Neurologic disorders: Parkinson's disease, Huntington's chorea, Wilson's disease, traumatic brain injury, stroke, infections, multiple sclerosis, and epilepsy.
- Endocrine diseases: thyroid disorders (hypothyroidism and hyperthyroidism), adrenal gland disorders (Cushing's and Addison's disease) and diabetes.
- Infectious and inflammatory diseases: infectious mononucleosis, systemic lupus erythematosus, acquired immune deficiency syndrome (AIDS), and pneumonia.
- Miscellaneous: cancer (especially pancreatic), cardiac disease especially after a myocardial infarction, liver disease, renal disease, and vitamin deficiencies (vitamin B_{12}, thiamine, and folate).
- Pharmacologic agents: antihypertensive medications and other cardiac drugs, sedatives and hypnotics, steroids and other hormones, antibacterials, and antifungals.
- Depression as a symptom can be present in a variety of psychiatric disorders. The common psychiatric conditions associated with mood symptoms are alcohol and drug dependence, anxiety disorders, dementia, delirium, adjustment disorder with depressed mood, and bereavement.

E. Evaluating the severity of problems

- The foremost decision a physician must make is whether to treat the patient in an outpatient setting or as an inpatient. The indications for hospitalization include uncertainty of diagnosis, suicide or homicide risk, inability to care for oneself, and lack of a social support system. Not infrequently patients with mood disorders refuse hospitalization on a voluntary basis. This may necessitate involuntary psychiatric hospitalization.

F. Managing the patient

- The mainstay of treatment of major depression is antidepressant medication. Antidepressants include tricyclic and tetracyclic antidepressants, monoamine oxidase inhibitors (MAOIs), and selective serotonin reuptake inhibitors (SSRIs). SSRIs are considered first-line treatment because of better tolerability and improved side effect profile. These drugs include citalopram (Celexa), fluoxetine (Prozac), fluvoxamine (Luvox), paroxetine (Paxil), sertraline (Zoloft), and escitalopram (Lexapro). SSRIs are associated with fewer side effects and are particularly safe for patients with multiple medical problems. Onset of action is typically 2 to 4 weeks. Common side effects associated with the SSRIs include gastrointestinal side effects and sexual dysfunction. The most serious side effect is the serotonin syndrome characterized by agitation, myoclonus, hyperpyrexia, hypertension, abdominal cramps, and even death. Other medications include serotonin-norepinephrine reuptake inhibitors such as venlafaxine (Effexor) and duloxetine (Cymbalta). Other medications include bupropion (Wellbutrin) and mirtazapine (Remeron).

- The choice of an antidepressant for a particular patient is determined by a history of response to a particular agent and the side effect profile of the medication. Until the introduction of Prozac, the tricyclic antidepressants were used most frequently. These drugs include amitriptyline, nortriptyline, imipramine, desipramine, and doxepin. These drugs differentially prevent reuptake of norepinephrine and serotonin. The common side effects of tricyclic antidepressants include dry mouth, inability to urinate, constipation, hypotension, cardiac arrhythmias/conduction delays, and sexual dysfunction. Most of the tricyclic antidepressants have a 2- to 3-week onset of action. Patients are usually started on a low dose that is gradually increased over a few weeks, according to clinical response and tolerance of side effects. The efficacy of SSRIs is probably similar to the tricyclic antidepressants. The monoamine oxidase inhibitors (MAOIs) are usually not first-line treatment for depression because of the possibility of serious side effects. The drugs most commonly used are phenelzine, tranylcypromine, and isocarboxazid. MAOIs may be particularly useful for depressed patients who present with atypical features of marked anxiety, excessive sleep, and increased appetite. Patients taking MAOIs have to be on a special tyramine-free diet. These patients must avoid consumption of aged cheese, red wine, pickled herring, chocolate, and other tyramine-containing food. If MAOIs are given and tyramine is not avoided, patients can develop severe hypertension, which can lead to complications including death. Although a hypertensive crisis is the most serious side effect, hypotension is the most common side effect of the MAOIs. The most common mistake when using an antidepressant drug is using too low a dose for too short a time. Unless adverse effects prevent it, the dose of an antidepressant should be raised to the maximum recommended dosage and maintained at that level for at least 4 weeks before a drug trial is considered unsuccessful. However, if a patient is improving clinically on a low dose, then the dosage should not be raised unless clinical improvement stops. In those patients who fail to respond to a particular antidepressant, a different class of antidepressant medication should be tried. In treatment-resistant patients, a trial of a combination of antidepressants as well as lithium, thyroid hormone, or other adjunctive therapies should be considered. ECT is recommended for medication-resistant or acutely suicidal patients or patients with depression with psychotic features.

- Lithium, divalproex (Depakote), and atypical antipsychotics such as olanzapine (zyprexa) and quetiapine (seroquel) are standard treatments of manic episodes. Most manic patients, however, may require polypharmacy or benzodiazepines at the initiation of treatment to control psychotic symptoms and agitation. Noncompliance is a particularly difficult problem in the treatment of manic patients, and the clinician should always be aware of this potential cause for lack of response. Other treatments include carbamazepine and lamotrigine (Lamictal). Patients with bipolar disorder benefit from prophylactic treatment with any of the medications just mentioned. Drug interactions should be considered when multiple medications are used.

- Extensive research has shown that a combination of pharmacotherapy and psychotherapy is the most efficacious treatment for mood disorders. Interpersonal and cognitive therapists have developed approaches specifically for the treatment of depression. Insight-oriented psychoanalytically based psychotherapy, family therapy, and occasionally behavior therapy can also be useful.

VII. Personality Disorders
    A. Basic science
- The etiology of personality disorders is likely multifactorial including developmental and genetic factors; psychoanalytical theory is by far one of the best recognized theories to explain the etiology of personality disorders. Freud believed that personality traits were the product of fixation at a particular stage of psychosexual development.

    B. History and physical examination
- Although the general medical history and physical examination should be performed in all individuals, there are no pathognomonic findings in patients with isolated personality disorders. The psychiatric history is discussed in the following sections.

    C. Formulating the diagnosis
- All personality disorders demonstrate enduring and inflexible patterns of experiences and behavior that are inconsistent with cultural expectations. These disruptions must occur in at least two of the following areas: cognition, affectivity, impulsivity, and interpersonal relationships. The enduring pattern is inflexible and pervasive across a broad range of personal and social situations. It also leads to distress or impairment in social and occupational or other important areas of functioning. A pervasive pattern of maladaptive functioning must be present. The existence of a few isolated personality traits is not sufficient to make a diagnosis of a personality disorder. The symptoms often begin in adolescence or early adulthood. They cannot be accounted for by another mental disorder, substance abuse, or a general medical or neurologic condition that affects CNS function.
- Personality disorders are divided into three primary clusters that contain disorders with similar symptoms.
- Cluster A disorders include paranoid, schizoid, and schizotypal personality disorders. As a group, individuals with a cluster A diagnosis are suspicious, eccentric, and socially isolative.
- Cluster B diagnosis individuals are distinguished by impulsive, dramatic behaviors and a decreased capacity for empathy. This cluster includes antisocial, narcissistic, borderline, and histrionic personality disorders. Substance abuse and mood disorders are common comorbid conditions, especially with borderline and antisocial personality disorder.

- Cluster C diagnosis individuals are typically excessively anxious, fearful, or perfectionist. Avoidant, dependent, and obsessive-compulsive personality disorders are included in the C cluster. Individuals with a cluster C diagnosis may suffer from a comorbid anxiety or mood disorder.
- In this review, only key features of each disorder will be emphasized.
  1. Paranoid personality disorder
     - The prevalence in the general population is between 0.5% and 2.5% (2% to 10% in the outpatient setting and 10% to 30% in the inpatient setting). It is far more common in males than females. Interestingly there is a higher incidence in minority groups, immigrants, and the deaf.
     - The core feature of paranoid personality disorder is persistent, pervasive, inappropriate mistrust of people. These individuals are typically cold and aloof and are prone to becoming excessively angry. Their preferred defense mechanisms include projection, denial, and rationalization. The diagnosis differs from delusional disorder and schizophrenia by the absence of frank delusion; also, patients with paranoid personality disorder have good reality testing.
  2. Schizoid personality disorder
     - The prevalence in the general population is between 1% and 7.5%. It is twice as common in males as females. Schizoid personality disorder includes persons who are socially withdrawn exhibiting decreased emotional responsiveness and ability to relate to others. They frequently do not experience their lack of intimate relationships as disturbing and prefer solitary activities. They tend to withdraw from social situations and so seem indifferent to the world around them.
  3. Schizotypal personality disorder
     - This disorder affects about 3% of the general population and appears to be more prevalent in first-degree relatives of schizophrenic patients. Schizotypal personality disorder is similar to schizoid personality disorder in that these persons are socially isolated. They experience discomfort with interpersonal relationships and demonstrate odd and eccentric behavior, speech, and thoughts. They may experience perceptual disturbances such as telepathy, ideas of reference, clairvoyance, or magical thinking to a degree that is outside cultural references. They may present with frank psychotic symptoms, but these are brief and lack severity in comparison with schizophrenia. The prognosis is guarded; some clinicians believe that schizotypal personality disorder is a precursor of schizophrenia, and nearly 10% of these patients commit suicide.
  4. Antisocial personality disorder
     - The prevalence is approximately 3% for males and 1% for females. About 75% of the prison population carries this diagnosis. Antisocial personality disorder is characterized by a pervasive disregard and violation of the rights of others with little or no remorse. Individuals with this diagnosis often behave impulsively and irresponsibly. They exhibit outbursts of anger and frequently have legal difficulties. This pattern of behavior must have started prior to age 15 (history of

conduct disorder); however, the diagnosis requires that the patient be at least 18 years of age.

5. Borderline personality disorder
   - The prevalence is around 2% to 3% of the population with 2:1 female:male ratio. It is the most prevalent personality disorder (12% to 15%). This individuals have a higher rate for comorbid psychiatric disorders (mood disorders, eating disorders, substance abuse, PTSD). By the age of 30 years, 10% of these patients will have committed suicide.
   - Borderline personality disorder is similar to antisocial personality disorder in that there is a history of a pattern of instability and lack of control over impulses. In addition, individuals with this disorder suffer from disturbed interpersonal relationships, self-image, and affect (especially anger). They may frequently threaten or attempt suicide and make excessive, often manipulative demands in close interpersonal relationships or of care providers. They may complain of chronic feelings of emptiness and boredom and may suffer from dissociative or transient psychotic episodes.

6. Histrionic personality disorder
   - Prevalence is around 2% to 3% of the general population. Histrionic personality disorder is characterized by a pattern of excessive attention seeking and exaggerated emotional responses, which are frequently superficial and fleeting. These patients also have a very poor frustration tolerance.

7. Narcissistic personality disorders
   - The best estimates are less than 1% of the general population.
   - The key feature is overwhelming pathologic self-absorption. The disorder is further characterized by a sense of uniqueness, grandiosity, entitlement, and decreased empathy and exploitation of others. They lack of empathy of others and tend to exploit others to meet their self-serving needs.

8. Avoidant personality disorder
   - It is diagnosed in 1% to 10% of the general population and is equally prevalent in males and females. Avoidant personality disorder includes patients who exhibit a pattern of feelings of inadequacy, excessive sensitivity to criticism or evaluation, and social inhibition. Unlike the person with schizoid personality disorder, these individuals desire close relationships and are distressed by their interpersonal difficulties. This patients use pathologic avoidance as means of self-protection.

9. Dependent personality disorder
   - This disorder occurs in 2% to 4% of the general population. Females are more commonly diagnosed than males. Patients with a history of separation anxiety disorder or chronic illness may be predisposed. Dependent personality disorder is often coexistent in individuals with a diagnosis of avoidant personality disorder. These patients have an extreme fear of abandonment and a strong desire for others to take care of them. They frequently rely on others to make decisions and require excessive reassurance to do so on their own.

10. Obsessive-compulsive personality disorder
   - This disorder is a common diagnosis in the general population, more frequent in males than females. Obsessive-compulsive personality disorder is characterized by a preoccupation with perfection, orderliness, rules, and interpersonal control, which, because of rigidity, ultimately interferes with efficiency, task completion, flexibility, and personal relationships.

D. Evaluating the severity of problems
   - Nearly all patients with personality disorders are treated as outpatients.

E. Managing the patient
   - Individuals with a cluster A personality diagnosis frequently do not seek psychiatric treatment. Psychotherapy is the treatment of choice. Low-dose antipsychotic medications may be helpful with paranoid and schizotypal personality disorders when these patients develop brief psychotic decompensation. There is little evidence that individuals with antisocial personality disorder respond to conventional psychiatric treatment. Unfortunately these patients respond better when placed in confined settings such as prison where physical constraints can substitute for their moral deficits.
   - Cluster B disorders may respond to limit setting, a clear explanation of required expectations for treatment, and strict adherence to professional boundaries by all health care providers. Individuals who suffer from narcissistic, borderline, and histrionic personality disorders can improve with psychotherapy. Dialectical behavioral therapy has been proved very effective for the treatment of borderline personality disorder. A variety of medications such as tricyclic antidepressants, SSRIs, monoamine oxidase inhibitors, neuroleptics, anticonvulsants, and benzodiazepines have been useful in persons suffering from borderline personality disorder. These medications help with mood instability, suicidality, impulsive behaviors, and dissociative and psychotic symptoms.
   - Individuals with a cluster C diagnosis generally respond well to cognitive behavioral therapy, group therapy, assertive training, and social skills training.
   - In individuals suffering from a personality disorder, one should be careful to avoid attributing all their complaints to the personality disorder. An attempt must be made to diagnose other comorbid psychiatric conditions, such as anxiety and mood disorders, which respond well to treatment.

VIII. Schizophrenia
   A. Basic science
   - The prevalence of schizophrenia is 1% worldwide. Risk factors include family history, obstetric complications such as fetal hypoxia and nutritional deficiencies, increasing parental age developmental difficulties, and CNS infections in childhood. The precise contribution of these factors and ways in which they interact is unclear.
   - Men and women are equally vulnerable. Increased activity of the neurotransmitter dopamine in the brain has been implicated etiologically, leading to the "dopamine hypothesis" of schizophrenia. Other

neurotransmitters are also likely to be involved. Imaging of the brain with various techniques suggests involvement of the frontal, prefrontal, and temporal areas of the brain in the development of the disorder. Evidence of genetic risk is clear but incompletely understood. Concordance among monozygotic twins is about 50%, implicating both genetic and environmental factors. The illness most often presents as the result of converging genetic, neurobiologic, and psychological vulnerabilities and psychosocial stressors.

B. History and physical examination
   - Schizophrenia is a clinical diagnosis made after a careful history and physical examination. It is a pervasive disorder that involves multiple areas of psychological function, may permanently change personality, and often leads to a gradual deterioration of motivation and ability to work, play, and relate to others. Psychological processes affected include disturbances in the content of thought (e.g., delusions); thought disorder (abnormal flow of ideas); perceptual disturbances (e.g., hallucinations); loss of ability to generate or regulate affect (e.g., flattening, blunting, gross inappropriateness); abnormal psychomotor behavior (e.g., odd mannerisms, agitation, catatonia); amotivation; and losses of a sense of self, volition, and relatedness.
   - Disturbances in the form and content of thought are central dimensions of the illness. Classically, schizophrenic thought is characterized by loose associations, meaning that the normal connections between ideas are lost. Other types of disordered thought found in schizophrenia include clang associations, neologisms, and thought blocking.
   - Delusions are false beliefs that are unshaken by reason. They may have a single theme or multiple themes, including religious, grandiose, somatic, and sexual preoccupations. Schizophrenic delusions tend to be bizarre; they are usually unconnected to mood and are termed mood incongruent. Ideas of reference (perceiving random events as intended to affect only oneself) and beliefs that people or supernatural forces can directly access or control thoughts are common.
   - Hallucinations in schizophrenia may involve any of the five senses, although most often these are auditory.
   - Many patients are plagued by a collection of symptoms called negative or deficit symptoms of schizophrenia. Anergy, amotivation, apathy, and ambivalence are typical to lesser or greater degrees. Negative symptoms are less likely to improve with antipsychotic medications than are positive symptoms such as hallucinations and delusions. Atypical antipsychotics appear to be more effective for the negative symptoms of schizophrenia. Physical examination is typically normal.

C. Laboratory and diagnostic studies
   - There are no pathognomonic features or specific tests to diagnose the illness. Evaluation should include careful assessment to exclude organic causes. Complete general physical and neurologic examinations and routine laboratory tests (including CBC, blood chemistries, thyroid and syphilis testing, sedimentation rate, urinalysis, and drug screen) are essential. Most psychiatrists today would agree that MRI and CT scans should be used to exclude masses,

vascular lesions, and evidence of white matter or degenerative processes in first presentations or if there are atypical features. If the psychosis starts before 18 years, copper and ceruloplasmin should be tested. Neuropsychological testing is frequently helpful to uncover underlying psychotic symptoms and cognitive impairment.

- Other mimics of schizophrenia include amphetamine- or cocaine-induced psychosis, subcortical dementias (e.g., Wilson's and Huntington's disease), and mood disorders (e.g., major depression and bipolar disorder with psychotic features). Other major psychiatric illnesses share features of schizophrenia, including schizoid, schizotypal, and paranoid personality disorders, the delusional disorders, and schizoaffective (symptoms of schizophrenia and periods of mood disturbance) and schizophreniform (have symptoms suggestive of schizophrenia but do not meet the criteria regarding symptom duration which is 6 months) disorders. Commonly used medications such as β-blockers and clonidine can cause hallucinations.

D. Formulating the diagnosis

- Schizophrenia typically presents in late adolescence or early adulthood. There are three distinct phases of the illness: prodromal, active, and residual. To diagnose schizophrenia a patient must meet two criteria: (1) an active phase of the illness with prominent psychotic symptoms lasting more than 1 month, unless symptoms are interrupted by effective treatment; and (2) a total duration of symptoms from all phases of at least 6 months.

- The active phase of the illness is defined by the active psychosis: the typical delusions, hallucinations, disorganized speech, grossly disorganized or catatonic behavior, negative symptoms (i.e., affective flattening, alogia, avolition).

- Prodromal and residual phases share many signs and symptoms. The prodromal phase may last many weeks or months, often so insidious as to be recognized only in retrospect. Individuals gradually become more aloof, perplexed, preoccupied, peculiar in behavior and beliefs, and less willing or able to participate in school or work. Attention to grooming, dress, and other social norms may be lost. Families may be more puzzled than worried. The residual phase is present when active phase symptoms are essentially absent, but oddities in speech and behavior and serious disturbances in social and role functioning persist. Negative symptoms are often prominent in this phase and represent much of the enduring disability of schizophrenia.

- The course of schizophrenia is variable. Common complications include major depression, chemical dependency, suicide, chronically poor social function, and homelessness.

- There are five subtypes of the disorder: paranoid, catatonic, disorganized, undifferentiated, and residual.

    1. Paranoid

        - The paranoid type is characterized by preoccupation with systematized delusions or auditory hallucinations with a single theme. Classic themes include persecution by agencies or supernatural forces and religious, scientific, and sexual ideas. This type carries the best prognosis.

2. Catatonic
   - The catatonic type shows prominent abnormalities of psychomotor behavior, such as posturing, mutism, stupor, catalepsy, purposeless excessive motor activity, extreme negativism, echolalia, or echopraxia.

3. Disorganized
   - The disorganized type is typified by grossly disorganized delusions and hallucinations of various themes, and disorganized speech and behavior, flat or inappropriate affect. This subtype carries the poorest prognosis.

4. Undifferentiated
   - The undifferentiated subtype is used to describe cases that do not clearly fit the other patterns.

5. Residual
   - The residual subtype describes individuals that no longer have active delusions, hallucinations, or other positive symptoms but are disabled with negative symptoms in an attenuated form.

E. Evaluating the severity of problems
   - Patients with homicidal or suicidal ideation require hospitalization.

F. Managing the patient
   - Pharmacologic interventions in the active phase are critically important to relieve the symptoms and improve the quality of life. Acute treatment usually includes antipsychotic medications, which are particularly effective in the treatment of positive symptoms such as hallucinations and delusions. Most antipsychotics block postsynaptic D_2 dopamine receptors. Newer atypical antipsychotics, such as clozapine, risperidone, olanzapine, aripiprazole, quetiapine, and ziprasidone, do not have this mechanism of action, creating uncertainty about their exact mechanism of actions. To establish acute antipsychotic effects, a dose the equivalent of 300 to 400 mg of chlorpromazine is usually needed. Benzodiazepines are useful adjuncts for sedation and may allow lower doses of antipsychotics to be effective in acute psychosis.
   - Many antipsychotics are available. They are arranged on a continuum from high potency (e.g., haloperidol fluphenazine) to midpotency (trifluoperazine), to low potency (e.g., chlorpromazine). High-potency agents have a low incidence of sedation, blood pressure, and anticholinergic effects but are more likely to cause extrapyramidal side effects and akathisia (a syndrome of motor restlessness). Low-potency agents conversely may cause considerable sedation, orthostasis, and uncomfortable anticholinergic side effects but less commonly muscular problems. Extrapyramidal side effects are often easily treated with anticholinergic agents (e.g., benztropine and trihexyphenidyl), by opting for a lower-potency agent or lowering the dose of the antipsychotic.
   - All antipsychotic side effects are important, but three are especially so.
     1. Acute dystonia
        - Acute dystonia is usually an early side effect that may be quite dramatic. Muscular males are particularly at risk. Signs may develop rapidly, including general muscular rigidity, torticollis, and oculogyric crisis. Laryngeal spasm can lead to airway obstruction. IM or IV diphenhydramine (25 to 50 mg) or IM benztropine (2 mg) will generally

rapidly reverse dystonia. Following an episode of acute dystonia, oral anticholinergic agents should be continued for at least several days to prevent recurrence.

2. Tardive dyskinesia
   - Tardive dyskinesia is a syndrome of involuntary movements typically involving muscles of the lips, face, and tongue but potentially affecting any skeletal muscle. Risk factors include high-potency antipsychotics, total dose and duration of exposure, older age, and female sex. If identified early, the dyskinesias most often remit with reduction or elimination of drug treatment. The movements may be permanent; 15% to 20% of patients exposed for more than 1 year will eventually show signs of tardive movements.

3. Neuroleptic malignant syndrome
   - This is a rare but potentially fatal side effect that may present at any time during antipsychotic treatment. It should be considered in any patient exposed to dopamine blockade or withdrawal of a dopamine agonist. Presentation includes fever, muscle rigidity, unexplained elevation of white blood cell counts and serum creatine kinase, and delirium. There is no definitive or reliable treatment beyond hydration and symptomatic management; however, bromocriptine and dantrolene can be helpful. Complications can lead to renal and hepatic failure, seizures, coma, and death.

- Psychotherapies focus on helping the patient and family understand the nature of the illness (psychoeducation), supporting them in learning to live with and around disabilities, coping with a chronic disease, managing life stressors, and connecting with and monitoring rehabilitation efforts. Also any effort toward compliance with medication will help the patient to have fewer relapses.
- Relapse prevention is a critical part of treatment. Antipsychotics clearly prevent return of symptoms and may need to be continued indefinitely. Family interventions aimed at decreasing undue amounts of expressed emotion, which lead to tension in the environment, have been associated with reduced rates of relapse.
- More than half the patients with schizophrenia have impaired insight into their illness, and may feel that the treatment is unnecessary, making the depot antipsychotics the best choice of treatment for them.
- Psychosocial treatment is a very important tool to add to the medication treatment. Between 25% and 50% of schizophrenics will continue to have very disabling symptoms and impaired social functioning. Assertive community treatment, in which patients are assigned to one multidisciplinary team (with a case manager, a social worker, a nurse, and a psychiatrist), has been shown to decrease the time spent in the hospital.

IX. Somatoform Disorders
   A. Basic science
      - Somatoform disorders consist of a group of disorders characterized by physical symptoms resembling medical disease but without organic disease or a known

pathophysiologic mechanism. Epidemiologic studies reveal a prevalence of 0.2% to 2% in females and 0.2% in males. Somatoform disorders include somatization disorder, conversion disorder, pain disorder, hypochondriasis, and body dysmorphic disorder. Syndromes that appear somatoform in nature but do not conform to the disorders just listed are usually termed undifferentiated.

- In somatization disorder, the patient has a long history of physical complaints affecting multiple organ systems (e.g., pain, gastrointestinal, genitourinary, pseudo-neurologic) that remain unexplained and lead to distress, disability, or medical care. The illness is chronic in nature and has a female preponderance. Onset is early in life. A fluctuating course is common, but complete remission is rare. Morbidity is significant in occupational, interpersonal, and medical spheres.
- Pain disorder is characterized by a preoccupation with pain for more than 6 months, without a clear organic explanation. Disability or distress is disproportionate to the pain. Low back pain is most common. The age of onset is usually in the 40s or 50s. The disorder often leads to depression or dysthymia.
- Patients with conversion disorder exhibit a loss of or alteration in physical functioning, suggesting a physical disorder (usually pseudoneurologic: pseudoseizures, pseudosyncopes, pseudoparaplegia, and mutism). The symptoms and examination findings cannot be explained by known anatomic pathways. The disorder is more common in females and often correlates with a known acute psychosocial stressor. The symptoms usually resolve spontaneously, although they may become chronic and result in substantial sequelae (e.g., chronic pseudoepilepsy, prolonged limb weakness leading to atrophy).
- Patients with hypochondriasis exhibit a long-standing preoccupation with, fear of, or belief that they have a serious disease. They exhibit a ruminative, anxious, obsessive quality to health concerns, with only temporary response to reassurance. It is slightly more common in men and peaks in the 40s and 50s. These patients may also be prone to depression.
- Body dysmorphic disorder patients have an excessive preoccupation with an imagined defect in appearance, causing marked distress and psychosocial impairment. They often pursue dental or surgical interventions to correct the "defect," leading to more dissatisfaction. In severe cases, morbidity is significant.

B. History and physical examination

- The evaluation of somatoform disorder must include a careful search for a possible medical explanation for the patients' symptoms. A lack of objective signs of disease matched with a disproportionate magnitude of distress or disability should alert the physician to the possibility of a somatoform disorder. Psychiatric disorders (such as depression and panic disorder which can masquerade as a somatoform disorders) should be identified and treated.
- It is essential to remember that somatoform disorders often coexist with medical illness and other psychiatric disorders. Many of these patients are resistant to psychiatric care. They should be informed about the possibility of a

psychological "component" to their symptoms early in the workup, thus minimizing the chances of resistance and denial. The exploration of family dynamics and a realization of the patient's unconscious motives will greatly assist in the diagnosis and management.

C. Laboratory and diagnostic studies
- The major goal of the patient is apparently to communicate distress through a recitation of symptoms.
- Patients with somatoform disorders often undergo extensive, unnecessary testing. Laboratory investigation should be performed as indicated by the history and physical examination.

D. Formulating the diagnosis
- There are some important points when making the diagnosis of somatoform disorders; it is important to distinguish medical from psychiatric disorders. Somatization disorders are more likely when there is a multiple organ involvement, early onset, chronic course and absence of any laboratory or radiologic or physical abnormalities.
- These disorders must be differentiated from other "somatizing" illnesses, such as adjustment disorder (with physical complaints), major depression with somatic complaints ("masked" depression), anxiety disorders with physical symptoms (particularly panic disorder and generalized anxiety disorder), and psychotic disorders. In the latter, somatic concerns are often bizarre and are impervious to logic or reason.
- Also important is the understanding that somatoform symptoms are not willfully or deliberately generated but are the product of unconscious conflicts or psychological needs. This clearly separates them from malingering (deliberate feigning for specific gain) and from factitious disorders.
  1. Factitious disorder
     - The patient's main goal is to produce or feign signs of medical and mental disorder and to assume the sick role.
     - Although these patients often feign illness when it is not present, they can present with legitimate serious medical disease, and therefore this possibility should not be dismissed.
     - Typically factitious disorder symptoms begin in early adult life. They have increased prevalence of borderline personality disorder, and there is also often a history of childhood abuse and frequent hospitalizations.
  2. Treatment
     - The goal is to provide care for the patient but not to focus on "the cure." The primary care provider should be encouraged to set clear limits with the patient: do not do more or less than you will for any other patient, set and always follow an agenda for each visit, prevent iatrogenesis, and focus on the diagnostic objective findings and not the patients' complaints. Psychiatric referral is always helpful to treat this disorder and its comorbidities.

E. Managing the patient
- Guidelines for treatment involve the development of a stable and trusting relationship with a primary physician who can then "centralize" the patient's care. A vital part of the physician's role is the reduction of iatrogenic morbidity

through reasonable workup and treatment. A negotiated contract involving an acknowledgment of the physician's inability to "cure" the patient, an invitation to more realistically redefine goals, and an ongoing reassurance that medical care will not be withdrawn despite negative objective findings is helpful. Occasionally, regular-interval, symptom-independent visits can help reduce the patient's need for renewed somatization to obtain care. It is always important to obtain collateral information to verify the facts and to avoid confrontation. A nonjudgmental attitude should be maintained at all times.

X. Substance Abuse
   A. Basic science
   - Adverse consequences of alcohol and drug use include not only their well-known medical sequelae but also psychiatric problems. Most psychiatric symptoms can be caused or exacerbated by alcohol or drugs.
   - About 10 million people in the United States have alcohol dependence. About 9 million report using marijuana regularly, 1.6 million report using cocaine, and less than 1 million use heroin. Slightly more than 1 million people report using hallucinogens, inhalants, or other drugs.
   - In response to equivalent doses of ethanol, women have higher blood ethanol concentrations than men, in part because of lower gastric mucosal alcohol dehydrogenase activity. Alcoholic women develop cirrhosis more rapidly than do alcoholic men.
   - Intravenous drug users are at risk for many infectious diseases, including human immunodeficiency virus (HIV), hepatitis, syphilis, gonorrhea, cellulitis, skin abscesses, endocarditis, pneumonia, and tuberculosis. Alcohol and drug users are also at risk for accidental and traumatic injuries.
   - Familial patterns are often noticed for both alcohol and drug dependence. Genetic factors are involved in the transmission of alcohol dependence and are suspected in the transmission of other substance dependence.
   B. History and physical examination
   - Most alcohol and drug users use more than one drug, and it is extremely common for drug users to deny their use. The clinician should ask about types of drugs used, amounts used, route of administration, age at onset of use for each drug used, means of obtaining drugs (or the money for them), history of tolerance, or withdrawal signs. The CAGE questionnaire is commonly used to assess alcohol dependence. It is also important to inquire about legal history and settings in which drugs are used, sequelae of use, family history, past treatments, and periods of abstinence. The clinician should determine whether there has been progression of use, including increasing severity of symptoms and increasing frequency and amounts used over time.
   - It is important to determine how long the patient has remained abstinent from drugs and alcohol and how he or she accomplished such abstinence. This will be helpful in deciding which treatment level the patient needs when referral is made. If during abstinence, psychiatric symptoms gradually improve without medication, these symptoms might be secondary to alcohol or drug use.

- Physical examination should include special attention to signs of active drug use (needle tracks) and signs of treatable but easily overlooked illnesses related to alcohol and drug use, such as Wernicke's encephalopathy or hyperthermia. The examiner should also look for rhinorrhea, changes in pupil size, nystagmus, cutaneous abscesses, piloerection (gooseflesh), tremor, and an altered level of consciousness.

C. Laboratory and diagnostic studies
- When evaluating a potential substance abuser, a urine drug screen should always be performed. Presence of drugs (or their metabolites) in blood or urine is diagnostic. Elevation of gamma glutamyl transferase (GGT) is a useful indicator of excessive drinking. Mean corpuscular volume (MCV) may be elevated in alcoholics as well. Creatine kinase (CK) levels should be done when cocaine-induced or PCP-induced rhabdomyolysis is suspected. Electrocardiograms and serial CK and troponin measurements can be helpful in evaluating the presence of myocardial ischemia in the cocaine user who complains of chest pain.

D. Formulating the diagnosis
- Substance use disorders are divided into substance abuse and substance dependence.
- Substance abuse includes impairment or distress from one or more of the following within 12 months: failure to fulfill social or familial role because of use, use in physically hazardous situations, legal problems related to use, and social or interpersonal problems related to use.
- Substance dependence includes three of the following symptoms within 12 months: tolerance, withdrawal, loss of control of use, efforts to cut down or control use, increased time spent to get or use drugs, activities given up because of drug use, and use despite medical or psychological consequences.

E. Evaluating the severity of problems
- Patients who have needed medical management for alcohol withdrawal in the past are likely to need it again in subsequent episodes of withdrawal. Patients with unstable vital signs or medically complicated withdrawal should be admitted for detoxification. Uncomplicated alcohol withdrawal can be accomplished on an outpatient basis.
- Consider psychiatric admission for severe withdrawal symptoms, patients whose substance abuse or overdose has caused psychotic symptoms, severe depression, suicidal risk, or has exacerbated a coexisting psychiatric illness. In emergency situations involving alcohol and drugs, the staff must rapidly assess the patient for vital sign instability and evidence of bleeding, head trauma, or coma. CNS depression is common with overdoses of sedative-hypnotics, opiates, and large amounts of alcohol.

F. Managing the patient
- Withdrawal symptoms can develop within a few hours of last use when substances with short half-lives are used. Withdrawal symptoms from substances with long half-lives may develop after a much longer period, sometimes weeks, and might be misdiagnosed.

- Alcohol and sedative-hypnotic withdrawal is serious and potentially life-threatening. Symptoms should be treated early with benzodiazepines, thiamine, folate, and multivitamins. One must continue to monitor vital signs and response to doses of administered benzodiazepines. Minor withdrawal syndrome can progress to major withdrawal syndrome and delirium tremens (anxiety, tremors, sweating, tachycardia, and visual hallucinations). Such progression can be prevented by administering appropriate doses of medication and providing supportive care. Waiting until symptoms become more severe or giving suboptimal doses of benzodiazepines can make major withdrawal more likely. Phenytoin is ineffective for prevention of recurrent alcohol-related seizures.
- Outpatient treatment for benzodiazepine withdrawal is appropriate for those patients who have been using low to moderate doses of benzodiazepines on a long-term basis. A slow benzodiazepine taper over several weeks or months is often recommended. For barbiturate or mixed sedative-hypnotic withdrawal, phenobarbital is often used.
- Opiate withdrawal is not life-threatening but may cause significant discomfort. For opiate withdrawal supportive care is usually all that is necessary. Administration of the α_2-adrenergic agonists clonidine or guanabenz can be effective, and methadone, naltrexone, and buprenorphine has been shown effective for detoxification. Nonsteroidal anti-inflammatory drugs can be given for abdominal cramping. It is seldom necessary to give opiate analgesics.
- Cocaine or other stimulant intoxication symptoms often resolve without any pharmacologic intervention. Severe agitation accompanying stimulant intoxication or withdrawal is often treated with benzodiazepines or with low doses of haloperidol. Cocaine withdrawal can include severe dysphoria and suicidal ideation, requiring psychiatric admission.
- Treatment of substance use involves abstinence while participating in a program of education about addiction, coping skills training, family support and education, and sometimes adjunctive medications. Patients are particularly vulnerable to relapse in the first 12 months of abstinence from alcohol or drugs. Adjunctive medications that can be helpful in maintaining abstinence include disulfiram and naltrexone for alcoholism, and naltrexone for opiate dependence.
- Psychosocial treatment includes individual, group, family, psychotherapy, therapeutic community, and self-help groups.

Rheumatology

I. Bursitis
   A. Basic science
   - A bursa is a thin sac-like structure lined with synovial tissue. The function is to reduce friction and protect the soft tissue structures from bony prominences. Repetitive trauma can lead to chronic bursitis in which the synovial lining proliferates and thickens, leading to the development of calcifications and adhesions. Bursitis may be caused by infection, trauma, and systemic diseases such as gout or rheumatoid arthritis.
   B. History and physical examination
   - Bursitis presents with local pain and may be associated with swelling and limited active range of motion of the affected joint or limb. Passive movement is usually not affected. Common sites of bursitis include the subdeltoid (or subacromial), olecranon, ischial, trochanteric, and prepatellar bursae (housemaid's knee) or the anserine bursa on the upper medical aspect of the tibia. Septic bursitis presents with warmth, erythema, and peribursal edema. Fever may rarely be present. The most common sites of septic bursitis are the olecranon and prepatellar bursae.
   C. Laboratory and diagnostic studies
   - The evaluation of acute olecranon or prepatellar bursitis should include bursal aspiration to rule out septic bursitis. A bursal fluid white blood cell (WBC) count exceeding 1000 cells/mm^3 indicates inflammation secondary to gout, rheumatoid arthritis, or infection. Septic bursitis usually has a high WBC count but as a rule the leukocytosis in septic bursitis is lower than in septic arthritis. The fluid should be examined under polarized microscopy for crystals and sent for Gram stain and culuture. *Staphylococcus aureus* is the most commonly identified organism. Imaging is recommended in the setting of trauma to exclude a foreign body.
   D. Formulating the diagnosis
   - The diagnosis of bursitis is suggested by the clinical presentation. Further diagnostic testing should be performed to exclude either infection or systemic disease, especially in recurrent or persistent bursitis. Aspirated bursal fluid should be sent for Gram stain, culture, crystals, cell count, and glucose.
     1. Subacromial bursitis
        - Subacromial bursitis presents with shoulder pain, particularly noted with abduction, under direct pressure, as when lying on the affected side, and with overhead activities such as reaching for objects or combing one's hair.

2. Trochanteric bursitis
   - Trochanteric bursitis causes pain over the greater trochanter. The pain is exacerbated by direct pressure over the trochanteric bursa, external rotation, and abduction against resistance. Pain may be present over the entire lateral aspect of the thigh.
3. Anserine bursitis
   - Anserine bursitis is often seen in middle-aged overweight women and is exacerbated by climbing stairs. The pain is felt just below the knee joint medially, although patients often state that they have knee pain.

E. Evaluating the severity of problems
   - Septic bursitis is more worrisome in immunosuppressed patients. Hospitalization and intravenous antibiotics should be considered for aggressive local infections or any signs of systemic infection.

F. Managing the patient
   - Patient education and elimination of precipitating factors such as repetitive aggravating movements is the initial step in the management of bursitis. Various measures of joint protection can be taken to avoid further traumatic injury. The use of ice, rest, and nonsteroidal anti-inflammatory drugs (NSAIDs) usually provides pain relief in mild cases. Injection of the bursa with a corticosteroid and local anesthetic is advised for more severe cases. Chronic bursitis may be treated with steroid injections but not more often than once every 3 months. Physical therapy helps to prevent joint contracture and conditions the joint to prevent reinjury. Septic bursitis is treated with antibiotics based on culture sensitivities and aspiration until the bursal fluid is cleared of infection. Septic bursitis must always be ruled out before injection with a steroid.

II. Calcium Pyrophosphate Deposition Disease (Pseudogout)
   A. Basic science
      - Calcium pyrophosphate deposition disease (CPPD) is defined as the deposition of calcium pyrophosphate crystals in articular cartilage, menisci, synovium, tendons, and ligaments. The etiology may be idiopathic, familial (autosomal dominant inheritance), or secondary to trauma, infection, or medical illness. Certain metabolic diseases are associated with CPPD including hyperparathyroidism, hypomagnesemia, hypophosphalemia, hemochromatosis, and possibly hypothyroidism.
   B. History and physical examination
      - The term "pseudogout" was initially used to describe the acute presentation of CPPD. However, CPPD can clinically mimic nearly any form of arthritis including gout, rheumatoid arthritis, osteoarthritis, ankylosing spondylitis, and neuropathic joint disease. Pseudogout often affects the elderly (average age approximately 70 years) and presents with pain, swelling, warmth, and erythema in one or a few joints. Constitutional symptoms such as fever and malaise may also be present. The most common location for pseudogout is the knee, followed by the wrist and ankle. The pubic symphyis is also a common site for CPPD, whereas the first metatarsophalangeal joint is more typical for

gout. Precipitants are similar to those for an acute gouty attack including trauma, infection, surgery, and medical illness.

C. Laboratory and diagnostic studies
- The synovial fluid in CPPD reveals rhomboid-shaped, weakly positive birefringent crystals on polarized light microscopy. The joint fluid is inflammatory in nature with white cell counts as high as 60,000/mm^3 with a neutrophil predominance. Infection may coexist with CPPD, so a Gram stain and culture should be performed. Chondrocalcinosis is the classic x-ray finding of calcified cartilage in which crystal deposits appear as punctate and linear densities in the articular cartilage. In patients younger than 55 years, routine screening for associated metabolic diseases should include a serum calcium, phosphorus, magnesium, alkaline phosphatase, thyroid-stimulating hormone, ferritin, and iron level.

D. Formulating the diagnosis
- Although pseudogout clinically resembles gout, CPPD can be a challenging diagnosis if it presents with features more characteristic of other forms of arthritis such as rheumatoid arthritis. A definitive diagnosis of CPPD implies that weakly positive birefringent crystals and the classic x-ray findings are both present, but the diagnosis is still probable with just one of these findings.

E. Evaluating the severity of problems
- Progressive CPPD can lead to joint degeneration with significant loss of function.

F. Managing the patient
- The treatment of CPPD is similar to that for gout (see details in Section V, Gout). Rest of the involved joint, joint aspiration, and intra-articular injection of corticosteroids is appropriate initial management. NSAIDs and colchicine are beneficial to reduce inflammation during an acute attack. Oral steroids are used if both NSAIDs and colchicine are contraindicated and multiple joints are involved. Treatment of any underlying metabolic disease usually does not alter the course of CPPD. There is no effective preventive measure to avoid disease progression or to remove deposited crystals in CPPD.

III. Fibromyalgia
A. Basic science
- Fibromyalgia is characterized by diffuse myalgias and marked fatigue. The cause of fibromyalgia is unknown. It is thought that abnormalities in pain perception lead to lower pain thresholds. Possible triggers include physical and emotional stressors, disturbed sleep, a variety of viral infections, and surgery.

B. History and physical examination
- The American College of Rheumatology (ACR) diagnostic criteria include both of the following:
  1. Widespread musculoskeletalpain for at least 3 months
  2. Tenderness in at least 11 of 18 specified tender points
- The clinician should apply pressure for a few seconds to the specific points and compare to control points, which are nontender. The 18 specific points are composed of 9 bilateral points that are mostly axial in location. The tender pressure points should be distinguished from trigger points seen in myofascial

pain; pressure on these areas elicits referred pain some distance from the point of pressure.

- Beyond muscle tenderness, the physical examination is normal. The onset of symptoms in fibromyalgia is often after a stressor or mild illness in middle-aged females. The pain is persistent, diffuse, and chronic and is usually worse at the end of the day. Patients typically complain of many nonspecific symptoms, but fatigue and sleep disturbances are almost always present. Exacerbations occur with exertion, stress, or lack of sleep. Many other conditions overlap with fibromyalgia, including irritable bowel syndrome, migraine headaches, interstitial cystitis, chronic fatigue syndrome, temporomandibular joint dysfunction, and mood disorders.

C. Laboratory and diagnostic studies
- The initial evaluation should include a complete blood count, sedimentation rate, thyroid-stimulating hormone, and muscle enzymes. Further testing should be based on clinical suspicion but is often not needed. Sleep studies may be indicated when the history suggests an underlying sleep disorder.

D. Formulating the diagnosis
- There is no gold standard test for the diagnosis of fibromyalgia. The diagnosis is based on the history and physical examination combined with the diagnostic criteria proposed by the ACR. Neither physical examination nor laboratory evaluation shows any evidence of joint or muscle inflammation.

E. Evaluating the severity of problems
- The symptoms of fibromyalgia fluctuate over time. Some patients become significantly debilitated owing to the chronic widespread pain of fibromyalgia.

F. Managing the patient
- The goal of treatment is to decrease pain and improve function. Some patients have spontaneous resolution of their symptoms, but a chronic pattern is more common. A multidisciplinary team approach tailored to the individual patient produces the best long-term results. Patient and family education is an important aspect of therapy. Patients benefit from acknowledgment that their pain is real and reassurance of the benign nature of the disease.
- Nonpharmacologic treatment options include exercise, physical therapy, massage therapy, tender point injections, biofeedback, hypnotherapy, behavioral therapy, and cognitive therapy. Pharmacologic treatment should start with a low-dose tricyclic antidepressant at bedtime, such as amitriptyline. Analgesics, including acetaminophen and tramadol, are beneficial, but the NSAIDs usually do not provide much pain relief. The SSRIs (selective serotonin reuptake inhibitors) and newer antidepressants may be helpful in treating coexisting mood disorders but have not shown drastic improvements in pain. Other pharmacologic options include cyclobenzaprine, anxiolytics, gabapentin, and sleep aids. Opioids should be avoided.

IV. Giant Cell (Temporal) Arteritis
A. Basic science
- Giant cell arteritis (GCA) is a medium-size and large vessel vasculitis which predominantly involves the branches of the carotids. The temporal artery is the

most common site. It affects women more than men and older individuals (>50 years old).

B. History and physical examination

- The onset of symptoms is usually gradual but can be sudden. Symptoms include headache, jaw or arm claudication, scalp tenderness, vision changes, and vision loss. Many nonspecific symptoms are common and include fever, myalgias, fatigue, fever, and weight loss. Polymyalgia rheumatica (PMR) occurs in about 50% of those with GCA at some point during their disease. Physical examination may reveal tender, erythematous, thickened, swollen, or pulseless temporal arteries. Other cranial arteries may be involved and have similar findings. A bruit may be present over the carotid, subclavian, brachial, or axillary arteries.

C. Laboratory and diagnostic studies

- The characteristic laboratory finding is an elevated erythrocyte sedimentation rate (ESR), which can be above 100 mm/hour. Other nonspecific laboratory findings include an elevated C-reactive protein (CRP), alkaline phosphatase, platelet count, and anemia. A biopsy of the involved artery is mandatory when the clinical suspicion is high.

D. Formulating the diagnosis

- All patients over age 50 with the classic symptoms and an elevated ESR should have a temporal artery biopsy as soon as possible. Temporal artery biopsy reveals necrotizing arteritis with granulomas and confirms the diagnosis.

E. Evaluating the severity of problems

- GCA can lead to visual impairment, which can progress to complete and irreversible vision loss secondary to ischemia if left untreated.

F. Managing the patient

- Referral to a surgeon for temporal artery biopsy should be done urgently. Corticosteroids should be started based on the history and physical examination when clinical suspicion is high and should not be delayed while awaiting biopsy results. The recommended starting dose of prednisone is 40 to 60 mg/day for at least a month. Higher doses are sometimes used in the setting of serious ophthalmic or neurologic compromise. ESR and CRP correlate with disease activity and can guide steroid tapering. Relapse can occur during the steroid taper and is more common in the first couple years after diagnosis. Most patients will require corticosteroids for at least 2 years.

V. Gout

A. Basic science

- Gout is an inflammatory arthritis caused by monosodium urate crystal deposition in joints. The cause is either overproduction or undersecretion of uric acid. Overproduction can be idiopathic or due to rare inherited enzyme deficiencies. Secondary causes of overproduction include excessive purine intake, lymphoproliferative disorders, hemolytic anemia, and psoriasis. Undersecretion can be idiopathic or secondary to renal insufficiency, dehydration, ketoacidosis, lactic acidosis, or medications (diuretics, salicylates, and cyclosporine). Gout is more common in middle-aged men than women.

B. History and physical examination
  - There are three clinical stages of gout:
    1. Acute gouty arthritis
    2. Intercritical stage
    3. Chronic tophaceous gout
  - The onset of an *acute gouty attack* is abrupt with severe pain and swelling, which often peak in severity over several hours. The affected joint is warm, swollen, erythematous, and exquisitely tender. Fever and malaise may be present.
  - Most initial attacks involve a single joint. Polyarticular involvement is uncommon as an initial presentation but is seen in recurrent attacks. Common locations are the lower extremity joints including the metatarsophalangeal joint of the great toe ("podagra"), ankles, and knees, although any joint can be affected. A classic example is a middle-aged male who wakes up after a night of heavy alcohol and meat consumption with a swollen great toe and is unable to bear weight on the foot because of severe pain.
  - Precipitants include surgery, infection, trauma, medical illness, dehydration, medications, and increased alcohol, fish, and meat consumption.
  - Recovery with desquamation of the overlying skin usually occurs within days to a couple weeks, even if left untreated. The *intercritical stage* is the asymptomatic period between acute attacks.
  - *Recurrent attacks* occur in about 90% of patients within 10 years and may result in tophi formation, joint deformity, and loss of function.

C. Laboratory and diagnostic studies
  - The synovial fluid shows needle-shaped, negatively birefringent crystals under polarized light microscopy. The joint fluid is inflammatory in nature with white cell counts as high as $60,000/mm^3$ with a neutrophil predominance. Infection may coexist with an acute gouty attack, so a Gram stain and culture should be performed. X-ray may show soft tissue swelling in an initial acute attack, whereas bony erosions and deformities are seen in more advanced disease.

D. Formulating the diagnosis
  - The history and physical examination usually suggest the diagnosis, which is confirmed by arthrocentesis. Uric acid levels can be misleading and are not used to make the diagnosis. A prolonged period of asymptomatic hyperuricemia precedes the initial acute gouty attack, but most people with elevated uric acid levels never develop gout.

E. Evaluating the severity of problems
  - Chronic hyperuricemia can be complicated by nephrolithiasis and urate nephropathy. Progression to the chronic tophaceous stage can be prevented with anti-hyperuricemic therapy and control of other associated comorbidities.

F. Managing the patient
  - Treatment of gout is divided into acute, prophylactic, and chronic therapy.
  - Acute gout: Rest, NSAIDs, and corticosteroids (PO or intra-articular) are the mainstay of therapy. Colchicine may also be used. Indomethacin is the drug of choice, but any NSAID can be used. NSAIDs are associated with

gastrointestinal intolerance, which may limit their use. Side effects of colchicine are nausea, vomiting, and diarrhea. Higher doses of colchicine can lead to bone marrow suppression, myopathy, and neuropathy. Oral colchicine is preferred over the IV route, as the IV route can result in life-threatening toxicity. Patients with renal insufficiency require dose adjustments with NSAIDs and colchicine. Corticosteroids (PO or intra-articular) can be used to terminate an acute gouty attack when both NSAIDs and colchicine are contraindicated. The intra-articular route is preferred over oral steroids if the attack involves a single joint, but infection should always be ruled out prior to administering steroids.

- Prophylaxis: NSAIDs or colchicine will prevent recurrent acute gouty attacks until the serum urate levels are normalized.
- Chronic suppression: Uricosuric medications (probenecid and sulfinpyrazone) or a xanthine oxidase inhibitor (allopurinol) will both lower serum urate levels with the goal of preventing and reversing complications of urate crystal deposition, nephrolithiasis, and nephropathy. Serum urate should be lowered to a goal of 5 to 6 mg/dL by a combination of pharmacotherapy and diet. Uricosuric agents increase renal excretion of uric acid and are used for underexcretors (<800 mg/24 hours). They should be avoided in patients with renal insufficiency or nephrolithiasis. Allopurinol decreases uric acid synthesis and is used in both overproducers and undersecretors. Antihyperuricemic therapy can precipitate or prolong an acute attack and should never be initiated during an acute attack. Chronic treatment should be started after complete resolution of the acute attack.

VI. Joint Effusion, Synovial Cysts, and Ganglia
   A. Basic science
      - *Joint effusion* is an accumulation of fluid in the synovium as a result of infection, systemic disease, or trauma.
      - Classification of joint effusion:
         1. Noninflammatory: osteoarthritis and trauma
         2. Inflammatory: rheumatoid arthritis, systemic lupus erythematosus, systemic sclerosis (scleroderma), crystal arthritis, and the spondyloarthropathies
         3. Infectious (septic): gonococci, staphylococci, streptococci, and less often gram-negative bacteria, especially in the immunocompromised host
         4. Hemorrhagic: trauma, anticoagulation therapy, and hemophilia
      Synovial cysts result from herniation of the synovial cavity. The knee is a common site for such herniation, which forms a fluid-filled sac in the popliteal fossa known as a Baker's cyst. An underlying joint effusion is present in these patients.
      A *ganglion* is a small cyst over a joint or tendon sheath which arises from herniation of synovial tissue from the underlying joint. Repetitive trauma may aggravate a ganglia and lead to enlargement. Ganglion cysts are most commonly found on the wrist and finger joints.
   B. History and physical examination
      - Joint effusions present with swelling, erythema, and pain to the affected joint. The underlying cause of the effusion dictates the severity of symptoms.

- A Baker's cyst is a palpable cystic swelling in the popliteal fossa. The amount of pain increases as the cyst englarges. Range of motion may be limited by a large cyst. A ruptured cyst will cause edema and pain mimicking thrombophlebitis. Ultrasonography of the lower extremity will aid diagnosis.
- A ganglion cyst is a palpable, firm, nontender, movable cystic swelling typically located over the dorsum of the wrist.

C. Laboratory and diagnostic studies
- Joint fluid aspiration and analysis should be performed when the cause of the effusion is unknown. The fluid should be sent for white cell count with differential, cultures, Gram stain, glucose, and protein. The fluid should be examined under polarized light microscopy for crystals.
- Characteristics of synovial fluid:
  - Normal joint fluid: highly viscous, transparent, colorless cells ($<200/mm^3$), polymorphonuclear cells (PMNs) below 10%, protein 1 to 2 g/dL, glucose similar to that in plasma.
  - Noninflammatory: highly viscous, transparent, yellow cells (WBCs 200 to $2000/mm^3$), PMNs less than 25%, protein 1 to 3 g/dL, glucose similar to that in plasma.
  - Inflammatory (no infection): low viscosity, translucent to opaque, yellow cells (WBCs 200 to $5000/mm^3$), PMNs above 50%, protein 3 to 5 g/dL, low glucose.
  - Septic: opaque, variable color and viscosity, WBCs above $50,000/mm^3$, PMNs more than 75%, protein 3 to 5 g/dL, very low glucose. Cultures are positive in septic arthritis.
  - Hemorrhagic: bloody, WBCs 200 to $2000/mm^3$, PMNs 50 to 75%, protein 4 to 6 g/dL, glucose similar to that in plasma.

D. Formulating the diagnosis
- The diagnosis of an effusion depends on the synovial fluid analysis. Physical examination and ultrasound will usually diagnose a synovial cyst. Transillumination is helpful to differentiate a ganglion from other solid tumors. Note that there is considerable overlap in the cell counts.

E. Managing the patient
- The treatment of a joint effusion depends on the underlying cause. Synovial cysts may be treated by aspiration and injection with corticosteroids. Treatment of a ganglion cyst is unnecessary in the absence of symptoms. Surgical removal is effective, although some will recur. See Chapter 20, Infectious Diseases, for details on septic joint effusion.

VII. Osteoarthritis
A. Basic science
- Osteoarthritis (OA) is the most common form of arthritis. The pathogenesis is complex and involves a combination of genetic, mechanical, biochemical, and metabolic changes in the articular cartilage and bone. OA is characterized by

degeneration of the articular cartilage and bone hypertrophy, especially at the articular margins. Inflammation is minimal. OA can be primary (idiopathic) or secondary.

- The cause of primary OA is unknown, but a number of factors may contribute to its development. These factors include obesity, age, poorly defined hereditary factors, and bone density. The incidence of primary OA increases with age and women (>60 years) are more commonly affected than men.
- The causes of secondary OA include trauma, rheumatoid arthritis, infectious arthritis, psoratic arthritis, congenital joint abnormalities such as Perthe's disease, and metabolic disorders such as hemochromatosis and Wilson's disease.

B. History and physical examination
- OA is characterized by a gradual onset of progressively worsening joint pain, which is exacerbated by activity and relieved with rest. As the disease progresses, pain at rest and at night can occur. Morning stiffness lasts less than 30 minutes, helping to distinguish OA from inflammatory arthritis, such as rheumatoid arthritis, in which morning stiffness usually lasts longer than 1 hour. As the disease progresses patients complain of stiffness on movement after prolonged inactivity such as sitting.
- OA is asymmetric and commonly affects the distal interphalanges (DIPs), proximal interphalanges (PIPs), carpometacarpal joint of the thumb, knee, hip, first metatarsophalangeal joint of the foot, and the cervical and lumbar spine. The elbow, wrist, and ankle are rarely involved in primary OA. Physical examination findings include joint tenderness without signs of inflammation, limited motion, crepitus, and joint effusion. Deformities due to osteophyte formation at the DIPs and PIPs are called Heberden's and Bouchard's nodes, respectively. Hip involvement is characterized by a gradual onset of groin or inner thigh pain. Pain may also be felt in the knee. A limp may be present and internal and external rotation is painful and limited.
- Knee OA causes pain and crepitus. An effusion may be present. Osteophytes may be palpable. Valgus or varus deformities may be due to loss of the lateral or medial meniscus.
- Symptomatic spine OA occurs most commonly in the cervical and lumbar spine. Local pain and stiffness may be associated with radicular pain caused by nerve compression by osteophytes. Spinal stenosis, most common in the lumbar spine, results from a combination of degenerative changes, osteophytes, soft tissue inflammation, and spondylolisthesis. Back, leg, and radicular pain are the result.

C. Laboratory and diagnostic studies
- There are no characteristic laboratory abnormalities in primary OA. X-ray findings include narrowed joint space, osteophytes, subchondral cysts, and sclerosis.

D. Formulating the diagnosis
- The diagnosis is based on the clinical history combined with the radiographic findings. X-rays can show evidence of OA but do not always correlate with

clinical severity. The absence of inflammation excludes many other forms of arthritis.

E. Evaluating the severity of problems
- Significant disability and loss of function are associated with OA. The course is slowly progressive but prognosis depends on the joint involved. Older patients with hand OA tend to progressively worsen with limited treatment options. Patients with advanced knee and hip OA may be candidates for joint replacement surgery.

F. Managing the patient
- The goal of therapy is to control pain, maintain function, and improve quality of life. Nonpharmacologic therapies include weight loss (especially for knee OA), exercise, heat, physical therapy, and devices to take pressure off the affected joint. Pharmacologic therapy begins with analgesics such as acetaminophen. NSAIDs can be tried if relief is not adequate with acetaminophen alone. Another option is tramadol alone or in combination with acetaminophen or an NSAID. Short-term use of opioids can be used with caution for exacerbations of pain when other agents are contraindicated.
- Intra-articular corticosteroid injections provide short-term relief of symptoms and are particularly useful during exacerbations of pain. Intra-articular hyaluronic acid derivatives may slightly improve symptoms in selected patients with knee OA.
- A popular alternative therapy is glucosamine and chondroitin sulfate, which appears to have some efficacy in alleviating pain and may slow disease progression.
- Finally, surgery (e.g., arthroscopy or joint replacement) is an option for treating severe joint damage or deformity that cannot be adequately treated medically.

VIII. Osteoporosis
A. Basic science
- A reduction in bone mass with disruption of bone architecture defines osteoporosis and predisposes the patient to fractures. Mineralization is preserved in osteoporosis and distinguishes it from osteomalacia. The rate of bone resorption exceeds the rate of formation in the remodeling process, resulting in decreased bone mass. Primary osteoporosis is related to aging and the hormonal state. Postmenopausal women are at highest risk. Secondary osteoporosis results from certain medications (glucocorticoids, heparin) or from other chronic medical conditions including hyperthyroidism, hyperparathyroidism, nutritional deficiencies, hypogonadism, multiple myeloma, malabsorption, liver, or renal insufficiency.
- Risk factors for osteoporosis:
  1. Increasing age
  2. Female gender
  3. Caucasian and Asian race
  4. Prior fracture

     5. Family history of osteoporosis

     6. Postmenopausal state (especially early menopause)

     7. Low body weight

     8. Sedentary lifestyle

     9. Cigarette smoking

    10. Excessive alcohol consumption

    11. Malabsorption syndromes

    12. Medications (e.g., steroids, heparin, and anticonvulsants)

B. History and physical examination
- Patients present with fractures and their sequelae, which are primarily responsible for the clinical manifestations seen in osteoporosis. The pain associated with a fracture may have an acute onset and result from routine activities or mild trauma. Severe pain generally subsides gradually within weeks and a dull chronic pain may persist at the site of fracture. Loss of height, increased thoracic kyphosis, and increased cervical lordosis are seen with vertebral fractures. Fractures usually occur in the anterior vertebrae, resulting in wedge-shaped vertebrae. Fractures can occur at any site, but vertebrae and hip are the most common sites.

C. Laboratory and diagnostic studies
- Blood tests are not helpful in diagnosing primary osteoporosis. The use of markers of bone turnover such as osteocalcin and hydroxyproline remains controversial. X-rays may reveal vertebral compression fractures.

D. Formulating the diagnosis
- The gold standard test for the diagnosis of osteoporosis is the dual energy x-ray absorptiometry (DXA). The T score compares the results to those of a young healthy adult of the same sex and race. T scores within 1 standard deviation are normal. A T score of −1 to −2.5 from the standard deviation of the young adult reference mean defines osteopenia. Osteoporosis is a T score less than −2.5 from the standard deviation. The Z score compares the results to an age- and sex-matched control and can guide whether a workup for secondary causes of osteoporosis is indicated.

E. Evaluating the severity of problems
- Hip fractures in the elderly carry a significant risk of morbidity and death. Efforts focused on prevention are critical.

F. Managing the patient
- Prevention of osteoporosis should begin at a young age with proper diet and exercise.
- Nonpharmacologic measures include a healthy diet with adequate calcium and vitamin D intake, weight-bearing exercise, and smoking cessation. Premenopausal women should get 1000 mg/day of calcium and 400–800 IU/day of vitamin D. The recommendation for postmenopausal women is 1500 mg/day of calcium and 800 IU/day of vitamin D.
- First-line agents for treatment include the bisphosphonates (alendronate, risedronate, and ibandronate) and raloxifene, a selective estrogen receptor modulator. The bisphosphonates both increase bone mass and decrease fracture risk. They are preferred for first-line treatment of osteoporosis

because raloxifene has not been shown to decrease hip fractures. The main side effect of the bisphosphonates is esophagitis. Patients should take the medication with a full glass of water in the morning while they are upright to avoid esophageal irritation.

- Estrogen replacement therapy (ERT) is an effective therapy to inhibit bone resorption but should not be used routinely for prevention or treatment of osteoporosis owing to increased risk of breast cancer, stroke, and deep venous thrombosis.
- Calcitonin is delivered in a nasal spray and inhibits bone resorption but is overall less effective in increasing bone mass and considered a second-line agent. However, calcitonin also has some analgesic properties, which may help for patients with acute pain due to fracture.
- Recombinant human parathyroid (teriparatide) is a newer option for the treatment of osteoporosis in high-risk patients. This drug effectively increases bone density and reduces fracture risk. It is, however, expensive and requires daily subcutaneous injection.

IX. Polymyositis/Dermatomyositis
   A. Basic science
      - Polymyositis (PM) and dermatomyositis (DM) are rare inflammatory myopathies, which occur more frequently in women. Although both are usually idiopathic, the pathologic picture differs. Immune complex deposition in vessels is seen in DM, but PM is a T cell–mediated muscle injury. The age of onset is typically in the 50s but it can develop at any age.
   B. History and physical examination
      - Symmetric proximal muscle weakness is gradually progressive over several months. Muscle atrophy can occur with prolonged disease.
      - The skin findings of DM:
         1. Gottron's sign: scaly erythematous papules on extensor surfaces of metacarpophalangeal joints (MCPs) and fingers
         2. Heliotrope rash: violet eruption on the upper eyelids, cheeks, and forehead with periorbital edema
         3. Shawl rash: erythematous, photosensitive, papular rash located over the anterior chest, neck, and shoulders in a V-shaped (shawl) distribution
         4. "Mechanic's hands": periungual erythema with painful cracking of the skin at the fingertips
      - Patients may also present with polyarthritis, Raynaud phenomenon, interstitial lung disease, esophageal involvement, and cardiac involvement.
   C. Laboratory and diagnostic studies
      - Serum muscle enzymes (creatine kinase [CK], lactic acid dehydrogenase [LDH], aspartate aminotransferase [AST], alanine aminotransferase [ALT], and aldolase) are elevated in PM/DM. Electromyography (EMG) shows myopathic changes with increased irritability and decreased amplitude. Antinuclear antibody (ANA) is usually positive. Anti-Jo-1 antibody is also present in about one third of patients with PM/DM.

D. Formulating the diagnosis
   • DM/PM can overlap with other connective tissue diseases and can mimic other forms of myopathy. A lack of distal muscle involvement helps to distinguish PM/DM from other causes. Although the characteristic EMG findings support the diagnosis, a muscle biopsy confirms the diagnosis and excludes other causes of myopathy.
E. Evaluating the severity of problems
   • Factors associated with a poor outcome include delayed diagnosis, severe muscle weakness, and involvement of respiratory, esophageal, or cardiac muscle. An increased risk of malignancy is seen with both dermatomyositis and polymyositis, but the risk is higher with DM.
F. Managing the patient
   • Corticosteroids are the cornerstone of therapy with a goal of improving muscle strength and normalizing muscle enzymes. Refractory cases may respond to azathioprine, methotrexate, or intravenous immunoglobulin (IVIg).

X. Polymyalgia Rheumatica
   A. Basic science
      • The pathogenesis of polymyalgia rheumatica (PMR) is not completely understood but a clear association with giant cell arteritis (GCA) is recognized with a similar genetic susceptibility pattern involving the same HLA-DR4 antigen. Approximately 15% of patients with PMR have GCA. Other associated diseases include rheumatoid arthritis, polymyositis, and malignancy. Similar to GCA, PMR is a disease of the elderly and is rarely diagnosed under the age of 50. Women are affected more than men.
   B. History and physical examination
      • PMR presents subacutely with symmetric proximal muscle pain and stiffness. The shoulders, neck, and hip girdles are involved. Patients will often complain of difficulty with activities such as combing their hair, getting dressed, climbing stairs, and rising from a chair. Associated symptoms include fatigue, fever, malaise, and weight loss. The gelling phenomenon (stiffness after a period of inactivity) is a common complaint.
      • Physical examination may reveal limited range of motion in the shoulders, neck, and hips. Although patients may complain of weakness, muscle strength is preserved unless there is atrophy from disuse in prolonged disease.
   C. Laboratory and diagnostic studies
      • Similar to GCA, the characteristic laboratory finding in PMR is an elevated erythrocyte sedimentation rate (ESR) greater than 40 mm/hour. An ESR above 100 mm/hour is not uncommon. Other laboratory findings are nonspecific as in GCA. No radiographic evaluation is needed. A temporal artery biopsy is indicated if any symptoms or signs of GCA are present (see GCA section).
   D. Formulating the diagnosis
      • PMR should be considered in elderly patients who present with a consistent clinical history and an elevated ESR. No other active disease process should be present to explain the findings. A trial of low-dose steroids with rapid clinical response confirms the clinical diagnosis.

E. Evaluating the severity of problems
- Patients with PMR who complain of new onset headache, temporal artery tenderness, jaw claudication, or visual impairment should be promptly evaluated for GCA. Treatment with steroids should immediately be started or escalated and a temporal artery biopsy should be arranged.

F. Managing the patient
- PMR is usually self-limited but may persist for several years. Patients often respond dramatically to low-dose corticosteroids, such as prednisone 10 to 20 mg/day. The corticosteroids should be continued for several weeks after symptoms resolve and then tapered very slowly to avoid relapse. ESR correlates with disease activity and is helpful in guiding the steroid taper in conjunction with the clinical symptoms. Continued follow-up and monitoring for signs of GCA is necessary.

XI. Rheumatoid Arthritis
A. Basic science
- Rheumatoid arthritis (RA) is a chronic systemic inflammatory disease of unknown cause. Genetic susceptibility and an environmental trigger lead to disease expression. The disease has a female predominance with an onset usually between the second and fifth decades of life.

B. History and physical examination
- Patients usually present with a gradual onset of symmetric polyarticular arthritis with pain, stiffness, swelling, joint effusions, and limited range of motion to the affected joints. Morning stiffness lasting at least 1 hour and stiffness after periods of inactivity (gelling) are very common. Although the hand joints are most often involved in early disease, the distal interphalangeal joints (DIPs) are spared in RA. The joints most affected are the metacarpophalangeal (MCP), proximal interphalangeal (PIP), wrist, elbows, knees, ankles, and feet. The lumbar spine and sacroiliac joints are usually spared in RA. The cervical spine may be affected and instability can lead to atlantoaxial subluxation and myelopathy.
- The clinical course of RA typically fluctuates, but most patients suffer from a progressive course over time. Persistent active disease leads to irreversible structural damage including flexion deformities, subluxation, fibrosis, and ankylosis. Ulnar deviation, swan neck, and boutonniére deformities are typical changes of advanced disease in the hand. Extra-articular manifestations include rheumatoid nodules, scleritis, episcleritis, interstitial lung disease, pleuritis, pleural and pericardial effusions, pericarditis, myocarditis, vasculitis, and polyneuropathy. Rheumatoid nodules are typically found over bony prominences or extensor surfaces, especially the elbow, but can develop at any location. Sjögren's syndrome manifest by ocular and oral dryness also occurs in RA. Finally, patients may have a variety of nonspecific symptoms including malaise, myalgias, fever, weight loss, and fatigue.

C. Laboratory and diagnostic studies
- Rheumatoid factor is positive in 80% of patients with rheumatoid arthritis but is not a specific marker as it is seen in many other conditions. Anti-CCP

(cyclic citrullinated peptides) antibodies are more specific for RA. Anti-Ro (SSA) and anti-La (SSB) are seen in Sjögren's syndrome. Inflammatory markers including ESR and CRP are helpful in monitoring disease activity and differentiating from noninflammatory conditions, such as osteoarthritis or coexisting fibromyalgia.

- Other nonspecific laboratory findings include anemia of chronic disease, leukocytosis, thrombocytosis, and inflammatory synovial fluid. X-rays of the hand show joint space narrowing, erosions, and deformities with more advanced disease. These typical x-ray findings may not be present at initial presentation.

D. Formulating the diagnosis
- The American College of Rheumatology diagnostic criteria for RA (4 of the 7 criteria must be present):
   1. Morning stiffness lasting at least 1 hour for 6 weeks
   2. Swelling of three or more joints for 6 weeks
   3. Swelling of the hand joints (MCP, PIP, wrist) for 6 weeks
   4. Symmetric joint swelling for 6 weeks
   5. Rheumatoid nodules
   6. Positive rheumatoid factor
   7. Typical erosive changes on hand x-rays

E. Evaluating the severity of problems
- Significant deformity and joint destruction from erosion of cartilage and bone occur in untreated and refractory cases. Surgical intervention is sometimes required to relieve pain and restore function caused by structural damage. Cervical spine x-rays are prudent prior to elective intubation in patients with RA to exclude C1-C2 instability, which if present can result in cervical cord compression secondary to cervical vertebrae subluxation.

F. Managing the patient
- Patient education and nonpharmacologic measures (rest, exercise, and physical therapy) are important, but pharmacotherapy is the mainstay of treatment. The goal of therapy is to relieve pain, restore function, and prevent joint damage. Early aggressive control of inflammation with disease-modifying antirheumatic drugs (DMARDs) is critical as it will slow the progression of joint destruction and preserve function. The best combination of medications is unclear, but most patients with moderate to severe disease do require multiple medications.
- Pharmacotherapy in RA:
   1. NSAIDs
      - NSAIDs offer symptomatic relief but have no impact on the course of disease. Monitor for gastrointestinal (GI) and renal side effects. Selective cyclooxygenase-2 (COX-2) inhibitors have less GI toxicity but an increased risk of cardiovascular events.
   2. Corticosteroids
      - Corticosteroids provide symptomatic relief by reducing inflammation at disease onset and with subsequent flares. They are given orally or intra-articularly. Long-term side effects limit prolonged use.

3. DMARDs
- DMARDs have a slower onset of action. The choice of DMARD depends on activity of disease and side effect profile.
  a. Methotrexate
     - Methotrexate is a very effective folic acid antagonist used as first-line DMARD therapy for RA. Side effects include myelosuppression, hepatotoxicity, pneumonitis, diarrhea, mouth ulcers, nausea, and alopecia. Folic acid supplementation daily is essential when methotrexate is given. The CBC and liver and renal function should be monitored regularly.
  b. Hydroxychloroquine
     - Hydroxychloroquine is effective for mild RA alone or in combination with other DMARDs for more aggressive disease. Monitoring for ocular toxicity requires annual ophthalmology consultation.
  c. Sulfasalazine
     - Sulfasalazine is effective for mild RA or in combination with other DMARDs for treating more aggressive disease. Side effects are nausea, vomiting, and diarrhea. CBC should be monitored because myelosuppression is a side effect.
  d. Leflunomide
     - This pyrimidine synthesis inhibitor can be used in combination with methotrexate. It may cause hepatotoxicity.
4. Anticytokines biologic agents
   a. Anti-tumor necrosis factor alpha agents (etanercept, infliximab, adalimumab)
      - These drugs constitute second-line therapy and are usually added on to methotrexate for persistently active disease. Side effects include immunosuppression with risk of serious infection, congestive heart failure, demyelinating disease, and malignancy.
   b. Anakinra
      - This is an IL-1 receptor antagonist that also causes immunosuppression.
      - Other agents used less commonly include azathioprine, cyclosporine, penicillamine, gold, and minocycline.
5. Other biologic agents recently approved: rituximab, abatacept

XII. Seronegative Spondyloarthropathies
A. Basic science
   - Ankylosing spondylitis (AS), psoriatic arthritis (PA), and reactive arthritis represent a group of inflammatory arthropathies that are strongly linked with HLA-B27 and affect the spine and peripheral joints in an asymmetric fashion. The pathogenesis is unclear but likely involves a combination of genetic, environmental, immunologic, and infectious factors. Genitourinary or gastrointestinal bacterial infection may precede the development of reactive arthritis. Organisms that have been implicated include *Chlamydia, Shigella, Salmonella, Yersinia,* and *Campylobacter.*

B. History and physical examination
- AS presents with low back pain and morning stiffness for at least 3 months which improves with exercise but not with rest. Extra-articular manifestations include uveitis, aortitis, and apical pulmonary fibrosis. Men are affected more commonly than women and age of onset is typically in the third and fourth decades of life. Physical examination shows limited range of motion in the lumbar spine, limited chest expansion, and tenderness of the sacroiliac (SI) joint.
- PA presents with a similar inflammatory arthritis with joint pain and stiffness that improves after exercise. The spine and DIPs are commonly involved. Psoriatic plaques, dactylitis (sausage-shaped digits), and characteristic pitting of the nails are seen. Psoriasis usually precedes the development of arthritis. Women and men are equally affected and age of onset is in the fourth and fifth decades.
- Reactive arthritis presents with an abrupt onset of asymmetric synovitis following an episode of infectious diarrhea or urethritis. Males are affected more than females. Clinical findings overlap with the other spondyloarthropathies including inflammatory back and joint pain and dactylitis. Reiter's syndrome is a form of reactive arthritis with a classic triad of symptoms: uveitis, urethritis, and arthritis. Skin lesions called keratoderma blennorrhagica can occur on the palms and soles and mimic psoriasis. Genitourinary mucosal lesions can be seen.
C. Laboratory and diagnostic studies
- The spondyloarthropathies lack autoantibodies. Laboratory findings are nonspecific except for the presence of HLA-B27. There is a strong association between sacroiliitis and HLA-B27 in these disorders, especially with ankylosing spondylitis. The synovial fluid is inflammatory in nature. X-rays show sacroiliitis and eventual fusion of the SI joint. In PA, a classic "pencil-in-cup" deformity is seen at the DIP joints on x-ray.
D. Formulating the diagnosis
- AS is diagnosed by a clinical history of inflammatory back pain and sacroiliitis on x-ray. A positive HLA-B27 serology adds further support for the diagnosis. A positive family history is an important component of the history.
- PA is diagnosed by a clinical history of psoriasis and inflammatory arthritis affecting the spine and distal joints with supporting radographic evidence. Disease activity does not correlate with the extent of skin involvement. A positive culture or serology indicative of an associated bacterial infection supports the diagnosis of reactive arthritis.
E. Evaluating the severity of problems
- The seronegative spondyloarthropathies can progress and cause significant disability because of decreased mobility and pain. Fusion of the vertebral column known as "bamboo" spine is a sign of advanced disease and sacral joint fusion in AS. Arthritis mutilans is a destructive form of PA with severe deformities.
F. Managing the patient
- Physical therapy, posture training, and exercise are important components of therapy. NSAIDs are beneficial as first-line therapy to control pain in these

disorders. Sulfasalazine was previously used more commonly in AS but is now being replaced by the tumor necrosis factor (TNF) alpha inhibitors (etanercept, infliximab, adalimumab), which are very effective. Intra-articular corticosteroids are beneficial during flares of disease. Sulfasalazine and methotrexate are beneficial in PA and reactive arthritis but the TNF alpha inhibitors are gaining popularity in these disorders as well.

XIII. Systemic Lupus Erythematosus
   A. Basic science
      • Systemic lupus erythematosus (SLE) is a multisystem inflammatory autoimmune disorder that occurs mainly in young women. Men with SLE often have a worse prognosis than women and a higher incidence of renal involvement. The cause is unknown. A combination of genetic, hormonal, immune, and environmental factors play a role in forming antibodies and creating immune complexes. Certain medications (e.g., hydralazine, procainamide, and isoniazid) manifest a mild reversible form of a lupus-like illness with antibodies to histone.
   B. History and physical examination
      • The clinical course of SLE is variable and depends largely on which organs are involved. Any organ may be affected. Common sites of involvement include the skin, joints, kidneys, lungs, and nervous system. Acute exacerbations are typically followed by full or partial remission. Constitutional symptoms are very common and include fever, fatigue, malaise, and weight loss. Both Raynaud's phenomenon and Sjögren's syndrome can be seen in SLE.
      • Clinical manifestations
       1. Skin
         • Malar ("butterfly") rash, discoid (rounded slightly raised scaly rash with atrophic center) rash, photosensitivity, and alopecia. There may be small, painless ulcerations in the mouth.
       2. Renal
         • Renal involvement is generally the most serious organ involvement and manifests as proteinuria, hematuria, urinary cellular casts, and renal failure.
       3. Musculoskeletal
         • Musculoskeletal involvement includes arthralgias, myalgias, and nonerosive arthritis. Joint symptoms occur in most patients with SLE and often are present early in the disease, most commonly in the hands, wrists, and knees.
       4. Pulmonary
         • Pleuritis, pleural effusion, pneumonitis, interstitial lung disease, alveolar hemorrhage, and pulmonary hypertension may occur.
       5. Cardiac
         • Pericarditis, (most common cardiac manifestation) pericardial effusion, myocarditis, endocarditis, and coronary artery disease may occur.
       6. Central nervous system (CNS)
         • These features include seizures, psychosis, organic brain syndrome, stroke, headaches, delirium, cranial nerve palsies, peripheral neuropathies, and mood disorders.

7. Gastrointestinal
  • Peritonitis, hepatitis, colitis, abdominal pain, nausea, vomiting, and diarrhea may occur.
8. Vascular
  • Vasculitis, thrombosis, hypercoagulable state with recurrent miscarriages, and thrombotic events are possible.

C. Laboratory and diagnostic studies
  • Several autoantibodies are present in SLE. The antinuclear antibody (ANA) in high titers is the most sensitive diagnostic test for SLE but it is not specific. Anti-dsDNA and anti-Sm antibodies are very specific for SLE and should be checked if the ANA is positive. Other antibodies seen in SLE include anti-Ro (SSA) and anti-La (SSB) which are associated with Sjögren's syndrome. Anti-histone antibodies are found in drug-induced SLE. Complement levels (C3, C4) are typically low during disease exacerbation and are used to follow disease activity. The antiphospholipid antibodies (lupus anticoagulant and anti-cardiolipin) and a false positive VDRL test can also be seen in patients with SLE. Hematologic abnormalities in SLE include leukopenia, lymphopenia, thrombocytopenia, and anemia.

D. Formulating the diagnosis
  • ACR SLE classification criteria (4 of the following 11 criteria must be present):
    1. Malar rash
    2. Discoid rash
    3. Photosensitivity
    4. Oral or nasal ulcers
    5. Arthritis: nonerosive involvement of at least two peripheral joints
    6. Serositis: pleuritis or pericarditis
    7. Renal disorder: proteinuria (>0.5 g/day) or cellular casts
    8. Hematologic disorder: leukopenia, lymphopenia, hemolytic anemia, or thrombocytopenia
    9. Neurologic disorder: seizures or psychosis
    10. Positive anti-dsDNA, anti-Smith antibody, or anti-phospholipid antibodies
    11. Positive ANA

E. Evaluating the severity of problems
  • The major causes of death in SLE are infection (due to immunosuppression), renal failure, CNS involvement, and premature coronary artery disease. Severe lupus nephritis may advance to end-stage renal disease requiring hemodialysis or possible kidney transplantation.

F. Managing the patient
  • The assessment of disease activity requires frequent monitoring of the clinical history, physical examination, and laboratory values. Anti-dsDNA, ESR, and CRP typically rise while complement levels fall with worsening disease activity. These markers are useful in guiding treatment.
  • No treatment for SLE is curative; hence, the goal of treatment is to reduce the severity of acute attacks and to minimize end organ damage. NSAIDs are the first line of treatment for musculoskeletal symptoms and serositis but should not be used in patients with nephritis. Antimalarials (e.g., hydroxychloroquine)

are also beneficial for musculoskeletal symptoms and skin involvement. Patients should be monitored for ocular toxicity while on hydroxychloroquine. Corticosteroids are added for more severe disease with significant organ involvement and can be used alone or in combination with other immunosuppressants. Cyclophosphamide is commonly used with steroids for lupus nephritis or vasculitis. Other immunosuppressants used in SLE include methotrexate, mycophenolate, and azathioprine.

XIV. Systemic Sclerosis (Scleroderma)
  A. Basic science
    • The pathogenesis of scleroderma is not well understood. This chronic disorder characteristically causes thickening of the skin and may affect internal organs such as the gastrointestinal tract, heart, and kidneys.
    • Scleroderma is classified based on distribution of skin lesions and internal organ involvement:
      1. Systemic: cutaneous sclerosis with internal organ involvement
        a. Diffuse cutaneous disease: thickening of skin on extremities, trunk, and face (skin fibrosis is extensive including proximal extremities)
        b. Limited cutaneous disease: thickening of skin on distal extremities and face (skin fibrosis does not extend proximally beyond the knees or elbows). Associated with CREST syndrome (calcinosis, Raynaud phenomenon, esophageal dysmotility, sclerodactyly, telangiectasias) and pulmonary hypertension
      2. Localized: cutaneous sclerosis without internal organ involvement. Several forms include linear, en coup de sabre, localized and generalized morphea.
  B. History and physical examination
    • The clinical findings vary depending on the type of scleroderma and specific organ involvement, but all have thickened sclerotic skin lesions that typically begin in the hands and face. Other skin findings include sclerodactyly, calcinosis, edema, telangiectasias, and nail fold capillary dilatation.
    • Raynaud's phenomenon is an early sign in systemic scleroderma and presents with vasospasm of the extremities due to cold or emotion. Puffiness of the fingers and hands are also seen early in the disease. The characteristic color changes of the extremity include an initial pallor (white), acrocyanosis (blue), and hyperemia (red). Digital ulcers are caused by ischemia.
    • Gastrointestinal involvement is very common and may present with reflux, dysphagia, odynophagia, early satiety, diarrhea, or malabsorption.
    • Most GI symptoms are secondary to reflux, strictures, and abnormal motility.
    • Pulmonary involvement presents with dyspnea and cough due to interstitial lung disease or pulmonary hypertension. Pulmonary hypertension is the leading cause of death in systemic sclerosis.
    • Musculoskeletal symptoms are common, including arthralgias, decreased mobility, and contractures.
    • A sudden onset of hypertension and acute renal failure raises serious concern for a scleroderma renal crisis.

C. Laboratory and diagnostic studies
- Circulating autoantibodies present in scleroderma include anti-Scl-70 (diffuse cutaneous/ILD), anti-centromere (limited cutaneous/CREST), anti-RNA polymerase, and anti-U3-RNP. ANA is positive in over 90% of cases. With renal involvement, proteinuria and elevations in the blood urea nitrogen (BUN) and creatinine are seen. With pulmonary involvement, interstitial fibrosis is seen on chest CT, and pulmonary function tests (PFTs) show a restrictive pattern.

D. Formulating the diagnosis
- The clinical findings highly suggest scleroderma and the serologic tests help strengthen the diagnosis. The autoantibodies have a low sensitivity, so the diagnosis is not excluded if these tests are negative. Nail fold capillary testing (i.e., examining the capillaries of the nail fold under microscopy) has been shown to aid in the diagnosis. Further organ-specific testing is guided by symptoms and adds support to the diagnosis. Localized scleroderma is diagnosed clinically and can be confirmed by skin biopsy if needed.

E. Evaluating the severity of problems
- Diffuse cutaneous systemic scleroderma has a worse prognosis than limited systemic scleroderma. However, a subset of patients with the limited cutaneous systemic form can develop pulmonary hypertension (about 10%), which has a very poor prognosis.

F. Managing the patient
- Treatment options are somewhat limited in scleroderma. No therapy effectively reverses the fibrotic changes in scleroderma, but efforts are made to slow progression and provide symptomatic relief. Routine monitoring with PFTs, electrocardiogram (ECG), cardiac echocardiogram, and renal function testing should be performed annually. Further evaluation is often required based on specific organ involvement.
- Treatment of Raynaud's phenomenon includes avoidance of triggers (cold exposure) and smoking cessation. Sustained-release calcium channel blockers (amlodipine, nifedipine) are the initial drugs of choice for Raynaud's phenomenon.
- Proton pump inhibitors are used to treat gastroesophageal reflux and the prokinetic agent metoclopramide is used for motility disorders.
- Cyclophosphamide and prednisone are used in interstitial lung disease. Oxygen, calcium channel blockers, bosentan (an inhibitor of the potent vasoconstrictor endothelian 1), and prostacyclin analogs are used in pulmonary hypertension.
- Aggressive antihypertensive treatment with ACE (angiotensin-converting enzyme) inhibitors to control hypertension and decrease the rate of renal damage progression is critical.

XV. Wegener's Granulomatosis
A. Basic science
- Wegener's granulomatosis (WG) is a systemic granulomatous vasculitis of the small and medium-sized arteries which predominantly affects the respiratory

tract and kidneys. Necrotizing granulomatous inflammation is seen on biopsy in WG. Microscopic polyangiitis (MPA) is a similar type of systemic vasculitis that mimics WG clinically but lacks granulomas on biopsy.

B. History and physical examination
   - WG presents with upper airway involvement in over 90% of patients and is characterized by rhinorrhea, oral and nasal ulceration or perforation, otitis, sinusitis, hemoptysis, cough, and dyspnea. Constitutional symptoms including fever, malaise, weight loss, myalgias, and arthralgias are common. Ocular (conjunctivitis, scleritis, retro-orbital mass), skin (papules, purpura, and subcutaneous nodules), and CNS involvement can also occur.

C. Laboratory and diagnostic studies
   - The presence of antineutrophil cytoplasmic antibodies (ANCA) is highly suggestive of WG, especially in the presence of glomerulonephritis; c-ANCA is seen in WG and p-ANCA is seen in MPA. Urine will reveal an active sediment with proteinuria, hematuria, and red blood cell casts if there is renal involvement.
   - The other laboratory findings in WG are nonspecific with elevations of inflammatory markers (ESR, CRP), normocytic anemia, leukocytosis, and thrombocytosis. Chest x-ray findings may include nodules, infiltrates, and alveolar and pleural opacities.

D. Formulating the diagnosis
   - The clinical and laboratory findings suggest WG. A tissue biopsy confirms the diagnosis and is typically taken from a site of active disease. Biopsy confirmation of the diagnosis revealing necrotizing granulomatous inflammation is important because the treatment of WG is associated with significant toxicity.

E. Evaluating the severity of problems
   - WG is a life-threatening disease with mortality rates near 100% for untreated disease.

F. Managing the patient
   - The combination of cyclophosphamide and corticosteroids are used to induce remission of WG. Once remission is achieved, a less toxic immunosuppressant is substituted for cyclophosphamide, and the steroids are tapered. Methotrexate and azathioprine are the most common agents used for maintenance therapy of WG. Relapse is not uncommon and is recognized by the clinical symptoms in conjunction with a rising c-ANCA titer. The treatment of MPA is similar to that of WG.

Orthopedics

CHAPTER 9

I. Approach to Joint Pain
  A. Basic science
   - Joint pain is a common condition for which patients seek medical evaluation. A thorough history and physical examination are imperative to generate a proper differential diagnosis, as there are numerous causes of joint pain. Pain can be referred from underlying or surrounding organs, or caused by bones, ligaments, muscles, nerves, or inflammatory processes.
  B. History and physical examination
   - The exact location, quality, acuity of onset, duration, and exacerbating and relieving factors of pain are important in trying to limit the causes of pain and create a workable differential diagnosis. Systemic symptoms such as fever and chills may be a sign of a more diffuse process. Associated weakness or sensory or neurologic deficits may also alter the differential diagnosis. A history of trauma and the mechanism of injury can provide valuable information as to the underlying disorder. Past medical, surgical, and family history are important for a complete evaluation and may provide insight to patients at higher risk for particular illness or disorder.
   - Physical examination consists of inspection to look for asymmetry, erythema, ecchymosis, atrophy, or swelling of the affected joint with comparison to the unaffected side if possible. The patient should be asked to localize the area of maximal discomfort with this region being examined last. It is also important to examine one joint above and below the symptomatic joint to eliminate possible distracting diagnosis. Next, palpate the bony prominences and soft tissue landmarks. Comparison should be made with the unaffected side if possible. This is followed by functional testing of the joint, passive range of motion, strength testing and a gait assessment, and neurologic screening as appropriate. Finally, depending on the joint involved, a series of specialized maneuvers may be utilized in an attempt to isolate a particular anatomic structure to further refine the ultimate diagnosis.
  C. Formulating the diagnosis
   1. Joint stiffness
    - "Stiffness" is a common complaint encountered by health care providers and can have several different causes. "Stiffness" can actually have many different meanings to patients, making the history and physical examination vital to the evaluation process.

- Patients often complain of stiffness when they actually have a joint effusion. The effusion results in a decreased range of motion. Stiffness can also be caused by inflammation in tendon sheaths such as in trigger finger.
- Stiffness can result from connective tissue or muscle hypertrophy such as in the formation of flexion or Dupuytren's contracture, or from muscle spasm after a soft tissue injury.
- Exacerbating and relieving factors are also important; stiffness due to rheumatoid arthritis is often worse in the morning, and stiffness secondary to osteoarthritis is worsened by inactivity and actually improves with exercise.

2. Joint swelling/effusion
    a. Basic science
        - An effusion or swelling in a joint is an important sign of a pathologic process. All joints normally contain a small amount of fluid, but a deviation from normal joint stasis must occur for an effusion to develop. Joint effusions should evaluated by their location, number of joints involved, and type of fluid. Increased blood flow to the joint for any reason can cause an effusion.
    b. History and physical examination
        - The history and physical examination are key to the workup of an effusion. For example, a history of traumatic injury would suggest an anatomic cause of the swelling and some disruption of bone, cartilage, muscle, or ligament. However, a painless effusion of one or more joints without trauma or swelling that comes and goes would suggest a systemic process. The presence or absence of pain, morning stiffness, prior illness, medication use, and additionally systemic symptoms can be helpful. Physical examination can be important as well. The presence of rashes, nodules, or a significantly swollen, warm joint with pain on passive range of motion would suggest an infection.
    c. Laboratory and diagnostic studies
        - Analysis of joint fluid should be obtained when the cause of a joint effusion is unknown despite a thorough history and physical examination. Aspiration is also necessary in the evaluation of a possible septic joint. It can be utilized to relieve pain and pressure.
        - Routine analysis consists of complete blood count (CBC) and differential, Gram stain and culture, and crystal analysis. Characteristic features of a septic joint include a white blood cell count greater than 50,000 with more than 75% neutrophils and low glucose. The synovial fluid from an inflammatory condition typically displays a white blood cell (WBC) count of 2000 to 50,000, neutrophil count of greater than 50%, and only mildly decreased glucose concentration. Lastly, a noninflammatory synovial fluid would display a white blood cell count of less than 2000, neutrophil count of less than 25%, and near-normal glucose value.
        - The diagnosis of gout can be made from the finding of negatively birefringent needle-shaped crystals. Pseudogout would produce positive birefringent crystals.

- Further laboratory testing such as erythrocyte sedimentation rate (ESR), C-reactive protein, and antibody testing (ANA, RF) may be helpful to confirm a suspected diagnosis.
  d. Formulating the diagnosis
  - A host of conditions can cause monoarthritis including trauma, crystal disease such as gout and pseudogout, septic joint, and osteoarthritis. Oligoarthritis is characterized by the involvement of two to four joints. Common conditions that cause this include osteoarthritis, arthritis associated with inflammatory bowel disease, Reiter's syndrome, and psoriatic arthritis. Involvement of greater than five joints is common in rheumatoid arthritis, reactive arthritis, systemic lupus erythematosus, and the seronegative spondyloarthrities.

3. Internal derangement of the knee
   a. Basic science
   - Internal derangement of the knee is a generic term used to describe an injury or abnormality of the ligamentous structures, cartilage, or menisci of the knee. Many of these injuries occur together. Damage to one of the four ligaments of the knee is usually traumatic and can involve the medial collateral ligament (MCL), lateral collateral ligament (LCL), or posterior cruciate ligament (PCL). An anterior cruciate ligament injury (ACL) may be traumatic or nontraumatic. A tear of the meniscus also can be a traumatic event, especially in younger patients. In older patients with degenerative changes of the joint, less force is required to produce a tear, and injuries may occur during somewhat routine maneuvers.
   b. History and physical examination
   - The evaluation of the stability of the ligaments of the knee is performed by utilizing specialized maneuvers. Lachman's test and anterior drawer test are most useful for accessing the stability of the ACL. Increased translation of the injured knee versus the unaffected knee or loss of a firm end point would indicate a tear. Varus and valgus testing at 0 degrees and 30 degrees of flexion is used to access the stability of the lateral collateral ligament and medical collateral ligament, respectively. Increased pain or "opening" of the knee with varus or valgus testing would indicate an injury to the respective ligament. The posterior cruciate ligament injury is accessed by the posterior drawer test which again would demonstrate increased translation. Meniscal injury can be assessed with the McMurray's test which produces a click, pop, or increased pain along the joint line as a flexed knee is extended under stress.
   c. Formulating the diagnosis.
     (1) Anterior cruciate ligament injury
     - The anterior cruciate ligament is a knee stabilizer that prevents anterior translation of the tibia on the femur. An injury to the anterior cruciate ligament is one of the most dreaded injuries in sports. Most injuries involve a twisting motion of the knee where the foot is fixed, hyperextended, or during an abnormal landing

after a jump. Patients often report feeling or hearing a "pop." Swelling, ecchymosis, and pain follow. Patients complain of instability of the knee. Their leg "gives out" while cutting (e.g., sudden movements). Concurrent damage to the meniscus is common while damage to other ligaments is possible. Bone bruising almost always accompanies the injury. Females are at greater risk than males.

- Physical examination is significant for a painful swollen knee. Limitations in flexion and extension are normally noted acutely due to swelling. Medial joint line tenderness is common due to meniscal injuries or bone bruising. The Lachmans test and anterior drawer test will show increased translation. McMurray's testing may also be positive if the meniscus is affected. Neurovascular status should also be accessed as an injury to these structures can occur in association with significant knee injury. Diagnosis can be clinical if early in the injury. Assessment of the patient is more difficult after a significant amount of swelling is present. Patients may need to be re-examined after improvement in the swelling. X-rays are helpful to rule out a fracture but a magnetic resonance imaging (MRI) scan is useful to confirm the diagnosis and to evaluate the other structures of the knee for damage.
- Treatment of an ACL injury initially involves immobilization, crutches, ice, elevation, compression, pain control, control of swelling and physical therapy. Patients should be referred to a specialist to consider possible surgical repair.

(2) Posterior cruciate ligament
- Injuries to the PCL are much less common and are usually caused by a significantly directed posterior force. Patients may present with pain, swelling, and instability. Concomitant injuries are common. Physical examination is significant for swelling contributing to decreased range of motion. A "sag" can be observed when the patient is supine with knees flexed to 90 degrees compared to the unaffected side (the abnormal position of the tibia posterior to the femoral condyles). The posterior drawer test is positive for increased translation. Diagnosis is usually made clinically. Assessment of the patient is more difficult after a significant amount of swelling is present. Patients may need to be re-examined after improvement in the swelling. X-rays are helpful to rule out a fracture but an MRI is useful to confirm the diagnosis and to evaluate for additional structural damage to the knee. Initial treatment of a PCL injury involves immobilization, crutches, ice, elevation, compression, pain control, control of swelling and physical therapy. Surgery is usually not required, but these patients should be referred to a specialist.

(3) Collateral ligament injuries
- An injury to the medial collateral ligament occurs due to a force directed to the lateral knee which is transmitted across the knee to

the MCL. An injury to the lateral collateral ligament is due to a force directed to the medial knee which is transmitted across the knee to the LCL. Patients present with pain and swelling. Ecchymosis and stiffness may also be present. Physical examination reveals pain along the medial femoral condyle and medial tibia for an MCL injury and lateral femoral condyle and fibula for an LCL injury. Varus or valgus testings show increased pain and may display "opening" of the joint. Diagnosis is clinical. X-rays are helpful to rule out a fracture. An MRI scan may be necessary to confirm the diagnosis and evaluate for other potential injuries. Initial treatment involves immobilization, crutches, ice, elevation, compression, pain control, control of swelling, and physical therapy. High-degree sprains may require a brace. Although few patients require surgery, a specialist should be involved in the treatment process to rule out associated injuries especially in high-level sprains.

(4) Meniscal injuries
- The medial and lateral meniscus are C-shaped rings of cartilage that function as shock absorbers in the knee. Injury to the meniscus can occur in association with other injuries to the knee, or can occur with twisting motions. Patients present with joint line pain, clicking, or inability to fully flex or extend the knee. They may or may not recall a specific event that was the start of their symptoms. Physical examination reveals swelling, joint line tenderness, or loss of flexion or extension. McMurray's test is positive for a click. Diagnosis is clinical but can be confirmed by MRI. X-rays are helpful initially to rule out fracture after a traumatic injury. Treatment consists of activity modification, ice, elevation, and anti-inflammatory medication. Patients with significant locking or loss of range of motion should be referred immediately to a specialist to consider arthroscopic surgery. Patients that do not settle down with conservative measures should also be referred for possible intervention.

(5) Juvenile rheumatoid arthritis
- Rheumatoid arthritis in children is a generalized systemic disease of which arthritis is but one component. The average age of onset is 6 years but may range from 1 to 14. The many variants of this disease may be grouped into three categories: pauciarticular, polyarticular, and systemic. The systemic variety is the most severe type, and involvement of multiple organ systems is common. Patients present with painful, swollen joints. In the systemic type they may also complain of fever, rash, ocular complaints, or systemic involvement.
- Physical examination is significant for tender, swollen joints. Fever, hepatosplenomegaly, generalized lymphadenopathy, pericarditis, rash, subcutaneous nodules, ocular inflammation, and amyloidosis may occur in the systemic variety. Laboratory evaluation consists of a CBC (normal to elevated WBCs), ESR, or C-reactive proteins

(elevated), and antinuclear antibodies may be detected. Joint aspiration may be appropriate in the case of effusion without injury. Radiographs should be obtained. Soft tissue swelling, capsular distention, and periarticular osteopenia are the initial findings. With progression of the disease, articular space narrowing and juxta-articular erosions occur. A suspected inflammatory arthritis involves prompt referral and evaluation. A multidisciplinary approach is imperative, involving pediatricians, rheumatologists, orthopedic surgeons, hematologists, physical and occupational therapists, psychologists, and social workers. Treatment is aimed at controlling the inflammation causing the joint damage, correction of joint contractures, and prevention of growth deformities of the bones.

II. Congenital Musculoskeletal Deformities
 A. Congenital muscular torticollis
   • Congenital muscular torticollis refers to a unilateral contracture of the sternocleidomastoid muscle, resulting in the head being tilted toward the side of the shortened muscle and the chin rotated toward the opposite side. The exact cause of the fibrosis producing this contracture is not completely understood. Presentation usually occurs at birth or during the first few weeks of life. The patient's mother notes an inability to rotate the chin to the affected side or tilt the head toward the contralateral side.
   • Physical examination reveals limitations of head tilt and rotation with chin rotated away from the contracted sternocleidomastoid and ipsilateral ear rotated toward the affected shoulder. A palpable mass may be found within the affected muscle. X-ray evaluation is not required for diagnosis.
   • Patients should be referred to a specialist for treatment and to rule out other confounding diagnosis. Treatment generally consists of passive stretching of the contracted sternocleidomastoid. Surgical intervention is reserved for those cases discovered late or those not responding to stretching as secondary facial and head abnormalities may develop.
 B. Developmental dysplasia of the hip (DDH)
   • DDH refers to a wide spectrum of abnormalities of the hip, ranging from simple instability to frank dislocation. Most patients have some degree of ligament laxity. DDH is a relatively common condition, occurring in 2.5 to 10 infants per 1000 live births, with females affected six times more often than males. Caucasians also appear to be more affected than African Americans. A combination of environmental and genetic factor are believed to be the cause of this abnormality. Cases that are initially unrecognized in infancy may develop a limp later in life, which may be the presenting complaint.
   • A thorough evaluation of the hips during the newborn period is essential for making this diagnosis. Physical findings are age dependent. The Ortolani and Barlow tests are the two most important maneuvers to test for hip stability. The Barlow test should be done first because it is a sign of dislocation of the femoral head from the located position. The Ortolani test is a sign of reentry of the femoral head into the acetabulum from the dislocated position. Other

findings that may indicate hip disease include asymmetric gluteal creases, which may be a signal of an already-dislocated hip. Hip abduction may also be limited in these patients. The physical examination is most important key to diagnosis. Ultrasound is utilized in infants to assess the amount of femoral head coverage by the acetabulum in cases of dislocatable hips. X-ray evaluation is usually not indicated in infants but may be appropriate in older patients when this diagnosis is being considered.

- Any suspected abnormality of the hips should prompt an urgent orthopedic referral. Delay in treatment can increase the severity of the condition. In hips that can be located, early treatment consists of a Pavlic harness, which keeps the hips in an abducted and flexed position. In older patients, a brace, cast, or surgical procedure may be required to locate the hips.

C. Other congenital deformities

- Numerous additional congenital deformities can occur both in the upper and lower extremities and include congenital dislocations of the radial head, knee, or patella; bowing of bones including the tibia; or deformities of the digits including extra digits (polydactyly), fused digits (syndactyly), short digits (first metatarsal), or absent bone or digits. Treatment is aimed at restoring normal alignment when possible and limiting disability. Referral to a specialist should occur at the time of diagnosis in order to optimize timing of any interventions.

III. Disorders of the Back and Spine

A. Basic science

- Low back pain is the most frequent cause of worker disability in America, resulting in substantial decreased productivity and days lost from work. Approximately 90% of all people will have complaints of lower back pain at some time in their life. Most cases of low back pain resolve within 2 weeks and approximately 85% to 95% resolve within 6 to 12 weeks. In most instances, the exact pain generator is not identified. These cases are often referred to as mechanical back pain as they are attributable to injuries to the back musculature or ligamentous structures.
- A small proportion of acute low back pain may have serious pathologic conditions as its underlying cause. Some examples of these more serious conditions include fractures, neoplasms, infections, and other conditions with the potential to produce neurologic compromise.

1. Mechanical lower back pain

- Mechanical lower back pain can be called by many different names including lumbar strain, lumbago, or lumbosacral sprain.
- Generally patients can identify an episode of activity, twisting, or lifting that is unusual or can relate using improper body mechanics.
- Pain may be of sudden onset or more commonly is delayed. Pain is localized to the lower back and buttock region but may radiate into the posterior thigh. This is different from true radicular pain, which radiates below the knee. The low back pain is reproduced by movement, twisting, or bending.

- Historical features that would suggest an alternative diagnosis or a need for further workup include age above 50 or below 18 years of age, previous history of malignancy, history of significant weight loss, systemic symptoms such as fever or chills, history of recent surgical procedure, immunocompromised, night pain, intravenous drug use, back pain for more than 4 weeks, and pain not relieved with standard treatment. The history should attempt to rule out potentially serious spinal conditions.
- Significant trauma should raise suspicion for fracture. Constitutional symptoms such as weight loss, fever, and chills may indicate infection or neoplasm. Significant pain not associated with activity may also be indicative of saddle distribution numbness with bowel and bladder dysfunction (cauda equina syndrome).
- The examination begins with careful observation of the patient. A survey of the skin condition, with note of any abrasions, ecchymosis, lacerations, or swellings, should be taken. Careful palpation of the spine should be performed, with attention to severe tenderness, crepitus, deformity, and paraspinal muscle spasm. Often several areas may be tender, and multilevel involvement may be present.
- A complete neurologic evaluation is often necessary. This should involve not only the bilateral lower extremities but the perineal area as well. Careful motor and sensory testing of each radicular and dermatome level, with comparison to the uninvolved side, is mandatory.
- Motor testing should be based on the five-point strength scale (0 = no active twitch, 1 = visual or palpable twitch, 2 = contraction with gravity eliminated, 3 = contraction against gravity, 4 = submaximal strength, and 5 = maximal strength). Motor groups of the lower extremity include L2-L3 iliopsoas (hip flexors), L4 quadriceps (knee extension), L5 extensor hallus longus (great toe extension), and S1 gastrocnemius/soleus (ankle plantar flexion). Dermatomal sensory charts are available in many texts. Specific isolated areas include L2 proximal anterior thigh, L3 middle anterior thigh, L4 anterior shin, L5 medial dorsal foot, S1 lateral dorsal foot, S2 plantar foot and posterior leg, and S3-S4 perianal area. Reflexes, including patellar (L4), Achilles (S1), and bulbocavernosus (lower sacral), are also tested.
- Physical examination generally reveals pain that is localized to the lower back, buttock, or posterior thigh area. Pain increases with activity or bending. Placing the sciatic or femoral nerve under stretch is a useful test for irritability. A positive straight leg raise, indicated by reproduction of the radicular symptoms, is useful in testing the sciatic nerve. Hip extension similarly tests the femoral nerve. Straight leg raise should be negative and neurologic examination is normal with no evidence of atrophy, weakness, or sensory findings.
- Further diagnostic workup including x-rays and advanced imaging is usually not initially indicated in the absence of any red flags and a short duration of symptoms (less than 4 to 6 weeks). An MRI scan is usually the imaging test of choice. Additionally, laboratory studies are usually not

indicated; however, in cases in which infection or neoplasm is a concern, CBC, ESR, and other studies may be needed.

- Treatment of presumed mechanical back pain consists of a period of "relative rest." That is, the patient may partake in activities of daily living but should avoid activities that exacerbate the pain. Ice, nonsteroidal anti-inflammatory drugs (NSAIDs), and acetaminophen are useful for pain relief. Narcotics are rarely needed except in the treatment of severe pain for a short duration of time. Muscle relaxants can be helpful in the initial stages of injury (the first 2 to 3 days), particularly if the patient has trouble sleeping at night because of pain and displays a significant amount of spasm on physical examination. Physical therapy may also have a role both in the acute phase and in attempting to modify factors that helped contribute to the injury in the first place. Increased strength, flexibility, and improved ergonomics may help decrease the number and severity of reinjuries in the future.

2. Cauda equina syndrome
  - Cauda equina syndrome is a surgical emergency. Fracture, disk herniation, infection, and tumor can cause sudden compression of nerve roots causing significant neurologic compromise. Patients complain of lower back pain, which can radiate into the bilateral lower extremities. Patients also can display decreased anal sphincter tone, urinary retention, erectile dysfunction, and saddle anesthesia.
  - Neurologic symptoms can be rapidly progressive. Patients often complain of paresthesias and inability to ambulate because of weakness. Patients should be immediately referred to a spine specialist for emergency elevation as prolonged nerve compression can lead to permanent deficits. An emergent MRI is the imaging modality of choice. Treatment often requires surgical decompression.

3. Sciatica/radicular symptoms
  - Radicular symptoms can occur with low back pain and are caused by irritation of the nerve root. These usually manifest as electric-type sensations in a certain nerve root distribution. Numbness and weakness may be related by the patient as well. Sciatica refers to radicular symptoms within the sciatic nerve distribution. Ninety percent of cases of radiculopathy involve the L5 or S1 nerve roots. Radicular pain is often increased with sitting and can improve with standing.
  - Physical examination is revealing for low back pain that extends below the knee. Patients may also display weakness and decreased reflexes of the affected nerve root. A straight leg raise is positive in approximately 80% of patients with a herniated disk. A straight leg raise is performed by placing a patient in the supine position and elevating the patient's symptomatic leg. A positive test will reproduce radicular pain below the knee when the leg is moved in an arc from 30 degrees to 70 degrees. The occurrence of back pain does not constitute a positive test. A contralateral straight leg raise involves symptoms in the affected leg while the asymptomatic leg is elevated. This test is less sensitive than the straight

leg raise. Initially imaging studies are rarely warranted except when red flags are present to exclude a confounding diagnosis.

- Treatment is similar to that for mechanical lower back pain. Initial treatment involves relative rest, anti-inflammatory medication, and physical therapy. Patients who have progressive neurologic findings or intractable pain may become candidates for surgical decompression. Computed tomography (CT) or MRI may be helpful to delineate anatomic defects in patients in whom surgery is a consideration.

4. Spondylolysis/spondylolisthesis

- An additional cause of lower back pain that is most common in children and adolescents is spondylolysis. Males tend to be more affected than females. Spondylolysis is a fracture through the pars interarticularis of the vertebral body. They are most common in the fourth and fifth lumbar vertebrae. The defect is caused by repetitive trauma to the spine and is considered more of a stress fracture than a direct traumatic injury. Patients who undergo activities that place them in extension or hyperextension are at risk.

- Symptoms are variable ranging from completely asymptomatic to constant pain even at rest. Pain is localized to the lower back but can radiate to into the buttock and posterior thigh bilaterally. Physical examination may reveal muscle spasm (especially the hamstrings) and point tenderness along the vertebral body. Pain is often exacerbated by lumbar extension and single leg stand. Muscle strength and neurologic examination are otherwise unremarkable. X-ray evaluation is a relatively poor method for identifying a pars defect. Bone scan (with SPECT [single-photon emission CT]), CT, or MRI is often required to confirm the diagnosis if initial x-rays are negative.

- Treatment is aimed at improving symptoms and consists of relative rest, ice, and NSAIDs. A back brace may be utilized in patients who are symptomatic at rest or with minimal activity. Physical therapy may be helpful in order to prevent recurrence. Severe cases or cases refractory to medical management may be candidates for surgical intervention.

- In contrast to spondylolysis, spondylolisthesis is a fracture of both pars interarticularis of the vertebral body with concomitant anterior slippage of one vertebra on another. Patient demographics and presentation are similar to those of spondylolysis. In addition to muscle spasm and localized tenderness, a palpable step-off of the vertebral bodies may be noted. Diagnosis is confirmed on x-ray with the lateral the view being the most important. Flexion and extension views may be necessary if spinal instability is considered. Initial treatment options are similar to those for spondylolysis but are based on the degree of vertebral slippage. The amount of slippage is graded from 1 to 5 in which a grade 1 slippage reflects displacement of less than 25% of the vertebral body and grade 5 represents complete displacement. Patients who fail medical management in terms of uncontrolled pain, increased slippage, or spinal instability should be referred for surgical evaluation.

5. Spinal stenosis
   - Spinal stenosis is a degenerative process affecting patients older than 50 years of age. The lumbar spine is the most affected. Narrowing of the spinal canal causes nerve root compression. Patients complain of achy low back pain, buttock pain, and thigh pain. Pain may be bilateral, and radiates into the lower extremities (past the knee). Patients can also complain of weakness, fatigue, and paresthesia. Historically, pain increases with activity such as walking and is relieved with sitting. Patients are often symptomatic while standing at rest. Forward flexion at the hips relieves pain and patients often report that they do better when grocery shopping compared to other activities because they can lean over the cart.
   - Physical examination is remarkable for painful lumbar extension with possible decreased range of motion. Patients may exhibit a stooped posture, weakness, minor sensory findings, and altered reflexes. A complete neurologic examination is important to rule out cauda equina syndrome. Additionally, a thorough vascular examination is needed to evaluate for vascular claudication which is often the competing diagnosis. MRI or CT scan is needed to evaluate the degree of stenosis.
   - Treatment is aimed at maintaining functional level and decreasing pain. Activity modification is often used to avoid particularly painful positions. NSAIDs and other analgesics may be necessary to help relieve pain. Physical therapy is hallmark of treatment and is used to strengthen the surrounding soft tissues and help relieve pressure in extension. Patients who fail conservative measures have significant limitations in activity, or severe neurologic deficits can be considered for surgical intervention.
6. Kyphosis/scoliosis
   - Kyphosis is an exaggerated outward curvature of the spine and appears as an exaggerated "hump" when patients are viewed in the sagittal plane. In contrast, scoliosis is an exaggerated lateral curvature of the spine (>10 degrees) and is best viewed by standing directly behind a patient. The thoracic and lumbar spine are most commonly affected. These two conditions can occur together, a term called kyphoscoliosis. Both conditions occur in children and adults although the causes are somewhat different in each group. Kyphosis most often presents in adolescents or older adults. Adolescent kyphosis is most commonly caused by congenital vertebral defect or postural habits. In adults, compression fractures from osteoporosis is the leading cause, although secondary causes can occur both in adolescents and adults and include other disease processes such as juvenile rheumatoid arthritis, congenital or vertebral abnormalities, or neuromuscular disease. Childhood scoliosis affects males and females equally although females tend to be more severely affected. The most common cause of scoliosis in children is idiopathic although it can be secondary to other disease processes such as Marfan syndrome, congenital or vertebral abnormalities, or neuromuscular disease. In adults, scoliosis can be caused by worsening of congenital disease or degenerative changes of the spine (fracture, disk degeneration, slippage).

- Most children with kyphosis and scoliosis are asymptomatic and are picked up on routine screening examinations. Adult patients typically present with thoracic or lumbar pain, asymmetry which may have progressed, and loss of height. Physical examination should include palpation of the spine and thorough inspection of symmetry to included scapula, iliac crest, and flexion and extension testing. The curvature in scoliosis is worse in flexion and therefore the forward bend test is the best screening tool and is often used in children and adolescents. They should also be viewed from the side to evaluate for kyphosis. Differences of more than 5 degrees should be further evaluated.
- Diagnosis is confirmed by posteroanterior (PA) and lateral x-rays. Treatment is dependent on the age at time of diagnosis, underlying cause, and degree of curvature and disability. In general, most patients with kyphosis and scoliosis should be referred to establish the cause of the curvature. Adolescents with kyphosis scan be treated with observation, physical therapy, back brace, or may require surgical stabilization depending on progression and symptoms. Adult patients are treated with physical therapy, anti-inflammatory medications, and back braces. Patients with severe pain or neurologic symptoms not responsive to conservative measures, worsening curvature, spinal instability, or respiratory compromise due to kyphosis may be candidates for surgical intervention (fusion, vertebralplasty, rod stabilization).
- Children and adolescents with scoliosis are often followed for progression of disease if the curvature is mild. More severe curvature (>50 degrees) is treated with bracing and possibly surgery for patients with significant progression or respiratory compromise. In older patients with more of a degenerative disease, treatment is more conservative and includes physical therapy and anti-inflammatory medications. Patients with pain or neurologic symptoms not responsive to conservative measures, worsening curvature, and spinal instability may be candidates for surgical intervention (fusion, vertebralplasty, rod stabilization).

7. Intervertebral disk disorders
   - Intervertebral disk can also be the cause of back pain including infections of the disks, disk degeneration, and disk herniation. Normally, intravertebral disks act as shock absorbers for the vertebral bodies. The disk is a gel-like material (nucleus pulposus) that is encapsulated by a fibrous ligament (anulus fibrosus) which keeps the gel in place. A disruption of this ligamentous structure can cause the gel to exude from its normal location. This can occur in the cervical, thoracic, or lumbar disks but tends to occur more at the lumbar level because of the increased size and load placed on the disks and vertebral bodies. Herniation of the L4-L5 disk is the most common followed by L5-S1. Patients ages 30 to 50 appear to be the most affected. Physical examination may reveal tenderness over the region of the involved disk and muscle spasm. The straight leg raise will be positive in the majority of cases. Patients may exhibit weakness, sensory deficits, and abnormal reflexes depending on

the degree or nerve compression associated with the herniation. CT, CT myelogram, and MRI are often helpful to visualize the herniated disk although treating physicians must be aware that many patients have asymptomatic disk herniation and care must be taken to correlate the anatomic defect with the patient's symptoms and physical findings. Electromyographic (EMG) testing may be utilized in the workup of patients with significant weakness to rule out competing diagnosis and to attempt to localize the level of nerve impingement.

- Multiple treatment modalities exist and can be utilized depending on the patient's individualized symptoms. It is important to stress that most patients do improve with conservative treatment in 4 to 12 weeks. Surgery is reserved for patients with intractable pain or progressive neurologic deficit despite conservative treatment. Acutely, disk herniation is treated with rest, ice, anti-inflammatory medications, and muscle relaxants and traction if a significant degree of spasm is present. Patients may also benefit from massage, heat, aggressive pain control, and possibly steroids. Physical therapy is helpful to control recurrences by strengthening the supports of the spine.

- Degenerative disk disease is another cause of back pain and can occur at any level but most commonly affects the lumbar spine. Pain is the dominant symptom and neurologic involvement is absent in contrast to disk herniation. Onset is often gradual. Aging produces degradation of the gel-like nucleus pulposus leading to less shock absorption and loss of disk height. The surrounding ligaments also degrade owing to excessive wear and tear changes, and higher risks for slippage of the vertebral bodies and disk herniation are present. Treatment consists of anti-inflammatory medication, pain control, and physical therapy. Surgery can be considered in patients who failed conservative measures, have intractable pain, or experience progressive neurologic symptoms.

8. Other causes of back pain
  a. Osteoarthritis
    - Osteoarthritis can affect any joint in the body. The spine, particularly the thoracic and lumbar spine, is no exception. Degenerative changes can lead to osteophyte formation, foraminal stenosis, and facet joint changes. Patients over 50 years of age are the most affected. They report pain and stiffness that improves with exercise. Diagnosis is confirmed by x-ray. Treatment of osteoarthritis of the spine is similar to treatment of other joints and includes pain control and a generalized strengthening and flexibility program to maximize soft tissue support and maintain patient functionality.
  b. Infection
    - Infections of the spine are relatively rare but can be very serious and lead to permanent neurologic compromise. Infections can occur of the bone (osteomyelitis), intravertebral disk (diskitis), or epidural space. Infections of the epidural space are particularly worrisome as they can lead to compression of the nerve roots and cauda equina syndrome.

These require emergent evaluation. Osteomyelitis can occur in any bone. Spinal involvement usually involves the lumbar or sacrum although any level can be involved. Patients of any age can be involved. Those with diabetes, immunocompromise, overlying infections, or recent procedures tend to be at greater risk for infection. Patients present with a sharp or localized tenderness. Fever or systemic symptoms may or may not be present. Initial x-rays are usually unremarkable but may be positive if symptoms have been present for more than 2 to 3 weeks. MRI or bone scan is often needed to confirm the diagnosis. Inflammatory markers such as sedimentation rate and C-reactive protein are usually elevated. Treatment is based on available microbiologic data. Most infections are caused by *Staphylococcus* and *Streptococcus* species and other organisms may be involved as well. Diskitis is a similar condition that actually involves an infection of the intervertebral disk. Although it can occur at any age, young children can be affected. Diagnosis and treatment is similar to that for osteomyelitis.

c. Malignancy
- Malignancy of the spine must also be considered in patients over 50 years of age with lower back pain. Patients complaint of a dull aching or throbbing pain which may be progressive in nature and is unrelieved by activity or position. The pain may be worse at night or with recumbence. Patients with a history of previous cancer, weight loss, new onset of kidney disease (myeloma), or unexplained fever require further evaluation. Neurologic signs or symptoms may or may not be present. CT or MRI may be necessary in patients with a high index of suspicion.

d. Rheumatologic considerations
- Several rheumatologic conditions can cause low back or sacroiliac joint pain and deserve mention. The seronegative spondyloarthropathies include ankylosing spondylitis, Reiter's syndrome, inflammatory bowel disease associated arthritis, and psoriatic arthritis. These diagnoses should be considered in patients with systemic complaints, multiple joint involvement, atraumatic joint swelling, patients with a family history of seronegative spondyloarthropathies, eye, or skin manifestations. Patients often present at a younger age than typical for back pain (in their teens and twenties). They may complain of stiffness, which improves with activity. X-ray may reveal pronounced enthesitis or sacroiliac involvement for a patient's given age. Patients should be referred to a specialist for further workup to establish a diagnosis and to rule out other organ system involvement. Treatment ultimately will be determined by the exact diagnosis but often includes a regular exercise program.

e. Sacroiliac joint dysfunction
- The sacroiliac (SI) joint can also be a cause of low back pain. As previously mentioned, the SI joint is often a site of involvement in the seronegative spondyloarthropathies. In addition, a strain, sprain, or

"dysfunction" of the SI joint has been reported to limit or alter motion at the SI joint, thus altering mechanics and causing pain or a functional leg length discrepancy. Because of the wide variation in symptoms, and difficulty in isolating the joint, a great deal of controversy exists in the diagnosis of sacroiliac disorders. Treatment is aimed at restoring normal movement and function of the joint. A period of relative rest is followed by a core stabilization program. Anti-inflammatory medications may be helpful for pain control.

IV. Disorders of the Shoulder
  A. Rotator cuff impingement/tear
   • The rotator cuff is a group of four muscles—the supraspinatus, infraspinatus, subscapularis, and teres minor—which help to stabilize the humeral head in the glenoid fossa. This group of muscles is responsible for the wide variety of movements available at the shoulder joint. Anatomically, the rotator cuff is limited to a small space, which decreases in size with the arm elevated. Patients can develop inflammation of the rotator cuff tendons from repetitive compression on the acromion or coracoacromial ligament. Adults over age 40 are at the highest risk for rotator cuff problems. Rotator cuff impingement or tendonitis involves inflammation of the tendon(s). Tears of the rotator cuff tendons can also occur and can be difficult to differentiate. Inflammation of the bursa can occur concomitantly.
   • Patients can present with acute or chronic anterior shoulder pain. Acute presentation can be caused by a fall, trauma, lifting a heavy object, or a rotator cuff tear. Pain is described as achy, dull, and increases with overhead activity. A significant amount of night pain may be present and could likely represent a tear. Physical examination is remarkable for a painful arc of motion with abduction. Internal and external rotation may also be limited due to pain. In severe instances, the patient may have difficulty lifting the shoulder. The biceps tendon in the bicipital groove of the humerus may also be involved. Rotator cuff impingement signs include the Hawkins sign, Neers sign, "empty can test," and subscapularis lift test. Resistance testing may be painful but should not be significantly weak, especially with any one particular maneuver. Significant weakness may indicate a rotator cuff tear. The diagnosis is generally clinical. A diagnostic injection using only anesthetic can be helpful in distinguishing patients who have tendonitis from those with a tear. A patient with tendonitis and weakness on examination will have improved strength on re-examination after injection and improvement in their pain. A patient with a rotator cuff tear will not. X-rays are helpful to rule out other potential causes of shoulder pain such as osteoarthritis. An MRI is the best method for visualizing the rotator cuff tendons and should be considered in patients with a suspected large rotator cuff tear or a patient who is not improving with conservative treatment.
   • Treatment is aimed at treating the inflammation and returning the patient back to a normal functional level. Initially, most patients can be treated with activity modification, ice, and anti-inflammatory mediation. Physical therapy is the most important part of treatment and should focus on restoring range of motion and strength. Patients with significant pain and disability may benefit

from an initial cortisone injection or this can be reserved for patients not responding to initial management in milder disease. Many patients with small rotator cuff tears can respond to conservative management. Patients who fail initial treatment, are considering surgical intervention, or have suspected or large cuff tears should be referred for possible surgical intervention.

B. Adhesive capsulitis
- Adhesive capsulitis or frozen shoulder is the loss of range of motion of the shoulder due to fibrosis of the joint capsule. Patients older than 40 and diabetics are at highest risk. This condition can occur alone or with other shoulder injury such as rotator cuff impingement or tears that lead to prolonged immobility.
- Patients present with a long-standing history of shoulder pain followed by an inability to move the shoulder. Physical examination reveals significantly reduced range of motion both actively and passively. Abduction tends to be the most affected. The patient may or may not have pain with active range of motion but should not have significant pain with passive range of motion.
- Diagnosis is clinical. X-ray evaluation is relatively unremarkable. Treatment consists of anti-inflammatory mediations and physical therapy to reduce pain and restore range of motion. Patients with significant limitation in pain or range of motion may benefit from an initial cortisone injection or this may be reserved to patients who fail to respond to initial treatment. In general, physical therapy is the key to treatment; however; it may take months to years before patients have returned close to their baseline status.

C. Labral tear
- The labrum is a rim of cartilage that surrounds the glenoid, deepening the socket and supporting the humeral head. This cartilage can be torn by a fall, dislocation or subluxation, or repetitive trauma as in a throwing athlete.
- Patients complain of pain, often related to the position of their arm, clicking or grinding, and weakness. Physical examination may reveal a clicking sensation with certain arm positions, and joint laxity. O'Brien's test is a maneuver whereby the affected limb is extended outward and the thumbs are rotated down. Pain with resisted motion is considered positive for labral damage. X-rays are helpful to rule out competing diagnosis but do not show the labrum. An MRI arthrogram is the test of choice for evaluating a labral tear. Patients with a suspected tear should be referred to a specialist for evaluation and treatment which is usually surgical.

V. Fractures
A. Basic science
- Fractures are caused by either high-energy impact to the bone itself or excessive overload of the bone by its connecting structures, resulting in disruption of the bony architecture. Because of increased pliability of bones in children, the potential for deformation of the bone beyond its elastic threshold is possible without a true cortical break. This results in a buckle or greenstick fracture, in which the cortices are not completely disrupted. In adults, bones are less elastic and disruption of the cortices is observed instead.

- Many classification systems exist to describe fractures. One important distinction to make is to categorize fractures into open and closed because of the difference in management. An open fracture is one in which the integrity of the skin overlying the fracture site is compromised. Open fractures are at significant risk for infection and usually require surgical intervention to restore alignment and irrigate the affected area. Closed fractures are those in which the overlying skin remains intact. Closed fractures can be further evaluated in terms of alignment, displacement, angulation to determine optimum treatment. The Salter-Harris classification system is also commonly used to describe the anatomic location of a fracture in terms of its relation to open growth plates. The physis, or growth plate, is the weakest area of bone in children and therefore a common site of injury. Type I Salter-Harris fractures involve fracture though the physis. Type II fractures involve the physis and metaphysis, the portion of bone proximal to the joint. Type III fractures involve the physis and epiphysis, the end of the long bone. Type IV fractures involve all three structures, the physis, metaphysis, and epiphysis. These fractures tend to be the most serious. Type V fractures are actually a compression of the growth plate.

B. History and physical examination
- Patients with a fracture almost always present with a history of a traumatic event. Physical examination reveals an area of localized tenderness, which can be severe. A deformity of the bone or "step off" can be apparent if the fracture is displaced. More severe fractures can present with deformity of the joint itself or alteration of the joint angle. Swelling is also present. A neurologic and vascular examination should be performed to rule out damage to these vital structures as any abnormality would necessitate immediate intervention. Most acute fractures can be confirmed with x-ray evaluation. Occasionally, fractures are not observed acutely on initial radiographs but evidence of healing fractures can be apparent on repeated radiographs 7 to 14 days later. In addition, specific fractures such as scaphoid fractures are poorly visualized on x-ray and may need further imaging studies such as CT or MRI to delineate the fracture.

C. Formulating the diagnosis
1. Fractures of the facial bones
- Fractures of the facial bones are relatively uncommon. They include mandibular fractures, maxillary or Le Fort fractures, nasal bone and cartilage fractures, orbital floor or blowout fractures, and zygomatic arch fractures. All these fractures are caused by significant direct trauma. Physical examination can reveal asymmetry, ecchymosis, epistaxis, focal tenderness, bony step-off, crepitus, and limitations or asymmetric opening and closing of the jaw. Initial evaluation should also include evaluation of the cervical spine, as this injury can coexist, and assessment of ABCs. Initial management includes protection of the airway and control of bleeding. Conscious patients can sit up and lean forward. Unconscious patients may require airway protections and intubation. Diagnosis is made by evaluation with panoramic or facial series radiographs. CT or MRI may be required, depending on the severity of injury. Treatment depends on the affected site,

size of fractures, and displacement. Mandibular fractures are often treated with intramaxillary fixation.

2. Fractures of vertebral column
   - Fractures of the spinal column are classified by location into cervical, thoracic, and lumbar. Cervical spine injuries can be life-threatening and cause significant morbidity due to neurologic compromise. High-energy injuries, such as motor vehicle accidents, and axial compression injuries are the most common causes of fractures. Cervical spine injuries should be suspected in all unconscious, intoxicated, or trauma patients with neck pain. Patients can complain of focal tenderness or radicular symptoms with weakness, numbness, or tingling down the extremities. C5 is the most commonly fractured vertebra, accounting for approximately 50% of all vertebral fractures.
   - Physical examination reveals focal midline tenderness, often with muscle spasm. The transverse process should be palpable. A step-off would be an indication of a displaced fracture. A neurologic examination should be performed to document focal weakness, loss of sensation, and reflexes of the bilateral upper and lower extremities. Initial management of injuries includes immobilization of the cervical spine with a hard cervical collar and spine board and the ABCs with protection of the airway (if required). Initial x-ray evaluation includes anteroposterior (AP), lateral, oblique, and odontoid views. It is important to verify that all seven cervical vertebrae are in view on the x-ray series. Suspected spinal cord injuries are often treated with steroids to help reduce cord edema. All fractures should be evaluated by a specialist. If the initial x-ray series is negative, CT and MRI are often useful to evaluate further for fractures.
   - Thoracic spine injuries are caused by the same mechanisms as cervical spine injuries. In addition, the thoracic spine is commonly involved in less traumatic fractures in patients with poor bone quality such as those with osteoporosis. Patients present with midback pain that increases with motion. Physical examination reveals focal midline tenderness. A step-off may be noted at the level of the fracture. A neurologic examination to include motor, sensory, and reflexes is important to exclude spinal cord injury or peripheral nerve involvement. Generally, the diagnosis is established with AP and lateral radiographs. Initial management of any acute spine injury involves immobilization with a rigid collar and spine board. Isolated thoracic vertebral fractures of the spinous process can be treated with a brace or corset for symptom control. Compression fractures can be treated with activity modification, bracing, pain control, and physical therapy. Patients with multiple compression fractures, neurologic compromise, severe kyphosis, or instability, or who fail to respond to medical management may be candidates for surgical intervention such as spinal fusion or kyphoplasty.
   - Lumbar spine fractures are caused by the same mechanisms as cervical and thoracic spine fractures. Patients present with lower back pain, which increases with motion. Physical examination reveals focal midline

tenderness. A step-off may be noted at the level of the fracture. A neurologic examination to include motor, sensory, and reflexes is important to exclude spinal cord injury or peripheral nerve involvement. Generally, the diagnosis is established with AP and lateral radiographs. Initial management of lumbar spine fractures is similar to that for cervical and thoracic spine. Treatment options for lumbar vertebral fractures are similar to those of the thoracic spine.

3. Rib fractures
   - Rib fractures are caused by direct trauma. The fourth through seventh ribs are the most commonly fractured. Patients complain of pain and often breathe more shallowly to prevent chest wall expansion. Displaced rib fractures can be problematic as they can cause a pneumothorax, hemothorax, or laceration to the liver or spleen. Physical examination reveals focal tenderness, ecchymosis, and possible step-off. Diagnosis is made by x-ray evaluation. Nondisplaced rib fractures are treated with pain control and respiratory support if needed. Any complicating injuries should also be addressed. Displaced rib fractures or multiple rib fractures that cause a flail chest may require surgical intervention.

4. Fractures of the upper extremity
   - Fractures of the upper extremity are extremely common. They can involve any joint or bone. In general, nondisplaced, nonangulated fractures can be treated with immobilization. Angulated, displaced, or intra-articular fractures should be referred to a specialist for further evaluation. Patients present with pain, swelling, and ecchymosis. A complete neurovascular examination of the affected extremity is important to rule out concomitant injury. Diagnosis is confirmed on radiograph. Treatment centers around analgesia, ice, and splinting followed by more definitive immobilization as swelling allows. Physical therapy is later utilized to restore range of motion and strength. Displaced fractures should be reduced as soon as possible by a qualified specialist. All open fractures should be emergently referred as well. Any fracture that fails to heal (nonunion) after appropriate conservative treatment should also be referred. Examples of some common fractures follow.
   - The clavicle is one of the most commonly fractured bones, usually from a direct blow. Most occur in the middle third of the clavicle and can be treated conservatively in a sling or figure-of–eight sling followed by physical therapy. Fractures of the scapular are rare and are usually associated with other injuries. Shoulder dislocation can lead to fracture of the glenoid while significant trauma can cause fracture of the scapular body or spine. Both can usually be treated with sling immobilization if no other significant injures are present (rare).
   - Proximal humerus fractures can involve the greater and lesser tuberosity, or the anatomic or surgical neck. Treatment involves a shoulder immobilizer initially, followed by physical therapy to restore range of motion, then strength. Humeral shaft fractures can involve damage to the radial nerve. Patients with neurologic injuries should be immediately referred. Most

humeral shaft fractures can be managed in a coaptation splint, followed by functional brace, and later physical therapy in the absence of significant displacement or angulation. Fractures of the distal humerus are rare.

- Fractures of proximal ulna (olecranon) are usually caused by a direct blow or fall. Olecranon fractures that are nondisplaced can be immobilized in a splint; displaced fractures should be referred for surgical intervention. Isolated nondisplaced ulna shaft fractures can often be treated in a splint and cast. Fractures of the radial head also occur from falls. Nondisplaced fractures can be treated by immobilization followed by early physical therapy to prevent stiffness. Displaced fractures should be referred as they may require aspiration and surgery. Fractures of the distal radius are extremely common and problematic as even small amount of angulation or displacement can cause loss of function. Nondisplaced fractures can be splinted initially, then casted, and advanced to a brace. Most displaced or angulated fractures require surgical fixation to prevent loss of wrist motion.
- Fractures of the scaphoid are among the most commonly missed fractures. Fractures occur from a fall on an outstretched hand. Patients complain of central wrist pain. On examination they display pain over the anatomic snuffbox and decreased range of motion of the wrist. X-rays can be negative initially and may require further imaging for evaluation. These fractures should be treated by a qualified specialist.
- The most common fracture of the hand is the fifth metacarpal (boxer's fractures) although fractures can occur in any of the metacarpals. Nondisplaced fractures can be treated in a splint or cast. Displaced fractures may require intervention to prevent deformity and loss of function. Most phalangeal fractures with significant displacement or angulation can be treated with cast immobilization.

5. Fractures of the lower extremity
- Similar principles apply to most fractures of the lower extremity. Fractures that are nondisplaced, nonangulated, and not intra-articular can usually be treated with immobilization. All other fractures should be referred for possible surgical intervention.
- Proximal femur fractures can be at the femoral neck or intertrochanteric. They often occur after a fall in elderly patients or patients with poor bone quality. Almost all proximal femur fractures are treated operatively and hence should be referred emergently. Similarly, distal femur and shaft fractures are caused by a significant trauma such as a motor vehicle accident. These fractures also require prompt surgical fixation and hence emergent referral.
- Fractures of the tibia plateau can result from direct trauma (from medial or lateral force plus axial load) or insufficiency fracture (in elderly patients). Displaced fractures require prompt referral for surgical consideration. Nondisplaced fractures can be treated with immobilization. Tibial shaft fractures can also be treated in a long-leg cast if there is no significant angulation or displacement. Fractures of the medial malleolus can be treated conservatively; however; any widening of the ankle mortise, associated

lateral malleolus fracture, displacement, angulation, or joint instability would require surgical evaluation.

- Fibular fractures are also common and can be problematic. Proximal fibular fractures due to an ankle injury should be referred for possible surgical intervention as they may become unstable. Isolated proximal and distal (lateral malleolus) fibular fractures that do not involve the joint line can be treated with immobilization. On the other hand, distal fibular (lateral malleolus) fractures that are associated with instability, joint line involvement, widening of the ankle joint, or additional injuries should be referred for possible surgical stabilization.

- Fractures of the midfoot are relatively rare and usually associated with significant trauma; they should be referred to a specialist for further evaluation and treatment. Fractures of the metatarsals are more common and can usually be treated with immobilization. The fifth metatarsal fracture can be more problematic requiring more prolonged immobilization or surgical fixation depending on the location of the fracture. Earlier referral may be appropriate if questions exist, displacement is present, or multiple metatarsals are involved. Phalangeal fractures can be handled in a similar manner. Nondisplaced or angulated fractures can be buddy taped for immobilization. Significant displacement or angulation may warrant surgical intervention.

VI. Miscellaneous Causes of Limb Pain
   A. Carpal tunnel syndrome
   - Carpal tunnel syndrome is the most common compression neuropathy of the upper extremity. Middle-aged females are most commonly affected. Affliction with this disorder is responsible for substantial decreased work productivity and increased lost days from work. The carpal tunnel is a fibro-osseous canal on the palmar aspect of the wrist through which pass nine flexor tendons (four from the flexor digitorum superficialis, four from the flexor digitorum profundus, and the flexor pollicis longus) and the median nerve. The median nerve carries motor function to the muscles of the thenar eminence (flexor pollicis brevis, abductor pollicis brevis, opponens pollicis), the two most radial lumbricals, and sensation to the most radial $3^1/_2$ fingers. Extrinsic or intrinsic pressure to the median nerve is responsible for the symptoms of this syndrome. Patients classically complain of pain, tingling, or numbness in the thumb, index, long, and radial aspect of the ring fingers. Symptoms are often first noticed at night and will awaken the patient from sleep. Activities that cause repetitive flexion or extension at the wrist will also precipitate symptoms. In advanced or severe cases, symptoms may become persistent and lead to continuous numbness or motor weakness.

   - Physical examination may reveal decreased sensation to light touch and two-point discrimination within the median nerve distribution. Atrophy and weakness of the muscles of the thenar group may be present. A positive Tinel's sign (reproduction of the symptoms with tapping on the nerve at the wrist) and Phalen's test (reproduction of the symptoms with forced wrist flexion) may be found. Although the diagnosis is clinical based on the quality and distribution of symptoms, nerve conduction studies are often useful to confirm the diagnosis and to examine the severity of compression in patients considering surgical intervention. Neither x-rays nor routine laboratory evaluation is generally indicated. Thoracic outlet syndrome, mononeuropathy or polyneuropathy, cervical radiculopathy, intraspinal canal lesions, multiple sclerosis, hypothyroidism, diabetes, and collagen vascular disorders may produce similar symptoms or contribute to a secondary form of carpal tunnel syndrome.

- Patients with mild, intermittent symptoms should be managed with activity modification, anti-inflammatory drugs, and wrist splinting in the neutral position. Wrist splinting is particularly important at night to prevent the normal wrist flexion that occurs during sleep. Patients who do not improve can be referred for possible steroid injection into the carpal tunnel. Patients with chronic symptoms or evidence of significant sensory deficit or muscle wasting may require earlier surgical referral as they may be candidates for a surgical carpal tunnel release.

B. Slipped capital femoral epiphysis (SCFE)
- SCFE describes a condition whereby the proximal femoral epiphysis slips off the metaphysis. This occurs through the physis and usually results in the epiphysis being posterior and inferior to the normal location. Adolescents who are overweight and active are most commonly affected. Males are affected more than females. Occasionally, SCFE can be associated with endocrine disorders. Patients may present acute or chronic pain. The pain is activity related and is localized to the hip region. Most commonly in the acute scenario, patients are unable to bear weight, which is what brings them to medical attention. Some precipitating trauma can usually be elicited.
- Physical examination reveals a limited and painful range of motion. Occasionally, the pain is difficult to localize and the patient may refer the pain to the thigh, knee, or ankle instead of the hip. Loss of internal rotation is the most pronounced finding. Therefore, the most comfortable position for patients is with the hip held in external rotation. A leg length discrepancy is usually noted. Diagnosis is confirmed by radiographs that demonstrate the slip. The severity is based on the degree of slippage. SFCE is an emergent condition and requires immediate referral to an orthopedist.

C. Legg-Calve-Perthes disease
- Legg-Calve-Perthes disease is a condition of the hip that involves aseptic necrosis of the femoral head with subchondral fracture. The fracture marks the onset of the clinical course, which then progresses through bone resorption and repair. Some patients have a self-limited course; others develop collapse of the femoral head and early arthritis. The condition most commonly affects males between the ages of 4 and 10. Patients present with the complaint of a painful limp for several weeks to months. The pain is usually aggravated by activity and may be referred to the groin, knee, or thigh.
- Physical examination reveals a limited and painful range of motion and an antalgic gait on the affected side. Loss of abduction is the most pronounced

finding in contrast to SFCE in which internal rotation is the movement most affected. Diagnosis may be confirmed by radiographs if they demonstrate areas of necrosis, sclerosis, resorption, or repair. X-rays may be negative early in the disease, necessitating an MRI at times to make the diagnosis. The goals of treatment center around maintenance of the range of motion and preservation of femoral head coverage by the acetabulum.

D. Enthesopathy, tendonitis, and tendinosis
- Enthesopathy is the pathologically inflamed state that occurs at the site of insertion of soft tissue such as tendons, fascia, and joint capsules onto bone. Repetitive microtrauma and overuse of the muscle are contributing factors that lead to this chronic inflammatory state. Fibrosis and calcium deposition may occur. Adults over age 40 and patients with chronic inflammatory conditions such as the seronegative spondyloarthropathies are at increased risk. Although any site of tendon insertion may be potentially involved, the plantar fascia and Achilles tendon are some common examples.
- In contrast, a tendonitis is an acute inflammation of a tendon but a tendinosis is a more chronic degeneration of the tendon. These are often due to overuse. Achilles, biceps, triceps, extensor tendons of the wrist, and patellar tendons are some of the more commonly involved tendons in overuse injuries.
  1. Achilles tendonitis
     - The Achilles tendon is the common insertion of the gastrocnemius and soleus muscles on the calcaneus. Inflammation can occur from overuse during activities such as running and jumping. Partial or complete tears can also occur. Patients present with pain along the course of the tendon, greatest at the start or conclusion of activity. Many patients report significant changes to their usual exercise routine or activity level. Physical examination displays pain along the course of the tendon, worst proximal to the insertion on the calcaneus. Pain is increased with passive dorsiflexion and resisted plantar flexion. Diagnosis remains clinical. Treatment consists of activity modification, anti-inflammatory medications, ice, and physical therapy programs that emphasize stretching. Heel lifts, orthodics, night splints, immobilization, and shock wave therapy may be useful in more severe cases. Refractory cases can be considered for surgical intervention.
  2. Plantar fasciitis
     - Plantar fasciitis is inflammation of the insertion of the plantar fascia on the calcaneus. It is caused by tightening, fatigue, and overuse. Patients who undergo a sudden increase in activity level, perform prolonged walking or standing, use unsupportive shoes, and are overweight are at increased risk. Females are more often affected than males. Patients complain of heel pain that has been gradually increasing. Pain is greatest with first steps in the morning and after prolonged inactivity and improves with continued activity.
     - Physical examination reveals tenderness of the medial calcaneal insertion of the plantar fascia. Patients may have "flat feet" or some other anatomic predisposition. Diagnosis is clinical. X-rays are not required unless other

injury is suspected. Treatment includes rest, ice, night splints, and anti-inflammatory medication. Orthotics are helpful to provide better support to the arch of the foot. Stretching is important for ultimate improvement. Severe symptoms may require cortisone injection, shock wave therapy, or surgery.

3. Patellofemoral pain
   - Patellofemoral pain is one of the most common causes of knee pain in adolescents. Pain is localized to the anterior knee pain and is caused by overuse and irritation of the patellar facets (femoral condyles) and posterior surface of the patella. Patients report pain that increases with increased activity, stair climbing, squatting, and moving from the sitting to standing position. Females are more often affected than males.
   - Physical examination reveals some tenderness over the femoral condyles. Some crepitus is noted with knee flexion, which may exacerbate the pain. No swelling or instability should be noted. Anatomic misalignment or poor tracking of the patella in the trochlear groove may be present in severe cases. Diagnosis is clinical but x-rays are helpful to demonstrate alignment of the patella and to rule out other causes of pain. Treatment is aimed at reassuring the patient, anti-inflammatory mediation, and physical therapy to balance out the muscles surrounding the knee. Neoprene sleeves are also helpful for some patients.

E. Chondral injuries
   - Articular cartilage surrounds the ends of bones and provides a smooth surface for bones to glide over each other. This cartilage is subject to damage from both traumatic injury and metabolic processes. As a result, the articular cartilage can soften (chondromalacia), crack, fissure, or fracture (osteochondritis dissecans). Patients may complain of mechanical symptoms such as locking or catching, swelling, or pain.
   - Osteochondritis dissecans describes the condition in which a segment of bone subjected to repetitive stress becomes ischemic and dies, leading to separation of the overlying cartilage and possibly a loose body. Children and adolescents are the most affected and the femur, humerus, and talus are the bones most often affected. Patients present with pain related to activity. They may complain of a catching or locking sensation if loose bodies are present. Physical examination reveals focal tenderness over the affected articular surface. A joint effusion and decreased range of motion also may be present. X-rays of the affected joint are often helpful and may show advanced or large defects. CT and MRI may be needed to demonstrate smaller or less advanced lesions if x-rays are negative. A high index of suspension is required in the appropriate population with nontraumatic pain or swelling.

F. Temporomandibular joint disorders
   - Temporomandibular joint disorders most commonly affect females ages 20 to 40. Causes of dysfunction include trauma, arthritis, or teeth grinding. Patients can present with headache, a popping sensation, tenderness, and abnormal alignment. Physical examination may reveal clicking with jaw closure,

tenderness over the joint line, and popping. Treatment is aimed at the underlying cause and can consist of analgesics, dietary changes, and dental appliance. Referral to a specialist or dentist if often advisable. Surgery is rarely indicated.

G. Osteoarthritis

- Osteoarthritis is the most common joint disease and will affect the majority of the population at some point in their life. Osteoarthritis is caused by an imbalance in the inflammatory response and synthetic function leading to inflammation, synovial fluid alternations, cartilage destruction, and bone abnormalities. Risk factors include advancing age, female sex, history of trauma, obesity, and family history. Weight-bearing joints tend to be the most affected, although any joint may be involved. Patients present with a dull achy pain, burning, stiffness, swelling, and decreased range of motion. Excessive activity tends to increase symptoms but inactivity tends to increase stiffness. Physical examination will verify these findings.

- Diagnosis is clinical. X-ray evaluation may reveal abnormal bone formation (osteophyte or spurs), joint space narrowing, subchondral cyst formation, and sclerosis.

- Treatments consists of analgesic medication, glucosamine and chondroitin preparations, regular but not excessive exercise or physical therapy (to include stretching and range of motion), and weight loss. Moderate disease can be treated with the use of braces and durable medical equipment for support and unloading, cortisone injections, and viscosupplementation. Joint fusion or replacement may be necessary for pain control and to restore function in advanced disease.

VII. Neoplasms of the Musculoskeletal System

- Musculoskeletal neoplasms are classified as either primary or metastatic. Neoplasms that arise in osseous, cartilaginous, or other mesenchymal tissues are considered primary sarcomas. Those that arise from distant sites and spread to these tissues are considered metastatic and are usually carcinomas.

A. Primary musculoskeletal neoplasms

- Primary musculoskeletal neoplasms are uncommon. They may be either benign or malignant, depending on their potential to metastasize. Benign musculoskeletal tumors are much more common than malignant ones. Certain tumor types occur more common in specific age groups. For example, rhabdomyosarcoma is the most common malignant soft tissue neoplasm in the first decade of life. It arises from skeletal muscle and is commonly located in the truncal regions.

- Osteosarcoma is the most common primary malignant bone neoplasm. It usually occurs before age 30 and arises within the metaphyseal region of long bones with the distal femur or proximal tibia most commonly affected, although it can occur anywhere. It is more common in males than females.

- Chondrosarcoma is the most common malignant cartilage neoplasm, which occurs most often within the pelvis, spine, scapula, femur, tibia, or humerus. Males age 30 to 60 are the most commonly affected.

- Ewing's sarcoma is malignancy that arises from precursor cells in the bone marrow. Males age 10 to 15 are the most commonly affected. Most patients demonstrate a translocation, which is responsible for the tumor.
- Malignant fibrous histiocytoma is the most common malignant soft tissue neoplasm in adults, typically occurring in the fifth to sixth decade of life.
- Multiple myeloma is the most common plasma cell neoplasm in adults. It arises from bone marrow precursor cells causing plasmacytosis and paraproteinemia.
- Giant cell tumor is a common benign tumor occurring in the epiphyseal region of long bones. Males aged 20 to 40 are most commonly affected.
- Osteochondroma is a common benign tumor arising from a remnant of the physis (growth plate). This is usually present in the metaphyseal or diaphyseal areas of long bones.
- Enchondroma is a common benign cartilaginous tumor arising in small tubular bones, typically the hands and feet. Most patients are asymptomatic.

B. Metastatic musculoskeletal neoplasms

- Metastatic neoplasms are the most common tumors of the musculoskeletal system, occurring up to 25 times more often than primary lesions. They typically arise from carcinomas in other areas of the body. The axial skeleton and proximal extremities are the most common areas involved. These neoplasms generally are lytic, destroying the bone with their growth. Some are able to form bone (prostate), although this bone is not normal. The origins of the most common metastatic carcinomas are breast, prostate, lung, kidney, and thyroid.
- In soft tissue neoplasms, patients may present with a painless, rapidly enlarging mass. This can create localized symptoms due to compression of nerves, blood vessels, and organs. Patients with bone involvement may complain of significant pain or may be asymptomatic. Pain typically is dull and achy, worse at night, and can be associated with fever and chills. In cases in which the neoplasm has significantly weakened the bone, pain may be associated with a pathologic fracture. The most likely source of the tumor varies with age. In some cases, a primary tumor can be difficult or impossible to identify.

C. Pathologic fracture

- A pathologic fracture is an atypical fracture that occurs in abnormal bone, meaning bone that has already been weakened by another process. Osteoporosis, osteonecrosis, bony cysts, and tumors can all contribute to the degradation in the quality of the bone.
- Pathologic fractures can occur with minimal to no trauma. Patients present with a sudden increase in pain in an area that may or may not have already been symptomatic. Physical reveals significant tenderness over the affected area.
- Diagnosis is confirmed by x-rays although these fractures can be more subtle and require CT or MRI for verification.
- Treatment may be more complicated than routine fracture care, depending on the size of the fracture and its location. Therefore, patients should be referred to a specialist for treatment options. Patients also should undergo full evaluation as to the cause of the pathologic fracture if this is not known or

obvious, as some patients with cancer can present with a pathologic fracture as their first manifestation.

VIII. Soft Tissue Injuries
  A. Contusions
    1. Basic science
- A contusion is a soft tissue injury caused by direct trauma. All soft tissues, including muscles, tendons, and adipose tissue, can be involved.
- Large or serve contusions can involve extravasation of a significant amount of blood into the local tissues. With a significant traumatic injury, a build-up of pressure in the soft tissues can occur as a result of the increased amount of fluid and blood. This increased pressure can cause nerve damage, impede vascular supply to distal areas, and cause necrosis of soft tissue (e.g., compartment syndrome).
- Compartment syndrome most commonly involves the lower extremity. Compartment syndrome is a medical emergency and must be treated with an urgent fascia release to prevent irreparable damage.

    2. History and physical examination
- Patients with contusions complain of pain, swelling, and stiffness at the traumatic site. Physical examination reveals a tender focus of soft tissue. A sense of fullness and ecchymosis may be present.

    3. Managing the patient
- Most contusions can be treated with rest, ice, compression, elevation, and NSAIDs. Patients with large, severe, or repetitive contusions are at risk for heterotrophic bone formation called myositis ossificans. Myositis ossificans commonly involves large muscle groups such as the quadriceps and biceps and are caused by the deposition of calcium 3 to 6 weeks after a severe traumatic injury. Physical examination is remarkable for a discrete palpable tender mass or nodule in the area of injury. Patients may display decreased range of motion owing to loss of the elastic properties of the affected soft tissue. The diagnosis can be confirmed by observation of the calcified hematoma at the site of pervious injury on x-ray evaluation. Treatment for myositis ossificans is the similar to that for contusions; however, stretching is emphasized and modalities such as transcutaneous electrical simulation (TENS) are often avoided. Ultimately, most of the calcium deposition is reabsorbed over the next 6 months, but surgery is occasionally required to excise the heterotrophic bone deposits that continue to be painful or cause limitations in range of motion or function.

  B. Sprains and strains
    1. Basic science
- Sprains and strains are exceedingly common soft tissue injuries. A sprain is defined as a stretching or tearing of the connective tissue support of a joint, the ligaments, or joint capsule. A ligament is a collagen-containing connective tissue with two bony attachments that spans a joint, thus providing stability. The joint capsule is a less defined collagen-containing connective tissue that surrounds a joint providing protection and stability.

- In contrast, strains are a stretching or tearing of the muscle most commonly at the musculotendinous junction. The severity of a sprain or strain is directly related to the amount of tearing and the resultant instability of the involved joint. Both injures can occur at any age and can be precipitated by a traumatic event. Sprains are most common in adolescents and young adults, and strains are more common in adults. Sprains can occur at any joint, although ankle and knee injuries are the most common. Strains are most common in the larger muscle groups.

2. History and physical examination
   - An exact mechanism of injury is helpful to identify structures at risk. However, similar mechanisms of injury can result in various injury patterns based on age, genetics, and an individual's fitness level. Patients complain of pain, swelling, stiffness, and ecchymosis. The patient is often unable to use the affected limb. A complete physical examination of the involved area can be revealing. Skin changes, such as swelling, ecchymosis, and abrasions, should be noted because they are often more apparent with sprains than strains, which can be less obvious and are anatomically less superficial. Both active and passive range of motion should be examined and are often decreased secondary to pain and swelling. An inability to produce any active motion would identify a complete muscle rupture. Resistance testing of the affected structure will also prove to be painful and help narrow the differential diagnosis. Joint stability should be tested and may be compromised in severe sprains or if fractures are present. Neurologic testing and vascular status should also be noted.

3. Laboratory and diagnostic testing
   - In general, the diagnosis of a sprain or strain is made by a careful history and physical examination. X-ray evaluation is necessary only when a fracture is suspected. Further imaging of joint structures and soft tissues with CT or MRI are reserved for patients with severe injuries, to confirm a suspected diagnosis, and in patients who do not respond to initial treatment.

4. Formulating the diagnosis
   - Two of the more common disorders are described here.
     a. Ankle sprain
        - Ankle sprains are one of the most common musculoskeletal injuries, with inversion injures being more common than eversion. Pain and swelling occur because of stretching, partial tearing, or complete tearing of the soft tissues and ligaments that stabilize the ankle (anterior talofibular, calcaneofibular, posterior talofibular, anterior tibiofibular, and deltoid ligaments). Patients report a traumatic twisting of the ankle followed by pain, swelling, ecchymosis, and an inability to move or decreased movement. Examination confirms these findings. Patient's ability to bear weight should be assessed, as patients who are unable to do so may signify a more significant injury. Palpation of the ankle joint, fifth metatarsal, medial and lateral malleolus, and fibular head should be assessed because significant pain

should be an indication for prompt referral. Lastly, the syndesmosis should be checked by the squeeze test and dorsiflexing the foot and externally rotating. Increased pain with these maneuvers would also prompt immediate referral and x-ray evaluation.

- Diagnosis is generally clinical. X-rays are required to rule out fracture with a more significant injury. Treatment options include activity modification, ice, anti-inflammatory medication, brace or immobilization, and later physical therapy for minor injuries that require crutches, complete cast immobilization, and a longer therapy course for severe injuries. Fractures may be surgically or nonsurgically treated depending on the location, stability of the fracture, and amount of angulation or displacement.

   b. Acromioclavicular sprain (shoulder separation)

- The acromioclavicular (AC) joint is the connection between the distal clavicle and the acromion of the scapula. Trauma to the shoulder either in the form of a direct blow or fall can injure the ligament. Patients can present with pain over their AC joint which increases with movement. Physical examination reveals pain, swelling, and ecchymosis. Strength and range of motion may be limited by pain. Depending on the degree of injury, a palpable step-off may be present between the acromion and clavicle. Cross-arm adduction increases pain.
- Diagnosis is made based on history and examination; however, x-rays are needed to ensure there is no fracture. Treatments consist of ice, analgesics, and possibly shoulder immobilization in a sling, depending on the severity of injury. Physical therapy should begin once the shoulder is pain-free at rest and should include range of motion exercises, stretching, and strengthening. Surgery is only required in severe cases or in patients who do not improve with conservative measures.

5. Managing the patient

- Treatment for other sprains and strains depends on the severity of injury. Minor sprains and strains can be treated with rest or activity modification, ice, compression, and elevation. NSAIDs are often used to relieve discomfort. In addition, patients with moderate strains will require a period of immobilization followed by a period of rehabilitation to restore range of motion, flexibility, and lastly strength. Patients who display significant instability (joint "opens" with maneuvers that stress the joint) should be immobilized and referred for orthopedic evaluation; some of these patients may require surgical repair.

C. Dislocations, subluxations, and separations

1. Basic science

- A dislocation is the total separation of the bony articular surfaces of a joint. In contrast, subluxation is an incomplete separation of the articular surfaces that make up a joint. In general, dislocations are caused by a significant amount of trauma and can occur at any joint. Commonly dislocated joints include glenohumeral, patella, elbow, wrist, distal interphalangeal (DIP), knee, hip, metacarpophalangeal, metatarsophalangeal, and midfoot. Subluxations usually require significantly less energy to occur.

2. Formulating the diagnosis
   a. Shoulder
      - Because of the extensive range of motion of the glenohumeral joint, the glenohumeral joint is relatively unstable and relies on soft tissue structure for support. This large range motion and relative instability is reflected in the fact that it also is the most commonly dislocated joint. The most common cause of shoulder dislocations is a fall on an outstretched hand. Subluxation of the shoulder is also a common injury and some patients can even voluntarily sublux or dislocate their shoulder. Most shoulder dislocations occur with anterior displacement. Patients with increased laxity (glenohumeral translation) are at increased risk for subluxation and dislocation.
      - Patients present in the acute setting with pain and an inability to move the shoulder. Patients tend to keep the arm in the abducted externally rotated position for anterior dislocations and adducted and internally rotated for posterior dislocations. Physical examination will reveal tenderness around the entire shoulder. This may be relatively mild in patients with subluxation who have returned into anatomic alignment or severe in patients who remain dislocated. Patients with subluxation can then attempt active range of motion with abduction, internal rotation, and external rotation. These maneuvers may be too painful to perform in the patient with an acutely dislocated shoulder who had been reduced and will not be possible in a patient who has not been reduced but may help to establish the diagnosis. A complete neurovascular examination is also important in the affected limb as the axillary nerve (among other structures) can be injured with dislocations. Recent injuries will have a positive apprehension sign as patients become uncomfortable and nervous when the affected limb is placed in 90 degrees of abduction and is externally rotated.
      - Treatment is aimed at restoring anatomic alignment. In most instances, a subluxed shoulder is self-limited and will spontaneously reduce. For dislocations, a qualified orthopedist can immediately perform a reduction if the diagnosis is known. Confirmatory x-ray is required to verify complete anatomic reduction and better evaluate for fracture. The heeling process can take 4 to 12 weeks to complete.
   b. Elbow
      - Radial head subluxation or nursemaid's elbow is one of the most common orthopedic injuries in young children. Almost all cases occur between 1 and 4 years of age. It is caused by a sudden axial traction on a wrist while the elbow is extended and pronated. The annular ligament becomes trapped between the radial head and the capitellum, preventing reduction of the radial head.

- Children are usually brought to the emergency room with complaints of pain at the affected extremity. The caregiver (nursemaid) may relate a forceful pull on the extremity. They may report a period of disuse of the involved extremity by the child as well. Physical examination often reveals the child holding the painful extremity. The arm is in a pronated and slightly flexed position. There is local tenderness over the radiocapitellar joint. Supination of the forearm is limited and resisted. Radiographs may be helpful to confirm the diagnosis and to rule out other injuries such as fracture and frank dislocations. X-ray may reveal a volarly subluxed radial head.
- Treatment is aimed at restoring anatomic alignment. In some instances, the subluxation is reduced unknowingly by the x-ray technician while trying to obtain a true AP view of the elbow with the forearm in supination. If not, reduction is accomplished by gentle flexion of the elbow to 90 degrees with subsequent rapid, full supination. The examiner's thumb may aid by pushing the radial head back into position. A clunk may be palpated during the reduction. Immediate relief of pain and resumed use of the extremity can then be noted. Approximately 50% of children will begin to use the arm within minutes; the remaining half may need up to 24 hours.
- If the radial head does not spontaneously relocate, further treatment by a specialist is necessary, as a delay in reduction increases the difficulty of relocation.
- Frank dislocations of the elbow can also occur in both adults and children and are usually caused by a fall on an outstretched hand. Most patients report extreme pain and inability to use the affected arm. Because of the close proximity of the brachial artery, median and ulnar nerves, these structures are at high risk for injury. Therefore, a complete neurovascular examination must be performed. Patients with any abnormalities must be emergently treated.
- If a qualified orthopedist is immediately available, reduction should be performed as soon as possible because reductions are much easier to perform before the onset of significant swelling. However, if no such provider is available, patients should be referred urgently to the emergency department for treatment. The diagnosis can be confirmed by x-ray evaluation, which is also necessary to rule out associated fractures. Reductions are often performed under anesthesia by a qualified provider. Confirmatory x-ray is usually required to verify complete anatomic reduction and better evaluate the fracture.
  c. Hip dislocations
  - Dislocations of the hip are relatively rare. They are caused by a significant amount of trauma such as a motor vehicle accident. Patients with a suspected dislocated hip will need urgent evaluation as they may also have other significant injuries.

    d. Patellar dislocation/subluxation
- Patellar dislocation/subluxation occurs when a flexed knee is forcibly extended. Patients complain of severe knee pain, and there is a noticeable deformity. Most subluxations and even dislocations reduce spontaneously. Manual reduction may be necessary in some instances. Risk factors for patellar subluxation/dislocation include abnormal alignment, shallow trochanteric groove (or hypoplastic condyles), poor muscle balance, and previous history of patellar instability.
- Treatment is aimed at restoring anatomic alignment and improving strength and function. In most instances, a subluxed patella is self-limited and will spontaneously reduce. Dislocations are often reduced immediately and should be performed as soon as possible. Initial treatment consists of ice, pain management, and immobilization. Rehabilitation is then performed to recover range of motion and flexibility, and finally, the patient undergoes a balanced strengthening program. Patients with recurrent events despite adequate rehabilitation may be candidates for surgical stabilization.

    e. Dislocation of the digits
- Dislocations of the joints of the hand are relatively common events. Most are due to a traumatic hyperextension injuries. The proximal interphalangeal joint is the most common site of dislocation but can also occur at the distal interphalangeal joint or metacarpophalangeal joint. Dislocation of the carpal joints and midfoot are rare and should be referred to a specialist if suspected. Many of these injuries are handled immediately by bystanders or the patient themselves. Most of these injures can be reduced by applying axial traction and counterforce. Bony landmarks should be evaluated for potential fractures. Stability of the joint should be tested as well as active range of motion but not resisted motion. Diagnosis can be confirmed on x-ray, which are performed to rule out fracture. Treatment consists of ice, pain control, and immobilization.

D. Bursitis
   1. Basic science
- A bursa is a fluid-filled sac located in various areas throughout the body and functions to decrease friction over bony prominences. The bursa acts as a cushion between a bony prominence and soft tissues such as tendons. Occasionally, when this bursa can become inflamed, painful, and swollen, the condition is called bursitis. Most bursitis is caused by trauma or overuse of the affected limb. Some of the most commonly affected bursae include the acromial bursa, olecranon bursa, trochanteric bursa, prepatellar bursa, and pes anserine bursa.

   2. Formulating the diagnosis
    a. Pes anserine bursitis
- The pes anserine bursa lines beneath the insertion of the semitendinosus, gracilis, and sartorius (pes anserine) tendons on the tibia. They insert medially and inferior to the medial joint line. Patients

present with pain on flexion and extension of the knee. Physical examination reveals tenderness over the insertion of the pes anserine with localized swelling. Diagnosis is clinical. Treatment is aimed at treating the inflammation and consists of activity modification, anti-inflammatory medication, ice, and physical therapy. Severe cases can be treated with a steroid injection.

b. Prepatellar bursitis (housemaid's knee)

- The prepatellar bursa lies anterior to the patella and superior to the insertion of the patellar tendon. Patients present with pain on kneeling which can be severe. Pain also occurs with flexion and extension of the knee. Physical examination reveals superficial swelling and tenderness over the patella. Diagnosis is clinical. Treatment is aimed at treating the inflammation and consists of activity modification, anti-inflammatory medication, ice, and physical therapy. Severe cases can be treated with a steroid injection.

c. Trochanteric bursitis

- The trochanteric bursa lies along the lateral superior thigh, anterior to the greater trochanter of the femur and beneath the iliotibial band. Patients present with "hip pain," trouble sleeping on their side at night, and pain with running, walking, and biking which is worse after periods of inactivity. Inflammation occurs because of friction of the iliotibial band on the grater trochanter. Physical examination reveals tenderness over the greater trochanter. Diagnosis is clinical although x-rays may be helpful in ruling out other causes of pain if the diagnosis is unclear. Treatment is aimed at treating the inflammation and consists of activity modification, anti-inflammatory medication, ice, and physical therapy. Severe cases can be treated with a steroid injection.

d. Subacromial bursitis

- The subacromial bursa lies inferior to the acromion and superior to the rotator cuff. Patients present with shoulder pain, trouble sleeping on their side at night, and pain with overhead activities. Bursitis often occurs concomitantly with rotator cuff injury. Physical examination reveals a pain arc with abduction, positive rotator cuff impingement testing, and mild weakness (secondary to pain). Diagnosis is clinical although x-rays may be helpful in ruling out other causes of pain. A subacromial anesthetic injection may also be helpful to rule out a significant rotator cuff tear but will not differentiate impingement. Treatment consists of activity modification, anti-inflammatory medication, ice, and physical therapy. Severe cases can be treated with a steroid injection.

e. Olecranon bursitis

- The olecranon bursa lies between the olecranon process and the extensor tendon. Patients can present with acute onset of pain, swelling, and limited flexion or extension either after a traumatic event, or a more gradual painless onset from repetitive microtrauma. Physical examination reveals swollen painful fluid collection. The skin should be inspected for any disruption, discharge, warmth, erythema, and other signs of infection. Diagnosis is clinical. Aspiration should be performed if infection is suspected and the sample sent for Gram stain and culture. Treatment consists of activity modification, anti-inflammatory medication, ice, and compression. The bursa should be aspirated if infection is possible or range of motion is severely limited owing to the size of the bursa. Patients with infection need prompt drainage and antibiotic management. Severe or re-accumulating noninfected cases may benefit from a steroid injection.

10

Dermatology

I. Acne Vulgaris
   A. Basic science
      - Acne vulgaris is a disease of the hair follicle and associated sebaceous gland, seen primarily in adolescents.
      - The etiology of acne is multifactorial:
         1. Abnormal, denser keratinization within hair follicles, resulting in follicular plugging
         2. High rate of sebum secretion
         3. *Propionibacterium acnes,* an anaerobic diphtheroid
      - The first event is follicular plugging leading to comedo formation. This is followed by distention and rupture with the release of proinflammatory agents. *P. acnes* plays a role in the inflammation. The inflammatory reaction can lead to eventual scarring.
      - Androgens play a role in sebum production and acne formation. Excess systemic androgens, as in disease states (e.g., polycycstic ovarian syndrome), or increased localized concentrations can worsen acne.
   B. History and physical examination
      - Acne is primarily seen in adolescents; onset usually occurs after age 8 and can persist into late adulthood. Severe disease is more common in males. Infants, usually less than 3 months old, can present with acne (i.e., acne neonatorum). Primary site includes the face; back, chest, and shoulders can also be involved.
      - Characteristically several types of lesions can be seen. Lesions can be noninflammatory or inflammatory. The comedo is the prototypic noninflammatory lesion; comedones can be open (blackheads) or closed (whiteheads).
      - Closed comedones can progress to inflammatory lesions. Inflammatory lesions include papules, pustules, and large fluctuant nodules. Inflammatory lesions may become scarred. Healing may lead to hyperpigmentation; lightening requires weeks to months (longer in darkly pigmented individuals).
      - Acne-like eruptions can be caused by the following:
         1. Medications (systemic and topical steroids, lithium, phenytoin)
         2. Mechanical irritation (acne mechanica)
         3. Occupational exposure (tars, cutting oils, chlorinated hydrocarbons)
         4. Cosmetics and hair care products
         5. Sun exposure

C. Laboratory and diagnostic studies
  * There are no routinely used diagnostic studies in the evaluation and treatment of acne.
D. Formulating the diagnosis
  * The diagnosis is clinical. The presence of polymorphic acne lesions in an adolescent or young adult is virtually diagnostic. The presence of monomorphic lesions should raise suspicion of drug-induced, mechanical, or occupationally induced acne. The sudden worsening of preexisting acne should raise concern about possible gram-negative folliculitis (proliferation of gram-negative organisms due to prolonged antibiotic use for acne). The differential diagnosis also includes rosacea, folliculitis, perioral dermatitis, and sarcoidosis.
E. Evaluating the severity of problems
  * Clinical evaluation of the severity of inflammatory lesions and potential for and existence of scarring is crucial. Patients with suspected gram-negative folliculitis should be cultured.
  * Onset of acne at an older age or severe, persistent acne in females should raise concern about androgen excess, either of adrenal or ovarian origin. Severe, persistent acne in prepubescent children should raise similar concerns. Endocrine consultation may be indicated.
F. Managing the patient
  * Many treatments for acne vulgaris exist; three general categories are topical agents, systemic agents, and surgical approaches.
  1. Topical therapy
     * First-line topical agents in current use include topical retinoids such as tretinoin and tazarotene; agents with retinoid activity such as adapalene; benzoyl peroxide; and antibiotics. Topical retinoids work by reversing abnormal keratinization; it is the treatment of choice for comedonal acne. Benzoyl peroxide has a bacteriostatic effect on *P. acnes.* The topical antibiotics used frequently are clindamycin and erythromycin; they exert antibacterial and anti-inflammatory effects and can be used in combination with benzoyl peroxide.
  2. Systemic therapy
     * Systemic antibiotics are indicated for most inflammatory lesions. Tetracycline and erythromycin are first-line agents. Doxycycline or minocycline can be used as alternatives for tetracycline. A dermatologist should manage nodular cystic acne with systemic retinoids as indicated. Accutane (13-cis-retinoic acid) inhibits sebaceous gland activity and can markedly improve severe acne. Potential side effects include teratogenic effect on the fetus, dry skin and mucous membranes, musculoskeletal complaints, headaches, elevation in liver function tests (LFTs), hypertriglyceridemia, and the risk of future scarring at sites of trauma or surgery, and others. Its use requires regular laboratory and clinical monitoring. Accutane is contraindicated in women who are pregnant or those who might become pregnant during treatment.

3. Surgical treatment
- Surgical approaches are used during all stages of acne, from comedo extraction to dermabrasion and excision of scars.

II. Actinic Keratosis
   A. Basic science
   - Actinic keratosis is a precancerous lesion consisting of proliferation of atypical keratinocytes that develops in response to prolonged ultraviolet (UV) light exposure. They have the potential to transform into squamous cell carcinoma.
   B. History and physical examination
   - An actinic keratosis presents as 2- to 6-mm, flat, rough, red or tan patches on sun-exposed skin (head, neck, dorsal hands, and forearms), mostly in fair-skinned individuals.
   - Immunosuppressed individuals, such as renal transplant patients, are at high risk.
   C. Laboratory and diagnostic studies
   - Lesions larger than 1 cm, nodularity, and ulceration raise the suspicion of squamous cell carcinoma and require biopsy.
   D. Formulating the diagnosis
   - Clinical inspection is usually sufficient to establish the diagnosis.
   E. Evaluating the severity of problems
   - The range of risk of progression of actinic keratosis into squamous cell carcinomas varies from less than 1% to 20%. These are clinical markers for chronic sun damage and predict future development of squamous and basal cell cancers; therefore, regular skin checks are important.
   F. Managing the patient
   - Cryosurgery (most commonly used method), topical 5-fluorouracil (for extensive lesions), and electrosurgery are used to treat actinic keratoses. Sun protection with wide-brimmed hats, sun-protective clothing, and topical sun block reduce the development of new lesions.

III. Atopic Dermatitis
   A. Basic science
   - Atopic dermatitis is a genetically determined skin disorder seen in up to 20% of the population. Factors such as antigens, mechanical friction, and irritating materials produce an excessive reaction characterized by itch. It is frequently associated with hay fever, asthma, serum IgE elevation, and peripheral eosinophilia.
   B. History and physical examination
   - Atopic dermatitis occurs at any age but usually starts before 5 years of age. There are three stages: infantile, childhood, and adult. Acute skin lesions are intensely itchy red papules and vesicles. Chronic lesions are thick scaly plaques. White dermatographism (a white streak left in the skin after pressing on the skin) is a characteristic finding.

- Infantile atopic dermatitis frequently involves the face, scalp, and extensor areas (the forearms and over the knees and legs), which are rubbed and subject to friction during crawling.
- In later childhood (ages 2–12 years), the dermatitis involves the flexor areas (posterior neck, antecubital and popliteal fossae). A symmetric prominent fold beneath the lower eyelids (Dennie-Morgan lines) and periorbital darkening (allergic shiners) may be seen.
- Most adults will have "sensitive skin," and a small minority will continue to have full-blown flexural eczema throughout life. In adulthood, nummular (coin-shaped) skin patches are common, especially during the winter season. Other adult manifestations include itchy ill-defined skin patches and hand dermatitis.
- A family or personal history of atopy (dermatitis, hay fever, and asthma) is common. The history needs to focus on aggravating factors such as irritating clothing, skin care products, wet work, frequent hot-water baths or showers, and overheating from prolonged wearing of occlusive gloves.

C. Laboratory and diagnostic studies
- Patch testing for contact allergens is appropriate in recalcitrant cases of atopic dermatitis.

D. Formulating the diagnosis
- Diagnosis is established clinically. It is based on the physical appearance and duration of the lesions, as well as a family history of atopy. Contact dermatitis (a dermatitis that results from direct skin contact with an offending agent) needs to be ruled out.
- Secondary infection with yeast, dermatophytes, or bacteria needs to be excluded. A potassium hydroxide (KOH) preparation (microscopic examination of the skin scrapings after a KOH soloution is applied) will help rule out a yeast or dermatophyte infection.

E. Evaluating the severity of problems
- Severity is correlated to the extent of dermatitis, presence of infection, and resultant impairment (e.g., inability to use hands or to walk due to severe inflammation). Hospitalization is rarely necessary, and only after failed outpatient management. Cataracts may develop in patents with protracted atopic dermatitis. Secondary staphylococcal or streptococcal infection is common.

F. Managing the patient
- Topical steroids are the first line of therapy. Recently two topical macrolide immunomodulators, tacrolimus and pimecrolimus, have been used with good results.
- Other steps in management:
  1. Use of mild soap and frequent emollients
  2. Treatment of secondary infections
  3. Search for irritants and allergens
  4. Tepid compresses for acute/crusted lesions
  5. Oral antihistamines (diphenhydramine, hydoxyzine) for itching (Topical antihistamines should be avoided because contact dermatitis may result.)

6. UVB phototherapy for extensive involvement
7. Oral corticosteroids or other immunosuppressants have been used as a last resort for severe, unresponsive, generalized atopic dermatitis.
8. A short course of hospitalization to remove the patient from environmental etiologic factors is sometimes indicated.

IV. Basal Cell Carcinoma
  A. Basic science
   • Basal cell carcinoma is a malignant tumor arising from the basal keratinocytes of the epidermis. It is the most common skin malignancy, accounting for 900,000 cases annually in the United States. It is common among fair-skinned whites but is unusual in blacks, Hispanics, and Asians. It is locally destructive and invasive; however, metastases are extremely rare (<0.1% of cases).
  B. History and physical examination
   • Chronic sun exposure is the most common predisposing cause for basal cell carcinoma. Other factors include fair skin, North European decent, and exposure to ionizing radiation. Certain hereditary diseases carry an increased risk for basal cell carcinomas (albinism and xeroderma pigmentosum).
   • Basal cell carcinoma is slow growing; it occurs most commonly on the face, especially the nose. The most frequent type of basal cell carcinoma is nodular. It presents as a raised, translucent to yellowish papule or nodule. Overlying telangiectasia and a rolled border are characteristic. As it enlarges, the center of the lesion ulcerates and necroses (rodent ulcer). Occasionally, basal cell carcinomas are pigmented with blue-black coloration. These lesions must be differentiated from melanoma.
  C. Laboratory and diagnostic studies
   • Biopsy and histologic examination are mandatory when basal cell carcinoma is suspected.
  D. Formulating the diagnosis
   • Consider the diagnosis of basal cell carcinoma when seeing persistent nodulocystic or noduloulcerative lesions. Skin biopsy is required for diagnostic confirmation.
  E. Evaluating the severity of problems
   • Basal cell carcinoma is locally invasive and disfiguring but metastasizes extremely rarely. When metastasis does occur, regional nodes, lungs, and bones are most commonly involved.
  F. Managing the patient
   • Basal cell carcinoma can be treated with surgical excision, electrosurgery and curettage, cryosurgery, and Mohs' microscopically controlled surgery. Mohs' surgery is indicated for recurrent or poorly defined basal cell carcinoma and lesions in anatomic areas such as the eyelid, canthi, and nasolabial or postauricular folds. Topical imiquimod is a recent nonsurgical method for treating basal cell cancers. It is a biologic response modifier that elicits local cytokine production.
   • Preventive efforts include sun protection with comfortable clothing, hats, and sunblock that provides both UVA and UVB photoprotection.

V. Common Warts (Verruca Vulgaris)
  A. Basic science
    • Warts are benign epithelial tumors caused most frequently by human papillomavirus, a double-stranded DNA virus.
  B. History and physical examination
    • Common warts may appear at any age but are most common in older children. A majority regress spontaneously within 1 to 2 years. However, warts may persist for many years and may also reappear after periods of dormancy.
    • Common warts are raised, firm, brown, or tan papules and nodules and most commonly appear in areas subject to trauma such as fingers, elbows, and knees.
  C. Laboratory and diagnostic studies
    • If there is concern about potential malignancy, the wart should be removed and sent for histologic evaluation.
  D. Formulating the diagnosis
    • Common warts are easily recognized by their verrucous appearance.
  E. Evaluating the severity of problems
    • Some papillomaviruses may cause malignant warts (i.e., cutaneous warts in immunosuppressed and transplant patients). Suspicious lesions should be referred to a dermatologist.
  F. Managing the patient
    • Most common warts spontaneously regress. Treatment modalities are numerous, but recurrences after treatment are common:
      1. Having the patient apply salicylic acid/ lactic acid/collodion solution daily
      2. Cryotherapy
      3. Electrodesiccation
      4. Laser vaporization

VI. Contact Dermatitis
  A. Basic science
    • Contact dermatitis can be irritant or allergic (type IV delayed hypersensitivity reaction).
  B. History and physical examination
    • Patients will usually present with acute or chronic skin irritation and inflammation that is usually well demarcated and localized to the site of contact with the allergen. Poison ivy and nickel (jewelery, watches) are common allergens. Topical antibiotics (neomycin, bacitracin), clothing, rubber and latex products, dyes, cosmetics, and drugs are other potential causes. Often the patient has used a skin medication for years before developing an allergy.
    • Symptoms vary according to the severity of reaction. Redness, irritation, itching, and sometimes blister formation are observed. The dermatitis is usually well demarcated and occurs where the allergen contacts the skin. Once the cause is removed, the dermatitis generally disappears within several weeks.
  C. Laboratory and diagnostic studies
    • If the source of irritation is unclear, patch testing with a standard group of allergens should be considered to rule out allergic contact dermatitis.

D. Formulating the diagnosis
- A detailed history of exposures, in combination with characteristic skin changes, suggests contact dermatitis. Confirmation is made with patch testing.

E. Evaluating the severity of problems
- Severe reactions can cause facial and eyelid swelling. In rare cases the physician must pay close attention to the patient's respiratory status.

F. Managing the patient
- The allergen should be removed from the skin. Unless the allergen is removed from the skin, treatment will be ineffective. In known poison ivy exposure the skin should be washed immediately with soap and water. Gently washing the skin and applying topical corticosteroids can manage mild reactions. If the reaction is severe (or facial swelling occurs), systemic corticosteroids should be given. Patients should be educated regarding allergen avoidance.

VII. Dermatophyte Infections
A. Basic science
- Dermatophytes are fungi that exclusively invade the dead tissues of the skin, nails, or hair. There are several species of fungi with similar pathogenicity; infections are classified according to the site involved.

B. History and physical examination
- Infection is classified according to the area infected:
  1. Tinea unguium/onychomycosis: nail fungal infection (thick, discolored, crumbling nails)
  2. Tinea corporis: ringworm of the body (annular red plaques with raised borders and central clearing)
  3. Tinea pedis: ringworm of the feet, athlete's foot (itching and inflammation occurring between the toes, areas of maceration, with raised blister-like lesions, occurs more often in warm weather)
  4. Tinea cruris: ringworm of the groin, jock itch (areas of maceration, pain, and erythema in the crotch: more common in males; recurrence is common; associated with tight clothing and the summer season)
  5. Tinea capitis: ringworm of the scalp (patches of dryness, scaling and hair loss, or boggy inflammation of the scalp; occurs most commonly in children)

C. Laboratory and diagnostic studies
- Hair or scale from affected areas in a potassium hydroxide (KOH) preparation may demonstrate the fungus when viewed under the microscope.

D. Formulating the diagnosis
- The diagnosis is made clinically in combination with the result of microscopic analysis and fungal culture.

E. Evaluating the severity of problems
- Most dermatophyte infections are superficial and may be treated with topical antifungals; however, some infections may become widespread or resistant to therapy. Nail infections are especially difficult to eradicate.

F. Managing the patient
- Most dermatophyte infections are superficial and may be treated with topical antifungals such as miconazole, clotrimazole, terbinafine, and ketoconazole.

Extensive tinea corporis, resistant tinea pedis, tinea unguium/onychomycosis, and tinea capitis require systemic therapy with oral agents (griseofulvin, terbinafine, ketoconazole, itraconazole). Griseofulvin and the azoles are contraindicated during pregnancy.

VIII. Genital Warts
  A. Basic science
   - Genital warts (condylomata acuminata) are lesions of epithelial proliferation due to infection by human papillomavirus (HPV), a double-stranded DNA virus.
   - There are more than 100 HPV types. Genital warts are most often associated with HPV 6 and 11. An association of HPV with epithelial dysplasia and carcinoma has been shown. There is a frequent association of HPV 16 and 18 with cervical dysplasia and carcinoma of the cervix, vulva, and penis.
   - Genital warts are highly contagious and are acquired by contact, either during sexual intercourse or passage through an infected birth canal. The incubation period after exposure lasts weeks to months.
  B. History and physical examination
   - A history of other sexually transmitted diseases may be elicited. The existence of genital warts in the mother of an affected infant may be demonstrated.
   - Condyloma acuminatum occurs on both skin and mucus membranes. Genital lesions in men are often initially at the frenulum or coronal sulcus, and in females at the posterior introitus. Perianal and rectal lesions are seen predominantly in those who practice anal intercourse. Oral lesions may occur via sexual transmission.
   - Genital warts can vary widely in appearance from single to multiple, coalesced, flesh-colored to pink or gray papules with a ridged, moist surface, to large cauliflower-like growths. Genital warts are usually asymptomatic.
  C. Laboratory and diagnostic studies
   - Subclinical lesions may be demonstrated by surface whitening with dilute acetic acid (acetowhitening). A biopsy will aid diagnosis and is essential when dysplasia or carcinoma is suspected.
  D. Formulating the diagnosis
   - The diagnosis of genital warts is made clinically. The differential diagnosis includes condylomata lata of secondary syphilis, squamous cell carcinoma, and benign growths.
  E. Evaluating the severity of problems
   - The demonstration of externally located genital warts mandates internal examination. Females should undergo a thorough pelvic examination with a Pap smear to look for dysplasia. Anoscopy should be performed when perianal involvement exists. Urethral visualization should be done if urethral lesions are suspected. Sexual partners should be evaluated. Young children with condylomata should be evaluated for sexual abuse, particularly if new lesions appear after age 2.
  F. Managing the patient
   - Local destructive approaches:

1. Cryotherapy with liquid nitrogen
2. Application of 20% to 50% trichloroacetic acid
3. Electrocautery
4. Application of podophyllotoxin 0.5% twice daily for 3 days in weekly cycles
   - Podophyllotoxin is contraindicated in pregnancy.
- Patients should be examined regularly until complete disappearance of the lesions. Carbon dioxide laser ablation can be used for larger, recalcitrant lesions. The vapor produced by laser ablation should be evacuated because it contains potentially infectious viral DNA. Surgical excision is occasionally required and may be the treatment of choice either for large, pedunculated lesions or when dysplasia is suspected. Imiquimod is a topical immunomodulator recently approved for treatment of genital warts.

IX. Impetigo
   A. Basic science
      - Impetigo is a superficial skin infection, which presents as nonbullous (70%) and bullous forms. The former is usually due to group A beta-hemolytic streptococci. *Staphylococcus aureus* is the sole cause in several cases and causes bullous impetigo.
      - Newborns can develop group B streptococcal infection.
      - Children and young adults are most commonly affected; the prevalence is highest in late summer and early fall. Impetigo is highly contagious; it is acquired either from persons with impetigo or from bacterial carriers. Minor trauma is needed for infection to occur. It is found most commonly on the face (especially the nasolabial and perioral areas), extremities, and trunk.
      - Poststreptococcal glomerulonephritis can complicate impetigo. Chronic carrier states can occur with colonization of the nasopharynx.
   B. History and physical examination
      - A history of exposure to affected individuals and crowded living situations may be elicited. The initial lesion is a vesicle or pustule that very rapidly forms a plaque with honey-colored crust and surrounding redness. There are no constitutional symptoms. Bullous impetigo presents as superficial blisters on normal appearing skin. Regional lymphadenopathy may occur.
   C. Laboratory and diagnostic studies
      - Culture and Gram stain of early vesicles (or the base of older lesions) will demonstrate gram-positive organisms. Antistreptolysin O (ASO) titers are usually negative.
   D. Formulating the diagnosis
      - The clinical picture of honey-colored crusted lesions is very suggestive and cultures are usually not needed. The differential diagnosis includes the following:
        1. Chickenpox (presents with more extensive distribution)
        2. Herpes zoster (has a prodromal burning or tingling sensation, more hemorrhagic crusting, and a dermatomal distribution)
        3. Acute contact dermatitis

  E. Evaluating the severity of problems
- Impetigo usually responds to treatment without complications, although untreated patients may develop a carrier state.
- In less than 5% of cases, streptococcal impetigo can result in acute poststreptococcal glomerulonephritis.

  F. Managing the patient
- Topical treatment with mupirocin ointment (Bactroban) is often effective for localized infections.
- Systemic antibiotics (e.g., penicillin, erythromycin, or an oral first-generation cephalosporin) are the treatment of choice for widespread or complicated cases. Patients with recurrent infections should be evaluated and treated for nasal or perineal carriage of *Staphylococcus aureus.*

 X. Keloids and Hypertrophic Scars

  A. Basic science
- Keloids and hypertrophic scars result from hyperproliferation of fibrous tissue following skin injury. Hypertrophic scars develop only at the site of original injury, whereas a keloid extends beyond it. In normal scars, fibroblasts are arranged parallel to the skin surface. In keloids and hypertrophic scars, there is a whorled arrangement of fibroblasts. Keloids are more common in dark-skinned individuals.

  B. History and physical examination
- Keloids and hypertrophic scars are more common on the upper back, shoulders and chest, and on the ear lobes after ear piercing. Hypertrophic scars are raised scars that follow the lines of original injury, such as surgical excision. Keloids can itch and be painful, and range in color from flesh-colored to hyperpigmented, from pink to purple.

  C. Laboratory and diagnostic studies
- Biopsy may be, but is rarely, used to identify keloids.

  D. Formulating the diagnosis
- The diagnosis is made by appropriate history and physical examination.

  E. Evaluating the severity of problems
- Discomfort, disfigurement, and restriction of movement due to contractures are the main concerns. Ulceration and hyperesthesia can also occur.

  F. Managing the patient
- Hypertrophic scars and smaller keloids can be injected with steroids.
- Larger keloids can be excised with steroid injection at the edges. Larger lesions can be grafted with pressure dressings applied to both the donor and graft site.
- Silicon gel sheets have been tried for both keloids and hypertrophic scars.

 XI. Malignant Melanoma

  A. Basic science
- Malignant melanoma is a tumor arising from melanocytes. Melanomas generally present as pigmented lesions of various size and shape. These lesions

can invade and metastasize to distant organs so rapidly that the patient may die within months of diagnosis. Patient prognosis is correlated with the depth of the melanoma. Early detection and removal of the tumor are critical to the treatment of malignant melanoma. Melanoma is responsible for 2% of all cancer deaths.

- In the United States over 40,000 new cases are diagnosed annually.
- The incidence has been increasing and is attributed to ultraviolet radiation exposure of lightly pigmented skin. Body sites that receive intermittent high-intensity sun exposure (trunk of men and lower extremities of women) are at increased risk for development of melanoma.
- Other risk factors:
  1. Family history of melanoma or atypical nevi
  2. Atypical/dysplastic nevus syndrome
  3. Personal history of melanoma
  4. DNA repair defect (i.e., xeroderma pigmentosum)
  5. Immunosuppression
- Sites of primary lesions besides the skin include the eye, meninges, oral mucosa, urethra, and anus. Sixty percent of malignant melanomas arise in normal skin; 40% develop from pigmented moles.
- Melanoma is much less common in blacks and Asians. The most frequent sites are the soles, mucous membranes, palms, and nail beds.
- There are four major types of melanoma:
  1. Superficial spreading melanoma (70%)
     - Patients generally notice an asymptomatic brown or black macule with irregular borders. They may also notice enlargement or irregular coloration of a mole. It is seen most commonly on the trunk of men and the legs of women.
  2. Nodular melanoma
     - Nodular melanoma is the second most common type and presents as an asymptomatic blue or black nodule. Patients may seek medical attention because of rapid growth.
  3. Lentigo maligna melanoma
     - Lentigular maligna melanoma arises on photodamaged skin of older individuals. It is usually 1 to 3 cm and is a flat, slowly growing, irregularly pigmented brown-black spot.
  4. Acral lentiginous melanoma
     - Acral lentiginous melanoma is the most common melanoma in Africans and Asians. These lesions have an irregular border and pigmented tan-brown-black component. These are seen on acral sites such as the nail bed, digits, palms, and soles.
B. History and physical examination
   - The cardinal indication of melanoma is a persistent, changing, pigmented lesion. Amelanotic melanoma presents as a skin-colored or tan lesion and may cause confusion in diagnosis. Patients are instructed to look for the **ABCD** of moles: **a**symmetry, irregular **b**order, **c**olor change, **d**iameter greater than 6 mm.

- Rapid enlargement, ulceration, bleeding, and pain are a few additional signs that should prompt immediate attention.

C. Laboratory and diagnostic studies
- Excisional biopsy should be done on all highly suspicious lesions. There is no evidence that incisional biopsy causes spread of tumor.
- Two methods are used to histologically measure melanomas: Breslow's thickness (measures thickness of tumor) and Clark's level (measures depth of invasion from surface of skin).

D. Formulating the diagnosis
- Diagnosis is established by careful histologic examination.

E. Evaluating the severity of problems
- The staging of melanoma is categorized into local, regional, or distant disease and strongly correlated with survival. Sentinel node biopsy is being tried to identify regional metastatic disease. Liver chemistries and scanning of the chest and abdomen and MRI are indicated for staging in patients with suspected spread of melanoma.
- Breslow's thickness and tumor ulceration (microscopic) are major prognostic indicators. For tumors less than 1 mm in thickness, 5-year survival rate is approximately 95%, compared to 3% to 14% for patients with distant metastasis.

F. Managing the patient
- Melanomas are treated by surgical excision. Staging is essential for managing the patient.
  1. Primary melanoma (stages I and II)
     - Primary melanoma refers to localized disease with no evidence of regional lymph node involvement. Therapy for stage I melanoma generally consists of wide surgical excision. Patients should be checked two to four times per year for at least 2 years and every 6 months to annually thereafter (physical examination should include medical history, skin and lymph node examination, laboratory and radiographic studies as indicated).
  2. Regional metastasis (stage III)
     - Stage III indicates regional node involvement. Therapy includes wide surgical excision and regional lymph node dissection. Immunotherapy with interferon-alfa has been tried for high-risk stage II and stage III melanoma.
  3. Distant metastasis (stage IV)
     - Stage IV indicates that distant metastases are present. Therapy for distant metastasis is surgical excision along with adjuvant radiation, chemotherapy, and immunotherapy. Dacarbazine is the most widely used single agent. Symptomatic treatment for relief of pain and discomfort should be given.

XII. Psoriasis
A. Basic science
- The essential pathogenic event in psoriasis is increased epidermal cell proliferation. The disease affects 2% to 4% of the population.

B. History and physical examination
- Psoriasis can occur at any age; however, onset is common during the young adult years. A family history of psoriasis is common.
- The onset of psoriasis is usually gradual. Precipitating events for the development of psoriatic lesions include trauma, infection (especially with beta-hemolytic streptococci), emotional stress, and hypocalcemia. Precipitation or worsening can also be drug-induced; known culprits include lithium, antimalarials, interferon, and β-blockers. Rapid taper of systemic steroids can precipitate pustular psoriasis.
- The classic lesion of psoriasis is a sharply demarcated red plaque with a silvery scale. If gently scraped, the scale can be removed, leaving bleeding points (Auspitz sign). These plaques are usually found on extensor surfaces (i.e., knees and elbows).
- The nails are frequently involved (i.e., pitting of the nail beds). Scalp involvement with thick, large, flaky scales is also common. Erosive seronegative arthritis may be associated.

C. Laboratory and diagnostic studies
- Skin biopsy is important when the diagnosis is uncertain. Biopsy utilizing direct immunofluorescence is indicated when lupus is in the differential diagnosis.

D. Formulating the diagnosis
- The diagnosis is made both by history and by clinical inspection of the lesion. Presence of scalp and nail involvement helps confirm the clinical impression. Drug eruptions and several other skin disease states may present with similar physical findings, making biopsy necessary.

E. Evaluating the severity of problems
- Some forms of psoriasis, such as erythroderma and pustular psoriasis, can be life-threatening. A dermatology consultation and inpatient management may be essential in certain cases. Major complications of severe psoriasis include sepsis and electrolyte imbalance from secondary fluid losses with widespread and severe disease.

F. Managing the patient
- Topical treatment should be tried first.
- Topical agents:
  1. Topical corticosteroids
  2. Calcipotriol (a vitamin D analog)
- First-line drug therapy for stable, mild psoriasis:
  3. Coal tar and its derivatives
  4. Anthralin
- Severe psoriasis is treated with the following:
  5. Phototherapy, narrow band UVB, 311 to 313 nm (is considered optimal)
  6. Psoralens and high-intensity ultraviolet A light (PUVA)
  7. Retinoids
  8. Methotrexate (if extensive, recalcitrant and disabling)
  9. Cyclosporin (for severe disease)

- Recently, antibodies against T-lymphocyte surface molecule (alefacept), and anti-TNFα agents (etanercept) are being used for moderate to severe psoriasis with good results. Etanercept is useful for psoriatic arthritis as well.

XIII. Pyogenic Granuloma
  A. Basic science
    - Pyogenic granuloma is a localized growth of granulation tissue surrounded by a collar of skin (epithelium). The lesion generally develops at a site of injury and represents a fibrovascular response to trauma.
  B. History and physical examination
    - Patients generally report a history of trauma to the involved area. Pyogenic granuloma presents as a smooth red nodule. Central ulceration and bleeding are common. Pyogenic granuloma is most frequently seen in young adults on the face, hands, forearms, palms, soles, and oral mucosa. Recurrence is common.
  C. Laboratory and diagnostic studies
    - Biopsy is required for definitive diagnosis.
  D. Formulating the diagnosis
    - Pyogenic granuloma must be differentiated from malignant melanoma or other vascular tumors. Excisional biopsy provides the definitive diagnosis.
  E. Evaluating the severity of problems
    - This is a benign lesion.
  F. Managing the patient
    - Surgical excision serves both diagnostic and therapeutic purposes. These lesions can also be treated by curettage and electrodesiccation of the base.

XIV. Scabies
  A. Basic science
    - Scabies is an intensely pruritic skin eruption caused by the mite *Sarcoptes scabiei.* The fertilized female mite tunnels under the stratum corneum into the viable epidermis and lays eggs within the burrowed skin. Eggs mature and larvae are released in 3 to 5 days. The larvae become adults in 10 to 14 days and group around the hair follicle. Lesions result from hypersensitivity to the mite. Scabies is spread by skin-to-skin contact with infected carriers. Because the mite can survive 1 to 5 days off the human body, clothing and bed linens may act as fomites.
    - In immunosuppressed patients, thousands of organisms may be present, creating a crusted form of scabies known as Norwegian scabies.
  B. History and physical examination
    - The main symptom of scabies infection is intense itching. Itching is intensified at night. Because the mite may live away from its host for up to 5 days, a history of contact with known scabies carriers is not necessarily elicited.

- Scabies is commonly present on the hands, feet, axillae, breasts, periumbilical region, hips, buttocks, and genitalia. The primary lesions consist of raised threadlike lines (burrows) and small erythematous papules.
C. Laboratory and diagnostic studies
  - Diagnosis is confirmed by demonstration of mites, eggs, or fecal pellets on microscopic examination of skin scrapings obtained from a lesion. Several lesions should be scraped to collect material because it can be very difficult to get a positive scraping.
D. Formulating the diagnosis
  - Itching and the presence of dermatitis in close contacts may help establish the diagnosis. Once microscopic analysis of skin scrapings demonstrates the scabies mite, the diagnosis is confirmed.
E. Evaluating the severity of problems
  - Scabies is highly infectious, especially where skin-to-skin contact is present (e.g., within a household, parent-child interactions, and body contact sports such as wrestling). Itching can be very distressing. In areas of excoriation, secondary streptococcal infection may occur.
F. Managing the patient
  - Despite a negative scraping, treatment may be required, especially if persistent, generalized itching with a scabies-like eruption is present.
  - Treatment is aimed at eradicating the mite:
    1. Permethrin 5% cream or lindane (Kwell) is used. Crotamiton and 10% sulfur in petrolatum have also been used. Topical treatment should be repeated in 7 days to ensure complete clearance. Ivermectin is an oral antiparasitic agent effective against the mite.
    2. Close contacts need to be treated simultaneously.
    3. Clothing and linens should be washed in hot water, or dry cleaned, or isolated in closed plastic bags for 5 days to prevent reinfection from fomites.
    4. Pruritus should be treated with systemic antipruritics.
    5. Secondary infections need to be treated with appropriate antibiotics.

XV. Squamous Cell Carcinoma
  A. Basic science
    - Squamous cell carcinoma is a malignancy that arises from keratinocytes. It can arise suddenly or from preexisting lesions such as actinic keratoses. Squamous cell carcinoma is the second most common skin cancer in the United States, accounting for 80,000 to 100,000 cases per year.
    - Cutaneous squamous cell carcinoma causes tissue damage by direct tumor invasion. Cutaneous squamous cell carcinomas rarely metastasize.
    - Approximately 30% of oral (lingual and mucosal) squamous cell carcinomas metastasize before diagnosis is made.
  B. History and physical examination
    - Squamous cell carcinoma occurs most frequently on sun-exposed skin areas of fair-skinned people, particularly those of Northern European ancestry living in sunny areas. Men, particularly farmers and sailors, are more frequently affected.

- Squamous cell carcinoma can arise from a preexisting lesion such as an actinic keratosis. Immunosuppressed individuals and those with severe photodamage are at particular risk for developing squamous cell carcinoma. The appearance of squamous cell carcinoma is variable. In the early stage, squamous cell carcinoma presents as a smooth, red-pink raised lesion with a crusted surface. As the lesion develops it may become irregular, wart-like, and ultimately ulcerative. Other potential squamous cell carcinoma sites include the following:
  1. The oral cavity (i.e., the floor of the mouth, the side of the tongue, and the soft palate)
     - Oral squamous cell carcinoma is associated with leukoplakia; about 4% of leukoplakia lesions develop into squamous cell carcinoma.
  2. The vulva
     - Squamous cell carcinoma can present as a small, wart-like lesion or as erosion with itching and bleeding.
  3. The scrotum
     - The patients may have a wart-like papule or a friable nodule.
  4. The penis
     - The initial lesion can be a well-defined red patch with an irregular border.
  C. Laboratory and diagnostic studies
  - Biopsy is necessary for diagnosis.
  D. Formulating the diagnosis
  - Asymptomatic but persistent oral lesions should undergo biopsy 2 weeks after any irritating factors have been eliminated.
  - Clinical differential diagnoses include basal cell carcinoma, fungal infections, and other skin malignancies. Skin biopsy will provide definitive diagnosis.
  E. Evaluating the severity of problems
  - Squamous cell carcinomas arising on sun-exposed areas are less aggressive than those arising on mucocutaneous surfaces, or on areas affected by radiation dermatitis. The rate of metastasis from lesions arising in sun-damaged skin is between 0.5% and 3%; as larger lesions invade the deeper dermis, the rate of metastasis increases.
  F. Managing the patient
  - Therapy depends on the age of the patient and on the size and location of the lesion. Treatment methods commonly used include the following:
    1. Surgical excision
    2. Curettage and electrodesiccation (of smaller lesions on sun-exposed areas)
    3. Irradiation (in older and debilitated patients)
    4. Mohs' microscopically controlled surgery (for difficult, recurrent, or ill-defined lesions)

XVI. Varicella Virus Infection
  A. Basic science
  - The varicella zoster virus causes varicella (chickenpox) and zoster (shingles). The virus is a double-stranded DNA virus that belongs to the herpesvirus

family (human herpesvirus 3). It is very contagious. Respiratory secretions usually transfer primary varicella, though the vesicular fluid of chickenpox and zoster lesions may also transmit the disease. The incubation period is approximately 14 days after which the skin lesions of chickenpox appear. After the skin clears, the virus may remain alive, dormant in dorsal root ganglion cells for several decades.

- Reactivation of the virus is spontaneous or due to a decrease in cellular immunity. If spontaneous, the reactivation usually occurs after the age of 50. The reactivated virus replicates in sensory nerve ganglia, causing local inflammation, destruction and pain, or sensory distrubances. After replication, the virus travels down sensory neurons into the skin. This results in the cutaneous eruption of zoster. The virus may reactivate and produce pain without causing skin lesions.

B. History and physical examination
- Patients with zoster usually have a history of chickenpox. Coexisting immunosuppressive conditions may be noted (e.g., malignancy, AIDS, and the use of immunosuppressive drugs). Events that may hasten reactivation of the virus include trauma, stress, fever, surgery, and sunburn.
- With zoster, a prodromal syndrome of sharp or lancing pain or tingling, burning, fever, headache, malaise, and tenderness at the site of future skin lesions is often noted. After 1 to 4 days, grouped vesicles on a red base appear. The eruption is unilateral and is usually confined to one dermatome. The most commonly affected dermatomes are thoracic, cervical, trigeminal, and lumbosacral. Clearing occurs within 2 to 4 weeks. Patients may have tender regional adenopathy.
- Involvement of the first branch of the trigeminal nerve is of special concern, as 50% of these patients will develop ophthalmic involvement. Lesions of the tip of the nose suggest potential eye involvement and warrant an urgent ophthalmology consultation (Hutchinson's sign).

C. Laboratory and diagnostic studies
- A Tzanck smear performed by scraping the base of a vesicle or pustule and staining should reveal multinucleated giant cells. Cell culture and tests for viral antigens are specific and serve to distinguish varicella zoster from other herpesviruses. However, the most useful laboratory test is direct immunoflourescence of the lesions.

D. Formulating the diagnosis
- The diagnosis is based on the history (prodromal pain) and physical findings (vesicles in a dermatomal distribution). The prodromal pain syndrome can be confused with multiple conditions including myocardial infarction, cholecystitis, pleuritis, and otitis.

E. Evaluating the severity of problems
- Potential complications of zoster depend on the site of reactivation and the host's immunologic status. Patients with cranial nerve V_1 involvement should be evaluated early by an ophthalmologist. An otorhinolaryngologist should evaluate patients with ear involvement.

- The existence of distant lesions removed from the site of primary disease suggests disseminated disease. Immunocompromised patients are at increased risk for disseminated disease that may lead to pneumonitis, hepatitis, pericarditis, and neurologic involvement. Secondary bacterial infections and skin necrosis can occur.
- The most common complication of zoster is persistent pain after the skin clears (postherpetic neuralgia). Over one third of the patients with zoster will experience persistent pain for some time (50% of cases resolve in 3 months and 75% of cases within 1 year).

  F. Managing the patient
- Acyclovir has been shown to halt the progression of skin lesions, increase viral clearing from vesicle fluid, and reduce disseminated disease. It also helps to decrease the incidence and duration of postherpetic neuralgia. Intravenous acyclovir is indicated in immunosuppressed patients or patients with serious complications. Systemic corticosteroids may lessen the incidence of postherpetic neuralgia but should be used with caution.
- Local symptomatic therapy includes analgesics, cool compresses, and calamine lotion. Postherpetic neuralgia is treated with analgesics, topical capsaicin, tricyclic antidepressants (e.g., amitriptyline), gabapentine, nerve blocks, and biofeedback.

XVII. Yeast Infections (Candidiasis)
  A. Basic science
- *Candida albicans* exists as part of normal human flora. The organism is usually found in warm, moist areas of the body (between skin folds and on mucous membranes). The organism may become pathogenic if host defenses weaken or if the environment becomes favorable to the organism (such as following use of oral antibiotics).

  B. History and physical examination
- Candidiasis of the skin usually begins in intertriginous zones (between opposing skin surfaces where friction and moisture occur). The lesions appear as red, well-demarcated patches of various sizes. Small, red satellite pustules usually surround the lesions. Common sites of infection include the inner aspect of the thighs, the axillae, inframammary area, and the gluteal and inguinal folds of infants (diaper rash).
- Oral candidiasis (thrush) appears as white plaques on the tongue and buccal mucosa. The plaques can be scraped from the tongue. In infants and young children, oral candidiasis is both common and benign. In adults, however, persistent oral candidiasis should raise the suspicion of HIV infection.

  C. Laboratory and diagnostic studies
- Yeast and pseudohyphae can be demonstrated microscopically from scrapings treated with potassium hydroxide, or Gram stain.

  D. Formulating the diagnosis
- The diagnosis is made clinically. Confirmation involves microscopy. In unusual cases, histologic examination of the skin specimen is necessary.

E. Evaluating the severity of problems
    - Superficial candidiasis is common in infants. The infection is benign and easily treated. HIV patient can develop persistent candidiasis, which may be refractory to therapy.
F. Managing the patient
    - Topically applied nystatin and imidazoles (e.g., miconazole, ketoconazole) are the drugs of choice for yeast infections of the skin and mucous membranes.
    - For diaper rash, nystatin powder, or imidazole creams are used. Frequent diaper changes to keep the skin dry are also important.
    - Oral candidiasis is treated with nystatin liquid. The patient is instructed to "swish and swallow" the liquid.
    - Oral fluconazole is indicated for extensive disease.

11

Endocrinology

I. Adrenal Disorders
  A. Cushing's syndrome
    1. Basic science
      - Cortisol is the primary functional glucocorticoid produced by the adrenal cortex. In the normal physiologic state, cortisol production is regulated by adrenocorticotropin (ACTH) release from the pituitary. ACTH in turn is released under the influence of corticotropin-releasing hormone (CRH) from the hypothalamus.
      - Cushing's syndrome occurs whenever excessive cortisol is secreted by the adrenal glands either as a result of autonomous adrenal production (adrenal adenoma or carcinoma), excess production of ACTH (pituitary or ectopic) or CRH, or administration of excess exogenous glucocorticoids. Cushing's disease refers specifically to hypersecretion of pituitary ACTH.
      - The most common cause of Cushing's syndrome remains iatrogenic, that is, exogenously administered glucocorticoid. The spontaneous syndrome is more common in women, particularly in the third and fourth decades.
    2. History and physical examination
      - Patients relate a history of fatigability, weakness, mood changes, and easy bruising. Women may note menstrual irregularities and features of androgen excess including hirsutism, acne, and male pattern baldness.
      - Hypertension is often present. Clinical manifestations of hypercortisolemia include truncal obesity, impaired glucose tolerance, hirsutism, acne, abdominal striae, and osteoporosis.
    3. Laboratory and diagnostic studies
      - Screening tests in patients with clinical evidence of cortisol excess include the measurement of 24-hour urinary free cortisol (preferred) or the overnight low-dose (1 mg) dexamethasone suppression test. A diurnal variation in plasma cortisol (which peaks around 8:00 AM) is normally present; its absence is an indicator of Cushing's syndrome, but this is not a very sensitive or specific test.
      - If a screening test suggests hypersecretion, the next step is to determine whether the patient has Cushing's syndrome. The low-dose dexamethasone suppression test (dexamethasone 0.5 mg every 6 hours for 2 days) will distinguish patients with a false positive screen (cortisol suppresses) from those with Cushing's syndrome (cortisol does not suppress). The next steps are to do high-dose dexamethasone suppression (either 8 mg overnight or 2 mg every 6 hours for 2 days) and a serum ACTH level. If the ACTH is

elevated, and there is cortisol suppression with the high dose, this is most likely a pituitary source of cortisol excess (Cushing's disease). If the cortisol does not suppress and the ACTH is low, then this is likely an adrenal adenoma or carcinoma. If the cortisol does not suppress and the ACTH is elevated (usually several times the upper limits of normal), then this is most likely ectopic ACTH. Anatomic localization should then proceed to confirm the most likely source of the ectopic production. If the suppression tests are uncertain and ACTH is in the normal range or elevated (suggesting a pituitary source) or the biochemistry suggests a pituitary source, but imaging studies are not confirmatory, then petrosal sinus sampling may be helpful. CRH testing may also help distinguish normal from abnormal ACTH pituitary secretion.

4. Formulating the diagnosis
   - As just noted, it is useful to perform biochemical testing to formulate the diagnosis before proceeding to anatomic studies. It is useful to group patients into ACTH-dependent (Cushing's disease and ectopic ACTH syndrome) and ACTH-independent (adrenal tumors) categories. Measurable plasma ACTH virtually excludes primary adrenal disease as the cause.

5. Evaluating the severity of problems
   - Adrenal carcinoma forecasts a poor prognosis. Similarly, the outlook for patients with small cell lung cancer (the most common source of ectopically produced ACTH) is poor.

6. Managing the patient
   - The mainstay of treatment for Cushing's disease is transsphenoidal microadenectomy. Pituitary irradiation is an option for nonsurgical candidates. Postoperative patients should be treated for adrenal insufficiency and evaluated for recovery of corticotropic pituitary function in the postoperative period. Most patients with ACTH-producing microadenomas will recover a normal hypothalamic-pituitary-adrenal axis. If they have permanent hypofunction, they will need chronic glucocorticoid replacement including increased doses for periods of stress and illness. In addition, such patients will often need replacement of other hormones regulated by the anterior pituitary (L-thyroxine, sex steroids).
   - Surgical resection is the treatment for ectopic sources of ACTH. Surgery is also the primary treatment for functioning adrenal adenomas and all adrenal carcinomas. Medical adjuncts are available for adrenal carcinomas and include mitotane, aminoglutethimide, ketoconazole, and metyrapone.

B. Adrenocortical hypofunction
   1. Basic science
      - The adrenal cortex secretes three classes of hormones: glucocorticoids, mineralocorticoids, and androgens. Glucocorticoids and mineralocorticoids are associated with clinically significant deficiency syndromes. Adrenocortical hypofunction describes the condition in which steroid output from the adrenal cortex is insufficient to meet the body's needs. Adrenal insufficiency is most commonly due to primary adrenal disorders.

The most common cause of primary adrenal insufficiency is autoimmune destruction of adrenal hormones. Infection (especially tuberculosis), hemorrhage (often associated with anticoagulant use), and metastatic invasion also cause primary adrenal insufficiency. Secondary adrenal insufficiency due to pituitary hypofunction may occur as a result of pituitary tumors, pituitary apoplexy or autoimmune pituitary failure, and suppression of the hypothalamic-pituitary-adrenal (HPA) axis from exogenous glucocorticoid use.

- The most common cause of primary adrenal insufficiency (also known as Addison's disease) is idiopathic atrophy; an autoimmune mechanism is thought to be responsible. There is an increased incidence of other endocrine and autoimmune processes in these patients including hypothyroidism, type 1 diabetes mellitus, hypogonadism, and hypoparathyroidism.
- Secondary adrenal insufficiency is due to insufficient ACTH secretion, either from exogenous glucocorticoid use (most commonly) or from primary pituitary disorders. Unlike patients with primary adrenocortical insufficiency, these patients often have normal or near-normal levels of aldosterone; whereas ACTH stimulates aldosterone secretion, aldosterone production also occurs in response to renin-angiotensin stimulation from volume depletion and hyperkalemia.

2. History and physical examination
- Early adrenal insufficiency may present with only mild constitutional symptoms of fatigue and malaise. With more advanced adrenal insufficiency, the most common symptoms are weakness, hyperpigmentation, weight loss, anorexia, nausea, and vomiting. Less often, patients complain of abdominal pain, salt craving, diarrhea, constipation, and syncope. Patients with secondary adrenal insufficiency do not have hyperpigmentation, nor do they complain of symptoms attributable to hypoaldosteronism. The medical history should include questions regarding the duration of symptoms, because hyperpigmentation and weight loss are seen only in the more chronic cases. Patients with AIDS (acquired immunodeficiency syndrome) are at risk for a necrotizing infection of the adrenal gland caused by cytomegalovirus and other opportunistic pathogens.
- The physical examination is often remarkable for hypotension and orthostasis. Hyperpigmentation, when present, is seen diffusely, including areas shielded from sun exposure; mucous membranes may be pigmented as well.

3. Laboratory and diagnostic studies
- Early in the course of adrenal insufficiency, basal glucocorticoid and mineralocorticoid output may be normal, but secretion during periods of stress may be inadequate. In general, glucocorticoid deficiency occurs before mineralocorticoid deficiency. Because glucocorticoid deficiency is associated with impaired free water clearance, hyponatremia may occur earlier than hyperkalemia. Hyperkalemia is a result of mineralocorticoid

deficiency. Glucocorticoid deficiency is best elicited through the ACTH stimulation test, in which plasma cortisol is measured 30 to 60 minutes after the administration of intravenous cosyntropin, an ACTH analog.

4. Formulating the diagnosis
   - The diagnosis of adrenal insufficiency is established by demonstrating an inadequate response to ACTH stimulation testing. In primary adrenal insufficiency, the serum ACTH is elevated and the serum aldosterone level is below normal. In secondary adrenal insufficiency, the serum ACTH is low with a correspondingly low cortisol level. However, serum aldosterone concentrations are normal.

5. Evaluating the severity of problems
   - Adrenal crisis is the acute exacerbation of chronic adrenal insufficiency. It occurs in patients with chronic adrenal insufficiency during periods of severe stress (e.g., surgery) or septicemia (e.g., the Waterhouse-Friderichsen syndrome). However, the most frequent cause is abrupt withdrawal of exogenous glucocorticoids in glucocorticoid-dependent patients. Affected individuals complain of severe abdominal pain, nausea, and vomiting; they become somnolent and hypotensive.
   - Treatment consists of rehydration with normal saline and treatment with stress doses of glucocorticoids. Glucocorticoid treatment is best accomplished with a 100-mg bolus of hydrocortisone, followed by 50 to 100 mg intravenously every 8 hours. Separate mineralocorticoid is unnecessary in patients receiving these high doses of cortisol replacement therapy.

6. Managing the patient with chronic glucocorticoid deficiency
   - Treatment consists of glucocorticoid replacement in all patients and mineralocorticoid replacement in many patients. A typical glucocorticoid regimen consists of hydrocortisone 25 mg in the morning and 12.5 mg in the afternoon or evening; this regimen mimics the normal diurnal variation of steroid secretion. Patients with hypoaldosteronism (i.e., with primary adrenocortical insufficiency) should also receive a source of mineralocorticoid; usually, fludrocortisone is given once daily in dosages from 0.05 to 0.1 mg. Patients should be given explicit instructions to supplement glucocorticoid during periods of stress or illness, usually by doubling the dose for 2 or 3 days. Monitoring of replacement usually relies on control of clinical symptoms. ACTH levels are not a good measure of replacement therapy and typically are mildly elevated in patients on adequate glucocorticoid replacement. Suppression of ACTH levels may result in clinical features of excessive cortisol (cushingoid features).
   - Complications of therapy include electrolyte disturbances and sometimes hypertension (excess mineralocorticoid replacement); therefore, electrolyte levels should be checked periodically. Hyponatremia suggests inadequate glucocorticoid replacement. Hypokalemia and hypertension suggest excessive mineralocorticoid replacement.

C. Pheochromocytoma
  1. Basic science
     - Pheochromocytoma is a rare tumor composed of chromaffin cells that is capable of secreting biogenic amines and peptides including epinephrine, noreepinephrine, and dopamine. Most occur in the adrenal medulla while the rest occur in the thorax or abdomen. About 10% are bilateral and 10% are malignant.
  2. History and physical examination
     - The classic triad consists of headache, diaphoresis, and palpitations. However, the signs and symptoms are variable and some patients may be asymptomatic. The hypertension may be paroxysmal or sustained. Pheochromocytoma should be suspected if hypertension is very difficult to treat. Pheochromocytomas are associated with multiple endocrine neoplasia (MEN) IIA and IIB.
  3. Laboratory and diagnostic studies
     - Screen with 24-hour urine for metanephrine, VMA (vanillylmandelic acid), and catecholamines. The metanephrine test is the least sensitive to medicines. It is very sensitive and specific when it is collected while the patient is symptomatic, off medicines, and resting. If the 24-hour urine catecholamine test is inconclusive in a patient with suspected pheochromocytoma, fasting serum catecholamines should be collected. A level above 1000 pg/mL is suggestive and above 2000 pg/mL is diagnostic. When elevations of catecholamines are not clearly definitive for a pheochromocytoma, clonidine suppression tests may be useful.
  4. Formulating the diagnosis
     - The diagnosis is usually made based on biochemistry. Magnetic resonance imaging (MRI) (preferable) or computed tomography (CT) of the adrenals should be done to locate the tumor. Metaiodobenzylguanidine (MIBG) scintography (a norepinephrine analog) can be used; MIBG concentrates in the adrenals and in pheochromocytomas. This test is used when other imaging is not definitive. Some pheochromocytomas are found only during surgical exploration.
  5. Evaluating the severity of problems
     - Metastases from a slow growing pheochromocytoma may remain unapparent for several years. Therapy is rarely curative. They respond poorly to radiotherapy and chemotheraphy. Treatment here is usually palliative.
  6. Managing the patient
     - The treatment is surgical. Patients are treated preoperatively with phenoxybenzamine (α-blocker) to control blood pressure and propanolol is used as needed for tachycardia. Adequate volume replacement reduces risk of postoperative hypotension. Follow-up biochemical testing and, as indicated, radiologic testing are done postoperatively.

II. Diabetes Mellitus

A. Basic science

- Diabetes mellitus is a chronic disorder that is characterized by a relative or absolute deficiency of insulin secretion and activity. There are several classification systems of diabetes; most systems recognize type 1 (formerly called insulin-dependent diabetes mellitus), type 2 (formerly called non–insulin-dependent diabetes mellitus), gestational diabetes, and diabetes secondary to other causes (e.g., pancreatic disease or drugs).

- The onset of type 1 diabetes typically occurs before age 30, although there is a second peak in the fifth decade of life. Pancreatic β cells are gradually destroyed by autoimmune mechanisms. Eventually there is insufficient insulin to maintain glycemic control. There is genetic association with alleles in the major histocompatibility complex on the short arm of chromosome 6. Monozygotic twin studies typically show a 30% to 50% concordance rate. However, it is likely that type 1 diabetes has a polygenic cause with both environmental risk factors and protective genetic components. Viral causes and association with exposure to cow's milk have been proposed as immunologic triggers, but the exact mechanisms remain unproved. Although the immunologic process causing β cell destruction takes place over a period of years, the development of symptoms may be abrupt. Common symptoms include polydipsia, polyphagia, polyuria, and associated weight loss. Dependence on exogenous insulin and susceptibility to ketosis are characteristics of type 1 diabetes.

- Most patients with type 2 diabetes are diagnosed after age 40, although childhood onset of type 2 diabetes mellitus is now becoming increasingly common. Type 2 diabetes is clearly genetic as monozygotic twins have concordance rates of greater than 90% after age 55 years. Except for selected autosomal dominant forms of type 2 diabetes, the exact genetic loci for type 2 diabetes mellitus are not yet well characterized. Although the exact pathogenesis remains unclear, hallmarks of this disease include insulin resistance and a progressive decline in β cell function (nonimmunologically mediated). In patients who have a genetic predisposition to develop diabetes it is now quite clear that increasing calorie intake (especially the "Western" diet) and decreasing exercise are associated with increased prevalence of diabetes mellitus. Most type 2 diabetic patients are asymptomatic. When symptoms occur, they are often gradual and include polyuria, polydipsia, and weight loss. Some patients may never have symptoms and may not come to attention until end-organ damage (e.g., retinopathy, nephropathy, neuropathy) has occurred.

- Gestational diabetes mellitus (GDM) is present in up to 2% of pregnancies. Glucose tolerance becomes most impaired in the third trimester. Maintenance of euglycemia is particularly important in the prevention of fetal morbidity and death, especially related to large fetal size. Most women with GDM do not require treatment for diabetes immediately after pregnancy, although women with GDM are at increased risk of developing type 2 diabetes mellitus in the future.

- Secondary forms of diabetes include pancreatic disease associated with a pancreatectomy, chronic pancreatitis, cystic fibrosis, and hemochromatosis as well as disorders associated with increased counterregulatory hormones such as Cushing's syndrome (including exogenous glucocorticoids) or acromegaly. When these disorders are associated with significant β cell loss (e.g., pancreatitis/pancreatectomy), insulin therapy is usually required for adequate glycemic control.

B. History and physical examination

- A recent history of weight loss, polydipsia, polyphagia, and polyuria in an adolescent or young adult suggests the diagnosis of type 1 diabetes. These patients are often at or below normal weight. Most type 2 diabetic patients are obese. They may present with complaints similar to those of the type 1 diabetic or may have nonspecific symptoms such as fatigue or pruritus or may be completely asymptomatic.
- In patients with long-standing diabetes mellitus (of any type), some end-organ complications may be evident on physical examination (e.g., retinopathy, neuropathy, peripheral vascular disease). Hypertension is common in type 2 diabetes mellitus and is often associated with evidence of diabetic nephropathy (e.g., proteinuria).

C. Laboratory and diagnostic studies

- Because plasma glucose levels are subject to fluctuations during periods of illness, severe stress, or drug ingestion, hyperglycemia must be documented on more than one occasion. Specifically, fasting plasma glucose (FPG) values in excess of 126 mg/dL on two separate occasions are diagnostic. However, patients with FPG below these levels may have diabetes based on glucose-stimulated PG values. Thus, the diagnosis of diabetes mellitis may be made by using the 2-hour oral glucose tolerance test; the 2-hour plasma glucose >200 mg/dL is diagnostic. A random glucose level over 200 mg/dL, accompanied by symptoms of diabetes, is diagnostic.
- Hemoglobin (Hgb) A_{1c} is an assay that reflects glycemic control over the preceding 2 months; the result is expressed as a function of total hemoglobin as a percentage. After the diagnosis of diabetes mellitus has been made, home glucose monitoring kits using finger stick capillary glucose determinations are used to monitor glycemic control and to adjust oral glucose lowering medications or insulin. Additionally, type 1 diabetic patients should routinely test their urine for ketones any time they have significant hyperglycemia.

D. Formulating the diagnosis

- The diagnosis of diabetes mellitus is established by the aforementioned abnormal fasting or stimulated glucose levels glucose levels. GDM criteria are based on somewhat lower glucose levels. Individuals who have FPG levels between 100 and 125 mg/dL have impaired fasting glucose (prediabetes), and those who have stimulated 2-hour values between 140 and 199 mg/dL have impaired glucose tolerance (prediabetes).
- Other illnesses (Cushing's disease, cystic fibrosis, pheochromocytoma, etc.), medications (thiazide diuretics, glucocorticoids etc.), and severe stress can

precipitate hyperglycemia. Stress-related hyperglycemia may improve with the resolution of the stress, but may also unmask the risk for future diabetes— much the same as GDM.

E. Evaluating the severity of problems

1. Acute complications

- The acute metabolic consequences of diabetes mellitus include diabetic ketoacidosis and hyperglycemic hyperosmolar nonketotic coma. Diabetic ketoacidosis (DKA) occurs most commonly in type 1 diabetes mellitus, but may occur in type 2 diabetes mellitus. DKA results when there is insufficient insulin and lipolysis with release of organic acids. Insulinopenia is the most common cause in type 1 diabetes; in type 2 diabetes mellitus, a relative deficiency in insulin accompanied by high levels of glucagon (and other stress hormones) will also result in ketoacidosis. In hyperosmolar nonketotic coma (HHNKC), there is also relative insulinopenia, but ketosis is absent or mild. The increased glucose concentrations cause an osmotic diuresis producing losses of sodium, potassium, and phosphate. Profound dehydration may occur with either DKA or HHNKC. Criteria for the diagnosis of DKA are hyperglycemia, hyperketonemia, and metabolic acidosis. Although infection and failure to take insulin are usual inciting events, often no precipitating cause is found for DKA. In HHNKC inciting causes also include myocardial infarction, sepsis, or use of medications such as glucocorticoids or thiazide diuretics. Initial treatment should include regular insulin (administered intravenously) and normal saline. There is usually a large total body potassium deficit, though patients may present with hyperkalemia. Acidosis usually corrects with rehydration (and the addition of glucose as glucose levels come down). Bicarbonate is not usually needed, but should be given with severe acidosis.

- Hyperosmolar nonketotic coma occurs over a period of days, during which time there is progressively worsening hyperglycemia, dehydration, and hyperosmolality (>325 mOsm/L). This form of diabetic coma is seen more often in the elderly, and unlike DKA, ketonemia and acidemia are not prominent features. The inciting event should be sought and corrected; initial resuscitation is similar to that for DKA. Normal saline should be used initially, although the majority of replacement fluid may be 0.9% or 0.45% normal saline in some cases of marked hypernatremia in which the total body water deficit may be greater than that of the sodium deficit.

2. Chronic complications

- The chronic complications of diabetes include macrovascular disease, microvascular disease, and neuropathies. In diabetes mellitus, macrovascular disease is a result of dyslipidemia, hypertension, clotting abnormalities, and other features of insulin resistance related to the risk for accelerated atherosclerosis. Diabetes mellitus increases the risk for atherosclerotic vascular disease by two- to fivefold inclusive of coronary, cerebral, and peripheral vascular disease. "Silent" coronary ischemia is not uncommon, and patients who present with atypical angina, dyspnea on exertion, or nausea with exertion may already have advanced coronary artery disease.

- The microvasculature of diabetics reveals diffuse capillary basement membrane thickening; nephropathy and retinopathy are two common manifestations of this vascular pathologic process. Rigorous glycemic control reduces the risk for onset and progression of retinopathy, nephropathy, and neuropathy. Laser therapy has a major role in the treatment of retinopathy. Annual ophthalmologic follow-up is appropriate. Diabetic nephropathy is accelerated in the face of hypertension, so blood pressure control is important. Agents that block the renin-angiotensin-aldosterone system including angiotensin-converting enzyme (ACE) inhibitors and angiotensin receptor blockers (ARBs) reduce the risk for progression of nephropathy beyond their blood pressure lowering effects.
- Diabetic neuropathy worsens in proportion to the duration and magnitude of hyperglycemia. The most common form of neuropathy is a symmetric distal polyneuropathy. The loss of sensation is a leading cause of neurotrophic foot ulcers. Loss of sensation can be detected using monofilament testing. Patients should be taught to inspect their feet and wear appropriate footwear as prescribed in the face of callus formation or any foot deformity. Charcot changes constitute the most severe foot deformities. Polyradiculopathy is associated with painful lower-extremity paresthesias. Besides intensifying glycemic control, treatment with B-complex vitamins, phenytoin, carbamazepine, amitriptyline, gabapentin, duloxetine, and capsaicin have all been used with modest success.
- Autonomic neuropathy may involve the gastrointestinal (e.g., gastroparesis) and cardiovascular (e.g., resting tachycardia, abnormal beat-to-beat variation, orthostatic hypotension) systems and may lead to abnormal papillary reflexes and gustatory sweating.

F. Managing the patient
 1. Medical nutrition therapy
    - The importance of the diet in diabetes cannot be overemphasized. The American Diabetes Association has made recommendations regarding the distribution of total energy intake with reduction in weight to help improve metabolic control. Saturated fat calories should not exceed 10% of total calories. Protein intake should be limited to 0.8 g/kg in those with nephropathy. Carbohydrate and mono/polyunsaturated fat account for the rest of the caloric intake with individualization of content based on weight loss and glycemic control.
 2. Insulin therapy
    - All type 1 diabetic patients need insulin therapy. The regimen requires basal and bolus therapy adjusted to caloric intake and exercise. There is increasing use of long- and short-acting insulin analogs with insulin adjustments based on measures of glucose control and carbohydrate intake. Patients with type 2 diabetes who require insulin may be started on simpler regimens such as a two-injection-per-day regimen of intermediate-acting human recombinant insulin. Often the evening dose of insulin may be higher than the morning dose in order to suppress hepatic glucose

production and to control fasting hyperglycemia. Rigorous glycemic control in type 2 diabetes often requires three or more daily injections.

- Often short-acting (regular) or rapid-acting (lispro, aspart, or glulisine) insulin is added before meals to adjust for daily dietary variations. An attempt is made to maintain fasting and preprandial glucose levels between 80 and 120 mg/dL. One-hour postprandial glucose values should ideally be less than 160 mg/dL. Premixed insulins may also be used for convenience in patients with visual or cognitive impairment or limited manual dexterity. Sites of insulin injection should be varied because use of the same site leads to tissue lipohypertrophy and impaired absorption.
- Hypoglycemia is an important side effect of insulin use (discussed later in this chapter). Long-standing diabetes, a recent hypoglycemic event, and agents such as β-blockers are associated with reduced ability to detect the adrenergic symptoms of hypoglycemia. Hypoglycemic unawareness often is the limiting factor for rigorous glucose control.

3. Oral glucose-lowering agents

- Oral glucose-lowering agents are used in type 2 diabetic patients who are not controlled adequately by diet and exercise alone. There are currently four general classes of agents that work by different mechanisms. Sulfonylureas (and short-acting insulin secretagogues such as nateglinide and repaglinide) stimulate insulin production from the pancreatic β cell. Biguanides (metformin) have their major effect on suppressing hepatic glucose production and limited effect on reducing peripheral insulin resistance. Thiazolidinediones (TZDs) have their major effect on reducing peripheral insulin resistance. Alpha-glucosidase inhibitors slow absorption of glucose from the gut by inhibiting the brush border enzymes that break down disaccharides and larger carbohydrate molecules; their major effect is to reduce postprandial hyperglycemia. Typically the sulfonylureas, metformin, and TZDs will reduce $HgbA_{1c}$ by approximately 1% to 1.5% at maximal doses. The short acting insulin secretagogues and alpha-glucosidase inhibitors will reduce $HgbA_{1c}$ by about 0.5% to 1.0%. Agents that work by different mechanisms generally have additive effects, so combination oral agent therapy is now common practice.
- Metformin is often the initial agent of choice in type 2 diabetes mellitus. Monotherapy is not associated with hypoglycemia. Weight gain is less of a problem with metformin than other agents. Metformin is contraindicated in the face of liver disease, decreased renal function (because of lactic acidosis risk), and heart failure. Following radiocontrast use, metformin should not be reinitiated until confirmation of normal renal function. TZDs are rapidly becoming an agent of first choice because of absence of hypoglycemia with monotherapy and some evidence of β cell protective effects. They can be used in the face of renal compromise, but should be used cautiously in liver disease and in the presence of heart failure. Weight gain and peripheral edema are common with the TZDs. Sulfonylureas have the greatest risk for hypoglycemia (either as monotherapy or in conjunction with other agents). They should be used cautiously in the face of renal and

hepatic disease (appropriate agents can be selected on the basis of clearance mechanisms). The alpha-glucosidase inhibitors do not have a risk for hypoglycemia when used as monotherapy. However, when used in combination with sulfonylureas, hypoglycemia may occur and patients must be instructed to treat hypoglycemia with glucose tablets or gel (the effects of disaccharides such as sucrose are impaired by the medication). Gastrointestinal symptoms of gas, flatulence, and bloating are limiting factors for alpha-glucosidase inhibitor use.

- Finally, two phenomena deserve mention: the dawn phenomenon and Somogyi effect. The dawn phenomenon is an increase in fasting blood glucose levels and insulin requirements before breakfast. The cause appears to be an inability to respond to normal nocturnal surges of growth hormone secretion with increased insulin secretion. The Somogyi effect represents rebound hyperglycemia in response to counterregulatory hormones (e.g., epinephrine, cortisol) during unrecognized hypoglycemic episodes.

III. Disorders of Calcium Balance
   A. Basic science
   - Calcium is an essential mineral for neuromuscular function and bone metabolism. Total serum calcium represents the bound (primarily to albumin) and free (clinically significant) fractions. Although the total serum calcium is often altered by changes in albumin concentration, the fraction of free calcium usually remains constant.
   - Hypercalcemia and hypocalcemia are disorders of calcium balance. Hypercalcemia, the more common of the two, is most often caused by primary hyperparathyroidism or malignancy. Other causes include sarcoidosis, vitamins A and D toxicity, thiazide diuretics, lithium ingestion, the milk-alkali syndrome, immobilization, and (the recovery phase of) acute renal failure. Parathyroid hormone (PTH) and vitamin D serve to raise serum calcium; calcitonin, a hormone secreted by the parafollicular cells of the thyroid, has weak actions that contribute to lowering serum calcium.
   - Hypercalcemia and hypophosphatemia are consistent features of hyperparathyroidism, although calcium values fluctuating from high normal to above normal ranges often characterize early hyperparathyroidism. Asymptomatic hypercalcemia due to hyperparathyroidism is often discovered incidentally on routine laboratory tests. Clinical manifestations of hyperparathyroidism include nephrolithiasis, constipation, mental status changes, and bone resorption. Solitary parathyroid adenomas represent the most common cause for hyperparathyroidism and present primarily between the third and fifth decades. Diffuse hyperplasia also causes hyperparathyroidism.
   - Malignancy (most often squamous cell tumors) is the second most common cause of hypercalcemia. Hypercalcemia is caused both by humoral mediators (in the absence of bone metastases) and by local destruction of bone by tumor. The most common humoral mediator is PTH-rp (PTH-related peptide).

Previous diagnoses of "ectopic" PTH were likely related to PTH-rp; assays can now readily distinguish PTH from PTH-rp.

- Hypercalcemia may also occur with a familial syndrome called familial hypercalcemic hypocalciuria. This syndrome is associated with normal or slightly elevated PTH levels and low 24-hour urinary calcium excretion (usually <100 mg/24 hour).
- Hypocalcemia, specifically low free-serum calcium, is caused by chronic renal failure, hypoparathyroidism (postsurgical or idiopathic), hypomagnesemia or hypermagnesemia, acute pancreatitis, malabsorption syndromes, vitamin D deficiency, and multiple blood transfusions (rare).

B. History and physical examination
- Clinical manifestations of hypercalcemia include the following:
  1. Renal (polyuria and nephrolithiasis)
  2. Gastrointestinal (anorexia, nausea, vomiting, and constipation)
  3. Neurologic (weakness, fatigue, stupor, and coma)
  4. Electrocardiogram (ECG) manifestations (shortened QT interval)
- Clinical manifestations of hypocalcemia include the following:
  1. Paresthesias and tetany (e.g., carpopedal spasm)
  2. Chvostek's sign (twitching of the facial muscles with tapping over the facial nerve)
  3. Trousseau's sign (carpal spasm with inflation of a blood pressure cuff over systolic blood pressure for 3 minutes)
  4. ECG manifestations (prolonged QT interval)

C. Laboratory and diagnostic studies
- Hypercalcemia usually becomes symptomatic when the calcium level exceeds 12 mg/dL. Elevated calcium levels in asymptomatic patients should be repeated to eliminate the possibility of laboratory error. Ionized calcium may be measured to determine the amount of free (or active) calcium. Parathyroid hormone should be measured; it will be elevated in patients with hyperparathyroidism and will be suppressed in malignancy-related hypercalcemia (assuming normal renal function). PTH levels may be in the normal range with hyperparathyroidism, but still be disproportionately high for the serum calcium level. When PTH levels are in the normal range, a 24-hour urine calcium should always be obtained to exclude familial hypercalcemic hypocalciuria. Routine chemistries and a complete blood count should be included in the workup; they can be useful in identifying patients with hematologic malignancies. Bone scans and x-ray examinations are indicated if evidence of bone involvement exists.
- Laboratory studies in patients with hypocalcemia should include serum ionized (free) calcium, magnesium, phosphorus, creatinine, and parathyroid hormone. Hypoalbuminemia is a frequent cause of low total calcium; however, the ionized fraction is typically unaffected.

D. Formulating the diagnosis
- Hyperparathyroidism and malignancy account for more than 90% of individuals with hypercalcemia. Over half of patients with hyperparathyroidism are asymptomatic; in contrast, patients with hypercalcemia secondary to a malignancy typically manifest evidence of malignancy before the discovery of

hypercalcemia. Additionally, most patients with malignancy-related hypercalcemia will live less than 6 months. Therefore, the duration of hypercalcemia and the presence of symptoms are the two historical factors that are most helpful in the diagnosis.

- The differential diagnosis for hypocalcemia includes disease states characterized by relative or absolute deficiency of PTH, magnesium, and vitamin D (including vitamin D deficiency associated with malabsorption syndromes).

E. Evaluating the severity of problems

- Severe hypercalcemia (>15 mg/dL) requires aggressive treatment with intravenous fluids and use of loop diuretics when patient is rehydrated. Intravenous bisphosphanates should be considered. If the cause of hypercalcemia is vitamin D–mediated, then glucocorticoids should be administered (this may also be the case with selected malignancies such as myelomas or lymphomas or in sarcoidosis). Invasive hemodynamic monitoring and frequent assessment of electrolytes are generally advisable. Dialysis may be necessary if hypercalcemia fails to respond to conventional therapy, although dialysis has limited effectiveness unless the cause(s) of hypercalcemia can be treated concomitantly.

- Severe hypocalcemia may cause laryngeal spasm, convulsions, and respiratory arrest. Repletion of calcium is best achieved with an intravenous solution of calcium gluconate; hypomagnesemia, if present, must also be corrected. If hypocalcemia is caused by vitamin D deficiency, then replacement with short-acting vitamin D is indicated.

F. Managing the patient

- The treatment of hypercalcemia should be directed at its cause. Nearly all patients with hyperparathyroidism should be managed surgically; exceptions to this approach are older (>70 years old) asymptomatic patients with normal bone mass and renal function who may be closely monitored.

- Acutely, the lowering of serum calcium is best achieved through saline diuresis; this serves to expand the intravascular volume. Once this has been achieved, a loop diuretic (e.g., furosemide) may offer additional benefit. Other effective therapies include pamidronate (inhibits osteoclasts, slow onset, lasts for weeks), calcitonin (rapid onset, useful in renal failure, rapid tolerance limits its use), oral phosphate (used in a chronic setting), and glucocorticoids (slow onset, useful in vitamin D toxicity including vitamin D toxicity associated with granulomatous diseases and some malignancies).

- Correction of chronic hypocalcemia due to hypoparathyroidism or renal failure is through replacement of calcium (e.g., $CaCO_3$) and vitamin D (e.g., calcitriol).

IV. Dyslipidemia

A. Basic science

- Lipoproteins are particles which have a hydrophobic core surrounded by a hydrophilic phospholipid outer layer. Chylomicrons (contain Apo B48, CII, A, and E) are a triglyceride-containing moiety; they are formed in the intestinal epithelium from dietary fats that get into the circulation via the lymphatic ducts. Chylomicrons attach to muscle and fat receptors, and CII activates lipoprotein lipase leading to formation of triglycerides (TGs) and free fatty acids (FFAs). The liver degrades the chylomicron remnants. Very low density lipoproteins (VLDLs) are synthesized by the liver and contain Apo B100, CII, and E. VLDLs also transport TGs to muscle and fat. Capillaries in fat contain lipoprotein lipase that is activated to hydrolyze TG from VLDL resulting in intermediate-density lipoprotein (IDL). VLDL remnants and IDL are taken up by the liver. Half the IDLs (contain Apo E and B100) stay in the plasma where they are converted to low-density lipoprotein (LDL). LDL contains Apo B100. HDL is formed as the result of LDL interaction with extrahepatic tissues.

B. History and physical examination
  - There are several familial hyperlipidemia syndromes; thus, attention to history is crucial. The physical examination is essentially unremarkable with the exception of xanthomas involving the tendons (very high LDL-C with familial hypercholesterolemia), palms (symmetric elevations of cholesterol and TG as well as VLDL-C to TG ratio > 0.3 with familial dysbetalipoproteinemia), and eruptive skin lesions (very high TG in chylomicrons and VLDL) in selected cases.

C. Laboratory and diagnostic studies
  - A fasting lipid profile is the test of choice including total cholesterol, TG, and HDL-C. LDL-C is calculated. If the sample is not fasting, only the cholesterol and HDL-C can be used for interpretation as TG may be elevated.

D. Formulating the diagnosis
  - LDL-C level is the main laboratory test used as a treatment target. Treatment targets are based on assessment of cardiovascular heart disease (CHD) risk.

E. Evaluating the severity of problems
  - LDL-C less than 100 mg/dL is optimal; 100 to 129 mg/dL is near optimal; 160 to 189 mg/dL is high; 190 and higher is very high. HDL-C less than 40 mg/dL is low and 60 mg/dL or greater is high.
  - Risk determinants are used in conjunction with LDL-C levels to determine treatment options. All patients with CHD are deemed to be "high" risk (target LDL-C < 100 mg/dL). If they also have associated risk factors such as diabetes mellitus, they are deemed "very high" risk (target LDL-C < 70 mg/dL).
  - Cardiovascular heart disease (CHD) risk equivalents include diabetes as well as other forms of atherosclerotic disease including peripheral arterial disease, abdominal aortic aneurysm, and symptomatic carotid artery disease. LDL-C target is below 100 mg/dL. Risk determinants include cigarette smoking, hypertension, low HDL-C, family history of premature CHD (less than 55 in men and less than 65 in women), and age (men 45 or older and women 55 or older). If the patient's Framingham cardiovascular risk score is 20% or higher for 10 years, LDL-C target is less than 100 mg/dL.
  - The goal for patients with CHD or CHD risk equivalents is LDL-C below 100 mg/dL. For patients with two or more risk factors the goal is less than 130 mg/dL. In patients with zero to one risk factor, the goal is less than 160 mg/dL.

F. Managing the patient
- Step II American Heart Association diet is the initial treatment of hyperlipoproteinemia. If diet is unsuccessful or lipoprotein is extremely elevated, drug therapy is used. In general, adding 30 to each LDL-C goal estimates the threshold in which drug treatment should be entertained for patients with increased TG or a corresponding elevation of non-HDL-C (VLDL-C + LDL-C) component.
- Several classes of drugs are used to treat hyperlipoproteinemia. Statins are first line for lowering LDL, and fibric acid derivatives are first line for lowering triglycerides. Bile resins or ezetimibe are a second-line treatment for elevated LDL, and nicotinic acid is second line for hypertriglyceridemia.

V. Hypogylcemia
A. Basic science
- Hypoglycemia is a clinical syndrome manifested by symptomatically low plasma glucose. It is useful to classify hypoglycemia as either postprandial or fasting.
- Postprandial hypoglycemia (reactive hypoglycemia) most commonly occurs in postgastrectomy patients in whom hypoglycemia results from insulin-glucose imbalance after rapid glucose absorption. Less often, hypoglycemia is seen in patients with rare enzymatic defects such as galactosemia and hereditary fructose intolerance. Occasionally other people may experience reactive hypoglycemia, which is likely an exaggerated insulin response to a carbohydrate load. It is not clear that this is truly a pathologic condition, but it is commonly treated with frequent feedings and by avoiding meals with a high carbohydrate load.
- Fasting hypoglycemia occurs when glucose use exceeds glucose production. Most commonly, this occurs during therapy of diabetes mellitus with either insulin, sulfonylureas, or the short-acting insulin secretagogues (see Section II, Diabetes Mellitus). Other medications, such as salicylates, sulfonamides, pentamadine, and alcohol (during periods of glycogen depletion) are also known offenders. Less frequently, severe liver disease, enzymatic defects, and tumors (e.g., insulinomas) are to blame.
B. History and physical examination
- Patients typically complain of either autonomic (sweating, anxiety, palpitations) or neuroglycopenic (lethargy, incoordination, headache) symptoms. The history should include questions about recent food, alcohol, and medication intake as well as the effects of exercise. Response to calorie ingestion is also helpful.
- Patients with insulinomas are more likely to have neuroglycopenic symptoms than adrenergic symptoms. Because these patients may also be amnesic for the hypoglycemic events, it is important to elicit a history of altered behavior from someone who has observed the hypoglycemic episodes.
- Physical examination findings associated with hypoglycemia are often remarkable but are generally too nonspecific to be diagnostic.

C. Laboratory and diagnostic studies
- The first diagnostic step in patients with suspected fasting hypoglycemia is the measurement of plasma glucose after an overnight fast; the fast is continued either until symptomatic hypoglycemia (<50 mg/dL) occurs or 72 hours have passed. Intermittent serial insulin (and perhaps C-peptide) levels should be obtained. In normal subjects insulin levels decrease as the glucose levels decrease. In patients with insulinomas, insulin levels typically stay higher than they should for the corresponding level of hypoglycemia. Any time during the test, if symptomatic hypoglycemia occurs, insulin levels should be obtained. It should be noted that fasting PG values below 50 mg/dL have been reported in normal healthy women, but corresponding insulin levels in these women is also low. In patients in whom surreptious or inadvertent (pharmacy drug substitution) sulfonylurea use is suspected, sulfonylurea levels should be obtained. However, this test may be negative even in the face of sulfonylurea-induced hypoglycemia.
- Although controversial, a 5-hour oral glucose tolerance test is sometimes used, during which time a symptom log is recorded by patients in whom postprandial hypoglycemia is suspected. This test will sometimes be positive in the face of an insulinoma. The diagnostic value of such testing is very limited and not recommended for general use.

D. Formulating the diagnosis
- Symptoms occurring after exercise or with no relation to meals suggest fasting hypoglycemia. The most common time for symptomatic hypoglycemia with insulinomas is actually late afternoon. The diagnosis is established when the criteria for Whipple's triad are met: symptoms of hypoglycemia, concomitant low plasma glucose, and relief of symptoms with normalization of plasma glucose.
- Symptoms that occur in relation to meals (>4 hours afterward) suggest postprandial hypoglycemia. The diagnosis of postprandial or "reactive" hypoglycemia can be established only after fasting hypoglycemia has been carefully excluded and symptomatic hypoglycemia has been documented after a "normal" mixed meal. As noted above, this may not be a pathologic condition.

E. Evaluating the severity of problems
- Severe hypoglycemia may be associated with seizures or coma. Prolonged hypoglycemia has been associated with permanent brain damage.

F. Managing the patient
- The initial management of serious hypoglycemia induced by insulin or other medications is use of either subcutaneous/intramuscular glucagon (for outpatients) or an IV bolus of glucose as a 50% solution (D_{50}). Once the patient is alert, he or she needs to take oral calories. If unable to eat, then parenteral glucose should be given until the patient is able to eat. Frequent measurement of plasma glucose may be necessary to ensure adequate replacement. The cause for hypoglycemia needs to be assessed and the medications, meal plan, or exercise regimen appropriately adjusted.
- Postprandial hypoglycemia is less easily managed, but eating frequent small meals high in protein and restricted in carbohydrates may be useful.

- Hypoglycemia due to insulin-producing tumors usually is treated with surgical removal of the tumor. In rare cases in which surgery is not possible, frequent caloric intake, diazoxide, and in some cases, somatostatin analogs may be used.

VI. Pituitary Disorders
   A. Anterior pituitary disorders
      1. Basic science
         - The pituitary gland is located in the sella turcica, below the optic chiasm. The anterior pituitary receives a mixture of peptide hormones and biogenic amines via its hypothalamic portal system. These include the following:
            a. Thyrotropin-releasing factor or hormone (TRH), which stimulates TSH (thyroid-stimulating hormone) and the lactotrophic hormone, prolactin
            b. Gonadotropin-releasing factor or hormone (GnRH), which, when released in a pulsatile fashion, stimulates LH (luteinizing hormone) and FSH (follicle-stimulating hormone) release
            c. Corticotropin-releasing factor or hormone (CRH), which stimulates ACTH (adrenocorticotropic hormone) and β-endorphin release
            d. Growth-hormone releasing factor or hormone (GHRH), which stimulates GH (growth hormone) release
            e. Somatostatin, which inhibits GH release
            f. Prolactin inhibitory factor (formerly called PIF), which is now known to be dopamine
         - Products released by the anterior pituitary are TSH, LH, FSH, ACTH, β-endorphin, GH, and prolactin (PRL). A pituitary disorder occurs when output is either excessive or insufficient or when a tumor is present.
         - Nearly all pituitary tumors are benign adenomas that are either "nonfunctional" or "functional." Most nonfunctional adenomas are small and do not cause symptoms. Functioning pituitary tumors may cause symptoms related to the specific hormone they produce. Pituitary tumors may produce GH, PRL, ACTH, TSH (rare), and gonodotropins (rare). These tumors may occur sporadically or as part of the multiple endocrine neoplasia syndromes, type 1 (MEN 1). MEN 1 consists of tumors involving the pituitary gland, the pancreas, and parathyroid glands. Prolactinomas are the most common functioning tumors.
         - Large pituitary tumors (whether functional or nonfunctional) may compromise production of trophic hormones. This mass effect generally affects GH and gonadotropins before affecting TSH and ACTH. This mass affect may result in increased PRL concentrations because of compression on the portal system and reduced exposure of the pituitary to dopamine. Large tumors may also compress either the optic chiasm (causing bitemporal hemianopsia) or the optic tracts (producing visual field cuts). Tumors may also compress the contents of the cavernous sinus (i.e., cranial nerves III, IV, V_1, V_2, and VI and the carotid artery), which are located lateral to the pituitary.

- Hypopituitarism may also occur as a result of autoimmune processes or pituitary apoplexy (a medical emergency). Hypopituitarism results in symptoms and signs associated with the deficiency of the target hormone. Similarly functioning pituitary adenomas result in symptoms and signs associated with hormone excess.
- In children, insufficient growth hormone results in growth retardation and hypoglycemia, whereas excess causes gigantism. In adults, insufficient growth hormone has few obvious effects while excessive growth hormone results in acromegaloid phenotype and impaired glucose tolerance.
- In women, hyperprolactinemia commonly results in galactorrhea and amenorrhea. Even microadenomas may produce sufficient prolactin to suppress gonadotropins. In men, prolactin galactorrhea is rare. Prolactinomas in men are usually detected based on decreased libido or impotence or may come to attention secondary to chronic headache or compression of adjacent structures. Prolactinomas in men are usually macroadenomas at the time of detection.
- TSH-releasing and gonadotropin-releasing hormone tumors are rare. The former usually presents with symptoms of hyperthyroidism in the face of a mildly elevated TSH.
- ACTH-secreting tumors cause Cushing's disease and are discussed earlier in Section I.
- Pituitary insufficiency is usually an insidious disorder characterized by the relative absence of one, several, or all the anterior pituitary hormones. Pituitary apoplexy represents spontaneous infarction or hemorrhage of a pituitary tumor that can lead to hypopituitarism. Pituitary apoplexy is often associated with a severe, sudden headache. Because of associated secondary adrenal insufficiency it is usually a medical emergency. Depending on the extent of hemorrhage/edema visual effects may also occur.

2. History and physical examination
   - Complaints of chronic headache concurrent with visual field cuts must prompt investigations to rule out a pituitary tumor. With clinically significant prolactin excess, inquiry must be made regarding pregnancy, use of drugs that inhibit dopamine (e.g., metoclopromide, phenothiazines and other antipsychotics), and hypothyroidism (elevated TRH stimulates both TSH and PRL).
   - Patients with pituitary insufficiency may have only mild symptoms, but are often fatigued, lethargic, and sluggish. There may be reduced pubic and axillary hair associated with sexual organ atrophy.
   - Apoplexy is associated with a severe headache, stiff neck, nausea, vomiting, depressed sensorium, and visual changes.

3. Laboratory and diagnostic studies
   - Studies in patients with suspected tumors based on symptoms and appropriate biochemical testing must include either CT or preferably MRI scans with pituitary cuts. In patients with GH-secreting tumors, insulin-like

growth factor 1 (IGF1, the functional mediator of GH) should be measured. Random GH is often also elevated. If IGF1 is equivocal, then a glucose challenge test with associated GH is the test of choice. In patients with acromegaly or gigantism, GH levels will fail to suppress following a glucose load.

- Patients with prolactin excess will demonstrate an increased serum prolactin. The degree of prolactin elevation correlates generally with the size of the tumor. Occasionally patients may have tumors that co-secrete GH and PRL.

- Routine chemistry panels should also be obtained in all patients with suspected pituitary dysfunction. Hyponatremia may be a result of secondary hypothyroidism and hypocortisolism because of associated impairment of free water clearance.

4. Formulating the diagnosis
   - The diagnosis of hormone excess or insufficiency is made by direct measurement of the hormone level and appropriate stimulation or suppression testing. Tumors are diagnosed by imaging studies (e.g., CT or MRI).
   - Patients at risk for hypopituitarism include those with a history of trauma, aneurysm, granulomatous disease, hemochromatosis, metastatic disease, infiltrative disease (e.g., histiocytosis X), type 1 diabetes mellitus (and other endocrine autoimmune disorders), and sickle cell anemia.

5. Evaluating the severity of problems
   - Patients with disorders of ACTH may develop serious electrolyte disorders, especially hyponatremia. Hyperkalemia does not occur with secondary adrenal insufficiency because aldosterone is also regulated via the renin-angiotensin system. Patients with large tumors or apoplexy (both rare) may develop intracranial problems requiring decompression.

6. Managing the patient
   - Children with GH deficiency are candidates for GH replacement therapy. For patients with GH excess the treatment of choice is usually surgery (transphenoidal approach is the most common). Other options for primary or adjunctive therapy include inhibitors of GH release (e.g., somatostatin analogs) and, less often, radiation or gamma knife therapy. High-dose dopaminergic agents such as bromocriptine are also an option in patients refractory to other therapies.
   - Prolactin-secreting tumors are usually treated with dopaminergic agents, most commonly bromocriptine. Patients who fail bromocriptine therapy are candidates for surgery. Patients who require surgery usually have more aggressive tumors and thus high relapse rates.
   - Management of hypopituitarism involves correction of the underlying cause. Hyponatremia responds quite rapidly to replacement of the deficient hormone along with fluid replacement. This is in contrast to the syndrome of inappropriate secretion of antidiuretic hormone, which responds to fluid restriction. Thyroxine, hydrocortisone, gonadal steroids, and GH (in

children) should be replaced. Mineralocorticoid replacement is not necessary with hypopituitarism.

B. Posterior pituitary disorders
1. Basic science
- Oxytocin and vasopressin (antidiuretic hormone, or ADH) are small peptides produced in the hypothalamus and released by the posterior pituitary. In the female, oxytocin is involved in breast milk release and uterine contraction; it has no known function in the male. ADH is the primary hormone responsible for maintaining serum osmolality. When serum osmolality increases, there is a rapid rise in ADH to help lower the serum osmolality by the retention of electrolyte-free water. Hypovolemia also results in the release of ADH and contributes to the hyponatremia seen with volume depletion. When ADH is secreted inappropriately it causes SIADH (syndrome of inappropriate secretion of antidiuretic hormone). When ADH is deficient, diabetes insipidus (DI) occurs. Of the two syndromes, SIADH is more common. SIADH may occur in the face of trauma, pulmonary disease, or malignancy. Because hypothyroidism and adrenal insufficiency amplify the effect of ADH, these disorders may mimic SIADH and should always be tested for.
- There are two main types of DI, including central (insufficient amounts of vasopressin are released) and nephrogenic (the distal nephron fails to respond to released vasopressin). Central DI occurs following head trauma, surgical intervention in the area of the hypothalamic/pituitary stalk, hypothalamic tumors (e.g., craniopharyngioma), metastatic malignancies, or infiltrative disorders of the hypothalamus (e.g., sarcoid, histiocytosis X). Nephrogenic DI is usually an acquired disorder. Psychogenic polydipsia is a psychiatric disease characterized by excessive free water ingestion. It can appear clinically like DI and should be ruled out by dehydration testing when clinically suspected.
2. History and physical examination
- Several drugs, including diuretics, chlorpropamide, carbamazepine, clofibrate, and vincristine have all been implicated as causes of SIADH. Trauma, pain, nausea, pulmonary tuberculosis, and small cell lung cancer are also potential causative factors. The physical examination is usually remarkable for the absence of edema.
- Diabetes insipidus may occur following head trauma, brain surgery, brain tumors, severe anoxia, and other tumors (e.g., breast cancer) that are metastatic to the pituitary; therefore, questions should be asked regarding a history of these events. Ingestion of ethanol, lithium, or phenytoin may cause transient DI. Patients with DI complain of intense thirst and increased urine output; frequently a history of nocturia is present. The physical examination may reveal evidence of hypovolemia and dehydration.
3. Laboratory and diagnostic studies
- Common laboratory findings in patients with SIADH include hyponatremia, hypo-osmolality in the presence of an inappropriately

concentrated urine (>100 mOsm/L), associated with a low blood urea nitrogen, and hypouricemia.

- In DI there is inappropriately dilute urine with low specific gravity. Often there is associated hypernatremia.

4. Formulating the diagnosis
    - The diagnosis of SIADH is made in the presence of appropriate laboratory findings only after eliminating the more common causes of physiologic vasopressin release, which include the use of diuretics, dehydration, and renal, anterior pituitary, thyroid, and adrenal disease.
    - The diagnosis of DI is made by demonstrating dilute urine in the presence of increased serum osmolality. Water deprivation may be used to demonstrate an inability to concentrate the urine. If administration of vasopressin significantly increases urine osmolality, central DI is confirmed. Failure to respond to vasopressin administration supports the diagnosis of nephrogenic DI.

5. Evaluating the severity of problems
    - Severe hyponatremia associated with SIADH may produce lethargy, headaches, seizures, and coma. Delirium or dementia may be manifestations of chronic hyponatremia.
    - Water deprivation in patients with DI may lead to profound dehydration and marked hypernatremia and result in altered mentation and coma.

6. Managing the patient
    - The treatment of SIADH is free water restriction. Although fluid restriction is not curative, it is effective in controlling hyponatremia. For patients with chronic SIADH who may be unable to tolerate fluid restriction for extended periods, demeclocycline, an inhibitor of ADH action, may offer benefit. Severely hyponatremic patients who manifest coma or seizure should receive a cautious infusion of hypertonic saline until the serum sodium has reached 120 mEq/L or the neurologic symptom has resolved; fluid restriction should then be carried out. In general, the sodium should be allowed to increase by 0.5 to 1 mEq/L/hour, but this can be increased to 1 to 2 mEq/L/hour in the presence of serious symptoms. The sodium should not be increased by more than 25 mEq/L in the first 48 hours. If serum sodium is corrected too quickly, central pontine myelinolysis may occur.
    - The treatment of patients with symptomatic central DI consists of administration of DDAVP (desmopressin), a vasopressin analog. Acutely DDAVP may be administered subcutaneously. Chronic therapy is usually by intranasal DDAVP. DDAVP is also available as an oral tablet. The treatment of nephrogenic DI is more difficult but includes adequate hydration, sodium restriction, thiazide diuretics, and indomethacin.

VII. Thyroid Disorders
   A. Hyperthyroidism
      1. Basic science
         - Hyperthyroidism is a pathophysiologic state resulting from an excess amount of free thyroid hormone in blood and tissues produced by a

hyperfunctioning thyroid gland. Thyrotoxicosis is a broader term describing a condition of thyroid hormone excess irrespective of thyroid gland function. Although there are many causes of this condition, Graves' disease is the most common. Other common causes include iatrogenic (overmedication), toxic nodular goiter, and thyroiditis (e.g., infectious or medication induced).

- Graves' disease is an autoimmune disorder characterized by the presence of a gamma immunoglobulin (IgG) called thyroid-stimulating immunoglobulin (TSI) that binds the TSH receptor. TSI serves to stimulate thyroid function. Graves' disease most often affects middle-aged women.
- Toxic nodular goiter refers to single or multiple autonomously functioning nodules. Toxic multinodular goiters are more common in older patients.
- Thyroiditis occurs in several variants and results in inflammation-induced release of thyroxine (T_4) and triiodothyronine (T_3).

2. History and physical examination
- Patient complaints often include nervousness, increased sweating, hypersensitivity to heat, palpitations, fatigue, increased appetite, weight loss, insomnia, weakness, and frequent bowel movements.
- Patients with Graves' disease may have a personal or family history of other endocrine autoimmune disorders.
- Dramatic physical examination findings are more common in younger patients. Signs of hyperthyroid disease in the elderly may be masked. The general signs include goiter, tachycardia, widened pulse pressure, warm moist skin, tremor, and eye signs (stare, lid lag, and lid retraction). Weakness is a common presentation in the elderly. There are certain signs specific to Graves' disease: infiltrative ophthalmopathy (often resulting in exophthalmos and ocular muscle weakness) and pretibial myxedema (a nonpitting edema in the pretibial region).

3. Laboratory and diagnostic studies
- When hyperthyroidism is suspected, serum TSH is often sufficient to make the diagnosis, but T_4 (free thyroxine index or free T_4) measurements should be made to help characterize the biochemical severity of disease. The presence of a normal TSH level almost always excludes the diagnosis of hyperthyroidism. Although most patients with hyperthyroidism manifest a high T_4, certain patients have only an elevated T_3.
- Rare cases of hyperthyroidism due to TSH-producing tumors have been reported. They have hyperthyroid symptoms and signs with elevated T_4 concentrations and mildly elevated TSH levels.

4. Formulating the diagnosis
- The diagnosis is usually evident from the history and physical examination and is confirmed by laboratory studies. Sometimes additional tests are necessary to distinguish various types of hyperthyroidism. Confirmation of Graves' disease may be done by obtaining measures of thyroid receptor antibodies. In some patients it may be difficult to distinguish clinically whether the patient has Graves' disease, multinodular goiter, or thyroiditis. A radioactive iodine uptake (using ^{131}I) will distinguish thyroiditis (low or

negative uptake) from Graves' disease (typically elevated uptake) or a multinodular goiter (normal to elevated uptake). If the thyroid gland is not palpable, then obtaining a thyroid scan will distinguish Graves' disease (homogeneous uptake on scan) from a toxic nodule (isolated area of increased uptake on scan) and a multinodular goiter (irregular pattern on scan).

5. Evaluating the severity of problems
   - The risk of atrial fibrillation is increased in patients with hyperthyroidism (especially the elderly) and deserves treatment. Severe hyperthyroidism may also precipitate heart failure, even in the absence of atrial fibrillation.
   - Thyrotoxic storm is a special complication of Graves' disease characterized by fever, tachycardia, marked weakness, mental status changes, and shock. It is often precipitated by an infection or stress.

6. Managing the patient
   - β-Blockers, such as propranolol, are useful adjuvants in treating patients with Graves' disease in that they ameliorate some of the adrenergic symptoms associated with hyperthyroidism. Radioiodine (^{131}I) is first-line therapy for patients with Graves' disease, although it often results in permanent hypothyroidism. An alternative to radioactive iodine therapy includes the antithyroid drugs propylthiouracil and methimazole. These agents inhibit thyroid hormone synthesis.
   - In patients for whom a more immediate response is needed, antithyroid drugs are considered first-line therapy. Once the patient is less thyrotoxic, then ^{131}I therapy may be administered after withdrawing antithyroid drugs. Surgery is rarely used to treat hyperthyroidism unless there are associated compressive symptoms (e.g., very large multinodular goiter) or in selected cases in which radioactive iodine or antithyroid drugs cannot be used effectively (e.g., with amiodarone-induced hyperthyroidism). Thyrotoxic storm is a medical emergency treated with supportive measures that include intravenous fluids, β-blockers, antithyroid medications, glucocorticoids, potassium iodide or ipodate sodium (administered after antithyroid drugs to block the release of thyroid hormones), and in some cases bile acid binding resins.

B. Hypothyroidism
   1. Basic science
      - Hypothyroidism is a hypometabolic state that results from a deficiency of thyroid hormone at the tissue level. The most common causes of hypothyroidism include Hashimoto's thyroiditis, thyroid ablation with radioactive iodine for hyperthyroidism, and surgical removal (usually for thyroid cancer).
      - Hashimoto's thyroiditis is an autoimmune disorder in which antibodies to thyroid peroxidase (often called antimicrosomal antibodies) result in a chronic inflammatory disorder and ultimately hypothyroidism. Hashimoto's disease is most common in young to middle-aged women. This disorder is frequently familial and coexists with other endocrine autoimmune diseases (e.g., type 1 diabetes mellitus, adrenal insufficiency, premature ovarian

failure) as well as systemic autoimmune processes such as pernicious anemia and vitiligo. It is occasionally associated with systemic lupus erythematosus, rheumatoid arthritis, and Sjögren's syndrome.

2. History and physical examination
   - The signs and symptoms of hypothyroidism are often insidious in onset and may be quite subtle. Patient complaints may include fatigue, weakness, cold intolerance, and constipation. In some cases paresthesias may occur in the hands and feet. Amenorrhea may occur in women because of associated hyperprolactinemia.
   - In more severe hypothyroidism patients may have slow dysarthric speech and a hoarse voice. Their skin is often dry, thick, and doughy; the face appears puffy and expressionless. The heart may be enlarged with a serous pericardial effusion. The hair tends to be dry and sparse. The reflexes reveal a prolonged relaxation time. In patients with Hashimoto's disease, a goiter is present with an irregular surface, which, over years becomes atrophic and fibrotic.

3. Laboratory and diagnostic studies
   - The single most useful test in making the diagnosis of hypothyroidism is the measurement of TSH. It is elevated without exception in patients with thyroid gland failure and allows the diagnosis to be made often before the thyroid hormones (T_4 and T_3) become low. Detection of antimicrosomal and antithyroglobulin antibodies often aids in the diagnosis of Hashimoto's thyroiditis but clinically are often not needed.

4. Formulating the diagnosis
   - The diagnosis depends on recognizing the clinical features along with appropriate laboratory evaluation.

5. Evaluating the severity of problems
   - Myxedema coma is a rare but serious complication of hypothyroidism. The coma is usually precipitated by some other cause in the face of hypothyroidism. Precipitating factors include cold exposure, infection, and trauma. Patients have severe hypothermia, hypoxia, hyporeflexia, seizures, and bradycardia. Treatment includes hormone replacement with either T_3 or T_4, in addition to gentle rewarming, respiratory support, glucocorticoids, and antibiotics when necessary.

6. Managing the patient
   - The preferred treatment for hypothyroidism is replacement therapy with L-thyroxine. Replacement doses average about 1.6 µg/kg body weight. The final appropriate dose is the dose which restores the serum TSH level to normal. Symptomatic improvement usually takes days to weeks.
   - In patients with symptomatic coronary artery disease it is prudent to begin replacement with 25 µg/day and increase the dose in similar increments every 1 to 4 weeks until the TSH has normalized.

C. Thyroid neoplasia
   1. Basic science
      - The majority of solitary thyroid nodules are benign. Of the malignant thyroid tumors, four major types exist: papillary, follicular, medullary, and anaplastic.

- Papillary carcinoma is the most common of the primary thyroid cancers. It is generally a slow-growing cancer. When it metastasizes, spread is usually via the lymphatics. Overall, mortality rate is quite low.
- Follicular carcinoma is the next most common variety; this tumor tends to metastasize earlier, usually by a vascular route. Again, mortality rate is low.
- Medullary carcinoma arises from the parafollicular C cells that produce calcitonin. It may occur sporadically or as part of another syndrome, such as the multiple endocrine neoplasia type II (MEN II). It metastasizes both locally via the lymphatics and to distant sites such as the lung, bone, and liver. Mortality rate is relatively low for most varieties of medullary carcinoma.
- Anaplastic carcinoma represents a small fraction of thyroid cancers. It is different from the other cancers in that its clinical course is distinctly aggressive, usually resulting in death within months of diagnosis.

2. History and physical examination
   - The history should contain questions regarding hyperfunction and hypofunction of the thyroid; a hyperfunctioning gland is less likely to be cancerous. The presence of pain, rapid rate of growth, and a change in voice are all suspicious for carcinoma. A history of head, neck, or upper chest irradiation is associated with increased risk for thyroid carcinoma later in life. Patients with a family history of MEN are also at great risk (for medullary carcinoma). Finally, nodules appearing in the young, in the elderly, or in males have an increased risk of malignancy.
   - Rarely, the physical examination may reveal features suggesting cancer: associated lymphadenopathy, a fixed, nontender lesion or one of stony-hard consistency.

3. Laboratory and diagnostic studies
   - The diagnostic approach to a solitary nodule should begin with fine needle aspiration (FNA). It is quite sensitive and specific with results often useful in directing management. FNA aspirations cannot consistently distinguish follicular adenomas from follicular carcinomas. Patients with FNA findings suspicious for malignancy or consistent with malignancy should be referred for thyroidectomy. Ultrasound may provide information on size and the presence of cystic elements, though it is rarely useful in differentiating benign from cancerous masses. Similarly, traditional laboratory studies offer little information to discriminate benign from malignant masses. The serum thyroglobulin is used to follow patients as a marker of recurrence of differentiated thyroid cancers after near total or total thyroidectomy and radioactive iodine ablation of the thyroid.

4. Formulating the diagnosis
   - The cornerstone of diagnosis remains FNA.

5. Evaluating the severity of problems
   - Lesions with distant metastases represent advanced disease and have a poorer prognosis, although long-term survival is well known even in patients with metastatic papillary and follicular thyroid cancers.
   - Anaplastic carcinomas generally have a poor prognosis.

6. Managing the patient
   - Benign lesions of the thyroid may be followed with serial clinical examinations and ultrasounds at 6- to 12-month intervals. Growth of the lesion justifies repeat FNA or consideration for surgery.
   - In general, malignant lesions are treated surgically. This is followed by ablative ^{131}I treatment. Evaluation for residual cancer is done using ^{131}I uptake and scans following thyroid hormone withdrawal or administration of recombinant TSH (Thyrogen). If there is evidence of residual tumor, repeated doses of ^{131}I are administered. Surgical intervention may also be necessary for tumor recurrence. Thyroxine administration is necessary to treat the associated hypothyroidism, but doses are higher than typical replacement doses. TSH levels are suppressed to reduce any effect of TSH stimulating tumor growth. Chemotherapy is generally ineffective in the treatment of most thyroid cancers. Local bony metastases of follicular cancers are often responsive to external beam radiation.

Nephrology and Urology

I. Acid-Base Disorders
- Whole body metabolism produces on a daily basis ~1 mEq/kg of nonvolatile acid (mostly sulfuric acid derived from sulfur-containing amino acids) and ~15,000 mmol of volatile acid (CO_2 which generates carbonic acid when combined with water).
- Body fluid pH is kept relatively constant at ~7.40 by pulmonary and renal excretion of CO_2 and hydrogen ions (H^+), respectively.
- Acid-base balance is assessed by measurement of a "blood gas" (typically arterial to obtain the partial pressure of oxygen [PaO_2] and to evaluate oxygenation status), which includes pH, partial pressure of CO_2 (PCO_2), and plasma bicarbonate concentration (HCO_3^-).
- The bicarbonate–carbon dioxide buffer system is used to assess acid-base balance:

$$\text{Dissolved } CO_2 + H_2O \leftrightarrow H_2CO_3 \leftrightarrow HCO_3^- + H^+$$

- At physiologic pH dissolved CO_2 is almost exclusively in the form of HCO_3^- and the presence of carbonic acid (H_2CO_3) is negligible.
- The ratio between the preceding reactants can be expressed by the Henderson-Hasselbalch equation:

$$pH = 6.10 + \log ([HCO_3^-] \div [0.03 \times PCO_2])$$

A. Definitions
1. Acidemia: pH less than 7.36
2. Alkalemia: pH greater than 7.44
3. Acidosis
   - Any process that tends to lower the plasma pH (by raising H^+ concentration). This can be achieved by a fall in HCO_3^- concentration or by an elevation in PCO_2.
4. Alkalosis
   - Any process that tends to raise the plasma pH (by lowering H^+ concentration). This can be achieved by an elevation in HCO_3^- concentration or by a fall in PCO_2.
5. Anion gap (AG)
   - Used primarily in the differential diagnosis of metabolic acidosis.

$$AG = \text{measured cations} - \text{measured anions}$$

$$AG = Na^+ - (Cl^- + HCO_3^-)$$

   - Note: even though routinely measured, K^+ is not included in this equation.

TABLE 12-1:
Primary Acid-Base Disorders

Primary Disorder	Primary Problem	pH	Pco₂	HCO₃⁻
Metabolic acidosis	Loss of HCO_3^- or gain of H^+	↓	↓	↓
Metabolic alkalosis	Gain of HCO_3^- or loss of H^+	↑	↑	↑
Respiratory acidosis	Hypoventilation	↓	↑	↑
Respiratory alkalosis	Hyperventilation	↑	↓	↓

↓ ↑, primary disturbance; ↑ ↓, compensatory response.

- In normal patients the AG is primarily determined by the negative charges on the plasma proteins (mainly albumin) → in hypoalbuminemia, for every 1 g/dL drop, subtract 2.5 mEq/L to the normal AG range (i.e., the "true" AG is greater than calculated).
- Normal AG ranges between 6 and 12 (varies depending on the normal ranges reported by each laboratory).
6. Δ AG / Δ HCO_3^- (delta/delta, or Δ/Δ)
   - Useful in assessing if multiple disorders are affecting HCO_3^-
   - Δ/Δ ≈ 1 to 2: typical AG metabolic acidosis (~1 : 1 relationship between ↑AG and ↓HCO_3^-)
   - Δ/Δ less than 1: AG metabolic acidosis + non-AG metabolic acidosis (i.e., ↓HCO_3^- greater than expected)
   - Δ/Δ greater than 2: AG metabolic acidosis + metabolic alkalosis (i.e., ↓HCO_3^- less than expected)
B. Primary acid-base disorders (Table 12-1)
   - Compensatory responses to primary acid-base disturbances are aimed at attenuating the pH shift from the normal value (7.40); however, they never fully compensate (or "overcompensate") for the primary disorder (i.e., if pH normal, consider mixed acid-base disorder, see Table 12-2).
C. Mixed acid-base disorders
   1. Consider the presence of two disorders if:
      a. Compensation is greater than or less than expected for a single disorder
         - Metabolic acidosis, but Pco_2 too low → concomitant respiratory alkalosis
         - Metabolic alkalosis, but Pco_2 too high → concomitant respiratory acidosis
         - Respiratory acidosis, but HCO_3^- too high → concomitant metabolic alkalosis
         - Respiratory alkalosis, but HCO_3^- too low → concomitant metabolic acidosis
      b. Normal pH in the presence of altered Pco_2 and HCO_3^-, or abnormal AG:
         - ↓ Pco_2 + ↓ HCO_3^- → respiratory alkalosis + metabolic acidosis
         - ↑ Pco_2 + ↑ HCO_3^- → respiratory acidosis + metabolic alkalosis

TABLE 12-2:
Rules of Compensation

Primary Disorder	Compensatory Response	Formula
Metabolic acidosis	Hyperventilation	$\downarrow P_{CO_2} = 1.25 \times \Delta\,HCO_3^-$ (rule of thumb, $P_{CO_2} \approx$ last 2 digits of pH)
Metabolic alkalosis	Hypoventilation	$\uparrow P_{CO_2} = 0.75 \times \Delta\,HCO_3^-$
Acute respiratory acidosis	Intracellular buffering (primary) + renal HCO_3^- retention (secondary)	$\uparrow HCO_3^- = 0.1 \times \Delta\,P_{CO_2}$
Chronic respiratory acidosis	Renal HCO_3^- retention + increased ammonium excretion	$\uparrow HCO_3^- = 0.4 \times \Delta\,P_{CO_2}$
Acute respiratory alkalosis	Renal HCO_3^- excretion + reduced ammonium excretion	$\downarrow HCO_3^- = 0.2 \times \Delta\,P_{CO_2}$
Chronic respiratory alkalosis	Renal HCO_3^- excretion + reduced ammonium excretion	$\downarrow HCO_3^- = 0.4 \times \Delta\,P_{CO_2}$

- Normal P_{CO_2} + normal HCO_3^- + $\uparrow$ AG → AG metabolic acidosis + metabolic alkalosis
- Normal P_{CO_2} + normal HCO_3^- + normal AG → non-AG metabolic acidosis + metabolic alkalosis *(or no disturbance)*.
  c. When $\uparrow$ AG and Δ/Δ below 1 or above 2 (see explanation for Δ/Δ)
  2. Consider the presence of three disorders when:
     a. Primary respiratory disorder (i.e., acidemia with $\uparrow P_{CO_2}$ or alkalemia with $\downarrow P_{CO_2}$), *plus*
     b. Primary AG metabolic acidosis (i.e., $\uparrow$ AG), *plus*
     c. Additional primary metabolic disorder (i.e., $\Delta/\Delta < 1$ or > 2)
  3. Any combination of acid-base disorders is possible *except* respiratory acidosis and respiratory alkalosis (hypo- and hyperventilation cannot coexist).
  D. Step-by-step approach to the analysis of acid-base disorders:
    1. Determine the primary (or main) disorder → check pH, P_{CO_2} and HCO_3^-.
    2. Calculate if degree of compensation is appropriate (if inappropriate → mixed disorder).
    3. Calculate the AG.
    4. Calculate the Δ/Δ if the AG is increased (to assess if more than one disorder is affecting HCO_3^-).
    5. Correlate the preceding information to clinical findings (history and physical examination) to determine whether the acid-base analysis is compatible with the patient's presentation.
  E. Metabolic acidosis (Tables 12-3 to 12-5)
    - Step-by-step approach to the analysis of metabolic acidosis:
      1. Calculate the AG (corrected for albumin level).

TABLE 12-3:
Causes of Increased Anion Gap (AG) Metabolic Acidosis

Category	Causes
Ingestions	**Methanol** (metabolized to formic acid)—also ↑ osmolal gap
	Ethylene glycol (metabolized to glycolic and oxalic acid)—also ↑ osmolal gap; look for Ca^{2+} oxalate crystals in urine, renal failure
	Aspirin/salicylates (metabolized to salicylic and lactic acid)—also respiratory alkalosis due to direct CNS effect
	Toluene (early) (metabolized to hippuric acid)—later stages present as non-AG metabolic acididosis (rapid excretion of hippurate into urine)
Renal failure (uremia)	Accumulation of organic anions (phosphates, sulfates)
Lactic acidosis	**Type A (hypoxic):** cardiogenic/septic/hemorrhagic shock, limb/bowel ischemia, seizures, carbon monoxide/cyanide poisoning
	Type B: diabetes, liver failure, leukemia/lymphoma, metformin, isoniazid
Ketoacidosis	Diabetes mellitus (DKA), alcoholism (AKA), starvation

TABLE 12-4:
Causes of Non–Anion Gap (AG) (Hyperchloremic) Metabolic Acidosis

Category	Causes
GI loss of HCO_3^-	Diarrhea, pancreatic/intestinal fistulas, enteric drains, ureteral diversion
Renal tubular acidoses (RTA)	**Type 1 (distal)** → defective distal H^+ secretion (idiopathic, familial [AR or AD], autoimmune [Sjögren's syndrome, rheumatoid arthritis], hypercalciuria, amphotericin B)
	Type 2 (proximal) → decreased proximal reabsorption of HCO_3^- (multiple myeloma [with or without Fanconi's syndrome], acetazolamide, ifosamide, amyloidosis, familial disorders)
	Type 4 (hypoaldosteronism) → ↑ K → ↓ urinary NH_4^+ excretion → ↓ urine acid carrying capacity
	▪ Adrenal—Addison's disease, heparin, low-molecular-weight heparin
	▪ Hyporeninemic—**diabetic nephropathy,** interstitial nephritis, **NSAIDs, ACE inhibitors,** HIV
	▪ Aldosterone resistance—K^+-sparing diuretics, cyclosporine
Dilutional acidosis	Rapid dilution of plasma with HCO_3^- free IVF (i.e., 0.9% NaCl)
Post-hypocapnia	Prolonged respiratory alkalosis → renal wasting of HCO_3^-
	Rapid correction of respiratory alkalosis → transient metabolic acidosis while the kidneys generate new HCO_3^-
Hyperalimentation	Total parenteral nutrition—amino acid solutions (i.e., arginine hydrochloride, lysine hydrochloride)
Early renal failure	Hyperchloremic state at early stages, followed by accumulation of organic anions (leading to AG metabolic acidosis, see above)

TABLE 12-5:

Findings in Non–Anion Gap (Hyperchloremic) Metabolic Acidosis

Category	UAG	Urine pH	Serum K⁺	FE$_{HCO_3^-}$
Gastrointestinal loss of HCO_3^- Hyperalimentation Post-hypocapnia Dilutional acidosis	Negative	<5.3	↓	—
RTA type 1	Positive	>5.3	↓	<3%
RTA type 2	Negative or positive	Variable*	↓ (rarely ↑)	>15%
RTA type 4	Positive	<5.3	↑	—

*Urine pH will be >5.3 after a bicarbonate load. FE, fractional excretion; RTA, renal tubular acidosis; UAG, urine anion gap.

2. If ↑ AG, → check for ketonuria (or serum ketones) → (+) in alcoholic ketoacidosis, diabetic ketoacidosis, starvation.
3. If ketones (–) → check lactate (lactic acidosis); blood urea nitrogen (BUN) and serum creatinine (uremia); blood and urine toxic screen + osmolal gap (OG > 10 in methanol, ethylene glycol intoxication).

$$OG = \text{measured } P_{osm} - \text{calculated } P_{osm}$$

$$\text{Calc. } P_{osm} = (2 \times Na^+) + (\text{glucose}/18) + (BUN/2.8) + (EtOH/4.6)$$

4. If normal AG → check urine anion gap (UAG), urine pH, serum K^+, and fractional excretion (FE) of HCO_3^- ($FE_{HCO_3^-}$)

$$UAG = \text{measured anions} - \text{measured cations} \rightarrow$$
indirect assay for urinary NH_4^+ excretion

$$UAG = (U_{Na} + U_K) - U_{Cl}$$

F. Metabolic alkalosis (Table 12-6)
   • Step-by-step approach to the analysis of metabolic alkalosis:
   1. Check volume status (depleted or replete) and urine chloride (U_{Cl})
      • U_{Cl} < 20 mEq/L + volume depleted → saline-responsive
      • U_{Cl} > 20 mEq/L + volume replete → saline-resistant (except current use of diuretics, see Table 12-6)
   2. If saline-resistant, check blood pressure (see Table 12-6 for differential diagnosis)
G. Respiratory acidosis
   • Decreased alveolar ventilation → hypercapnia
   • Etiologies
   1. Obstructive airway disease: asthma, COPD, mechanical airway obstruction, laryngospasm, obstructive sleep apnea
   2. CNS depression: opioid-induced, structural or ischemic CNS lesions involving the respiratory center
   3. Neural conduction disorders: amyotrophic lateral sclerosis, Guillain-Barré syndrome, high cervical spine injury

TABLE 12-6:
Causes of Metabolic Alkalosis

Category	Causes
Saline-responsive* (volume depleted and $U_{Cl} < 20\,mEq/L$)	**Gastrointestinal loss of H^+**—vomiting, NG drainage, villous adenoma **Diuretics (loop or thiazides)**—volume depletion → ↑ proximal $NaHCO_3$ reabsorption + ↑ aldosterone **Post-hypercapnia**—Respiratory acidosis → renal retention of HCO_3^- (compensation). Rapid correction of respiratory acidosis → transient metabolic alkalosis while kidneys excrete excess HCO_3^-
Saline-resistant (volume replete and $U_{Cl} > 20\,mEq/L$)	**Hypertensive** Endogenous mineralocorticoid excess—hyperaldosteronism, Cushing's syndrome, congenital adrenal hyperplasia Endogenous mineralocorticoid excess—licorice ingestion **Normotensive** Severe hypokalemia → transcellular K^+/H^+ shift Endogenous alkali—$NaHCO_3$, citrate, lactate, gluconate, acetate, massive transfusions (from citrate) Gitelman's syndrome—distal convoluted tubule dysfunction ≈ thiazide effect Bartter's syndrome—Loop of Henle dysfunction ≈ furosemide effect

*Exception is metabolic alkalosis seen with current use of diuretics → volume depleted and $U_{Cl} > 20\,mEq/L$ → saline-responsive (and stop diuretics).

4. Muscular disorders: polymyositis, muscular dystrophy, metabolic myopathies (acid maltase deficiency)
5. Parenchymal lung disease (often preceded by hypoxia → respiratory alkalosis from hyperventilation → eventual muscle fatigue → respiratory acidosis): pneumonia, interstitial lung disease, pulmonary edema
6. Diseases of the chest wall: flail chest, kyphoscoliosis, pneumothorax

H. Respiratory alkalosis
- Increased alveolar ventilation → hypocapnia
- Etiologies
  1. Hypoxia: high altitude, decreased PAO_2
  2. Parenchymal lung disease (leading to hypoxia): pneumonia, interstitial lung disease, pulmonary edema, pulmonary embolism
  3. Primary hyperventilation
     - CNS disease: stroke, tumor, trauma
     - Sepsis
     - Voluntary hyperventilation, anxiety
     - Pharmacologic/hormonal stimulation: salicylates, nicotine, xanthines, progesterone (pregnancy)
     - Hepatic failure
     - Mechanical overventilation

II. Acute Renal Failure
  A. Basic science
  - Acute renal failure (ARF) is defined as the rapid onset of decreased renal function, typically assessed by an increase in blood urea nitrogen (BUN) or serum creatinine.
  - The causes of ARF may be categorized as follows:
    1. Prerenal insults (30% to 60% of cases)
      - Prerenal damage can result from decreased perfusion to the kidney. It may be secondary to the following conditions:
        a. Hypovolemia (intravascular volume depletion, hemorrhage)
        b. Heart failure/cardiogenic shock
        c. Liver failure/cirrhosis
        d. Sepsis
        e. Renal vascular obstruction (renal artery stenosis, renal artery, or vein thrombosis)
        f. Medications (nonsteroidal anti-inflammatory drugs [NSAIDs])
    2. Intrinsic renal insults (40–70% of cases)
      - Damage to the kidney parenchyma may occur from the following:
        a. Ischemia (major hemorrhage, small vessel obstruction)
        b. Nephrotoxins (heavy metals, intravenous contrast material, antibiotics)
        c. Disease affecting the glomerulus (e.g., glomerulonephritis, hypertension)
      The areas of the kidney that may be damaged include the following:
        a. Glomerulus: acute glomerulonephritis, nephritic syndrome
        b. Tubules: acute tubular necrosis (ATN), ischemia, antibiotics, contrast agents
        c. Interstitium: acute interstitial nephritis (AIN), drugs
    3. Postrenal insults (<10% of cases)
      - Postrenal insults include several disease states:
        a. Urethral obstruction
        b. Bladder obstruction
        c. Bilateral ureteral obstruction
        d. Enlarged prostate
        e. Kidney stones
      - Once the initial insult has occurred, renal function can remain diminished. This may be due to:
      - Tubular debris causing obstruction
      - Continued decreased renal blood flow
      - Decreased glomerular permeability
      - Back leak of glomerular filtrate through damaged tubular cells
  B. History and physical examination
  - The first sign of renal failure in the hospitalized patient may be oliguria (<400 mL of urine output per day).
  - Patients may present with malaise, lethargy, fatigue, nausea, and itching. Renal failure may also be discovered incidentally on routine blood work or urinalysis.
  - History and physical examination should be directed at establishing the category of renal failure, because both prerenal and postrenal failure may be corrected immediately.

1. Prerenal failure
   a. Impaired cardiac function
      - History: congestive heart failure, myocardial infarction, cardiogenic shock
      - Physical examination: elevated jugular venous pressure, edema, lung rales
   b. Liver failure
      - History: hepatitis, cirrhosis
      - Physical examination: jaundice, ascites, other peripherial signs of possible liver disease (spider angiomas, palmar erythema, etc.)
   c. Renal vascular obstruction
      - History: usually asymptomatic but may cause back pain
      - Physical examination: bruit may be heard in renal artery stenosis
   d. Hypovolemia
      - History: hemorrhage, vomiting, diarrhea, recent major surgery (particularly cardiac valve or bypass surgery, aortic surgery)
      - Physical examination: tachycardia, hypotension, decreased capillary refill, orthostatic blood pressure changes
   e. Sepsis
      - History: fever, shaking chills, altered mental status, symptoms suggesting infection in a specific organ/system
      - Physical examination: hypotension, tachycardia, tachypnea, warm skin, toxic appearance, localized signs of infection in some cases
2. Postrenal failure
   - History: inability to urinate, straining to urinate, postvoid dribbling
   - Physical examination: palpable bladder, enlarged prostate
3. Intrinsic renal failure
   a. Glomerular diseases
      - History: sore throat, skin rash, weakness, fatigue, fever, edema, dark urine (blood), joint pain, foaming urine
      - Physical examination: hypertension, edema
   b. Tubulointerstitial diseases: direct toxicity
      - History: iodine-containing radiographic contrast agents, aminoglycoside antibiotics, antineoplastic drugs, amphotericin B, heavy metals, prolonged prerenal failure (sustained ischemia)
      - Physical examination: fever in some cases
   c. Tubulointerstitial diseases: hypersensitivity
      - History: NSAIDs, salicylates, penicillins, sulfa drugs
      - Physical examination: rash

C. Laboratory and diagnostic studies
   - Serum chemistries, BUN, creatinine, CBC (complete blood count), and urinalysis should be obtained. Urinary sediment should be examined, checking for red blood cells (RBCs), white blood cells (WBCs), and casts.
   - A renal ultrasound should be obtained to rule out postrenal failure (obstruction – hydronephrosis, hydroureters) and changes of chronic renal failure.

TABLE 12-7:

Differentiating between Prerenal Failure and Intrinsic Renal Failure

Measurement	Prerenal Failure	Intrinsic Renal Failure
BUN : serum Cr ratio	>20 : 1	<20 : 1
Urine Na	<20	>20
Urine osmolality	>500	<400
Urine specific gravity	>1.020	<1.010
Fractional excretion of Na (FE_{Na})*	<1%	>2%

*The FE_{Na} is calculated using the formula $FE_{Na} = (U_{Na}/S_{Na})/(U_{Cr}/S_{Cr})$.

- Heme positive dipstick without RBCs in the urine is generally indicative of rhabdomyolysis.
  D. Formulating the diagnosis
  - The physician must classify renal failure into prerenal, postrenal, or intrinsic renal categories. The workup should be performed in the following order:
    1. If obstruction is possible, a renal ultrasound should be ordered after thorough physical examination. A Foley catheter may also be placed.
    2. Once obstruction has been ruled out, the physician must differentiate between intrinsic renal disease and prerenal causes of ARF. Differentiation of these diseases may be aided by the parameters shown in Table 12-7.
       - These findings may not be accurate if the patient recently received diuretics.
    3. Urinary sediment
       a. Prerenal disease: normal sediment pattern (hyaline casts may be seen)
       b. Intrinsic renal disease
          - Acute glomerulonephritis: hematuria, RBC casts
          - Acute tubular necrosis (ATN): granular cell ("muddy brown") casts
          - Acute interstitial nephritis: WBCs, WBC casts, +/− eosinophils
  E. Evaluating the severity of the problem
    1. Severity of ARF depends on the urine output, electrolyte disorders, acid-base disturbances, volume status, and the cause of the renal failure.
    2. Major causes of death
       - Gastrointestinal hemorrhage
       - Sepsis
       - Heart failure
    3. Fluid and electrolyte complications during this phase include the following:
       - Hyponatremia (secondary to the kidneys' inability to excrete water)
       - Hyperkalemia (treat accordingly; see Section V, Hyperkalemia)
       - Metabolic acidosis (typically with an increased anion gap, secondary to the inability to excrete acidic metabolic end products)
       - Hyperphosphatemia (secondary to the inability to excrete phosphate)
       - Hypocalcemia (by-product of high blood phosphate levels)
       - Hypervolemia (secondary to oliguria)

4. Hematologic problems
- Anemia
- Platelet malfunction, coagulopathy
- Impaired phagocytic function

F. Managing the patient
1. Preventing acute renal failure is key.
   - Patients who are hypovolemic should be volume expanded to promote normal kidney perfusion. This is especially true of surgical patients before and after procedures and patients being exposed to intravenous contrast materials and chemotherapeutic agents.
   - Prevent hypotension during surgical procedures. When urine output falls the patient must be evaluated for volume status.
   - Use drugs such as allopurinol prior to chemotherapy in patients at risk for tumor lysis syndrome.
   - Patients on nephrotoxic drugs such as aminoglycosides should have drug serum levels monitored.
   - Medications potentially causing ARF should be used with caution with appropriate monitoring (NSAIDs, angiotensin-converting enzyme [ACE] inhibitors, aminoglycosides, penicillins, etc.).
   - If urinary obstruction is discovered, it should be corrected immediately.
2. If ARF does occur, treatment is geared toward reducing complications; always aim to remove the offending agent or correct the precipitating cause first.
   - The patient's daily weight, volume input/output, and serum electrolytes should be monitored.
   - Water overload manifests itself as a hyponatremia. If the patient is water overloaded, he or she should be water restricted.
   - Because of reduced ability to excrete potassium, all potassium intake should be limited.
   - Treat hyperkalemia accordingly (see Section V, Hyperkalemia).
   - Dosage and interval of administration of all medications that have renal excretion must be adjusted.
   - Patients with renal failure are prone to infections. Any sign of infection (e.g., increased temperature) should be treated aggressively. Blood and urine should be cultured. Any lines should be removed and the tips cultured, and a chest x-ray taken to determine the source of the infection.
   - Dialysis may be required in the following situations:
     a. Severe hyperkalemia
     b. Uremic pericarditis
     c. Uremic encephalopathy
     d. Refractory metabolic acidosis
     e. Severe volume overload (pulmonary edema)
   - If the process behind the ARF is a glomerulonephritis or vasculitis, treat accordingly with steroids or cytotoxic agents.
   - Because of reduced ability to excrete phosphate, phosphate binders (e.g., calcium acetate) are employed.

III. Benign Prostatic Hyperplasia
  A. Basic science
   - Benign prostatic hyperplasia (BPH) is a benign nodular neoplasia of the prostate that arises in the tissue surrounding the urethra. Enlargement of this tissue results in compression and narrowing of the prostatic urethra.
   - Compression of the prostatic urethra obstructs urine flow, causing the patient to retain urine. Retained urine predisposes the patient to urinary tract infections and kidney stones. Increased urinary tract pressures may lead to hydronephrosis, with potential for renal failure.
   - The predominant active hormone in prostate tissue is dihydrotestosterone, not testosterone.
  B. History and physical examination
   1. History
      - Prostatic hyperplasia becomes a common condition in the fourth or fifth decade.
      - Symptoms of obstruction are common (e.g., slow stream, hesitancy, a sensation of incomplete emptying, and postvoid dribbling).
      - Symptoms of bladder irritability are also common (e.g., frequency, urgency, and nocturia).
      - Hematuria may be associated with BPH, although more serious underlying causes must be excluded. The onset of symptoms is progressive but may be worsened by medications with anticholinergic or α-adrenergic effects.
   2. Physical examination
      - Physical examination of the prostate usually demonstrates an enlarged gland without hard nodules or localized tenderness. In patients with relatively advanced chronic obstruction, the bladder may be palpable or percussible. This indicates significant postvoid residual volumes.
  C. Laboratory and diagnostic studies
   - Assessment of BUN and creatinine is important. Increased levels may indicate renal failure due to prostatic obstruction.
   - A urinalysis should be sent to determine if hematuria, pyuria, or bacteria are present. These findings indicate other potential causes for the patient's symptoms.
   - Estimation of postvoid residual volume is important (>100 mL).
   - Imaging of the urethra with contrast to evaluate the anatomy of the prostate and exclude urethral strictures, stones, or tumor, which may cause irritative voiding symptoms, can be done.
   - Prostate-specific antigen (PSA) levels may be increased in patients with significant amounts of prostatic hyperplasia but usually less than 10 ng/mL.
   - Urodynamic studies should be reserved for patients with suspected neurologic disease or those who have failed prostate surgery or if considering surgical treatment.
  D. Formulating the diagnosis
   - BPH is the most common cause of decreased stream associated with irritative voiding in older men.

- BPH is a pathologic diagnosis and can only be confirmed by biopsy, resection, or extirpation surgery.
  E. Evaluating the severity of the problem
  - Patients with obstruction that has caused deterioration of renal function or hydronephrosis should undergo medical or surgical treatment.
  - Patients presenting with significant azotemia (renal failure) should be admitted. A significant postobstructive diuresis may occur following catheter drainage requiring fluid monitoring and intravenous replacement of electrolytes.
  - Urinary retention or recurrent urinary tract infections (UTIs) are indications for medical or surgical treatment.
  - Postvoid residuals exceeding 100 to 200 mL indicate the need for monitoring and treatment.
  F. Managing the patient
  - Patients should avoid medications with α-adrenergic or anticholinergic effects. These medications are commonly found in over-the-counter cold formulations. Avoiding caffeine and alcoholic beverages may reduce symptoms of frequency and urgency. The bladder should be emptied regularly to prevent overdistention of the bladder.
  - Monitoring the patient's symptoms is appropriate if the symptoms are not severe. For this purpose the International Prostate Symptom Score (IPSS) index can be followed every 1 to 6 months with yearly digital rectal examinations.
  - Medical therapies include treatment with alpha-blocking agents. Alpha-blocking agents relax the smooth muscle of the prostatic urethra.
  - Hormonal therapy with 5α-reductase inhibition (e.g., finasteride) prevents conversion of testosterone to dihydrotestosterone within the prostate. This causes the prostate to shrink over time.
  - Combination therapy with both alpha-blocking agents and 5α-reductase agents is more effective then using either agent alone.
  - Phytotherapy (e.g., *Serenoa repens* [saw palmetto]) has shown to be similar in efficacy to finasteride.
  - If medical treatment is unsuccessful at controlling the patient's symptoms, surgical intervention is indicated; multiple different surgical procedures are available.

IV. Chronic Renal Failure
  A. Basic science
    1. Chronic renal failure (or chronic kidney disease, CKD) is defined as 3 or more months of reduced glomerular filtration rate (GFR should be ≤ 60 mL/min/1.73 m^2) or kidney damage (abnormal pathologic findings or imaging, abnormal urine markers).
    2. The kidney acts as:
      - A filter removing toxins from the bloodstream
      - A regulator of the body's water, electrolyte balance
      - A regulator of acid-base homeostasis

- An activator of vitamin D, which promotes gut absorption of calcium
- A producer of erythropoietin, a hormone that stimulates RBC production

3. Most diseases that affect renal parenchyma gradually destroy the kidney. This leads to chronic renal failure, leading to loss of the usual kidney functions just listed.

4. Major causes of CKD include the following:
    a. Glomerulopathies
    - Diabetes mellitus (the most common cause); CKD within 7 to 15 years of proteinuria
    - Membranous nephropathy
    - Membranoproliferative glomerulonephritis (MPGN)
    - Focal segmental glomerulosclerosis
    - IgA nephropathy
    - Systemic lupus erythematosus
    - Amyloidosis
    - HIV-associated nephropathy and MPGN
    b. Tubulointerstitial disease
    - Drug hypersensitivity
    - Analgesic (NSAIDs) nephropathy
    - Multiple myeloma
    - Heavy metal poisoning
    - Thrombotic microangiopathies
    c. Hereditary diseases
    - Alport's syndrome
    - Autosomal dominant polycystic kidney disease (ADPKD) (mutation on chromosome 16)
    - Medullary cystic disease
    d. Obstructive nephropathy
    - Nephrolithiasis
    - Prostatic disease
    - Retroperitoneal fibrosis
    e. Vascular diseases
    - Hypertensive nephrosclerosis
    - Renal artery stenosis or ischemic nephropathy

5. CKD is a gradual process. The kidney attempts to compensate for loss of nephron function by increasing the workload of the remaining nephrons. This strategy works until less than 25% of nephrons are functioning. After this point is reached the kidneys lose the ability to eliminate toxins effectively. This leads to buildup of toxins, leading to a condition called the uremic syndrome. The uremic syndrome was so named because of the increase in measured serum BUN and creatinine levels, although it is accompanied by many other findings.

B. History and physical examination
    1. History
    - A significant number of patients may be asymptomatic at presentation.

- Common late symptoms include fatigue, malaise, pruritus, nausea, vomiting, anorexia, paresthesias, sensory deficits, and mental status changes.
2. Physical examination
   - Common findings include weight loss, wasting, edema, easy bruising, and hypertension (common). Urine output can be low, normal, or high.
   - Late findings include pericardial friction rub, pulmonary rales, uremic fetor, uremic frost, asterixis, and myoclonus.
C. Laboratory and diagnostic studies
   - Serum chemistries such as BUN and creatinine are elevated. Also common are high phosphate, low calcium, high parathyroid hormone, decreased active vitamin D, low bicarbonate (metabolic acidosis), and high potassium levels.
   - CBC may demonstrate anemia (typically normocytic, normochromic), and bleeding time may be prolonged (due to platelet dysfunction).
   - Urinalysis may show proteinuria (microalbuminuria is an early marker of diabetic nephropathy) and waxy casts. Specific gravity is usually approximately 1.010 (the serum specific gravity) because the kidney has lost its ability to concentrate urine (isosthenuria).
   - Renal ultrasound is useful in ruling out obstructive uropathy and morphologic abnormalities (such as polycystic kidneys). Typically kidneys are small and echogenic (exceptions are diabetic nephropathy, HIV-nephropathy, ADPKD, amyloidosis, and multiple myeloma).
   - A 24-hour analysis of urine for calculation of creatinine clearance is sometimes used to estimate the GFR, although more accurate means are available such as clearance of radiolabeled markers. However, various equations to estimate GFR are commonly used (such as the Cockcroft-Gault formula and the Modification Diet in Renal Disease [MDRD] formula).
   - Based on the GFR estimation, the National Kidney Foundation has classified CKD into five stages (Table 12-8).
D. Formulating the diagnosis
   - History, physical examination, serum chemistries, and analysis of urine sediment secure the diagnosis. In distinguishing between acute and chronic renal failure, previous serum chemistries (serum creatinine, especially) are most useful.

TABLE 12-8:
Staging of Chronic Kidney Disease

Stage	Description	GFR (mL/min/1.73 m²)
1	Kidney damage with normal or elevated GFR	≥90
2	Kidney damage with mildly decreased GFR	60–89
3	Moderately decreased GFR	30–59
4	Severely decreased GFR	15–29
5	Kidney failure (end-stage renal disease)	<15 (or dialysis/transplant)

GFR, glamerular filtration rate.

TABLE 12-9:

Treatment of Chronic Renal Failure Based on GFR

Stage	GFR (mL/min/1.73 m²)	Action
1	≥90	Diagnosis and treatment of underlying condition and comorbidities, cardiovascular disease risk reduction
2	60–89	Estimating progression
3	30–59	Evaluating and treating complications
4	15–29	Preparation for renal replacement therapy
5	<15	Replacement therapy (dialysis or transplant)

GFR, glomerular filtration rate.

- Renal biopsy may be helpful in defining specific lesions such as glomerulonephritis. However, once end-stage renal failure has developed, the results of biopsy are often nonspecific and not helpful.
- The cause of chronic renal failure should be ascertained to determine if the condition causing the renal failure may be stopped to slow progression of the disease. Some of the reversible conditions include infection, obstruction, nephrotoxic agents, congestive heart failure, and hypertension.

E. Evaluating the severity of the problem
- If the uremic syndrome is present, initiation of dialysis is warranted.
- Additionally, acute dialysis maybe needed in the presence of:
  1. Severe hyperkalemia
  2. Uremic pericarditis
  3. Uremic encephalopathy
  4. Refractory metabolic acidosis
  5. Severe volume overload (pulmonary edema)
- Severity of the chronic renal failure may be approached also by estimated GFR. According to the National Kidney Foundation, the measures discussed in Table 12-9 should be taken.

F. Managing the patient
  1. Emergency management
     - Institute acute dialysis as indicated previously.
  2. Chronic management
     - The main goal is to slow progression of the underlying disease and the renal dysfunction.
     - Early referral to a nephrologist should be considered.
     - Treatment should include the following:
       a. Strict control of hypertension (for patients with proteinuria >1 g/day or diabetes, the goal is ≤125/75 mm Hg; for all other patients, the goal is <130/80 mm Hg)
       b. Dietary measures:
          - Reduced phosphate intake (dairy foods are high in phosphate). Phosphate binders (e.g., calcium carbonate, calcium acetate) taken with meals decrease the absorption of phosphate.

- Protein intake restriction (not to exceed 1 g/kg/day)
- Salt and water restriction (if volume overloaded)
- Potassium restriction (for CKD stages 4 and 5)
- Vitamin supplementation for patients on dialysis (water-soluble vitamins)
- Vitamin D and calcium supplementation (for patients with elevated parathyroid hormone levels)
- Anemia treated by recombinant erythropoietin therapy and iron
- Use of ACE inhibitors (or angiotensin II receptor blockers) for patients with diabetes or proteinuria
- Avoidance of nephrotoxins (e.g., NSAIDs, radiocontrast agents)
- Pre-end-stage renal disease education for patients with CKD stage 4
- Prompt initiation of renal replacement therapy for CKD stage 5

V. Hyperkalemia
  A. Basic science
   - Hyperkalemia is an elevation of serum potassium above 5.0 mEq/L. The causes of hyperkalemia can be divided into four categories:
    1. Spurious (pseudohyperkalemia)
       a. Hemolysis during venipuncture
       b. Venipuncture from arm with K^+ infusion
       c. Repeated fist clenching during venipuncture (release of K^+ from muscles)
       d. Marked leukocytosis or thrombocytosis with release of K^+ (plasma K^+ should be normal)
    2. Increased load
       a. Increased exogenous intake (usually coupled with decreased excretion): oral or parenteral
       b. Endogenous release of intracellular K^+
          - Burns
          - Rhabdomyolysis
          - Massive cellular necrosis
          - Tumor lysis syndrome
          - Hemolysis
          - Internal bleeding
    3. Decreased excretion
       a. Renal failure (acute and chronic)
       b. Impaired renal secretion:
          - Interstitial nephritis
          - Sickle cell disease
          - Obstructive uropathy
          - Amyloidosis
       c. Type IV renal tubular acidosis (RTA): hyporeninemic hypoaldosteronism (often seen in patients with diabetic nephropathy and in HIV)
       d. Decreased mineralocorticoid activity
       e. Impaired excretion due to drugs

- ACE inhibitors
- Potassium-sparing diuretics (spironolactone, triamterene)
- Angiotensin II receptor blockers
- NSAIDs
- Cyclosporine
- Tacrolimus
- Trimethoprim

  4. Increased transcellular shift (redistribution)
    a. Acidosis
    b. Insulin deficiency
    c. Digitalis toxicity
    d. β-Adrenergic blockade
    e. Periodic paralysis
    f. Succinylcholine
    g. Arginine
    h. Fluoride intoxication

- The most significant source of potassium elimination is aldosterone-mediated renal excretion. Decreases in glomerular filtration rate, whether from intrinsic renal failure or a prerenal state, can impair the kidney's ability to handle a normal potassium intake. Similarly, adrenal insufficiency can result in hyperkalemia secondary to decreased aldosterone.

B. History and physical examination
- The patient should be questioned regarding dietary intake, medications, history of renal disease, previous hyperkalemia, and diabetes mellitus. An estimate of volume status and a full neuromuscular examination should also be sought (looking for evidence of numbness, weakness, paralysis).

C. Laboratory and diagnostic studies
- The diagnosis of hyperkalemia is made by the measurement of serum potassium from an unhemolyzed specimen. Depending on the urgency of the situation, one may want to confirm that the elevated level of serum potassium is genuine (plasma K^+ can be measured to avoid leakage of intracellular K^+ as clotting occurs). Measurement of serum blood urea nitrogen and creatinine (to estimate renal function), serum pH (to evaluate for acidosis), and glucose level (to evaluate for hyperglycemia and possible diabetic ketoacidosis) can all be useful in discovering the cause of hyperkalemia. Urinary potassium levels are often unhelpful.
- If hypoaldosteronism is suspected, an investigation of its stimulation, secretion, and effect is warranted.
- An immediate electrocardiogram (ECG) is indicated if the measured potassium is greater than 6.0 mEq/L. Characteristic ECG changes (e.g., peaked T waves, shortened QT interval, loss of P waves, and eventual QRS widening leading to sine-wave morphology) can be seen as the serum potassium level rises. ECG changes can occur very quickly and lead to ventricular fibrillation and cardiac arrest.

D. Formulating the diagnosis
- Increased intake, K$^+$-containing intravenous fluids, or medication-induced hyperkalemia can be elicited from the history.
- Metabolic disturbances causing potassium shifts to the extracellular space and renal failure are often apparent on routine laboratory tests.
- If no apparent cause is found, or dramatic hyperkalemia is present with a normal electrocardiogram, then pseudohyperkalemia should be suspected. After this is eliminated, a workup of aldosterone stimulation, release, and activity is warranted.

E. Evaluating the severity of the problem
- Any symptomatic elevation of potassium (particularly with ECG changes) requires emergent intervention.
- The level of hyperkalemia does not correlate well with the degree of ECG changes (i.e., ventricular fibrillation may occur at a K$^+$ level of 6.0 mEq/dL in acute hyperkalemia); therefore, measures to correct the hyperkalemia should be instituted even in the absence of severe ECG changes.
- Patients with chronic hyperkalemia (e.g., those with end-stage renal failure) tolerate higher potassium levels than those in whom the disturbance is acute.

F. Managing the patient
1. General measures include cardiac monitoring if ECG changes are present or for K$^+$ above 6.0 mEq/dL. All K$^+$ supplementation and medications that promote high K$^+$ levels should be withheld.
2. Symptomatic hyperkalemia requires urgent correction. The treatment falls into three categories: membrane stabilization, intracellular potassium shift, and K$^+$ removal from the body.
   a. Cardiac membrane stabilization can be achieved with 1 to 2 ampules of 10% calcium gluconate which will temporarily reverse ECG changes. This treatment is necessary only when ECG changes are present and the effect is short lived (30 to 60 minutes), so repeated doses may be needed.
   b. Intracellular K$^+$ shift treatments (all last a few hours)
      - Regular insulin (10 units IV) accompanied by 1 ampule of 50% dextrose if the patient is not extremely hyperglycemic will quickly drive much of the K$^+$ into the intracellular space.
      - Sodium bicarbonate (50 mEq IV), particularly in acidotic patients, accomplishes the same function.
      - Albuterol (10 to 20 mg), given as a nebulization, also has a temporary shifting effect.
   c. Potassium removal can be achieved by:
      - Renal losses from forced diuresis with a loop diuretic (furosemide) ± normal saline
      - Gastrointestinal (GI) losses with cation-exchange resins such as sodium polystyrene sulfonate (Kayexalate), which binds K$^+$ in the gastrointestinal tract
      - Hemodialysis or peritoneal dialysis are less immediate in their action but often necessary to definitively correct the potassium overload.

3. Chronic hyperkalemia can be controlled with use of loop diuretics, cation-exchange resins, exogenous mineralocorticoids, and dietary K^+ restriction if correction of the underlying problem is not possible.

VI. Hypernatremia
   A. Basic science
      • Hypernatremia is an elevation of the serum sodium greater than 145 mEq/L. Under normal conditions an intact thirst mechanism and access to free water prevent hypernatremia. Thus, whatever the underlying disorder, excess water loss can only cause hypernatremia when adequate water intake is suboptimal.
      • The causes of hypernatremia fall into two broad categories:
         1. Sodium retention (with increased total body sodium)
            • Oral route: sea water ingestion, improperly mixed infant formula
            • IV route: exogenous NaCl infusion (e.g., during cardiopulmonary resuscitation), repeated $NaHCO_3$ administration
            • Mineralocorticoid excess: usually not a cause for hypernatremia unless accompanied by decreased water intake
         2. Water deficit/hypotonic fluid loss (with normal or decreased total body sodium)
            a. Diabetes insipidus (DI): a deficiency in antidiuretic hormone (ADH) secretion (central or neurogenic) or ADH function (nephrogenic) resulting in renal free water losses and subsequent hyperosmolality. DI can be complete (usually with a urine osmolality (U_{osm}) <300 mOsm) or partial (with a U_{osm} = 300 to 600 mOsm); see discussion in this section under "Formulating the diagnosis" for further details on workup.
               • Central DI results from a process impairing the normal production or release of ADH.
               • Causes of central DI
                  • Neurosurgical procedures
                  • CNS trauma
                  • CNS tumors
                  • CNS granulomas (sarcoidosis)
                  • CNS infections
                  • Idiopathic
               • Nephrogenic DI occurs when production and release of ADH is normal but there is impaired or absent renal response to the hormone.
               • Causes of nephrogenic DI
                  • Drugs (e.g., lithium, amphotericin, demeclocycline)
                  • Hypercalcemia
                  • Severe hypokalemia
                  • Sickle cell anemia
                  • Amyloidosis
                  • Sarcoidosis
                  • Polycystic kidney disease
                  • Sjögren's syndrome

  b. Renal water loss: high urinary volume, U_{osm} = 300 to 600 mOsm
  - Diuretics
  - Osmotic diuresis
    - Glucose (diabetes mellitus)
    - Urea (post-ATN diuresis or postobstruction diuresis)
    - Mannitol
  c. Extrarenal water loss: low urinary volume, U_{osm} over 600 mOsm
  - Fever
  - Hyperventilation
  - Burns
  - Osmotic diarrhea
    - Vigorous exercise with profuse sweating
    - Newborns under radiant warmers
B. History and physical examination
  - Neurologic features may be the first and only symptoms of hypernatremia. Thirst, restlessness, lethargy, disorientation, weakness, seizures, coma, and eventually death may occur as the hyperosmolality worsens.
  - Patients with DI will complain of polyuria, polydipsia, and nocturia.
  - If hypernatremia is suspected, the patient's volume status must be ascertained:
    1. Hypervolemia points toward sodium excess (retention).
    2. Hypovolemia or euvolemia point toward water loss as the cause.
C. Laboratory and diagnostic studies
  - The diagnosis is usually made by routine serum sodium measurement. U_{osm} and the kidney's response to exogenous ADH help to determine the cause.
D. Formulating the diagnosis
  1. Suspicion of a hyperosmolar state is confirmed by basic serum chemistries. The plasma osmolality can be calculated or directly measured.
  2. The next step should be to measure U_{osm}.
    - If U_{osm} is greater than 600 mOsm, then the urine is (appropriately) maximally concentrated, and a source of extrarenal water loss or decreased intake should be sought (urine volume is usually low).
    - If U_{osm} is 300 to 600 mOsm, then at least a partial defect in ADH release or activity is present, or there is an osmotic diuresis or use of diuretics.
    - If U_{osm} is less than 300 mOsm, there probably is a complete defect in ADH release or activity is present.
  3. When DI is suspected, the patient should undergo a water deprivation test (only to be done if current serum sodium level is normal, otherwise proceed to vasopressin administration) followed by vasopressin (ADH) administration:
    - In a normal individual, the U_{osm} should increase to two to four times that of the plasma (P_{osm}) with 8 hours of water deprivation.
    - In an individual with DI the P_{osm} will increase to over 295 and U_{osm} remain below 300. Following this vasopressin is administered and the patient is allowed to drink as usual.
    - In central DI the U_{osm} increases by over 50% (response to ADH).
    - In nephrogenic DI the U_{osm} will not change (no response to ADH).

E. Evaluating the severity of the problem
- The presence of any neurologic symptoms requires urgent attention.
- Severity of symptoms usually correlate with the extent of hyperosmolality.

F. Managing the patient
1. The treatment of hypernatremia should be aimed at its cause.
2. Calculation of the free water deficit (in liters) is achieved by this formula:

Free H_2O deficit = 0.6 × ideal body weight
$$× [(\text{measured Na}/140) - 1] \ (×0.85 \text{ in women})$$

3. The type of fluid for rehydration depends on the patient's volume status.
- Hypovolemic patients may initially require normal saline (NS) followed by $^1/_2$ NS or $^1/_4$ NS.
- Euvolemic or hypervolemic patients are often better treated with D_5W.
- For chronic hypernatremia the rate of correction should not exceed 0.5 mEq/L/hour or 20 mEq/L/day (risk of cerebral edema).
4. The chronic treatment of patients with central DI can be achieved most conveniently with DDAVP (vasopressin) nasal spray every 12 hours. Drugs that lower urine output and a low-sodium/low-protein diet minimize polyuria. Drugs such as chlorpropamide and carbamazepine may increase the secretion of ADH in some patients.
5. In nephrogenic DI the defect is usually reversible. If it persists, the polyuria can be decreased by thiazides and a low-sodium/low-protein diet as in central DI. Other measures that may be beneficial include the diuretic amiloride and NSAIDs to decrease renal prostaglandins.

VII. Hypokalemia
A. Basic science
- Hypokalemia is defined as a serum potassium below 3.5 mEq/L. Hypokalemia can be divided into four broad categories:
1. Decreased intake: Potassium is ubiquitous in a normal diet; therefore, hypokalemia is rarely seen solely because of dietary deficiency.
a. Anorexia nervosa
b. Deficient diet in alcoholics
2. Increased intracellular shift: Redistribution occurs; total body K^+ remains normal.
a. Alkalosis
b. Insulin excess
c. β-Adrenergic excess (acute stress, intake of $β_2$-agonists)
d. New cell production (e.g., in patients receiving vitamin B_{12}, folate, or cellular growth factors; leukemia)
e. Hypokalemic periodic paralysis
f. Intoxications (barium, toluene, theophylline)
3. Increased renal losses
a. ncreased mineralocorticoid (aldosterone) effect
- Primary hyperaldosteronism (adrenal adenomas or carcinomas)
- Cushing's disease

- Ectopic adrenocorticotropic hormone (ACTH) (e.g., small cell carcinoma)
- Exogenous substances (e.g., glycyrrhizic acid in licorice)
- High renin states (as in decreased effective circulating volume seen in congestive heart failure and cirrhosis)
- Renovascular hypertension (with or without renal artery stenosis)
- Gitelman's syndrome (distal convoluted tubule dysfunction ≈ thiazide effect)
- Bartter's syndrome (loop of Henle dysfunction ≈ furosemide effect)
- Renin-producing tumors (e.g., renal cell carcinoma)
- Congenital androgenital syndromes
  b. Medications
  - Thiazide and loop diuretics
  - Penicillins
  - Aminoglycosides
  c. Salt-losing nephropathy
  d. Renal tubular acidosis (RTA type I or II)
  e. Magnesium depletion
  f. Liddle's syndrome (congenital defect in the distal nephron)
  4. Increased extrarenal losses
  a. Profuse sweating
  b. Dialysis
  c. Gastrointestinal losses
    - Diarrhea, contains high concentrations of K^+
    - Vomiting, mostly secondary to volume depletion and metabolic alkalosis
    - Laxative abuse
    - Fistulas
    - Villous adenoma
    - Zollinger-Ellison syndrome
B. History and physical examination
  - Patients with hypokalemia should have their medications reviewed. Diuretics are the most common cause of hypokalemia. The patient should also be questioned regarding intake and sources of potassium loss.
  - In the undiagnosed patient, symptoms of nausea, vomiting, muscle weakness (the most prominent manifestation), arrhythmias, glucose intolerance, polydipsia, and polyuria all warrant a serum potassium measurement.
  - Blood pressure measurement may help to differentiate hyperaldosteronism (i.e., in the hypertensive patient) from other causes of potassium loss.
C. Laboratory and diagnostic studies
  1. The diagnosis of hypokalemia is confirmed by serum potassium measurement.
  2. ECG changes of hypokalemia include increased ectopy (premature ventricular contractions, ventricular tachycardia or fibrillation), appearance of U waves, decreased T wave amplitude, depression of ST segment, and various degrees of AV block.
  3. The differential diagnosis of hypokalemia can be narrowed by urinary potassium measurement:

- In a euvolemic patient off diuretic therapy, potassium excretion of less than 25 mEq/day (or $U_K < 15$ mEq/L) suggests appropriate potassium conservation and an extrarenal or exogenous cause of hypokalemia.
- Conversely, values of over 30 mEq/day (or $U_K > 15$ mEq/L) imply renal wasting and either mineralocorticoid excess or a tubular defect.
4. If hypertension is present, hyperaldosteronism needs to be ruled out. Measure plasma renin and aldosterone levels to differentiate adrenal from nonadrenal causes. Only after an adrenal source has been confirmed should one proceed to imaging of the adrenal glands (CT or MRI).
5. If hypertension is absent and the patient is acidotic, consider RTA.
6. If hypertension is absent and the patient is alkalotic (or normal pH), check urine chloride:
   - If U_{Cl} is greater than 10 mEq/day consider hypokalemia secondary to diuretics or Bartter's or Gitelman's syndrome.
   - If U_{Cl} is less than 10 mEq/day consider hypokalemia secondary to vomiting.

D. Formulating the diagnosis
- Once identified by laboratory assay, the cause of hypokalemia can be discovered through a stepwise approach. As above, determination of U_K, and blood pressure measurement (hypertension or normo/hypotension) will be the most important tools in helping to arrive at the cause.

E. Evaluating the severity of the problem
- Potassium should be repleted to the normal range, but symptomatic hypokalemia, particularly with ECG changes, or K^+ less than 2.5 mEq/L should be corrected urgently. Uncorrected hypomagnesemia makes correction of hypokalemia difficult.

F. Managing the patient
- Because most potassium is intracellular, the total body deficit can be estimated only from the serum measurement. An approximation of the potassium deficit is 100 mEq for levels below 3.5 mEq/L, 200 mEq for less than 3.0 mEq/L, 300 to 400 mEq for a level below 2.5 mEq/L, and 400 to 600 mEq for less than 2.0 mEq/L. Potassium is most commonly combined with chloride in replacement preparations. Occasionally potassium citrate or potassium phosphate may be preferable in metabolic acidosis or phosphate deficiency, respectively.
- For nonemergent conditions ($K^+ > 2.5$ mEq/L) without cardiac manifestations, oral potassium is the preferable route of repletion. Owing to gastric upset, a maximum of 40 mEq per dose, and 160 mEq/day, is all that is commonly tolerated. An elixir can be used for rapid absorption, whereas long-acting tablets are better tolerated for chronic use.
- For emergent situations ($K^+ < 2.5$ mEq/L) with arrhythmias, intravenous repletion is indicated. Repletion at a rate of 20 mEq/hour (at a concentration ≤40 mEq/L) via peripheral vein or 40 mEq/hour (at a concentration ≤60 mEq/L) through central venous access is standard at most institutions (although greater concentrations can be administered in life-threatening circumstances). Too rapid repletion may precipitate cardiac arrhythmias.
- Treatment of the underlying cause, from correction of diarrhea to surgical removal of adenoma or change in medication, should always be attempted.

VIII. Hyponatremia
  A. Basic science
    - Hyponatremia is a serum sodium concentration less than 135 mEq/L. This state results from an excess of water relative to sodium and is almost always due to an increase in antidiuretic hormone (ADH).
    - The normal manifestation of excess water is a lowering of plasma osmolality (P_{osm}), which leads to a decrease in ADH. This decrease in ADH renders the collecting tubules of the kidney relatively impermeable to water reabsorption, resulting in a dilute urine and elimination of excess water. When this decrease in ADH does not occur, hyponatremia ensues.
    - This excess in ADH may be appropriate (e.g., hypovolemia or in hypervolemia with decreased effective circulating volume) or inappropriate (syndrome of inappropriate antidiuretic hormone secretion [SIADH]).
    - Hyponatremia can be classified into three categories according to the patient's tonicity (P_{osm}):
      1. Isotonic hyponatremia (also known as pseudohyponatremia) occurs as a result of a laboratory artifact secondary to a dilution of the aqueous phase by hypertriglyceridemia or hyperproteinemia (seen in multiple myeloma).
      2. Hypertonic hyponatremia is seen when another effective osmole is present in excess (e.g., glucose, mannitol, or glycine). In this situation there is a shift of water from the intracellular to the extracellular compartment with a resultant dilution of sodium.
      3. Hypotonic hyponatremia is true excess of water relative to sodium (see "Formulating the diagnosis" in this section for details).
  B. History and physical examination
    - The possibility of hyponatremia should be sought in patients with a history of volume loss (e.g., profuse vomiting, diarrhea, fever, diuretic use) or edematous states such as CHF, cirrhosis, or nephrosis. The history should also include a review of the common causes of SIADH.
    - The physical examination should include an assessment of volume status and observation for symptomatic hyponatremia (which presents as lethargy, disorientation, weakness, agitation, seizures, stupor, or coma). Unfortunately, the more severe neurologic manifestations of hyponatremia may be irreversible despite correction of the serum sodium.
  C. Laboratory and diagnostic studies
    - The diagnosis is usually obtained by screening serum chemistry. A measurement of P_{osm}, U_{Na}, and U_{osm} should be obtained in hyponatremic patients.
    - Additional laboratory studies may be needed as the search for a cause continues (see below).
  D. Formulating the diagnosis
    1. As described earlier (under "Basic science"), when approaching hyponatremia the first step is determining the tonicity of the patient's plasma (P_{osm}) and categorizing the hyponatremia as isotonic, hypertonic, or hypotonic.
    2. For isotonic hyponatremia, measurement of serum lipids and proteins should be sought.

3. For hypertonic hyponatremia, determination of another effective osmole must be sought.

4. For hypotonic hyponatremia the next step is to establish the patient's volume status.

- If hypovolemic (primary Na loss, secondary water gain) the U_{Na} will help distinguish renal ($U_{Na} > 20$ mEq/L, $FE_{Na} > 1\%$) from extrarenal losses ($U_{Na} < 10$ mEq/L, $FE_{Na} < 1\%$).

  a. Renal losses: diuretic use, hypoaldosteronism, salt-wasting nephropathy
  b. Extrarenal losses: GI losses (e.g., vomiting, diarrhea), insensible losses (e.g., burns, vigorous exercise)
    - If euvolemic (primary water gain), determine whether ADH is suppressed or not by measuring the U_{osm}.
    - If U_{osm} is greater than 100 mOsm, ADH is not suppressed and therefore is inappropriately high, that is, SIADH (typically $U_{Na} > 40$ mEq/L, low BUN, and low uric acid).
    - Causes of SIADH
      - Pulmonary disorders (e.g., pneumonia, asthma, COPD, pneumothorax)
      - CNS disorders (e.g., trauma, tumors, hemorrhage, hydrocephalus, infection)
      - Neoplasms (e.g., small cell carcinoma)
      - Medications (e.g., antipsychotics, antidepressants, antiseizure drugs)
      - Miscellaneous: pain, nausea, stress, postoperative state, HIV infection
      - Other causes of euvolemic hypotonic hyponatremia and adrenal insufficiency and hypothyroidism
    - If U_{osm} is less than 100 mOsm, ADH is suppressed. This situation occurs in psychogenic polydipsia when despite appropriate ADH suppression the ingestion of massive amounts of water (>12 to 20 L/day) overwhelms the diluting ability of the kidney resulting in hyponatremia.
  - If hypervolemic, determine whether there is decreased effective circulating volume ($U_{Na} < 10$ mEq/L, $FE_{Na} < 1\%$) as seen in cirrhosis, heart failure, and nephrotic syndrome; or ascertain if there is advanced renal failure ($U_{Na} > 20$ mEq/L)

E. Evaluating the severity of the problem
  - The presence of any neurologic symptoms requires urgent attention.
  - Severity of symptoms usually correlate with the extent of hypoosmolality.

F. Managing the patient
  1. There are two basic principles to the correction of hyponatremia: correct the plasma sodium at a safe rate and treat the underlying cause. If the patient is truly volume depleted then normal saline can be given; conversely, the volume-overloaded patient requires both sodium (1–3 g/day) and water (1–1.5 L/day) restriction.
  2. The sodium deficit can be estimated by multiplying the volume of distribution of sodium in the body by the sodium deficit per liter:

Na deficit = 0.6 × ideal body weight

$$× (140 - \text{measured } P_{Na}) \, (×0.85 \text{ in women})$$

- Too rapid correction can lead to central pontine myelinolysis (due to acute brain dehydration). It is generally assumed safe to correct the sodium at a rate less than 1.0 mEq/L/hour, and not greater than 12 mEq/L over the first 24 hours. Correction at a rate of 0.5 mEq/L/hour over the first 24 hours seems appropriately safe in a patient without severe neurologic symptoms. If stupor, seizures, or coma are present then more rapid correction is indicated. Use of hypertonic saline should be reserved for these situations only. In severe or refractory hyponatremia, the combination of normal saline and a loop diuretic may be cautiously employed to achieve a net loss of free water. Whatever the intended rate of correction, frequent checks of sodium and potassium are advisable during the initial treatment period.
- In SIADH and edematous states, water restriction is the first line of therapy. Patients with SIADH should have prolonged free water restriction if the underlying process cannot be corrected. The antibiotic demeclocycline inhibits the action of ADH and can be used when water restriction alone is insufficient.

IX. Kidney Stones (Nephrolithiasis)
  A. Basic science (~80% of stones)
    - Kidney stones are composed of any of the following compounds:
    1. Calcium
       a. The majority of kidney stones contain calcium oxalate (or calcium phosphate). These stones may be seen on x-ray (they are radiopaque).
       b. Several conditions may predispose to the development of calcium stones:
          - High levels of blood and urine calcium result from intestinal overabsorption of calcium (vitamin D intoxication, sarcoidosis), increased bone metabolism (primary hyperparathyroidism), and decreased renal reabsorption of calcium (type 1 renal tubular acidosis).
          - High levels of urine oxalate result from increased endogenous production and increased intestinal absorption (Crohn's disease or other ileal diseases).
          - In high levels of urine urate the urate crystals provide a nidus for calcium precipitation.
    2. Uric acid (~10% of stones)
       a. Uric acid stones form as a result of high levels of urine uric acid. In order for these stones to form there must be a low urine pH and low urine volume. These stones cannot be seen on x-ray (radiolucent).
    3. Cystine (rare)
       a. Cystine stones are formed as the result of a genetic disorder that leads to excessive amino acid excretion through the renal tubules. These stones may be seen on x-ray (radiopaque).

4. Struvite stones (magnesium ammonium phosphate) (~10% of stones)
   a. Also known as "triple phosphate" or "infection stones," these stones occur as the result of urea-splitting bacteria (*Proteus, Pseudomonas,* and *Klebsiella*) that produce a high urinary pH. Struvite stones are often large, filling the entire renal pelvis (i.e., staghorn calculi).
   b. Foreign bodies in the urinary tract can also lead to struvite stone formation.
B. History and physical examination
   1. History
      • Patients present with severe, intermittent, unilateral flank pain (renal colic) that radiates to the groin or testicle. Patients will often experience nausea, vomiting, and low-grade fever.
      • Patients may have a previous history of kidney stones. Many have a family history of kidney stones.
      • Patients should be questioned about previous urinary tract infections, medications, diet, bowel disease (Crohn's disease), gout, and renal disease.
   2. Physical examination:
      • Patients have various degrees of costovertebral tenderness. Patients are often writhing in pain.
C. Laboratory and diagnostic studies
   1. Urinalysis
      • Will usually demonstrate hematuria and crystals. It is important to check for the urine pH (urate stones typically appear in pH < 5.5; struvite stones in pH > 7.5).
   2. Serum chemistries
      • Increased BUN and creatinine indicate renal failure (rule out urethral obstruction or bilateral ureteral obstruction, or hypovolemia/prerenal acute renal failure). Serum parathyroid hormone should be measured if hypercalcemia is present. Elevated uric acid levels may point toward high urinary urate levels (although hyperuricosuria may still be present even with normal serum uric acid levels).
   3. X-ray (kidneys, ureter, bladder [KUB])
      • A significant number of stones (80% to 90%) can be seen on x-ray (notably, urate stones are radiolucent).
   4. Intravenous pyelogram
      • IVP will establish the diagnosis in patients with normal renal function.
   5. Abdominal ultrasound
      • Abdominal ultrasound may be used to visualize the urinary tract in cases of suspected obstruction.
   6. Noncontrast abdominal CT scan
      • This has become the imaging procedure of choice because it detects radiolucent and radiopaque stones, provides enough anatomic detail to rule out obstruction, and detects other possible causes for renal colic or abdominal pain that may mimic renal stones.
   7. If infection is possible a urine culture and CBC should be drawn.

8. Urine 24-hour collection for volume, pH, calcium, phosphate, oxalate, citrate, uric acid, sodium, and creatinine should be done outside the acute setting. If a stone is passed, it should be sent for composition analysis.

D. Formulating the diagnosis
   • History, physical examination, and results of blood/urine laboratory tests and imaging will yield the diagnosis.

E. Evaluating the severity of the problem
   1. Most kidney stones (80% to 90%) can be managed in the outpatient setting.
   2. Indications for hospitalization
      • Urinary obstruction
      • High fever or signs of infection
      • Intractable pain, nausea, or vomiting
      • Solitary or horseshoe kidney, nonfunctioning contralateral kidney, or urine extravasation

F. Managing the patient
   • Most stones smaller than 5 mm in diameter will pass spontaneously. Treatment includes oral hydration and narcotic analgesics. The nonsteroidal medication ketorolac is also an effective analgesic.
   • Patients with infection should be admitted to the hospital and started on IV antibiotics.
   • Patients with high-grade obstruction, persistent pain, and complicated infection may require drainage of the urinary tract.
   • Patients with unpassably large stones, located in the kidney, may require surgical treatment. Surgical treatment is often performed by extracorporeal shock wave lithotripsy (ESWL). With this method, shock waves are directed at the stone, resulting in stone fragmentation. Stone fragments are then passed spontaneously.
   • Surgical treatment of lower ureteral stones is accomplished through urethroscopy and direct extraction. Bladder stones are almost uniformly removed cystoscopically.
   • Patients with struvite stones should be treated with antibiotics to prevent progression of infection or recurrence of stone formation.
   • For cystine stones and uric acid stones the mainstay of therapy involves hydration and oral alkalization of the urine (typically with potassium citrate). Patients with cystine stones can also be treated with D-penicillamine or captopril to decrease the cystine excretion in the urine.
   • Because kidney stones are often recurrent further studies are necessary to uncover metabolic problems.

X. Nephritic Syndrome
   A. Basic science
      1. The nephritic syndrome is defined by the following:
         • Hematuria (often with dysmorphic RBCs and/or RBC casts)
         • Edema
         • Hypertension

- Proteinuria (usually <3 g/day)
- Renal failure

2. This disease state results from glomerular damage from many different processes, including primary renal diseases, or secondary to systemic processes.

3. Common causes of the nephritic syndrome
   a. Immune complex diseases
      - IgA nephropathy: the most common form of acute glomerulonephritis; normal C3 (complement) levels
      - Henoch-Schönlein purpura: most common in children; same lesion as IgA nephropathy plus systemic vasculitis; normal C3 levels
      - Acute poststreptococcal glomerulonephritis: develops 1 to 4 weeks after pharyngitis or impetigo; usually self-limited; + antistreptolysin O titers; low C3 levels
      - Endocarditis: typically blood cultures are positive; there is fever and evidence of valvular disease; low C3 levels
      - Systemic lupus erythematosus: + ANA titers; + anti-dsDNA; low C3 levels
      - Membranoproliferative glomerulonephritis (MPGN): low C3 levels; + C3 nephritic factor
      - Cryoglobulinemia: + cryoprecipitate; commonly associated with hepatitis C infection; low C3 levels
   b. ANCA (+) vasculitis
      - Wegener's granulomatosis: (+) c-ANCA (anti-PR3); typically has renal and pulmonary involvement
      - Microscopic polyangiitis: (+) p-ANCA (anti-MPO); renal compromise is more common than pulmonary involvement; systemic vasculitis
      - Churg-Strauss syndrome: (+) p-ANCA (anti-MPO); presents with asthma-like symptoms and eosinophilia
   c. Anti-glomerular basement membrane (GBM) diseases
      - Goodpasture's disease: pulmonary hemorrhage and glomerulonephritis; + anti-GBM
      - Anti-GBM disease: absence of pulmonary involvement with glomerulonephritis; + anti-GBM

B. History and physical examination
   1. History
      - Patients may complain of recent illness (e.g., "strep" throat or skin rash—impetigo), edema (typically periorbital or scrotal), dark or bloody urine, oliguria, or hemoptysis. Patients may also have a medical history of lupus or other autoimmune diseases.
   2. Physical examination
      - Physical examination may demonstrate hypertension, edema, and other disease-specific signs.

C. Laboratory and diagnostic studies
   - Urinalysis will demonstrate hematuria ± proteinuria. Sediment may demonstrate RBC casts or dysmorphic RBCs (pathognomonic for glomerulonephritis); WBC and granular casts are common.

- Serum chemistries may show high BUN and creatinine.
- Disease-specific laboratory studies should be ordered accordingly (as specified above).
- Definitive diagnosis may be obtained through renal biopsy. Biopsy specimens are analyzed by conventional (light), electron, and immunofluorescent microscopy.
- Typical patterns of glomerular injury:
  1. Granular staining (for immune complex diseases)
  2. Linear staining (for anti-GBM disease)
  3. Pauci-immune or minimal staining (for ANCA + vasculitis)
- D. Formulating the diagnosis
  - History, physical examination, and results of urinalysis help confirm the diagnosis of the nephritic syndrome. Demonstration of RBC casts is pathognomonic for glomerulonephritis.
  - About 50% of patients will have the diagnosis of nephritis made after an incidental finding of hematuria on routine urinalysis.
- E. Evaluating the severity of the problem
  - Rapidly progressive glomerulonephritis (RPGN) is a severe form of the nephritic syndrome associated with renal failure developing over weeks. Renal biopsy typical demonstrates crescents in over 50% of glomeruli. The overall prognosis of these patients is poor. RPGN does not usually respond to medical management and may lead to end-stage renal disease requiring renal replacement therapy.
- F. Managing the patient
  - Complications of the nephritic syndrome must be managed while the cause of nephritis is explored. Complications include hypertension (treated with antihypertensive medications), and edema (treated with diuretics, sodium restriction).
  - Disease-specific treatment
    1. Immune complex disease: questionable use of steroids ± alkylating agents for primary renal diseases (as for proliferative lupus nephritis); treat the underlying disease. Cryoglobulinemia may require plasmapheresis.
    2. ANCA (+) disease: immediate steroids + cyclophosphamide
    3. Anti-GBM disease: immediate steroids + cytotoxic agent. May benefit from plasmapheresis.

XI. Nephrotic Syndrome
  - A. Basic science
    1. Nephrotic syndrome occurs because the glomeruli lose the ability to retain protein. Pathologically it appears that either of two processes occur:
       - The glomerular epithelial cells (podocytes) lose surface charge. This leads to the inability of the kidney to retain small charged molecules.
       - The glomerulus loses the ability to act as a size selective barrier. Large, less densely charged molecules are unable to be retained in the vascular system.
    2. The classic features of nephrotic syndrome:
       - Edema

- Proteinuria (>3.5 g/day)
- Hypoalbuminemia (<3 mg/dL)
- Hyperlipidemia
3. Primary renal disease states that may lead to nephrotic syndrome:
   a. Focal segmental glomerulosclerosis (FSGS) (40%)
      - Most common cause in African American adults; HIV is associated with a "collapsing" variant of FSGS; heroin abuse is also an association.
   b. Membranous nephropathy (30%)
      - Membranous nephropathy is the most common cause in white adults; it is associated with multiple carcinomas (breast, lung, colon) and hepatitis B infection.
   c. Minimal change disease (20%)
      - This is the most common cause in children; it is associated with NSAID use and lymphoproliferative disorders.
   d. Membranoproliferative glomerulonephritis (MPGN) (5%)
      - Type I: associated with hepatitis C infection and cryoglobulinemia
      - Type II: "dense deposit disease" with C3 deposition (C3 nephritic factor)
   e. Mesangial proliferative glomerulonephritis (5%)
   f. Fibrillary-immunotactoid glomerulopathy
4. Systemic diseases that may lead to nephrotic syndrome:
   a. Diabetes mellitus
      - Overall diabetes is the most common cause of nephrotic syndrome; nodular glomerulosclerosis (Kimmelstiel-Wilson lesion) may be seen; kidneys are typically large.
   b. Amyloidosis
      - Kidneys are typically large.
   c. Systemic lupus erythematosus
   d. Cryoglobulinemia
      - Typically occurs with MPGN as outlined earlier.
B. History and physical examination
   1. History:
      - Patients may complain of weakness, anorexia, and edema. Often present are symptoms related to fluid retention (weight gain, abdominal distention, dyspnea, chest pain due to pericardial effusion). Patients often describe frothy urine. History of previous infectious diseases (e.g., syphilis, hepatitis, HIV) may indicate the cause of nephrotic syndrome.
   2. Physical examination:
      - Patients may be hypertensive and often have edema (typically periorbital or scrotal).
C. Laboratory and diagnostic studies
   1. Urinalysis and urine chemistries:
      - Significant proteinuria, typically 3 to 4+ on dipstick. On 24-hour urine collection proteinuria is greater than 3.5 g/day (urine should be sent for creatinine and total protein measurements). Also useful is estimating degree of proteinuria by random urine measurement of the protein to creatinine ratio.

- Lipiduria can be evidenced by the presence of fatty casts, oval fat bodies, or fat droplets on urine sediment ("Maltese cross" appearance under polarizing microscopy). Sediment may demonstrate broad, waxy casts.
  2. Serum chemistries
     - Hypoalbuminemia (<3 mg/dL in adults)
     - Hyperlipidemia
     - Azotemia may be present
  3. CBC may demonstrate anemia (caused by loss of erythropoietin production if process is chronic).
  4. Additional disease-specific tests may be required to aid in the diagnostic workup:
     - Complement levels
     - ANA, anti-dsDNA
     - Serum and urine protein electrophoresis (± monoclonal protein analysis)
     - Fat pad biopsy (in search for evidence of amyloidosis)
     - Diabetic testing (HbA_{1c})
     - Serologic testing for hepatitis (HBV, HCV), HIV
     - Serum cryoglobulins
  5. Renal biopsy may be needed to define the cause of nephrotic syndrome.
- D. Formulating the diagnosis
  - History, physical examination, and results of urinalysis will be diagnostic for nephrotic syndrome.
  - Additional disease-specific tests and renal biopsy will help narrow down the etiologic diagnosis.
- E. Evaluating the severity of the problem
  - Inability to control volume and electrolytes and bleeding diathesis (e.g., platelet dysfunction from uremia, hypercoagulable state) suggest severe disease. Patients with severe disease may require hemodialysis.
- F. Managing the patient
  - Complications of the nephrotic syndrome must be managed while the cause is explored. Complications include:
    - Hypertension and edema: treated with diuretics, salt restriction, and appropriate antihypertensives
    - Hyperlipidemia: low cholesterol diet and pharmacologic treatment
    - Proteinuria: ACE inhibitors slow the progression of proteinuria in all causes of proteinuria (best evidence in diabetes, even if normotensive). Use angiotensin II receptor blockers for ACEI-intolerant patients.
    - Thromboembolic events (occur due to loss of antithrombin III and other endogenous anticoagulants): use heparin and warfarin when indicated. Prevention in hospitalized and immobilized patients is key.
    - Infections: due to loss of immunoglobulins in urine
    - Multiple electrolyte abnormalities (particularly in the presence of azotemia): reduce fluid intake if hyponatremic; limit potassium and phosphorus-containing products if patient has renal failure.
  - Other general measures:
    - Protein supplementation in diet (1 g/kg/day)

- Avoidance of nephrotoxic medications (e.g., NSAIDs)
- Vaccines: influenza, pneumococcal, *H. influenzae*
- Specific treatment of the variety of primary renal causes of nephrotic syndrome; often includes corticosteroids and cytotoxic agents
  - Minimal change disease: usually responds to steroid therapy alone, often within 6 weeks of treatment; has an excellent prognosis in 80% to 90% of patients
  - Idiopathic membranous nephropathy: the mainstay of treatment; includes steroids and cytotoxic agents (including cyclophosphamide, chlorambucil, and cyclosporine)
  - The majority of patients with FSGS progress to renal failure regardless of medical treatment.
- The treatment of nephrotic syndrome caused by systemic disease (e.g., diabetes, amyloidosis, SLE, HIV) is directed at the underlying disease.

Obstetrics and Gynecology

I. Abnormal Pap Smear and Cervical Cancer Screening
   A. Basic science
   - The Pap (Papanicolaou) smear is a screening test used to detect premalignant lesions of the cervix. The introduction of the Pap smear has reduced the incidence of invasive cervical cancer by 50%. Pap smears are used to collect cells at the squamocolumnar junction of the ectocervix. This is the earliest site of neoplastic growth in the cervix.
   - Abnormal Pap smears can result from either dysplasia (i.e., precancerous change) or infection. Neoplastic changes can range in severity from atypia to carcinoma in situ. Cervical lesions found on Pap smear may resolve (either on their own or with treatment), remain dysplastic, or progress to invasive cancer.
   - Current guidelines recommend obtaining a Pap smear 3 years after starting intercourse or at least by age 21. Additionally, a Pap smear is usually obtained on pregnant women during the first trimester. Frequency varies from every 1 to 3 years, depending on risk factors and previous Pap smear results.
   - The reliability of the Pap smear as a screening tool is based on frequent sampling, because a single test can be falsely positive or negative. Yearly screening is usually done up to the age of 30 with a human papillomavirus (HPV) typing done to better evaluate an abnormal result (i.e., ASCUS: atypical squamous cells of undetermined significance). In women beyond 30 years of age, a Pap smear can be combined with HPV typing. If both the Pap and the HPV typing are negative, the frequency of screening can be reduced to every 3 years in women older than 30 years of age. Screening should continue until age 65.
   - Women who have had a hysterectomy for benign reasons do not need Pap smear screening. Women who have had a subtotal hysterectomy (cervix is left behind) or a total hysterectomy for precancerous or cancerous cervical lesions should continue to get Pap smear screening at regular, frequent intervals.
   B. History and physical examination
   - Screening is very important because cervical dysplasia rarely causes symptoms. The history may reveal risk factors significant for the development of cervical dysplasia, including the following:
     1. Early intercourse
     2. Multiple sex partners

3. A history of sexually transmitted diseases (STDs)

4. Tobacco use

- The physical examination may reveal abnormalities (e.g., genital warts) associated with cervical dysplasia and carcinoma. A Pap smear is obtained by rotating a spatula on the cervix to obtain cells from the squamocolumnar junction and using a brush which is inserted into the cervical os to obtain endocervical cells. The sample is then smeared on a microscope slide and fixed. The thin prep method utilizes a liquid transport medium into which the spatulas are immersed. Lesser cells are required for interpretation in this method.

C. Laboratory and diagnostic studies

- The Pap smear is only a screening test. Both false negative and false positive results can occur. Further evaluation of an abnormal result is required. This is usually done with colposcopy (a magnified examination of the cervix). Colposcopy provides a 10× to 16× magnification of the transformation zone.
- Colposcopy is considered adequate only if the entire transformation zone is seen. During the examination a dilute solution of acetic acid is applied to the cervix. Abnormal areas often appear white and may display prominent blood vessels in a mosaic pattern. A biopsy of abnormal areas should be obtained.

D. Formulating the diagnosis

- As stated earlier, a diagnosis of cervical dysplasia cannot be made by Pap smear alone. Confirmation with colposcopy and biopsy is required.

E. Evaluating the severity of problems

- The severity of the problem is determined histologically. Using the Bethesda system, a Pap smear is reported as normal, ASCUS (atypical squamous cells of undetermined significance), low grade SIL (squamous intraepithelial lesion), high grade SIL, or cancer.

F. Managing the patient

- Pap smears reported as normal will need repeat screening after 1 to 3 years, depending on risk factors and age. ASCUS reports are triaged based on HPV DNA subtypes. ASCUS patients with high-risk HPV DNA subtypes need a colposcopy for further evaluation, and HPV DNA negative patients will need a repeat Pap smear in 12 months. Dysplasias (low and high grade) proceed directly to colposcopy.
- Once an abnormality detected on a Pap smear is confirmed by colposcopy and biopsy, therapy must follow. The biopsy is reported as carcinoma in situ (CIN), normal, low-grade lesion (CIN-1) or high-grade lesion (CIN II or III).
- Low-grade lesions can be managed either expectantly with frequent follow-up in reliable patients of childbearing age. Treatments include ablation or excision of the affected area. This can be performed by cryotherapy, which uses liquid carbon dioxide to cool a probe applied to the cervix or carbon dioxide laser ablation. Excisional methods include cold knife conization and LEEP (loop electrosurgical excision of the cervix). The excisional methods have the advantage of providing a tissue sample for histologic evaluation.

- High-grade lesions are managed by LEEP procedure. However, other ablative or excisional procedures can also be done based on the ease and experience of the surgeon (cryotherapy, carbon dioxide laser, cold knife excision).
- Frequent follow-ups with Pap smear, HPV typing, or colposcopy are performed after treatment for cervical dysplasia. The prognosis is generally good. Larger size, higher grade, positive excisional margins and HPV positivity are associated with a higher rate of recurrence and progression to invasive cancer.
- The objective of management of an abnormal Pap smear during pregnancy is to rule out invasive disease. Colposcopy should be done and biopsies obtained if a high-grade lesion is suspected. The clinician should be prepared for heavier bleeding when performing biopsies on the cervix during pregnancy secondary to increased vasculature. Only when there is a concern of invasive cancer is excisional therapy performed during pregnancy.

II. Abnormal Uterine Bleeding
  A. Basic science
- The hypothalamic-pituitary-ovarian axis controls ovulation and mediates the cyclic changes within the uterine endometrium that manifest as the menstrual cycle. Menses normally occurs at regular intervals (usually every 28 days) for a defined period of time (2 to 7 days), beginning at puberty and lasting until menopause.
- Bleeding that is unexpected, irregular, prolonged, or excessive is called abnormal uterine bleeding (AUB). Although AUB may result from an organic cause (e.g., a fibroid), it most commonly occurs secondary to anovulation (or dysfunctional ovulation). In the absence of identifiable disease; such bleeding is called dysfunctional uterine bleeding (DUB).
- Anovulation (or dysfunctional ovulation) occurs for a variety of reasons, but does so most often after puberty and around menopause. In all cases of uterine bleeding an organic cause should be sought. Therefore, the diagnosis of DUB is one of exclusion. Common organic causes of AUB are listed in Box 13-1.
  B. History and physical examination
- A detailed history includes the amount and duration of current bleeding and the date of the last menstrual period. Methods of contraception and the use of medicines should be noted. The presence of pertinent diseases (e.g., blood dyscrasias, thyroid disorders) should be sought.
- A pelvic examination should be performed to rule out pregnancy, infection, cervical abnormality, adnexal mass, and uterine fibroid.
  C. Laboratory and diagnostic studies
- For excessive bleeding, a pregnancy test, thyroid function test(s), complete blood count (CBC), coagulation profile, and Pap smear should be ordered. The lack of ovulation may be confirmed by monitoring basal body temperature (increased temperature corresponds to increased progesterone levels seen at ovulation) or, more accurately, by checking serum progesterone levels in the midluteal phase (days 18 to 24 of the menstrual cycle).

BOX 13-1

COMMON ORGANIC CAUSES OF ABNORMAL UTERINE BLEEDING

In the Newborn and Child

Placental estrogen withdrawal (in the neonate)
Precocious puberty

In the Adult

Bleeding disorders (e.g., leukemia, hemophilia)
Spontaneous abortion
Ectopic pregnancy
Endometriosis
Cervical cancer
Leiomyoma
Ovarian cysts
Infection
Iatrogenic (intrauterine devices, medications, and hormones)

- A pelvic ultrasound may be helpful in eliminating ectopic pregnancy, fibroids, adnexal masses, endometrial thickening (due to atypia or cancer), adenomyosis (presence of endometrial tissue in the myometrium), and endometriosis as causes of uterine bleeding.
- Endometrial biopsy or dilatation and curettage should be performed in women over the age of 35 to rule out the possibility of endometrial cancer or premalignant lesions.

D. Formulating the diagnosis

- DUB is the cause of AUB in approximately 85% of patients. The differential diagnosis of AUB includes pregnancy complications, coagulation defects, thyroid or adrenal dysfunction, endometrial or cervical polyps, fibroids, adenomyosis, endometrial hyperplasia (or cancer), anovulation, endometritis, and the presence of an intrauterine device (IUD) (see Box 13-1).

E. Evaluating the severity of problems

- The most severe complication of abnormal menstruation is hemorrhage and acute anemia. Many patients will respond to oral estrogen in high doses or oral progesterone. IV estrogen maybe required in some cases. Invasive therapy (e.g., dilatation and curettage, hypogastric artery embolization, or hysterectomy) is rarely required.

F. Managing the patient

- Chronic mild to moderate menorrhagia can be managed with nonsteroidal anti-inflammatory drugs (NSAIDs) during the bleeding phase. NSAIDs decrease the bleeding flow 20% to 50% and relieve dysmenorrhea. Antifibrinolytics (tranexamic acid) may also be used for less severe cases.

- Patients with DUB usually respond to progestins (e.g., medroxyprogesterone or norethindrone) given during the luteal phase for several cycles. Alternatively, oral contraceptive pills may be given every 6 hours for 1 week; following this, patients can expect a heavy withdrawal bleed. The risk of recurrence is limited if the patient is maintained on a cycled oral contraceptive pill. Other medical management consists of progestin-containing IUDs, danazol (Danocrine), and gonadotropin-releasing hormone (GnRH) agonists. Patients with DUB who desire pregnancy may be treated with clomiphene (Clomid) to induce ovulation.
- Operative management for DUB is indicated for failure of medical management and includes hysteroscopic ablation of the endometrium, hypogastric artery embolization, and hysterectomy.

III. Abortion
  A. Basic science
    - Pregnancies that end spontaneously before the fetus has reached a viable gestational age are called abortions or miscarriages. This typically corresponds to pregnancies ending before 20 to 22 weeks of gestation.
    - Spontaneous abortion is the most common complication of early pregnancy; 10% to 20% of clinically recognized pregnancies and up to 70% of subclinical (unrecognized) or very early pregnancies end in miscarriage. Etiologic factors include chromosomal aberrations either de novo or inherited, congenital anomalies due to teratogen exposure, trauma and maternal factors such as uterine abnormalities, acute infection, endocrinopathy, coagulopathy, and other medical illness.
    - Risk factors associated with a higher rate of pregnancy loss include advanced age, previous miscarriage, multigravidity, smoking, alcohol use, cocaine use, low folate levels, and fever.
  B. History and physical examination
    - Vaginal bleeding is usually the first symptom of an abortion. The degree of vaginal bleeding and the loss of tissue must be ascertained by patient report. A complaint of suprapubic cramping and vaginal bleeding usually suggests a poor prognosis for continuation of the pregnancy.
    - Vital signs and orthostatics should be determined to ensure hemodynamic stability. If the fetus is more than 10 to 12 weeks old, a fetal heart rate should be heard (120 to 160 beats per minute) with an ultrasound stethoscope. The abdominal examination may reveal a palpable uterine fundus. Normally the uterine fundus reaches the level of the umbilicus at 20 weeks.
    - If the patient is undergoing an abortion, the speculum examination will reveal vaginal bleeding and cervical dilation. The bimanual examination should focus on uterine size (indicative of gestational age).

C. Laboratory and diagnostic studies
- A pregnancy test; complete blood count with differential, type, and screen; and a prothrombin time and partial thromboplastin time test should be ordered.
- Ultrasonography plays the most important role in diagnosing and managing a patient with a known intrauterine pregnancy and vaginal bleeding. Various parameters including presence of fetal heart, presence of a fetal pole, and size and appearance of gestational sac are used to correlate the patient's known gestational age with ultrasound findings. Serial ultrasound examination in a week's time may be performed for equivocal cases.

D. Formulating the diagnosis
1. Threatened abortion
   - Threatened abortion involves a pregnancy less than 20 weeks with uterine bleeding. The cervical os is closed. Pain, if present, is minimal. Half of the patients progress to abortion. Approximately 25% of all pregnancies have some degree of first trimester bleeding.
2. Inevitable abortion
   - Inevitable abortion is similar to threatened abortion except that the cervix is dilated, there is heavy uterine bleeding, or the membranes are ruptured. Menstrual cramps are present. Ultrasound may reveal a nonviable pregnancy in the process of being expelled.
3. Missed abortion
   - The fetus has died but it is retained in the uterus, usually for weeks.
4. Incomplete abortion
   - Incomplete abortion is similar to an inevitable abortion except that part of the products of conception is passed.
5. Blighted ovum
   - Ultrasound diagnosis reveals a gestational sac without fetal tissue.
6. Complete abortion (spontaneous abortion)
   - All tissue has been passed through the cervix. Uterine cramping and bleeding have resolved. The uterus is smaller than the gestational age reflects. Ultrasound reveals an empty uterus.
7. Therapeutic abortion
   - The pregnancy is terminated because of the patient's medical condition.
8. Elective abortion
   - A patient elects to terminate a gestation.

E. Evaluating the severity of problems
- Maternal hemorrhage with hypovolemic shock is the most serious problem complicating abortion. The potential for sepsis is present in women with an incomplete abortion and demands immediate recognition and treatment.

F. Managing the patient
- Avoiding alcohol and smoking during pregnancy is important in decreasing the risk of abortion. Adequate emotional support must be provided for patients who undergo spontaneous abortion or elective termination. Patients with a history of recurrent pregnancy loss should undergo a thorough evaluation to search for a possible cause (e.g., diabetes, lupus,

hypothyroidism). All pregnant patients with suspected abortion who are Rh negative (and do not have Rh antibodies) should receive RhoGAM (anti-D gamma globulin).

- Further management includes expectant, medical, or surgical methods. Expectant management is an option in early pregnancies (less than 13 weeks) with stable vital signs and no evidence of infection. Women can wait up to 4 weeks and come in for a medical or surgical procedure if they do not expel the products spontaneously.
- Medical management can be as effective as surgical management and consists of the administration of prostaglandin E1 analog called misoprostol intravaginally. It is performed in women who want to avoid an operative procedure and is contraindicated in septic abortions and with active hemorrhage. Patients can return home and wait for uterine contractions to expel the products of conception; they should be instructed to come to the hospital in case of severe bleeding. Patients opting for expectant or medical management should be made aware that they may require an operative procedure in the event of incomplete expulsion and continuing bleeding.
- Surgical procedures consist of dilatation and curettage (D&C) or dilatation and suction evacuation (D&E). Both techniques are performed in the first and second trimesters. Surgical management is the conventional method of managing missed and incomplete abortions and is indicated for women with active bleeding, signs of infection or those who want immediate and definitive treatment.
- Septic abortion: Patients in sepsis or other signs of infection require stabilization followed by immediate surgical evacuation and intravenous antibiotic therapy.
- Threatened abortion: If the patient is stable (not actively bleeding) and the fetus is viable, the patient is managed expectantly until the symptoms resolve or a diagnosis of nonviable pregnancy is made or she progresses to a complete, incomplete or missed abortion. There are no current obstetric interventions to prevent a first trimester spontaneous pregnancy loss. Bed rest and hormonal supplements have not proved to be effective. Coitus should be avoided.
- Inevitable abortion: The patient may choose expectant or medical or surgical management.
- Incomplete abortion: Patients are admitted to the hospital for evacuation of the remaining products of conception to prevent complications from bleeding and infection.
- Missed abortion or blighted ovum (less than 8 weeks' gestation): Expectant or surgical management is appropriate.

IV. Abruptio Placentae
  A. Basic science
  - Abruptio placentae refers to the premature separation of a normally implanted placenta after 20 weeks of gestation. The cause of the separation is the rupture of defective maternal vessels in the decidua at the site of placental

attachment resulting in the compromise of oxygen and nutrient delivery to the fetus.

- Blood may leak from the uteroplacental junction and pass into the vagina (external hemorrhage) or may remain trapped behind the placenta (concealed hemorrhage).
- The incidence of abruptio placentae in the general population is about 1 in 150 deliveries. Perinatal mortality rate is approximately 20%.

B. History and physical examination

- Several factors increase the risk of abruption including advanced age, multiparity, hypertension (chronic or pregnancy associated), external abdominal trauma, cocaine use, cigarette smoking, inherited thrombophilia (factor V_{Leiden} heterozygosity, prothrombin gene mutation, hyperhomocystinemia), multiple pregnancies, and polyhydramnios. Patients with a history of abruption also have a tenfold greater risk of a second placental abruption.
- The most common sign of placental abruption is vaginal bleeding. Abdominal pain, back pain, and increasing frequency of contractions are frequent symptoms. Physical examination reveals a rigid and tender uterus and a nonreassuring fetal heart tracing (nonstress test: NST). In unfortunate cases, NST revealing fetal distress or fetal death may be the first indication that an abruption has occurred.
- A speculum examination or digital vaginal or cervical examination should not be done in a third trimester patient with vaginal bleeding unless the location of the placenta is known. In the presence of placenta previa, a vaginal examination may worsen bleeding.

C. Laboratory and diagnostic studies

- Because of the risk of hemorrhage and disseminated intravascular coagulation (DIC), a type and screen, hematocrit, coagulation studies, and fibrinogen level should be obtained. Urine screen for cocaine metabolites should be checked.
- Ultrasound can be helpful in ruling out placenta previa, but most placental abruptions are not visible by ultrasound. Tetanic or high-frequency contractions suggest abruptio placentae.

D. Formulating the diagnosis

- The differential diagnosis of bleeding late in pregnancy includes normal labor, placenta previa, abruptio placentae, uterine rupture, and vasa previa. Placenta previa is associated with painless vaginal bleeding, whereas abruption is described as painful vaginal bleeding. Ultrasound may help in formulating the diagnosis. In some cases, however, the diagnosis cannot be confirmed until after delivery. In abruption the placenta will display a dark, adherent clot on its surface.

E. Evaluating the severity of problems

- Placental abruption can be life-threatening for both the fetus and the mother. Maternal complications include hemorrhage and hypovolemic shock, DIC, renal failure, and increased risk of cesarean delivery. Fetal risks include intrauterine growth restriction (IUGR), stillbirth, prematurity, and hypoxic damage because the placenta essentially functions as the fetus's lungs until birth.

F. Managing the patient
- Severe abruption warrants close monitoring including insertion of two large-bore IV cannulas, continuous monitoring of maternal vital signs and urine output, fetal heart rate monitoring, crystalloid replacement (± packed red blood cells and FFP or cryoprecipitate in DIC), frequent laboratory tests including CBC, coagulation profile and renal function. The definitive management is delivery, preferably by cesarean section.
- Mild abruption, defined as absence of fetal distress, DIC, hypotension, tender uterus, and concealed hemorrhage, can be managed conservatively with frequent monitoring in a hospital setting. This is especially done in cases that are remote from term in order to delay labor until steroids can be administered to accelerate lung maturation in the fetus. Tocolysis for preterm labor (a frequent complication) is generally contraindicated in the presence of abruption but can be used in selected cases that are less than 33 weeks gestation and with mild abruption in order to administer steroids. Delivery should occur in the event of fetal distress or evidence of maternal hemodynamic instability.

V. Amenorrhea
A. Basic science
- Normal menstruation depends on a functioning hypothalamic-pituitary-ovarian-gonadal (HPOG) axis. Amenorrhea (absence of menses) is a transient or permanent condition resulting from the dysfunction of the hypothalamus, pituitary, ovaries, uterus, or vagina. It is classified as follows:
  1. Primary amenorrhea: lack of menarche by age 16 in the presence of normal secondary sexual characteristics (i.e., growth spurt, breasts, pubic and axillary hair).
  2. Secondary amenorrhea: lack of three consecutive menstrual cycles or 6 months of amenorrhea in a previously menstruating woman.
- Amenorrhea is physiologic when it occurs before puberty, during pregnancy and lactation, and after menopause. If amenorrhea occurs at any other time, it is pathologic. The menstrual period is susceptible to outside influences; thus, missing a single period is of little consequence. In contrast, prolonged amenorrhea may be the first sign of declining health or a signal of an underlying condition such as a pituitary tumor. All young women should be evaluated for medical problems if there is no evidence of development of secondary sexual characteristics by age 13, or if there is no menses by age 16.
- See Box 13-2 for causes of primary and secondary amenorrhea.
B. History and physical examination
- History can provide many diagnostic clues in the evaluation of primary amenorrhea. It must be remembered that many causes of secondary amenorrhea can also cause primary amenorrhea. Younger patients should be questioned about family history of delayed puberty, suggesting a possible

BOX 13-2

COMPARISON OF CAUSES OF PRIMARY AND SECONDARY AMENORRHEA

Primary Amenorrhea

Pregnancy
Hypothalamic pituitary disease
  Functional hypothalamic amenorrhea
  Congenital GnRH deficiency
  Constitutional delay of puberty
  Hyperprolactinemia
  Other (infiltrative lesions of
    hypothalamus and pituitary)
Ovarian disease
  Gonadal dysgenesis (Turner's
    hyperprolactinemia
    syndrome—XO karyotype)
  Polycystic ovary syndrome
  Other (autoimmune oophoritis,
    chemotherapy or radiation
    induced ovarian failure)
Congenital anatomic lesions of
  uterus and vagina
  Imperforate hymen
  Transverse vaginal septum
  Vaginal dysgenesis or müllerian
    agenesis
Receptor abnormalities and enzyme
  deficiencies
  Complete androgen insensitivity
    syndrome
  5-α-reductase deficiency
  Congenital adrenal hyperplasia
    (rare variant)

Secondary Amenorrhea

Pregnancy
Hypothalamic disease
  Functional hypothalamic
    amenorrhea (stress, illness,
    anorexia, weight loss, exercise)
  Congenital GnRH deficiency
    (idiopathic or Kallmann's syndrome)
  Infiltrative diseases of the
    hypothalamus (hemochromatosis,
    tumors, sarcoidosis)
Pituitary disease
  Empty sella syndrome
  Thyroid disease
  Other (radiation, infiltrative lesions,
    etc.)
Ovarian disease
  Polycystic ovary syndrome
  Ovarian failure
Uterine disease
  Asherman's syndrome

GnRH, gonadotrapm-releasing hormone.

familial disorder. A history of recent stress or illness and change in weight, diet, and exercise habits suggests hypothalamic cause. Also important in the evaluation of primary amenorrhea is history about secondary sexual characteristics such as growth spurt, axillary and pubic hair, and breast development. Lack of development of secondary sexual characteristics suggests ovarian or pituitary failure or a chromosomal abnormality.

- The pattern of menstrual bleeding and associated symptoms are important in the differential diagnosis of amenorrhea. Breast tenderness or nausea may suggest pregnancy. Hot flashes and vaginal dryness may indicate menopause.
- Patients should be asked about signs of increased androgen release that may suggest an adrenal disorder. These signs manifest as male sex characteristics such as hirsutism, clitoromegaly, deepening voice, male pattern baldness, muscular hypertrophy, or a loss of female sexual characteristics.
- The patient should be questioned about galactorrhea (expression of milk in the nonpuerperal state). Other symptoms in hypothalamic-pituitary disease include headaches, fatigue, visual field defects, and polyuria-polydipsia.
- The medication history is important because many medicines can inhibit ovulation (e.g., phenothiazines, monoamine oxidase inhibitors, steroids).
- The patient should have a full physical examination (including pelvic examination). Anorexia, visual field defects, thyroid irregularities, galactorrhea, obesity, masses, and abdominal striae should be noted. Signs of androgen excess (e.g., hirsutism, acne, and clitoromegaly) should be looked for. Evaluation for classic physical features of Turner syndrome (low hair line, web neck, shield chest, and widely spaced nipples) should be noted. If Turner syndrome is suspected, the blood pressure should be measured in both arms to evaluate for coarctation of the aorta.
- The examination in the prepubertal patient should focus on the following:
    1. Height, weight, arm span (normal arm span is with 5 cm of the height and is reduced in Turner syndrome), and an evaluation of the patient's growth chart
    2. Degree and distribution of body hair
    3. Degree of breast development (Tanner stage I to IV)
    4. Expression of breast milk
    5. Development of genitalia (clitoromegaly may indicate adrenal tumor or hermaphroditism)

C. Laboratory and diagnostic studies
    1. The first step in the diagnosis of primary amenorrhea is to determine by physical examination or ultrasonography whether there are any anatomic abnormalities in the vagina, cervix, or the uterus.
    2. If the uterus is absent, serum testosterone levels and karyotyping should be obtained. These tests will help the clinician distinguish between abnormal müllerian development (46,XX karyotype with normal female testosterone levels) and androgen insensitivity syndrome (46,XY karyotype and male serum testosterone levels; i.e., levels that are elevated for a normal female).
        - Abnormal müllerian development (46,XX karyotype with normal female testosterone levels) is associated with vaginal and variable uterine agenesis

and is part of a rare syndrome called Mayer-Rokitansky-Kuster-Hauser syndrome. Imperforate hymen and vaginal septum are also less severe and easily surgically remediable disorders of müllerian development.

- Complete androgen insensitivity syndrome (46,XY with male testosterone levels) is an X-linked recessive condition in which 46,XY subjects appear as normal females. This syndrome results from a defect in the androgen receptors; individuals are resistant to the testosterone produced and fail to develop male sexual characteristics. 5α-Reductase deficiency (46,XY) is another disorder in which 46,XY individuals appear as females. In this condition the disorder lies in the peripheral conversion of testosterone to its potent metabolite dihydrotestosterone (DHT) via 5α-reductase. At birth, these neonates appear to be female or have ambiguous genitalia due to the lack of testes and prostate development consequent to absent DHT. They are recognizable during puberty when virilization occursbecause of the puberty-related rise in testosterone and development of testosterone-dependent processes such as voice deepening, increase in muscle mass, and male pattern hair growth.

3. If the uterus is present and there are no abnormalities of the vagina, an endocrine evaluation should be performed. This includes measurement of β-hCG (human chorionic gonadotropin) to exclude pregnancy and may include serum determination of follicle-stimulating hormone (FSH), luteinizing hormone (LH), prolactin (PRL), and thyroid-stimulating hormone (TSH).

- An elevated FSH indicates ovarian dysgenesis and primary ovarian failure. Karyotyping is then performed in this situation and may demonstrate partial or complete loss of an X chromosome (Turner syndrome).
- Low FSH levels point to hypothalamic-pituitary axis dysfunction and may be due to functional hypothalamic amenorrhea (stress, exercise, etc.) or congenital GnRH deficiency (Kallmann's syndrome; associated with anosmia).
- Prolactin and TSH levels are evaluated, especially in the presence of galactorrhea. Signs of hyperandrogenism should be evaluated by measuring levels of dehydroepiandrosterone sulfate (DHEA-S) and serum testosterone levels. Elevated levels may be due to androgen-secreting tumors or polycystic ovarian syndrome (PCOS).
- Patients with a low FSH levels or elevated PRL should be evaluated with a computed tomography (CT) or magnetic resonance imaging (MRI) scan of the pituitary and hypothalamus to evaluate for the presence of tumor.

4. The evaluation of secondary amenorrhea should begin with serum or urine β-hCG to exclude pregnancy. LH, FSH, TSH, PRL, testosterone, and DHEA-S are determined to rule out ovarian failure, PCOS, or androgen-secreting tumors, hyperprolactinemia, and thyroid disease.

- Elevated gonadotropins (FSH and LH) in women with clinically insufficient estrogen are consistent with ovarian failure; this is most commonly due to menopause. Normal or low gonadotropins are often present in women with anorexia, drug use, and severe illness or stress. FSH levels are typically higher than the LH levels in these cases.

- Cranial imaging is indicated in patients with hypogonadotropic amenorrhea and without a clear historical explanation or in those with headache or visual field defects. All women with elevated serum prolactin levels should also have cranial imaging of the pituitary to look for hypothalamic or pituitary tumor.
- PCOS is diagnosed in the presence of two out of three of the following criteria: menstrual irregularity due to oligo-ovulation or anovulation, clinical (hirsutism, acne, male pattern balding) or biochemical evidence (elevated serum androgens) of hyperandrogenism, and polycystic ovaries by ultrasound. LH levels are typically higher than FSH in PCOS, but this finding is not a required criterion for diagnosis.
- Women with normal FSH and PRL levels and a history of uterine curettage preceding the amenorrhea may have Asherman's syndrome, in which acquired uterine scarring results in amenorrhea. A progestin challenge test which does *not* result in bleeding is suggestive of the diagnosis; it is confirmed by hysterosalpingogram or hysteroscopy.

D. Formulating the diagnosis
- The diagnostic tests for primary and secondary amenorrhea are done as described earlier in this section.

E. Evaluating the severity of problems
- Amenorrhea may be the first manifestation of a pituitary, adrenal, or other tumor.

F. Managing the patient
- Treatment of amenorrhea is directed at correcting the underlying disease; helping the female achieve a pregnancy, if desired; and preventing long-term complications (e.g., osteoporosis with estrogen deficiency).
- Amenorrhea secondary to anatomic defects usually requires surgical intervention. Those with pituitary tumors should be referred to a neurosurgeon and an endrocrinologist.
- Hyperprolactinemia can be treated with dopamine agonists (e.g., pergolide and bromocriptine).
- Patients with premature ovarian failure should be counseled regarding the risks and benefits of hormone replacement therapy.
- Psychological counseling is important in patients with müllerian agenesis or a Y chromosome.
- Functional hypothalamic deficiency is usually reversible with weight gain and reversal of the underlying problem such as anorexia.
- Pulsatile GnRH can be used in patients with GnRH deficiencies who desire a pregnancy.
- Therapy of Asherman's syndrome consists of hysteroscopic lysis of adhesions followed by long-term estrogen administration to stimulate regrowth of endometrial tissue.
- Treatment of hyperandrogenism is directed toward achieving the woman's goal (e.g., relief of hirsutism, resumption of menses, fertility) and preventing

the long-term consequences of PCOS (e.g., endometrial hyperplasia, obesity, and metabolic defects such as insulin resistance/impaired glucose tolerance). For women with PCOS, the type of therapy depends upon whether fertility is desired. For treatment of hirsutism, oral contraceptives together with spironolactone are used. Oral contraceptives or cyclic progestins are used for endometrial protection. For women who desire pregnancy, weight loss and clomiphene citrate are used. For women with PCOS and impaired glucose tolerance or diabetes mellitus type 2, the management consists of conservative measures such as diet and weight loss followed by metformin.

- Advances with assisted reproduction technology make it possible for many women with primary amenorrhea to participate in reproduction. For women with gonadal dysgenesis, the use of donor oocytes and their partner's sperm with in vitro fertilization (IVF) allow the women to carry a pregnancy in their own uterus. For women with an absent uterus, use of their own oocytes in IVF and transfer of their embryos to a gestational carrier can allow these women to have genetically related children.

VI. Antepartum Fetal Surveillance
  A. Nonstress test
  - The nonstress test (NST) is the most widely used technique for antepartum assessment of fetal well-being. It is based on the observation that fetuses normally display oscillations and fluctuations of their baseline heart rate; when these are absent, there is an increased risk of perinatal morbidity and death.
  - Two fetal heart rate (FHR) patterns are identified: those that are associated with fetal well-being ("reactive") and those that may be associated with adverse fetal outcomes ("nonreactive"). The goals are to identify fetuses in which a timely intervention will prevent adverse outcomes and to avoid fetal neurologic injury.
  - Fetal monitoring is performed by using an external electronic fetal monitor which utilizes an ultrasonic beam. It is performed starting at about 28 weeks to allow for fetal cardioneurologic maturation; prior to this gestation accelerations do not occur.
  - The NST is utilized in high-risk pregnancies (e.g., diabetes mellitus, intrauterine growth retardation (IUGR), hypertension, postdated pregnancies, preeclampsia, and prior stillbirths) and in situations of perceived decreased fetal movement. Fetal compromise in postdated pregnancy is more often due to umbilical cord compression (secondary to decreased amniotic fluid volume) and not to uteroplacental insufficiency. For this reason, it is recommended that NST be performed twice weekly along with weekly ultrasound assessment of amniotic fluid volume.
  - A reactive test is one in which the fetal heart rate demonstrates at least two accelerations during 20 minutes of monitoring. Acceleration is defined as at least 15 beats per minute above baseline lasting at least 15 seconds.
  - A nonreactive NST is one that does not show such accelerations over a 40-minute period. The most common cause for a nonreactive test is a period of

quiet sleep or inactivity. Vibroacoustic stimulation may be utilized to change fetal state from quiet to active sleep. The predictive accuracy of a nonreactive NST is not nearly as high as that of a reactive test.

- Management of a nonreactive NST depends upon the clinical context. At term, delivery rather than further testing is warranted. Ancillary tests such as the contraction stress test and cordocentesis to assess cord pH (low pH indicates fetal acidosis secondary to hypoxemia) can be used to prevent premature iatrogenic delivery.

B. Ultrasonic assessment

- Ultrasonographic evaluation using the biophysical profile (BPP) or Doppler waveform analysis is used to assess fetal well-being. BPP involves measurement of fetal heart rate (NST) along with ultrasound assessment of fetal motor movement, fetal breathing movement, gross fetal tone, and amniotic fluid volume. Normally, there are at least three fetal movements and 30 fetal chest wall movements within 10 minutes. The largest pocket of amniotic fluid should measure at least 2 cm. In addition, the amniotic fluid is measured in each of the four quadrants of the gestational sac; the sum of these linear measurements should be between 5 and 20 cm.

- A normal ultrasonic assessment and a reactive NST together represent a normal biophysical profile. Doppler velocimetry analyses doppler waveforms in the umbilical artery and is only used to monitor intrauterine growth restricted fetuses.

C. Contraction stress test

- The contraction stress test (CST) attempts to detect uteroplacental insufficiency. A dilute solution of oxytocin is administered until three contractions occur within 10 minutes. Contraindications include preterm labor, high risk of preterm delivery, preterm premature rupture of membranes, placenta previa, and previous classical cesarean section or extensive uterine surgery.

- The CST is interpreted as negative if no late decelerations appear on the tracing when adequate contractions are present. The CST is positive if there are late decelerations present with the majority of contractions without uterine hyperstimulation. The test is also considered positive when persistent late decelerations are present before adequate contractions. A suspicious test is one in which there are inconsistent late decelerations or significant variable decelerations. In women having spontaneous uterine contractions, the CST is interpreted in the same way as described here.

- A negative CST has been associated with a good fetal outcome. A positive test usually indicates the need for delivery.

VII. Benign Breast Disease

A. Basic science

1. Benign breast disease represents a spectrum of disorders that can cause breast pain, breast lumps, or nipple discharge. The most common cause of breast nodularity and tenderness is fibrocystic change, which occurs in approximately 60% of premenopausal women. Hormones affect the growth

of breast tissue and can therefore influence lesions that produce breast disease:

- Estrogens stimulate the proliferation of ductal tissue.
- Progestins stimulate both proliferation and differentiation of the lobules.
- Androgens antagonize the effects of estrogen and progestins on the breast.

2. Benign breast lesions, which are discovered by breast palpation or mammography, have been subdivided into those that are associated with an increased risk of breast cancer and those that are not.

a. No increased risk of breast cancer:

- Fibrocystic changes: Fibrocystic changes consist of an increased number of cysts or fibrous tissue in an otherwise normal breast. According to current terminology fibrocystic changes alone do not constitute a disease state because they are so common.
- Fibrocystic disease: Fibrocystic disease is diagnosed when fibrocystic changes occur in conjunction with pain, nipple discharge, or a degree of lumpiness sufficient to cause suspicion of cancer. The disease is characterized by two types of cysts: small cysts lined by flattened cells; and larger cysts with an apocrine cell layer. These cysts are a consequence of blockage or dilatation of ducts. Breast pain is caused by stromal edema, ductal dilatation, and inflammation.
- Duct ectasia: Duct ectasia is characterized by distention of subareolar ducts and the presence within them of yellowish orange material with crystalline oval and round structures.
- Solitary papillomas: Solitary papillomas consist of a monotonous array of papillary cells that grow from the wall of a cyst into its lumen.
- Simple fibroadenomas: Simple fibroadenomas are benign solid tumors containing glandular as well as fibrous tissue. They usually present as a well-defined, mobile mass but may be multiple. The etiology is not known; a hormonal relationship is likely because they persist during the reproductive years, can increase in size during pregnancy or with estrogen therapy, and regress after the menopause.
- Other nonmalignant disorders of the breast include superficial thrombophlebitis of the thoracoepigastric vein (or Mondor's disease which may be spontaneous but is usually related to trauma; it may be associated with an underlying malignancy; mammography has been recommended in women over 35 years of age); mastitis or breast abscess (common in lactating women and usually caused by *Staphylococcus aureus* or *Streptococcus*); galactocele (a cystic area containing milk usually found after cessation of breastfeeding); fat necrosis (or panniculitis; often presents as a tender, firm mass that is caused by trauma); hamartoma; tubular adenoma (a tumor composed of ductal tissue); diabetic mastopathy (most commonly seen in women who have type 1 diabetes mellitus and is characterized by benign histopathologic characteristics showing keloidal fibrosis and lymphocytic lobulitis).

b. Increased risk of breast cancer
- Ductal hyperplasia: Ductal hyperplasia without atypia is the most common lesion associated with increased risk of breast cancer. The number of epithelial cells lining the basement membrane of ducts is increased; although the cells vary in size and shape, they retain the cytologic features of benign cells.
- Sclerosing adenosis: Lobular tissue can also undergo hyperplastic change with increased fibrous tissue and interspersed glandular cells.
- Diffuse papillomatosis: Diffuse papillomatosis refers to the formation of multiple papillomas.
- Complex fibroadenomas: Complex fibroadenomas are tumors that contain cysts greater than 3 mm in diameter, sclerosing adenosis, epithelial calcification, or papillary apocrine changes. They are associated with an increased risk of cancer when multicentric proliferative changes are present in the surrounding glandular tissue.
- Atypical hyperplasia: Atypical hyperplasia is a specific lesion of either ductular or lobular elements with uniform cells and loss of apical-basal cellular orientation. Both atypical ductal and lobular hyperplasias are associated with an increased risk of malignancy; atypical lobular hyperplasia is considered a preinvasive lesion. Both require excisional biopsy for diagnosis.
- Radial scars: Radial scars are benign breast lesions of uncertain pathogenesis that are usually discovered incidentally when a breast mass is removed for other reasons; occasionally they are large enough to be detected by mammography.

B. History and physical examination
- Breast disorders present as breast pain; nipple discharge that can vary in color from clear to milky, yellow, brown, green, gray, black, or bloody; and breast lumps palpated either by the patient or the physician during annual examinations. Information should be obtained from the woman about the nature and pattern of her symptoms and the relationship to her menstrual cycles, the timing of onset of breast lumps and their subsequent course, the color and location of nipple discharge, hormone use, and all prior treatments.
- The presence of risk factors for breast cancer should be determined. These factors include menarche before age 12 years, first live birth at younger than age 30 years, and menopause at age 55 years or later (each of which is associated with increased exposure to estrogen); the number of previous breast biopsies, the presence of atypical ductal hyperplasia on biopsy, the degree and rate of progression of obesity, nulliparity, increased age, the amount of alcohol consumed, and the number and ages of first-degree family members with breast cancer, with two such relatives having breast cancer at any early age connoting particularly high risk. The Gail model is a research-based set of criteria that utilizes these data to predict a 5-year and a lifetime risk of breast cancer.

- Breastfeeding, multiparity, regular exercise, low body mass index (BMI), oophorectomy before age 35, and aspirin use may protect against breast cancer.
- The classic symptom of fibrocystic breast disease is cyclic bilateral breast pain. Physical findings include engorgement, increased density, excessive nodularity, and fluctuation in the size of the cystic areas.
- Fibroadenomas are most common in adolescents and women in their 20s. They are painless and do not undergo cyclic changes. They are firm, smooth, rubbery, and mobile.
- Women should perform monthly breast self-examination after the age of 20. The self-examination should occur at the same time each month, within a few days after menses.
- A clinical breast examination by a physician should be performed starting after the age of 21. This examination should include inspection for contour, dimpling, symmetry, and nipple retraction or discharge. The breasts should be palpated in the supine and upright position. The axillae and supraclavicular regions should be palpated for lymphadenopathy. The classic characteristics of breast cancers on physical examination are single, immovable, hard lesions with an irregular border and measuring 2 cm or more.

C. Laboratory and diagnostic studies
- Current American College of Obstetricians and Gynecologists and American Cancer Society guidelines recommend that women have screening mammography every 1 to 2 years from age 40 to 49, and yearly beginning at age 50. Women at high risk for breast cancer should have an annual mammogram and biannual physical examination.
- Further evaluation of a breast mass is done by diagnostic mammogram, fine needle aspiration biopsy (FNAB), core needle biopsy, or excisional biopsy. The evaluation of palpable and nonpalpable lesions differs slightly, as discussed below.
- Diagnostic mammography is usually not helpful in women under the age of 35 because of their dense breast tissue. In these women, breast masses should be evaluated by FNAB if they feel cystic and are easily palpable. If fluid is obtained and is not bloody and the mass disappears completely, the patient can be reassured and followed in 4 to 6 weeks to check for recurrence. A recurrence suggests the need for surgical referral. Bloody fluid should be sent for cytologic examination. If the lump does not feel cystic, the patient may be referred for ultrasound. If ultrasound shows a solid mass, the patient should undergo either FNAB, core needle biopsy, or excisional biopsy, depending upon local expertise. Some experts suggest that if a solid lump is small (<1 cm in size) and is not clinically suspicious (e.g., is soft, not fixed, not new, and not changing), it is likely to be a fibroadenoma and the patient can be followed with physical examination every 3 to 6 months.
- Mammography is recommended as part of the evaluation of any woman age 35 or older who has a breast mass, primarily to search for other lesions that are clinically occult, but also to evaluate the mass in question. However,

mammography usually cannot determine whether a lump is benign. In addition, mammography misses 10% to 20% of clinically palpable breast cancers. Thus, a negative mammogram should not stop further investigation.

- Breast ultrasound is useful to distinguish solid from cystic masses. An attempt should be made to aspirate a cystic mass. If the fluid is clear or cloudy and no residual mass is palpated, follow-up 1 month later is recommended. The mass should not return within this time. If the aspirate is bloody or the cyst recurs within 1 month, biopsy is recommended. Aspiration of multiple macrocysts is not necessary. Fine needle aspiration cytology shouldn't be used to evaluate solid masses, especially those that do not feel cystic, are larger than 1 cm, and occur in women with significant risk factors for breast cancer or age older than 35.
- A core needle biopsy is different from FNAB; a larger needle is used with the former (14 to 18 gauge, compared with 21 gauge), thereby providing histologic material. Core needle biopsy is used most often for evaluating nonpalpable breast lumps in conjunction with either stereotactic mammographic equipment or ultrasound guidance.
- An MRI may be useful in women with complaints related to breast implants.
- Ductal lavage is a new procedure whereby ductal cells are collected using a microcatheter inserted into multiple individual ducts. It is currently an investigational procedure being used in women who have a high clinical risk of breast cancer.

D. Formulating the diagnosis
- The definitive diagnosis of benign breast disease remains histologic evaluation. Many women are candidates for fine needle aspiration biopsy. Absolute indications for open or excisional breast biopsy include positive fine needle aspiration biopsy, cystic masses with a solid component or bloody aspirate, masses with nipple discharge, and suspicious mammographic changes without a dominant nodule or discrete thickening.

E. Evaluating the severity of problems
- The most important differentiation in the evaluation of women with complaints related to their breasts is the differentiation between benign and cancerous breast disease.

F. Managing the patient
- Management of breast lumps depends on the diagnosis made after mammogram, fine needle aspiration, and histologic diagnosis. Lesions with an increased risk of malignancy or features such as hyperplasia or atypia are managed by excisional biopsy and regular follow-up. Women should also be trained in breast self-examination and should be examined by the physician and undergo mammography every year. Women with atypical hyperplasia are among those in whom tamoxifen is most likely to prevent breast cancer.
- Further management of lesions with a low suspicion of cancer is based on the symptoms. Patients with fibrocystic disease mainly present with breast pain. Breast pain is managed by switching to low fat diet, administering acetaminophen or NSAIDs, and usage of support bras. Vitamin E (<400 IU a day), evening primrose oil, decreased consumption of caffeine and tobacco,

and oral contraceptives containing androgenic progestins have also been used. Danazol can be used for severe symptoms. Bromocriptine and tamoxifen may be used when danazol fails, although use of bromocriptine is limited by its side effects. GnRH agonists is a last resort in women with severe breast pain refractory to all other measures; menopausal symptoms and rapid bone loss make it difficult to justify its use because the risks outweigh benefits.

- Controversy exists as to proper management of fibroadenomas. Many believe that these lesions have a characteristic ultrasound appearance and do not require biopsy, but only serial follow-up with ultrasound every 6 months to look for changes in appearance. Expectant management with ultrasound assessment is a reasonable approach as most fibroadenomas get smaller over time. Many surgeons recommend core biopsy to make a diagnosis and then advocate that no further follow-up is required. In contrast to previous recommendations, it is not necessary to perform an excisional biopsy to completely remove these lesions. Disadvantages of excisional surgery include scarring at the incision site, dimpling of the breast from the removal of the tumor, damage to the breast's duct system, recurrence and mammographic changes (e.g., architectural distortion, skin thickening, and increased focal density).

- Nipple discharge is usually benign. Increased risk of malignancy is associated with unilateral discharge, discharge from a single duct, bloody discharge, or presence of a mass on examination. Milky nipple discharge can be physiologic; however, galactorrhea secondary to hyperprolactinemia must be considered. Nipple discharge is further evaluated by mammogram and cytologic examination of the discharge.

VIII. Cervical Cancer
  A. Basic science
  - Cervical cancer accounts for one fifth of all female genital cancers; 90% of cervical cancers are squamous cell carcinomas, and 10% are adenocarcinomas. The incidence of invasive cervical cancer has decreased over the last 50 years, in large part due to the Pap test. The median age for invasive cervical cancer is 51, and for carcinoma in situ is 41.
  - HPV is the most important risk factor. HPV DNA, especially subtypes 16, 18, and 31, are isolated on almost all cases of cervical cancer. Other risk factors for cervical carcinoma include first sexual intercourse at an early age, multiple sexual partners, and smoking.
  B. History and physical examination
  - Precancerous changes and carcinoma in situ are asymptomatic and are detected by Pap smear screening.
  - Abnormal vaginal bleeding (including postcoital bleeding) is the most common presenting symptom. Malodorous vaginal discharge, pelvic pain and lower extremity edema are also common in advanced stages.
  - While there are no classic physical findings, a thorough pelvic examination is essential to determine the extent of the tumor.

C. Laboratory and diagnostic studies
- The workup of cervical cancer includes the following:
  1. Pap smear
  2. Colposcopy
  3. Biopsy of suspicious lesions
     - Cervical punch biopsy or endocervical curettage is most often used to diagnose invasive cervical cancer.
  4. Clinical staging of the cancer requires thorough physical and pelvic examination.
     - A metastatic survey (chest x-ray examination, intravenous pyelogram, cystoscopy, or colonoscopy) can also done to determine the extent of disease progression.

D. Formulating the diagnosis
- The following is an overview of the staging classification:
  1. Stage 0: the carcinoma is in situ, intraepithelial neoplasia.
  2. Stage I: the carcinoma is strictly confined to the cervix.
  3. Stage II: the carcinoma extends beyond the cervix but not into the pelvic wall. The carcinoma involves the vagina but not the lower third.
  4. Stage III: the carcinoma has extended to the pelvic wall. On rectal examination there is not cancer-free space between the tumor and the pelvic wall.
  5. Stage IV: the carcinoma has extended beyond the true pelvis or has clinically involved the bladder or rectum.

E. Evaluating the severity of problems
- The prognosis is proportional to the stage and histologic grading of the tumor.

F. Managing the patient
  1. The following are treatment options for carcinoma in situ:
     - Ablative therapies including cryotherapy and laser ablation
     - Excisional therapies including laser conization, cold knife conization, LEEP
     - Hysterectomy
  2. Conservative methods (sparing the uterus) are an option for younger women wishing to preserve their fertility. Among the various methods, excisional methods are preferred because of the lower recurrence rate and availability of tissue for histologic examination. In these cases, the patient should undergo a Pap smear every 3 months for the first year and at 6-month intervals thereafter.
  3. Invasive squamous cell cancer (stages I to IV)
     - Stage I and stage II and some stage III tumors can be cured. Treatment is mainly focussed on palliation of symptoms for late stage III and stage IV disease.
     - Surgery—Early stage I cancers (with a width of invasion <7 mm and depth <3 mm) can be treated with total abdominal hysterectomy and bilateral salpingo-oophorectomy. Younger women with early stage I cancer may opt for conization of the cervix or intracavitary radiation alone in

order to preserve their fertility; they require frequent follow-up. For late stage I disease (width of invasion >7 mmm and depth >3 mm, these are associated with higher incidence of lymphatic metastases) and some stage II diseases, radical hysterectomy and bilateral pelvic adenectomy are performed. Adjunctive chemotherapy or radiation may be needed.

- Radiation therapy—Radiation therapy is most often used for stage II to IV cancers. Treatment consists of applying cesium to the cervix for a total of 70 hours, called intracavitary brachytherapy. This is followed by external radiation to the pelvic wall lymphatics. Complications of radiotherapy are proctitis and cystitis.
- Chemotherapy—Cervical cancers respond poorly to chemotherapy. It is used mainly as a palliative option for stage IV tumors.
- Squamous cell carcinoma spreads via the lymphatics. Treatment is directed at destroying the primary cancer and all affected lymph nodes while sparing healthy tissue. Radiation therapy and surgery have been used alone and together to achieve these aims. Both radiation and surgery are equally effective (the 5-year cure rate for stages I and II is about 85%). The 5-year survival rate for recurrent disease is less than 5%.
- All patients should have long-term follow-up. Pelvic examinations, Pap smears of the vault, and periodic ultrasonography or CT scan should be performed.

IX. Contraception
  A. Natural family planning
   - Natural methods include periodic abstinence based on the last menstrual period (LMP method), also called the rhythm or calendar method (in which intercourse is avoided on days 10 to 19 of the menstrual cycle), and the ovulation method.
   - The ovulation method uses body temperature to predict the time of ovulation and fertility (increased temperature indicates progesterone release). The patient should be abstinent in the first half of the cycle. Sexual intercourse can proceed from the third day after the temperature spike until the end of the menstrual cycle.
   - Advantages: low cost and lack of medication side effects
   - Disadvantages: high failure rate
  B. Hormonal contraceptives
   - Hormonal contraceptives can be taken orally or transdermally, given as an injection or implant, or released from an intrauterine contraceptive device.
   1. Estrogen/progesterone combination pill
     a. The estrogen component of the pill inhibits FSH and the progestins are responsible for suppression of LH. Oral contraceptives also suppress ovulation and alter the properties of cervical mucus. Cervical mucus becomes thick, viscous, and hostile to sperm.
     b. Estrogenic side effects include nausea, cyclic weight gain, edema, and headache. Progestogenic side effects include depression, acne, and hirsutism.

    c. When prescribing oral contraceptives, one must be aware of serious potential complications. There is an increased risk of thromboembolism, myocardial infarction, and stroke. Women who smoke and are over 35 years of age on oral contraceptives are at greatest risk. Hepatomas have also been reported, but these are rare.

    d. Absolute contraindications to the pill:
- Previous history of history of venous thromboembolism
- Previous history of stroke
- Previous history of estrogen-dependent cancers such as breast or endometrial cancer
- Liver disease (severe)
- Undiagnosed vaginal bleeding
- Smokers older than 35 years
- Hypertriglyceridemia

    e. Relative contraindications include poorly controlled hypertension, anticonvulsant therapy, and classic migraine.

    f. Noncontraceptive benefits include protection against ovarian cancer, endometrial cancer (due to the progesterone component), and rheumatoid arthritis and decreased risk of pelvic inflammatory disease (PID) (although barrier contraception should still be used). Women with dysmenorrhea and menorrhagia also get symptomatic relief.

    g. Oral contraceptives are greater than 99% effective if taken properly.

2. Estrogen/progesterone combination patch and ring
- Hormonal contraceptives containing both estrogen and progesterone are also available as a weekly patch (Ortho Evra) or monthly intravaginal ring (Nuvaring). They are both associated with higher rates of compliance due to ease of use.
- Side effects and contraindications are felt to be similar to the pill. Local side effects such as application side redness and irritation for the patch and vaginitis with the ring can occur.
- The patch has limited efficacy in obese patients and should not be used in women heavier than 90 kg. It may be associated with a higher incidence of venous thromboembolic events.

3. Progesterone only pills (POPs)
- These pills contain only the progesterone component and are options for women who need to avoid estrogen. They include smokers older than 35 years, history of thromboembolic disease, cardiac disease, migraine headache, stroke, hypertriglyceridemia, hypertension, early postpartum period, and multisystem SLE. POPs are associated with higher rates of breakthrough bleeding and have higher failure rates.

4. Depo-Provera
- Depo-Provera is a depot intramuscular form of medroxyprogesterone acetate. The dose is 150 mg IM every 3 months. The mechanism of action is the same as with all progestin-only methods.
- Side effects include irregular vaginal bleeding, breast tenderness, weight gain, depression, and hair loss. The incidence of irregular bleeding is

30% within the first year. After several injections, most women become amenorrheic.

- One disadvantage is its association with infertility after discontinuing Depo-Provera. Delayed conception may persist for 9 months. The other disadvantage of Depo-Provera is the associated bone loss, which may be irreversible.
  - It is considered as effective as surgical sterilization.

5. Implantable contraceptives
   a. Norplant has been withdrawn from the market because of questionable contraceptive efficacy. A newer levonorgestrel releasing implant has been approved but is not widely used yet.

C. Intrauterine devices (IUDs)
- IUDs are either made of copper or release progesterone.
- Copper-containing IUDs induce a sterile inflammatory reaction within the uterine cavity that creates a toxic environment for sperm. They remain effective for up to 10 years.
- Progesterone-containing IUDs inhibit sperm survival and implantation. They also decrease menstrual loss and relieve dysmenorrhea and are particularly effective in women with these symptoms and in those on oral anticoagulants.
- Side effects include increased vaginal bleeding, perforation, infection, and displacement. Increased flow is the primary reason women discontinue use. Perforation is rare and occurs in 1 of every 1000 insertions. Infections are believed to be secondary to contamination at the time of insertion and due to high risk sexual behavior and sexually transmitted diseases (STDs). Women who are at low risk of STDs are not at higher risk of PID with use of an IUD. If a patient develops PID, antibiotics must be administered and the IUD must be removed. Therefore, it is prudent not to insert an IUD in a nulliparous woman so as not to impair future fertility. It is also recommended not to insert one in a woman with multiple sexual partners because of the increased risk of infection.
- If a pregnancy occurs with an IUD in place, spontaneous abortion will occur in approximately 50% of cases.
- The efficacy of the IUD is 98%.

D. Barrier methods
- Barrier methods of contraception include condoms, diaphragms, vaginal sponges, and cervical caps. All barrier methods protect against STDs, PID, and therefore cervical cancer.
- Condoms are made of latex or polyurethane (for latex allergy). Their effectiveness is about 85% and is user dependent.
- Diaphragms and cervical caps are dome-shaped and made of latex rubber with a metal spring. They cover the cervix and the anterior vaginal wall and act as physical barriers to sperm. They require fitting by a trained clinician and are only effective if used with spermicidal creams or jellies. Women must be instructed to leave the diaphragm in place for 6 hours after intercourse and must apply more spermicide for each act of repeated intercourse.

Cervical caps can be left in place for up to 48 hours. The effectiveness of the diaphragm is 85%.

- Vaginal sponges do not require fitting and can be left in place for up to 24 hours. They generally have higher failure rates and can be associated with the toxic shock syndrome.
- Spermicides include creams, jellies, foam, and suppositories and are ineffective if used without barrier methods. They do not in themselves protect against STDs or HIV.

E. Surgical sterilization

- These procedures are the most common and most effective form of contraception.
- Careful patient counseling should be provided prior to the procedure, which is considered effectively permanent.
- Female sterilization is performed by tubal obstruction either by ligation, electrocoagulation, or mechanical occlusion of the tubes done laparoscopically or by laparotomy. Hysteroscopic methods are also available. Failure rates are low and are about 18 per 1000 pregnancies. Higher failure rates can occur in younger women and in the postpartum period. Complications include anesthetic and surgical complications, failure, and higher risk of ectopic pregnancies in cases of failure.
- Male sterilization is performed by vasectomy. Vasectomies are safer, easier to perform, and less expensive than female sterilization. Semen analysis should be performed after the procedure to confirm azoospermia and other forms of contraception should be used for at least 12 weeks after the procedure.

X. Ectopic Pregnancy

A. Basic science

- Ectopic pregnancy refers to any pregnancy that implants at a site other than the endometrial cavity. The most common implantation site is within a fallopian tube. Rarely, an ectopic pregnancy may occur concurrently with an intrauterine pregnancy. This is termed a heterotopic pregnancy, which though uncommon, can occur with assisted reproductive technology.
- Ectopic pregnancy complicates 1% to 2% of all pregnancies. Most ectopic pregnancies occur among multiparous women (>50%); only 10% to 15% occur in primigravid women. Ectopic pregnancies are usually symptomatic 6 to 8 weeks after conception.
- Risk factors for ectopic pregnancy:
  1. High risk: previous ectopic pregnancy, previous tubal surgery, tubal pathology (PID), in utero DES (diethylstilbestrol) exposure.
  2. Moderate risk: previous STD, infertility and assisted reproduction techniques, multiple sexual partners, previous pelvic or abdominal surgery, smoking, vaginal douching, early age of intercourse (age <18 years).

B. History and physical examination

- Classically, women with an ectopic pregnancy present with a period of amenorrhea followed by:

    1. Unilateral abdominal pain
    2. Abnormal vaginal bleeding
    3. An adnexal mass
- Almost 50% of patients, however, are asymptomatic until rupture occurs. Rupture is usually accompanied by severe abdominal pain, shock, tachycardia, and shoulder pain secondary to hemoperitoneum. Other symptoms associated with ectopic pregnancy include rectal pressure, absence of menses, dizziness, breast tenderness, nausea, and passage of a decidual cast.
- The physical examination may reveal lateralized lower abdominal pain, vaginal bleeding, an adnexal mass, uterine size smaller than anticipated, cervical motion tenderness, and orthostatic vital signs (or other signs of hemorrhagic shock).

C. Laboratory and diagnostic studies
- In patients with a suspected ectopic pregnancy, the initial blood work should include a CBC, blood type, antibody screen and crossmatch, and quantitation of serum β-hCG levels.
- Patients who are hemodynamically unstable should proceed directly to the operating room after adequate fluid resuscitation. The diagnosis of ectopic pregnancy is made during laparoscopy (laparotomy is rarely required), at which time therapeutic procedures can be performed as well.
- In stable patients with a positive pregnancy test and signs and symptoms suggestive of ectopic pregnancy, an ultrasound must be performed. Ultrasound is used to identify the presence of an intrauterine pregnancy or an adnexal mass. Either transabdominal or transvaginal ultrasound may be used, although transvaginal is more sensitive in early pregnancy.
- An intrauterine gestation sac is usually identifiable by transvaginal ultrasound at serum β-hCG levels of 1500 to 2000 IU/L. Absence of an intrauterine gestation sac at serum β-hCG levels more than 2000 IU/L strongly suggest the possibility of an ectopic pregnancy. In these cases, serial measurement of β-hCG titers may be useful; in a normal pregnancy the titer doubles every 48 hours, whereas ectopic pregnancies rarely display normal increases in β-hCG.
- Other diagnostic modalities such as measurement of progesterone, laparoscopic diagnosis, and culdocentesis are rarely required. Measurement of progesterone is inaccurate and culdocentesis has a low specificity for the diagnosis of ectopic pregnancy.

D. Formulating the diagnosis
- The diagnosis of ectopic pregnancy is suggested by a positive β-hCG in a woman with an empty uterine cavity and an adnexal mass.

E. Evaluating the severity of problems
- Tubal rupture, intraperitoneal hemorrhage, and subsequent hypovolemic shock represent the most serious complications from an ectopic pregnancy. Therefore, women presenting to an emergency department with a suspected ectopic pregnancy should be evaluated urgently. Two large-bore intravenous lines should be secured early in the evaluation.

F. Managing the patient
- Multiple management strategies currently exist for ectopic pregnancy:
  1. Laparotomy with either conservative tubal surgery or salpingectomy
     - Laparotomy is indicated in hemodynamically unstable patients and in patients in whom a large hemoperitoneum is suspected. During laparotomy, a salpingectomy or salpingostomy can be performed. Obviously, greater fertility rates are seen with conservative surgery, but a 15% recurrence risk of ectopic pregnancies results.
  2. Laparoscopic surgery
     - Laparoscopic surgery is now the procedure of choice in stable patients. Studies have shown no difference in conservative procedures whether done laparoscopically or by laparotomy.
  3. Medical management (e.g., methotrexate)
     a. Medical treatment of ectopic pregnancy with methotrexate (MTX) is one of the most important developments in the management of this disorder and has supplanted surgical treatment in hemodynamically stable patients. MTX is a folic acid antagonist that inhibits DNA synthesis primarily in actively proliferating cells.
     b. Potential candidates
        - Asymptomatic patients
        - β-hCG level below 5000 IU/L
        - No fetal cardiac activity
        - Size less than 3 cm
     c. Contraindications
        - Hemodynamic instability
        - Contraindications to MTX, such as alcohol abuse, abnormal liver function tests, immunodeficiency, thrombocytopenia, or leukopenia.
        - A concern about patient compliance
     d. Presence of fetal heart or size greater than 3 cm or β-hCG level above 5000 IU/L is associated with a higher failure rate and need for prolonged monitoring and multiple doses of MTX.
        - Also, Rh-negative women with an ectopic pregnancy should receive RhoGAM.

XI. Endometriosis
  A. Basic science
     - Endometriosis is the presence and growth of uterine glands and stroma outside the endometrial cavity and myometrium. Implants of endometrium may occur anywhere in the body but do so most often in the ovaries and the dependent portions of the pelvis. There is a sevenfold increase in endometriosis among relatives of women with the condition.
  B. History and physical examination
     - Many women are asymptomatic. There is very little correlation between the severity of symptoms and the physical extent (stage) of endometriosis in the pelvis.

- Common symptoms include pelvic pain especially during menses, dyspareunia, abnormal bleeding, cyclic abdominal pain, and, rarely, urinary symptoms or rectal pain and bleeding.
- Infertility is often a major manifestation of the disease.
- Physical findings are variable; often there are no findings on physical examination. The most common finding is tenderness in the posterior fornix. Rarely, a fixed, retroverted uterus with scarring and tenderness posterior to the uterus may be seen. The characteristic nodularity (i.e., endometriomas) of the uterosacral ligaments and cul-de-sac of Douglas may also be felt on rectovaginal examination and may be tender. There may also be adnexal enlargement with tenderness.

C. Laboratory and diagnostic studies
- The definitive diagnosis of endometriosis is made by laparoscopy. Ultrasound may be helpful because it identifies endometriomas, which characteristically have irregular edges, and internal echoes produced by chronic intracystic bleeding. CA 125 is a test with a low sensitivity and specificity; it may be helpful in detecting and monitoring more severe cases. CT and MRI have a limited role.

D. Formulating the diagnosis
- The differential diagnosis should include pelvic inflammatory disease, ovarian neoplasia, and leiomyomas. A presumptive diagnosis may be made clinically but must be confirmed through laparoscopy or laparotomy.

E. Evaluating the severity of problems
- Endometriosis is classified as minimal, mild, moderate, and severe based on the size, depth, and location of the implants and associated adhesions on laparoscopy. The utility of the system is in providing a standard method for reporting operative findings; however, it does not correlate well with patient symptoms or with prognosis for fertility.

F. Managing the patient
- Treatment goals include preservation of fertility (when it is desired), symptom relief, and control of disease with medical therapy. Treatment options for endometriosis are noted here:
  1. Expectant management
     - Recommended for women who are perimenopausal or for women with minimal disease and minimal symptoms.
  2. Analgesia with NSAIDs plus expectant management
  3. Oral contraceptives (cyclic)
     - Oral contraceptives are an option for women with minimal disease who do not desire pregnancy currently; they help retard the progression of the disease. They are especially useful in adolescents because of the contraceptive benefit.
  4. Medical therapy with progestins, continuous combination oral contraceptives, GnRH analogs, and danazol
     - Medical therapies for endometriosis attempt to hormonally simulate pregnancy or menopause, the two physiologic states that inhibit or delay progression of endometriosis by interrupting cyclic ovarian hormone production.

- Progestins, alone or in combination with estrogen, mimic pregnancy; and GnRH analogs and danazol induce a state of "pseudomenopause." Progestins can be given either orally or as IM injections and have potential side effects such as bloating, weight gain, depression, and irregular bleeding; these are generally well tolerated.
- Continuous combination oral contraceptive therapy (continuous oral contraceptive pills without the week of placebo) is another safe and effective option and is generally well tolerated.
- GnRH analogs include nafarelin (intranasal spray) and leuprolide (IM) given for a duration of 3 to 6 months. Side effects include hot flashes, headaches, mood and sleep problems, depression, vaginal dryness, amenorrhea, and osteoporosis. Upon completion of GnRH therapy, the patient begins continuous combination hormonal therapy, as described above.
- Danazol is a testosterone derivative and acts by inhibiting pituitary gonadotropin secretion. Although it has efficacy comparable to GnRH agonists, it has considerable side effects including weight gain, hirsutism, acne, muscle cramps, decreased high-density lipoproteins, increased liver enzymes, hot flashes, mood changes, and depression.

5. Surgical therapy
    - Surgical therapy is divided into conservative and definitive treatment.
        a. Conservative procedures (via laparoscopy) include excision, vaporization, and coagulation of endometriotic implants, excision of ovarian endometriomas, and lysis of adhesions. In patients with extensive disease (e.g., cul-de-sac obliteration and dense scarring of the ovaries to the pelvic side walls), laparotomy may be preferable.
        b. Definitive therapy consists of total abdominal hysterectomy and bilateral oophorectomy and is indicated for patients with persistent pelvic pain after conservative management, or for patients who have completed childbearing.
        c. Approximately one third of the women treated conservatively will have recurrent endometriosis and require additional surgery within 5 years. Following definitive surgery (including bilateral oophorectomy), estrogen replacement therapy is recommended in premenopausal women and may be given with little risk of reactivating residual disease. However, many physicians delay estrogen replacement therapy for 3 to 6 months.

XII. Genetic Counseling
  A. Basic science
    - Approximately 2% to 3% of infants are born with a serious birth defect. Common indications for genetic counseling include the following:
      1. Maternal age above 35 years
      2. Previous child with birth defects or mental retardation or chromosomal anomalies

3. Family history of a hereditary condition (e.g., cystic fibrosis, hemophilia, trisomy 21), biochemical or metabolic conditions (e.g., phenylketonuria deficiency), chromosomal disorders (e.g., Down syndrome, chromosomal translocations), and early cancers.
4. Recurrent pregnancy loss
5. Abnormal maternal serum screening or antenatal ultrasound
6. Teratogen exposure during pregnancy
7. Ethnic background associated with an increased risk of a heritable disorder (e.g., Ashkenazi Jews).

B. History and physical examination
- A four-generation family history should be obtained. Known and suspected genetic conditions should be documented to identify genetic patterns.
- Ethnic and racial background should be identified. Many genetic abnormalities are associated with specific ethnic or racial groups (e.g., sickle cell anemia in African Americans, and Tay-Sachs disease in Jews).
- The physical examination of the prospective mother should include a search for obvious heritable defects.

C. Laboratory and diagnostic studies
- Maternal serum screening with the "quadruple test" between 16 and 18 weeks should be offered to all women. Standard prenatal tests include maternal serum α-fetoprotein, β-hCG, unconjugated estriol, and inhibin A measurement.
- Open neural tube defects and abdominal wall defects have been associated with elevated levels of α-fetoprotein. Abnormally low levels of α-fetoprotein and elevated levels of inhibin-A have been associated with Down syndrome. Results of this test depend on accurate gestational dating. Abnormal α-fetoprotein levels should be followed by an ultrasound and (possibly) amniocentesis.
- Low levels of α-fetoprotein and unconjugated estriol, or elevated levels of hCG, are associated with chromosomal abnormalities. These tests can identify Down syndrome in about 60% of cases. An abnormal serum screen should be confirmed by amniocentesis if a pregnancy termination is going to be considered.
- DNA and biochemical testing are available for many common conditions including cystic fibrosis, hemophilia, Tay-Sachs disease, and sickle cell anemia. Other genetic conditions may require family studies.
- Ultrasound examination offered between 16 and 20 weeks' gestation is a noninvasive procedure that assesses fetal growth and development. Ultrasound acts as a screen for physical birth defects such as neural tube defects. Certain findings (e.g., cystic hygroma) have been associated with chromosome abnormalities. Abnormal findings should prompt other investigations (e.g., amniocentesis).
- Chorionic villus sampling is available between 10 and 12 weeks' gestation. It is used in cases of suspected genetic abnormality. Chorionic villus sampling allows extremely early diagnosis of genetic diseases. The procedure involves placing a needle into the placenta to harvest chorionic cells for chromosomal,

biochemical, or DNA analysis. It is an outpatient procedure done under ultrasound guidance. It is associated with a fetal loss rate of 10%. Chorionic villus sampling cannot detect certain birth defects (e.g., neural tube defects). Women who have this test should also have a maternal serum screen at 16 weeks' gestation.

- Amniocentesis is available between 15 and 17 weeks' gestation. It is used in cases of suspected genetic abnormality. The procedure involves passing a needle into the amniotic sac to harvest amniotic fluid for chromosomal, biochemical, and DNA analysis. α-Fetoprotein testing of the fluid can identify the presence of a fetal neural tube defect. Amniocentesis performed in the second trimester is associated with lesser complications than chorionic villus sampling and is associated with a fetal loss rate of about 7.5%.

D. Formulating the diagnosis
- The diagnosis depends on the results of the specific prenatal test(s).

E. Evaluating the severity of problems
- Certain genetic abnormalities are largely asymptomatic, whereas others result in intrauterine demise or death shortly after birth.

F. Managing the patient
- Effective genetic counseling entails the following:
  1. Providing the family with the diagnosis
  2. Educating the family about the natural history of the condition including its effects on longevity, hospitalization, treatment costs, physical and mental development including ability to engage in daily activities independently, effect on reproductive performance and risk of occurrence in subsequent generations
  3. Screening other family members
  4. Educating the family about options available for this pregnancy
- The counselor must be supportive of the family throughout the decision-making process. Genetic counseling should be nondirective. The counselor should offer an unbiased and complete range of options (e.g., further testing, abortion, or carrying the fetus to term). It is important to have respect for the family's autonomy in making decisions.

XIII. Infections during Pregnancy
A. Basic science
- This section covers six infections commonly encountered during pregnancy: rubella, genital herpes, gonorrhea, chlamydia infection, syphilis, and HIV/AIDS (human immunodeficiency virus/acquired immunodeficiency syndrome).
  1. Rubella
     - Rubella may result in severe congenital malformations including microcephaly, cardiac structural defects, retinopathy, and deafness.
  2. Genital herpes
     - Genital herpes infections are classified as primary or secondary based on clinical or serologic evidence of prior infection.

- Primary infections are usually more severe for the mother and result in increased transmission to the fetus. Congenital infections causing fetal malformations are rare.
- Neonatal infections are acquired as ascending infections around the time of labor and delivery or because of direct contact during delivery. Infection of the newborn usually causes central nervous system (CNS) disease with a 50% mortality rate. Neurologic or ophthalmic sequelae are frequent among infants who survive infections.

3. *Neisseria gonorrhoeae*
- *Neisseria gonorrhoeae,* an aerobic gram-negative bacterium, has a prevalence rate of approximately 1% to 7% during pregnancy. There is an association between untreated gonorrhea and spontaneous abortion, preterm delivery, chorioamnionitis, and postpartum infections.

4. *Chlamydia trachomatis*
- *Chlamydia trachomatis* infection is the most common sexually transmitted bacterial disease in women. Perinatal transmission is associated with neonatal conjunctivitis and pneumonia. Vertical transmission occurs in approximately 50% of infants delivered vaginally by infected women.

5. Syphilis
- Syphilis is a chronic infectious process caused by the spirochete *Treponema pallidum.* The risk of congenital syphilis depends on the stage of maternal disease. In utero infection may result in stillbirth, intrauterine growth retardation, nonimmune hydrops, and premature labor. The spirochete may cause lesions in the lungs, liver, spleen, pancreas, and bones of the newborn.

6. Human immunodeficiency virus
- The rate of perinatal transmission of HIV is approximately 30%. Transmission is by transplacental infection or contraction of the virus at birth. There does not appear to be an increased rate of pregnancy complications such as preterm birth or restricted fetal growth in asymptomatic seropositive women.

B. History and physical examination
1. Rubella
- Rubella is usually asymptomatic in the mother. In symptomatic women, there is a 2- to 3-week incubation period followed by a prodromal phase lasting 1 to 5 days.
- Typical symptoms include low-grade fever, headache, malaise, anorexia, pharyngitis, and cervical adenopathy. A pink macular rash then appears and spreads quickly to involve the entire body.
- Fetal infection after maternal viremia leads to chronic infection, which affects organogenesis.

2. Genital herpes
- A primary infection with herpesvirus is characterized by painful vesicles on the vulva and perineum. Inguinal adenopathy and influenza-like symptoms may also occur. Recurrent infections generally have fewer lesions that shed the virus for shorter periods (2 to 5 days).

3. *Neisseria gonorrhoeae*
   - Women with gonococcal infection may display a mucopurulent cervical discharge or may be entirely asymptomatic.
   - Infections early in pregnancy may ascend and cause endometritis and spontaneous abortion. After 10 to 12 weeks ascending infections are not seen, but adherence of gonococci to chorionic membranes may cause premature labor or premature rupture of membranes.
4. *Chlamydia trachomatis*
   - Chlamydial infections may be associated with several clinical syndromes that include urethritis, mucopurulent cervicitis, and salpingitis, but most pregnant women have subclinical or asymptomatic infection.
5. Syphilis
   - The primary infectious lesion of syphilis is the chancre. It is a painless ulcer with a raised, indurated border that appears on the perineum, vulva, or cervix 2 to 3 weeks after exposure.
   - Between 6 weeks and several months after the appearance of the primary chancre, a systemic response is seen with fever and malaise. Skin manifestations include genital condylomata lata and red macules on the palms or soles.
   - Manifestations of late syphilis usually involve the cardiovascular and neurologic systems.
6. HIV
   - Individuals with HIV/AIDS develop lymphadenopathy, night sweats, fevers, opportunistic infections, and certain neoplasms.
   - Preliminary studies suggest that pregnancy does not appear to influence the progression of HIV infection in women.

C. Laboratory and diagnostic studies
   - Maternal serum is obtained to detect IgG specific for rubella. Absence of the rubella antibody indicates susceptibility to infection. The diagnosis of perinatal rubella infection in the newborn is supported by the presence of IgM in cord blood.
   - Virus isolation and tissue culture is the method used to diagnose herpes simplex virus.
   - Antepartum cervical sampling is the best method to detect gonorrhea and chlamydia.
   - The rapid plasma reagin (RPR) and venereal disease research laboratory (VDRL) serologic tests are commonly used to screen for syphilis. These tests lack specificity, and a direct treponemal test such as the fluorescent treponemal antibody absorption test (FTA-ABS) is used to confirm a positive result. Response to treatment may be followed by observing a decreasing serologic titer. (i.e., RPR or VDRL).
   - ELISA (enzyme-linked immunosorbent assay) is used as the initial screen for HIV. All positive results are followed by a Western blot test that identifies antibodies to specific viral proteins.

D. Formulating the diagnosis

- The diagnosis of each infection is made after considering the history, physical examination, and diagnostic test findings. Beyond diagnosing the maternal condition, specific techniques such as ultrasound, chorionic villus sampling, and cordocentesis may help to identify fetal infection.

E. Evaluating the severity of problems
- Each of the maternal infections (except HIV/AIDS) is usually mild and self-limited if properly treated. Fetal (and neonatal) outcomes depend on the developmental stage at the time of infection. Ultrasound may be helpful in evaluating growth restriction or congenital anomalies.

F. Managing the patient
- An attenuated live virus vaccine is available to provide immunity to rubella. All women are screened at the start of prenatal care. Seronegative (i.e., nonimmune) pregnant women are not given the vaccine during pregnancy; rather, the rubella vaccine is administered shortly after delivery. The impact of rubella on the fetus is most severe when acquired early in gestation. Fetal manifestations range from asymptomatic to congenital rubella syndrome to intrauterine demise.
- Unless previous herpes infection has been documented, all suspicious lesions should be cultured. An infant is at risk of acquiring herpes if the mother has an active lesion at the time of delivery. Maternal infection is also assumed if the woman is experiencing prodromal symptoms. If either prodromal symptoms or lesions are present, a cesarean delivery should be performed.
- Cervical sampling to screen for gonorrhea and chlamydia is usually performed at the first prenatal visit. A single intramuscular dose of ceftriaxone is recommended for treating gonococcal infection. A 7-day course of oral erythromycin is the first line of therapy for chlamydial infections in pregnant women. The sexual partner of any woman with chlamydia or gonorrhea should also be treated. Patients with positive cultures should be retested later in pregnancy to identify treatment failures or reinfection.
- A serologic test for syphilis is part of routine antenatal screening. Penicillin is the treatment of choice to eradicate maternal infection and to prevent congenital syphilis. Benzathine penicillin G cures early maternal infection and prevents neonatal syphilis in 98% of cases.
- The pregnant woman who has AIDS or is HIV positive must be appropriately counseled regarding the risks of fetal transmission. Antepartum and intrapartum use of zidovudine (AZT) has been shown to decrease the risk of transmission from 30% to 8%. Women with AIDS should be advised against breastfeeding. Women with a high viral load should be advised to undergo elective cesarean section to reduce the risk of fetal transmission.

XIV. Infertility
A. Basic science
- Infertility is the failure of a couple to achieve a pregnancy after 12 months of intercourse without contraception. Overall, infertility affects 15% of couples at any given time. For normal couples the probability of achieving a pregnancy during a single menstrual cycle is about 25%.

- Factors responsible for infertility include the following:
    1. Pelvic pathology (tubal disease and endometriosis)
    2. Male related disorders
    3. Ovulation disorders
    4. Cervical factor
    5. Coital disorders
    6. Unexplained or idiopathic
- After the age of 30, women show a substantial decline in fertility and an increase in spontaneous pregnancy loss. This is due to follicular loss secondary to age-related increase in chromosomal abnormalities in the oocyte and embryo.

B. History and physical examination

- Important historical information includes the duration of infertility, the age and general health of the partners, prior pregnancies and medical problems, and history of prior STDs, cigarette smoking, alcohol/drug use, and current medications. Inquiry should also be made about intercourse frequency and the use of lubricants (which may adversely affect sperm function).
- Questions for men include occupational history, history of mumps orchitis, hernias, testicular injuries, and operations. Sperm function can be affected by chemotherapeutic agents, cimetidine, and calcium channel blockers. The physical examination should focus on the sexual characteristics and the genitalia. Varicocele is the most common abnormality found on the male examination.
- For the female, the menstrual cycle history is critical. Anovulatory females may present with amenorrhea or dysfunctional uterine bleeding. A history of hirsutism, acne, or galactorrhea may point to a specific endocrine problem. A history of IUD use, particularly if associated with a pelvic infection, may suggest a tubal factor. Progressively worsening dysmenorrhea or dyspareunia may suggest endometriosis. The physical examination should include a detailed pelvic examination. Pelvic tenderness may suggest the presence of endometriosis, pelvic infection, or abdominal/pelvic adhesive disease.

C. Laboratory and diagnostic studies

1. Male factor
    - The initial diagnostic test is semen analysis. Parameters assessed include semen volume and sperm concentration, motility, and morphology.
2. Ovulatory factor
    - The simplest means to reasonably confirm ovulation is to document the basal body temperature. No increase in basal body temperature during the midcycle suggests anovulation. However, this method is cumbersome and not very accurate. A single serum progesterone level in the luteal phase showing levels more than 10 ng/mL is an accurate predictor of ovulation. If a patient does not show a midcycle progesterone increase, then she is anovulatory. Home urinary LH kits measure the urine LH surge which occurs 1 to 2 days before ovulation and can also be used to document ovulation.

- Anovulation or a history of irregular periods should be investigated with measurements of TSH, FSH, LH, PRL, and serum androgens. Patients with hypothalamic disturbances have low FSH and LH concentrations. Patients with ovarian failure have high FSH concentrations. A high prolactin concentration may suggest a prolactinoma. Patients with the polycystic ovarian syndrome often have high androgen concentrations.
    3. Tubal/peritoneal factor
    - Tubal disease is assessed by the hysterosalpingogram (HSG). HSG provides information about tubal obstruction and uterine cavity abnormalities. Laparoscopy is done if the HSG findings are abnormal or if peritoneal disease is suspected. Laparoscopy may reveal the presence of adhesions or demonstrate endometriosis.
    4. Cervical factor
    - Interactions between cervical mucus and sperm is an infrequent cause of infertility. The postcoital test is therefore not routinely performed in the initial evaluation.
- D. Formulating the diagnosis
    1. Male factor
    - The male is the cause of infertility in 30% to 40% of cases. Most cases involve defects in spermatogenesis due to primary (testicular disease) or secondary (hypothalamic or pituitary disease) hypogonadism.
    2. Ovulatory factor
    - Ovulatory dysfunction (generally anovulation) is the problem in 15% to 20% of cases.
    3. Tubal/peritoneal factor
    - About 30% of infertility cases are due to tubal/peritoneal factors. The two most common causes of infertility in this area are endometriosis and previous PID. *Chlamydia trachomatis*–induced PID may cause significant tubal damage in the absence of symptoms.
    4. Cervical factor
    - Infertility is attributed to cervical factors in 3% of cases.
- E. Evaluating the severity of problems
    - Couples affected by sterility should be provided with information about adoption.
- F. Managing the patient
    - Overall, about half of couples seeking infertility care ultimately achieve a pregnancy.
    - Anovulation is handled by treating the underlying defect. Patients with hypothalamic amenorrhea are best treated with gonadotropin preparations or pulsatile GnRH therapy. Hyperprolactinemia is treated medically with a dopamine agonist (e.g., bromocriptine). Patients with large pituitary tumors should be referred to a neurosurgeon. Patients with polycystic ovarian disease are initially treated with clomiphene citrate with or without metformin. If the response is unsatisfactory, gonadotropin preparations may be used.
    - Tubal/peritoneal factors generally require surgical therapy. Surgery ranges from laparoscopic ablation of endometriosis to tubal microsurgery.

Occasionally, infertility patients with endometriosis may benefit from medical therapy such as danazol (Danocrine) or a long-acting GnRH agonist.

- Couples failing to achieve pregnancy may opt to proceed with an assisted reproductive technology procedure (ART). All procedures involve oocyte retrieval after administration of a superovulation regimen.

  1. In vitro fertilization–embryo transfer (IVF-ET). Oocytes are inseminated in vitro 4 to 6 hours after retrieval. Embryo transfer into the uterus follows in 2 to 3 days.

  2. GIFT (gamete intrafallopian tube transfer). GIFT involves transferring both oocytes and sperm into the fallopian tube. Fertilization occurs within the fallopian tube. Women undergoing GIFT must have at least one normal, functioning tube.

  3. ICSI (intracytoplasmic sperm injection). ICSI is a newer advancement in the treatment of severe sperm abnormalities and is associated with high rates of fertilization. It involves the direct injection of a spermatid into the oocytes. It has a pregnancy rate per embryo transfer of 41%, a rate similar to patients with normal sperm.

     - Pregnancy rates are 17% for IVF-ET and 26% for GIFT. Complications associated with ART techniques include ovarian hyperstimulation syndrome, multiple gestation, preterm birth, and low birth weight.

XV. Leiomyoma

A. Basic science

- Leiomyomas are benign smooth muscle tumors. They are the most common pelvic tumor, affecting 20% to 25% of women of reproductive age. They are 10 times more common in black women. In the United States, leiomyomas are the most common indication for a hysterectomy.

- Leiomyomas often cause abnormal uterine bleeding, typically menorrhagia or hypermenorrhea (prolonged bleeding). Intermenstrual bleeding is not characteristic of myomas and must be investigated to exclude endometrial disease. Larger fibroids can be associated with urinary frequency, constipation, and dyspareunia secondary to pressure effects. Rarely, leiomyomas may degenerate, causing severe pain and peritoneal irritation.

- Submucous fibroids have been associated with subfertility. During pregnancy approximately one third of women experience increased growth of fibroids in the first trimester; the remaining women have stable or reduced tumor size. Adverse pregnancy outcomes including first trimester bleeding, abruption, intrauterine growth restriction, pain, preterm labor, retained placenta, dysfunctional labor, breech presentation, and increased risk of cesarean delivery can occur.

- Leiomyomas vary greatly in size, from microscopic growths to tumors weighing more than 100 pounds. It is common to find multiple tumors. Estrogen is thought to promote their growth.

- Histologically, leiomyomas have a characteristic whorled appearance, and each myoma is surrounded by a pseudocapsule (a layer of compressed muscle cells). This pseudocapsule is helpful by providing a surgical plane during excision (myomectomy).

B. History and physical examination
- Most women with leiomyomas are asymptomatic. Often leiomyomas are detected as enlarged, mobile uterus with an irregular contour on a routine pelvic examination or as an incidental finding during transabdominal ultrasonography. The most common symptom associated with leiomyomas is abnormal bleeding, typically abnormally heavy or prolonged menstrual bleeding. Pelvic pain, increasing in severity with menstruation, is another frequent symptom. The tumor may push on the bladder, causing urinary frequency and urgency.
- Reproductive problems such as infertility; recurrent, spontaneous abortions; and preterm labor have also been associated with leiomyomas.
- The pelvic examination may demonstrate an enlarged, firm, nontender, mobile, irregular uterus.

C. Laboratory and diagnostic studies
- Most leiomyomas are diagnosed through the physical examination. An ultrasound may help confirm the diagnosis. Hysteroscopy (a scope introduced into the uterus) can be used to diagnose leiomyomas directly. When abnormal bleeding presents, an endometrial biopsy should be performed to rule out endometrial hyperplasia or cancer. Baseline laboratory tests such as a pregnancy test should be performed.

D. Formulating the diagnosis
- Usually the diagnosis of leiomyoma is made after a pelvic examination. In the remaining cases, an ultrasound may be needed. The differential diagnosis includes pregnancy, adenomyosis, leiomyosarcoma, and ovarian neoplasia.

E. Evaluating the severity of problems
- Most women with leiomyomas are asymptomatic. A hematocrit should be obtained on patients with abnormally heavy menstrual bleeding to rule out anemia. In certain cases, an endometrial biopsy should also be performed to rule out endometrial hyperplasia.
- A uterine growth occurring after menopause is worrisome because of the potential for malignancy (e.g., leiomyosarcoma). In these circumstances, a hysterectomy should be performed.
- During pregnancy, degeneration of the leiomyoma is not uncommon. The patient may present with a low-grade fever, uterine tenderness, and mild peritoneal signs. These symptoms may mimic placental abruption and chorioamnionitis.

F. Managing the patient
- Most leiomyomas are asymptomatic. Patients without symptoms are managed by periodic pelvic examinations to follow the uterine growth rate. Medical or surgical management is indicated for symptomatic leiomyomas. Age, desire for fertility, and general health determine the treatment modality.
- Medical management consists of NSAIDs for symptomatic relief of menorrhagia and dysmenorrhea, oral contraceptives, progestins, danazol, and GnRH agonists. GnRH agonists reduce uterine volume by 50%. However,

myomas regrow after GnRH agonist therapy is stopped. Because of side effects such as decreased bone density, GnRH agonists should be used for no more than 6 months. They are primarily used 2 to 3 months preoperatively to facilitate surgery by reducing fibroid size, improving preoperative hematocrit, and reducing postoperative blood loss.

- Surgical management includes myomectomy, hysteroscopic endometrial ablation, and hysterectomy.
  1. The primary advantage of a myomectomy is that the uterus is preserved and the patient remains fertile. Myomectomy can be performed by laparotomy, laparoscopy, or hysteroscopy. Complications include recurrence and a risk of uterine rupture during pregnancy.
  2. Endometrial ablation can be performed in women who have completed childbearing and can be combined with hysteroscopic myomectomy in women who want to avoid hysterectomy. Hysteroscopic ablation using a rollerball, laser, or liquid nitrogen cryotherapy is commonly used.
  3. Uterine artery embolization is a procedure performed by interventional radiologists. Under fluoroscopic guidance, a catheter is inserted into the uterine arteries and an embolizing agent is injected.
  4. Hysterectomy is the definitive treatment for uterine myomas. In women who fail conservative medical management and no longer desire fertility, a hysterectomy should be considered.
- Use of oral contraceptive pills and hormone therapy in the postmenopausal age group is not contraindicated in women with a fibroid uterus. Oral contraceptive pills can cause a decrease in the size of fibroids in the premenopausal woman. However, estrogen therapy in the postmenopausal age group has been associated with continuation of symptoms due to some growth in the size of the existing myomas (not associated with development of new symptomatic fibroids).

XVI. Menopause and Hormone Therapy
   A. Basic science
   - Menopause is defined as the absence of menses for 1 year. Perimenopause refers to the 2 to 8 years preceding and 1 year following menopause when fluctuating ovarian function is common. The mean age of menopause is 51 years. The age at menopause is largely genetically determined. If menopause occurs before the age of 40, the diagnosis of premature ovarian failure is made.
   - The basic feature of menopause is depletion of ovarian follicles. This begins in utero and continues throughout life. As follicles are depleted, cyclic hormonal patterns are lost. Estradiol (E2) is the dominant estrogen produced by the dominant follicle during the monthly menstrual cycle and is the most potent natural estrogen. During menopause, estradiol and progesterone levels decline, resulting in increases in FSH and LH. Estrone (E1), a weak estrogen, becomes the most dominant form of estrogen during menopause. It is produced in small quantities by the ovary and adrenals but is mainly derived by the peripheral conversion of androstenedione in adipose tissue.

B. History and physical examination
- Symptoms of menopause relate to the lack of estrogen in multiple organ systems and include:
  1. Vasomotor symptoms—hot flashes
  2. Mood and sleep disturbances, hair loss
  3. Urinary symptoms including dysuria, frequency, stress incontinence, vaginal dryness
  4. Vaginal itching, burning, discomfort, dyspareunia, and bleeding secondary to atrophy
  5. Uterine descent, cystocele, rectocele, and enterocele
  6. Later onset disease processes such as osteoporosis

C. Laboratory and diagnostic studies
- Serum FSH and LH will be elevated in untreated postmenopausal women. Vaginal cytologic examination will reveal a low estrogen effect with a predominance of parabasal cells.
- Health maintenance tests include annual mammograms, annual to every third year Pap smears depending on risk factors, and a baseline bone density test after the age of 65 or earlier in the presence of risk factors.

D. Formulating the diagnosis
- Hot flashes, mood and sleep changes, and minor urinary symptoms are early symptoms and sometimes precede the onset of menopause. FSH levels fluctuate and are unreliable in the perimenopausal period. However, in the presence of prolonged amenorrhea with hot flashes, an FSH of 40 mIU/mL or more is diagnostic of menopause.

E. Evaluating the severity of problems
- Any episode of vaginal bleeding in the postmenopausal period needs investigation. Causes for postmenopausal bleeding include endometrial hyperplasia and carcinoma, endometrial polyps, cervical dysplasia, infections, atrophic vaginitis, estrogen therapy, fibroids or adenomyosis, and diverticulitis or urethritis. A thorough physical and pelvic examination with Pap smear must be performed. An outpatient endometrial biopsy should be performed to evaluate for endometrial cancer. Some physicians prefer to obtain a transvaginal ultrasound and perform a biopsy if the endometrial thickness is more than 4 mm (postmenopausal endometrium should be atrophic and less than 4 mm thick).

F. Managing the patient
- Hormone therapy (estrogen and progesterone therapy, formerly called "hormone replacement therapy") is no longer routinely recommended to all postmenopausal women. Menopause is treated on a symptomatic basis. Risks of hormone therapy include an increased risk of strokes, thromboembolic disease, gallbladder disease, endometrial cancer with unopposed estrogen use (without progesterone), and breast cancer.
- Absolute contraindications to hormone therapy include pregnancy, active venous thrombosis or pulmonary embolism, undiagnosed vaginal bleeding, active liver disease, active breast or endometrial cancer, and active cardiovascular disease. Relative contraindications include past history of

breast or uterine cancer, previous thromboembolism, gallbladder disease, uncontrolled hypertension, migraine headaches, uterine fibroids, seizure disorders, hypertriglyceridemia, and a history of cardiovascular disease.

- Benefits of hormone therapy include relief of hot flashes and mood disturbances, improvement in vaginal atrophy, and osteoporosis prevention.
- Hormone therapy is no longer used to prevent cardiovascular diseases and may increase a women's risk of cardiovascular diseases. Lifestyle changes; adequate control of hypertension, diabetes and hyperlipidemia; and antiplatelet therapy remain the cornerstone of cardiovascular disease prevention.
- Vasomotor symptoms can be bothersome in some patients and may not respond to conservative measures. Hormone therapy is currently indicated for the treatment of hot flashes and mood disturbances in women without risk factors and should be given at the lowest dose and for the shortest possible time, usually not for more than 5 years. Use of hormone therapy in the immediate postmenopausal period and in women with premature menopause or after hysterectomy in early life may have lesser complications than its use in the later postmenopausal period.
- Estrogen is available as oral estrogen, transdermal estrogen, intravaginal rings, or vaginal creams. Lower doses such as 0.45 or 0.3 mg may suffice. Women with an intact uterus should be given medroxyprogesterone acetate or micronized estrogen for 12 days in the cycle to produce withdrawal bleed for endometrial protection. Transdermal forms can be used in women who cannot tolerate oral pills due to nausea and in women with hypertriglyceridemia. Local (vaginal) preparations have minimal systemic absorption and can be used to relieve vaginal atrophic symptoms; these do not require progesterone therapy. Alternatives to hormone therapy for hot flashes (not FDA approved) include SSRIs, Venlafaxine, gabapentin, clonidine, and herbal products such as black cohosh, although none are as efficacious for vasomotor symptoms.
- Osteoporosis prevention can be achieved by daily intake of 1500 mg of elemental calcium along with 800 IU of vitamin D and weight-bearing exercise. Treatment options for osteoporosis include bisphosphonates, SERMs (selective estrogen receptor modulators, e.g., raloxifene), calcitonin, and parathyroid hormone.

XVII. Ovarian Cancer
  A. Basic science
    - Ovarian cancer occurs most often in women over 50 years of age. The lifetime risk of ovarian cancer is between 1% and 2%, but women with a *BRCA1* or *BRCA2* gene mutation carry a 45% or 25% lifetime risk of ovarian cancer, respectively.
    - About 90% of ovarian cancer originates from ovarian epithelial cells; 5% originates from germ cells, and 5% are sex-cord stromal tumors. Germ cell tumors are most common in the first two decades of life.

B. History and physical examination
- Ovarian tumors grow insidiously and are usually large before symptoms appear. The most common symptoms of ovarian cancer are vague and include abdominal discomfort, fullness, early satiety, fatigue, increasing abdominal girth, urinary frequency, and constipation.
- The etiology of ovarian cancer is poorly understood. The most significant risk factor is a positive family history, including family history of colon and breast cancer. Advanced age is also associated with an increased risk. High parity, oral contraceptive use, tubal ligation, and hysterectomy decrease one's risk of developing ovarian cancer.
- Pelvic examination is inefficient in detecting presymptomatic early ovarian cancer. However, symptomatic patients have a fixed ovarian mass. Abdominal examination may reveal ascites and an omental cake may be palpable in the upper abdomen.
- Adnexal mass in a younger woman may be caused by a physiologic ovarian cyst. The ovaries of postmenopausal women are not palpable. Therefore, any palpable mass in a postmenopausal woman is an ovarian tumor until proved otherwise.

C. Laboratory and diagnostic studies
- There is currently no effective mass screening method to detect ovarian cancer. Pelvic exam, CA 125, and transvaginal ultrasound have all been evaluated and have been proved to be ineligible screening tests to date.
- Patients with suspected ovarian cancer should have a workup that includes colonoscopy or barium enema to detect primary or metastatic colon cancer. Chest x-ray examination is required to detect metastatic lung cancer. A mammogram should be performed to detect a primary breast cancer that may have metastasized to the ovaries. A CT scan is used to detect liver and lymph node metastasis.
- CA 125 is a tumor marker elevated in most patients with epithelial ovarian carcinomas, but the test is not specific and may be elevated in a variety of other disorders. CA 125 is useful for assessing the response of ovarian cancer to chemotherapy.
- α-Fetoprotein, β-hCG, and LDH may be expressed by some germ cell tumors.

D. Formulating the diagnosis
- Ovarian cancer is diagnosed by histologic examination of the tumor. Ovarian cancer is surgically staged as follows:
  1. Stage I: growth limited to the ovaries
  2. Stage II: growth involving one or both ovaries with pelvic extension
  3. Stage III: growth involving one or both ovaries with extension outside the pelvis or positive lymph nodes
  4. Stage IV: growth involving one or both ovaries with distant metastases
- Higher stages are associated with a poor outcome. Five-year survival rates for ovarian epithelial cancer are as follows: stage I, 60% to 90%; stage II, 39% to 67%; stage III, 4% to 13%; and stage IV, 0% to 4%.

E. Evaluating the severity of problems
- Because of difficulty in detection before dissemination, ovarian cancer is the leading cause of death among women with gynecologic cancers.

F. Managing the patient
- Operative management is aimed at resection of as much tumor as possible. A total abdominal hysterectomy, bilateral salpingo-oophorectomy, node biopsy, omentectomy, and removal of all gross cancer (debulking) are performed whenever malignant disease is present. Both pelvic and periaortic lymph nodes should be sampled.
- Postoperative chemotherapy is employed in the treatment of stage II to IV ovarian cancer. Chemotherapy regimens often include multiple agents such as cisplatin, carboplatin, paclitaxel, doxorubicin, topotecan and gemcitabine in varying combinations.
- Intestinal obstruction secondary to advanced disease may benefit from palliative surgery. Prognosis is very poor in diffuse peritoneal carcinomatosis.

XVIII. Pelvic Inflammatory Disease
A. Basic science
- Pelvic inflammatory disease (PID) refers to acute infection of the upper genital tract structures in women, involving any or all of the uterus, fallopian tubes, and ovaries; this is often accompanied by involvement of the neighboring pelvic organs. By definition, PID is a community-acquired infection initiated by a sexually transmitted agent, distinguishing it from pelvic infections caused by medical procedures, pregnancy, and other primary abdominal processes.
- PID is most often caused by *Chlamydia trachomatis* and *Neisseria gonorrhoeae* (GC). Other endogenous organisms that can be involved include anarerobes, eneteric gram-negative rods, and streptococci.
- *Neisseria gonorrhoeae* is a gram-negative intracellular diplococcus. The organism is found within polymorphonuclear leukocytes.
- *Chlamydia trachomatis* is an obligate intracellular parasite. It is the most common cause of chronic PID and coexists with GC in up to one third of infections.
- PID occurs primarily in young, sexually active women. It is estimated that 5% of sexually active women in the United States have infection with *Chlamydia* or GC.

B. History and physical examination
- The classic presentation of PID is with lower abdominal pain associated with fever, increased white blood cell count, and purulent cervical discharge.
- More commonly, PID presents with progressively worsening lower abdominal pain beginning after menses, sometimes subtle and usually of less than 2 weeks' duration. Myalgia and fever may occur. The following are associated with an increased risk of PID: age less than 35 years, use of a nonbarrier contraceptive, new or multiple or symptomatic sexual partner, and previous history of PID.

- The physical examination may reveal a febrile patient who walks in a stooped position, taking small, shuffling steps. Lower abdominal examination may demonstrate mild guarding and rebound because peritoneal irritation adjacent to the site of infection usually occurs. Tenderness in the right upper quadrant occurs in 10% of cases due to the associated perihepatitis (Fitz-Hugh-Curtis syndrome).
- Pelvic examination reveals tender adnexa with or without masses, cervical motion tenderness, and a purulent cervical discharge.

C. Laboratory and diagnostic studies
1. All patients should have a pregnancy test and urinalysis. Specimens from the cervical os should be collected and sent for culture, rapid antigen test, Gram stain, and microscopy.
    - The definitive test for *Chlamydia* is a rapid, direct antigen test.
    - Gram stain may demonstrate gram-negative intracellular diplococci indicating GC infection. The definitive diagnosis of GC infection is by culture.
2. Other diagnostic modalities include the following:
    - Ultrasound is performed to rule out abscess and ectopic pregnancy (when suspected).
    - ESR and CRP are elevated in cases of PID.
    - Laparoscopy is performed if the diagnosis is uncertain. It directly visualizes the reproductive organs.
    - Abdominal x-ray examination or CT scan is performed if the diagnosis is uncertain.

D. Formulating the diagnosis
- All sexually active young women with the combination of lower abdominal, adnexal, and cervical motion tenderness should receive empiric treatment. The specificity of these clinical criteria can be enhanced by the presence of fever, abnormal cervical/vaginal discharge, elevated ESR, and serum C-reactive protein, and the demonstration of cervical gonorrhea or chlamydial infection.
- Beware of the wrong diagnosis. It is often difficult to differentiate PID from acute appendicitis, diverticulitis (in an older patient), endometriosis, ovarian torsion, ectopic pregnancy, pyelonephritis, and inflammatory bowel disease. Of note, a pregnancy test should always be done in a woman of reproductive age who presents with abdominal pain.

E. Evaluating the severity of problems
- Abscess (tubal, ovarian, or pelvic) may form during any stage of the disease. Perforation of an adnexal abscess may lead to peritonitis, endotoxemia, and shock (a surgical emergency).
- PID scars the fallopian tubes. Long-term complications include ectopic pregnancy, infertility, and chronic pelvic pain.

F. Managing the patient
- High-risk behaviors (e.g., numerous sexual partners, lack of barrier contraceptive use) should be identified and brought to the patient's attention. Patients with a history of an STD should be tested for *Chlamydia,* GC,

syphilis, hepatitis B and C, and HIV. Pap smears must be performed. The patient's partner should also be tested and treated (if necessary).

- Immediately after cervical specimens are collected, the patient should receive antibiotics. It is inappropriate to wait for culture results before beginning treatment. Early antibiotic therapy will decrease the risk of infertility.
- The following are recommended outpatient regimens (multiple antibiotics are given concurrently because the organisms often coexist):
  1. Ceftriaxone 250 mg IM single dose and doxycycline 100 mg PO bid and metronidazole 500 mg PO twice a day for 2 weeks; *or*
  2. Ofloxacin 400 mg PO twice a day or levofloxacin 500 mg once daily and azithromycin 2 g PO once and metronidazole 500 mg PO twice a day for 2 weeks.
- Patients should be seen again within 2 days. Admission to the hospital for intravenous antibiotic therapy is indicated if the diagnosis is uncertain; the patient is poorly compliant, has HIV, is pregnant, or fails outpatient treatment; or fallopian tube scarring or abscess has occurred.
- For inpatient treatment, antibiotics are given until the patient clinically improves and are then continued for an additional 24 to 48 hours. In the hospital, appropriate antibiotic regimens include intravenous ceftizoxime and intravenous doxycycline until improved (followed by oral doxycycline for a total of 14 days) or intravenous clindamycin and gentamicin.
- It must be remembered that patients with *Chlamydia trachomatis* infection and other STDs must have follow-up at 6 months with pelvic examination and cultures to document eradication of infection.

XIX. Placenta Previa
  A. Basic science
  - Placenta previa is a condition in which the placenta covers or adjoins the internal cervical os; it is a common cause of painless third trimester bleeding. A complete placenta previa completely covers the os; a partial placenta previa covers only part of the os, whereas a marginal placenta previa is a placenta lying in the lower uterine segment without covering the os.
  - The incidence of placenta previa is about 1 in 200. The incidence increases with age and parity. Other risk factors include previous cesarean delivery, uterine curettage for previous spontaneous or induced abortion, and multiple gestations.
  - Placenta accreta is a condition in which the placenta is adherent to the myometrium and occurs with a higher frequency in low lying placenta; it is a cause of postpartum hemorrhage.
  B. History and physical examination
  - Placenta previa classically presents with painless vaginal bleeding occurring around the 30th week. The bleeding is attributed to tearing of the placental attachments during formation of the lower uterine segment and effacement and dilatation of the cervix, which occurs around this gestational period. Many patients are diagnosed by ultrasound before vaginal bleeding occurs. Early ultrasound, however, is not a good predictor of placenta previa later in

pregnancy because 90% of low lying placentas in the first trimester resolve during later pregnancy.

- It is extremely important that placenta previa be excluded by ultrasound before a digital vaginal examination or speculum examination is performed. This simple manipulation can cause increased bleeding.

C. Laboratory and diagnostic studies

- The definitive diagnostic study is transabdominal ultrasound to determine placental location. In patients with bleeding, a hematocrit may be helpful in quantifying blood loss. A blood type, antibody screen, and coagulation studies should also be obtained. Continuous fetal monitoring should be done until the bleeding is stabilized or delivery occurs.

D. Formulating the diagnosis

- The diagnosis is established by a ultrasound examination that demonstrates placenta over the cervical os. Once placenta previa is excluded, other causes of bleeding late in pregnancy (e.g., placental abruption, cervical polyps or cancer, and cervical or vaginal trauma) are considered.
- Ultrasound should also evaluate for the presence of vasa previa (fetal vessels exposed in the placental membranes) and placenta accreta. Both of these coexist with placenta previa and early prediction can prevent catastrophic events such as fetal hemorrhage and death, and maternal hemorrhage later.

E. Evaluating the severity of problems

- The status of the fetus (based on fetal monitoring) and the hemodynamic stability of the mother are the main factors in evaluating the severity of problems.

F. Managing the patient

- The preterm patient with placenta previa who is not actively bleeding can often be observed at home with vaginal rest and close follow-up. Patients may be offered phlebotomy for autologous blood banking. There is an increased likelihood of preterm delivery. All mothers at less than 36 weeks' gestation should be offered antenatal steroids to promote fetal lung maturity in the event of preterm labor.
- Any patient with evidence of fetal or maternal compromise should be admitted to the hospital for close monitoring including insertion of two large-bore IV cannulas, continuous monitoring of maternal vital signs (and urine output), fetal heart rate monitoring, crystalloid replacement (± packed red blood cells), frequent laboratory studies including CBC, coagulation profile, and renal function test.
- Abdominal delivery by cesarean section is indicated in the presence of complete placenta previa or the presence of maternal or fetal compromise. The role of vaginal delivery is restricted to select cases of marginal placenta previa in advanced labor without excessive hemorrhage and a reassuring fetal heart tracing. From 5% to 10% of placenta previa may be complicated by placenta accreta (especially with a history of previous lower segment cesarian section) and may necessitate an abdominal hysterectomy in the event of severe postpartum hemorrhage.

XX. Preeclampsia and Eclampsia
   A. Basic science
      - Preeclampsia refers to the new onset of hypertension and proteinuria after 20 weeks of gestation in a previously normotensive woman. Eclampsia describes the development of grand mal seizures in a woman with preeclampsia. The seizures should not be attributable to another cause.
      - Preeclampsia is a state of endothelial dysfunction secondary to excessive amounts of circulating factors that are released by the diseased placenta. It complicates 5% to 7% of all deliveries, primarily nulliparas at the extremes of reproductive age.
      - The clinical presentation is mediated by arteriolar constriction and increased vascular sensitivity to pressors. Vasospasm leads to increased peripheral vascular resistance, hypertension, and vascular endothelial damage, followed by endothelial cell contraction. This results in interendothelial leakage, interstitial edema, hemorrhage, and ultimately end-organ necrosis.
      - Risk factors associated with the development of preeclampsia include primigravidas younger than age 20, past history of preeclampsia, preexisting chronic hypertension, multiple pregnancy, advanced maternal age, rheumatologic disease, pregestational diabetes and maternal age more than 35 to 40 years.
   B. History and physical examination
      - The hallmark symptoms reported by the patient with preeclampsia are headache, visual disturbances, rapid weight gain, increased edema, nausea, vomiting, right upper quadrant pain, and seizures (in eclampsia). The physical examination will reveal hypertension, generalized nondependent edema, hyperreflexia, right upper quadrant/epigastric tenderness (secondary to subcapsular liver hematoma), and oliguria.
   C. Laboratory and diagnostic studies
      - Hemoconcentration is produced by relative intravascular volume depletion. A peripheral smear is important to rule out hemolysis. Platelet count and coagulation studies (i.e., prothrombin time, partial thromboplastin time, fibrinogen, and fibrin degradation products) may all be abnormal secondary to consumption or DIC. Serum uric acid, blood urea nitrogen, and creatinine may be elevated because of development of a prerenal state. Evaluation for proteinuria may reveal levels over 300 mg per 24 hours. Antepartum surveillance of the fetus by serial ultrasound and biophysical profile or NST in cases of associated IUGR must be performed.
   D. Formulating the diagnosis
      - Preeclamptic/eclamptic hypertension is defined as a blood pressure (BP) above 140/90 mm Hg or an increase greater than 30 mm Hg in systolic BP, or greater than 15 mm Hg in diastolic BP over the baseline BP obtained in the first 20 weeks of gestation.
      - Chronic hypertension is defined as systolic pressure above 140 mm Hg, diastolic pressureat or above 90 mm Hg, or both, that antedates pregnancy, is present before the 20th week of pregnancy, or persists longer than 12 weeks post partum.

- Superimposed preeclampsia is diagnosed when a woman with chronic hypertension develops new onset proteinuria after 20 weeks of gestation. Women with chronic hypertension and preexisting proteinuria (before 20 weeks) are considered preeclamptic if there is an exacerbation of blood pressure to the severe range (systolic at or above 180 mm Hg or diastolic at or above 110 mm Hg) in the last half of pregnancy, especially if accompanied by symptoms or a sudden increase in proteinuria.
- Gestational hypertension refers to hypertension (usually mild) without proteinuria (or other signs of preeclampsia) developing in the latter part of pregnancy. If it resolves by 12 weeks post partum, then in retrospect, it is classified as transient hypertension of pregnancy. If the hypertension persists beyond 12 weeks post partum, then the diagnosis is chronic hypertension that was masked in early pregnancy by the physiologic decrease in blood pressure.
- Differential diagnosis of eclampsia includes cerebrovascular accident, hypertensive encephalopathy, pheochromocytoma, space-occupying CNS lesion, infection, metabolic derangement, thrombotic thrombocytopenic purpura (TTP), and use of illicit drugs.

E. Evaluating the severity of problems
- The mild preeclamptic will have a diastolic BP above 100 mm Hg, proteinuria greater than 300 mg/24 hours, or generalized nondependent edema. Development of diastolic BP above 110 mm Hg, proteinuria above 5 g/24 hours, signs of CNS irritation, right upper quadrant pain, oliguria, pulmonary edema, or the HELLP syndrome (hemolysis, elevated liver function tests, low platelets) will change the diagnosis to severe preeclampsia. Not all abnormalities must be present. Eclampsia is defined as any of the above plus seizure activity.
- Maternal complications include eclampsia, stroke, cardiac failure, pulmonary edema, acute renal failure, HELLP syndrome, disseminated intravascular coagulation, increased risk of operative delivery, and shock. Fetal complications include intrauterine growth restriction (IUGR), preterm labor, intrauterine death, prematurity, and increased perinatal morbidity.

F. Managing the patient
- Therapy for preeclampsia and eclampsia is based on the severity of disease and the gestational age of the fetus. Ultimately, the cure is delivery. Outpatient management of very mild preeclampsia is successful in compliant patients. Care consists of bed rest, daily home BP monitoring, baseline evaluation of CBC, platelet count, serum chemistries, and measurement of proteinuria. Patients are followed with twice-weekly tests of fetal well-being (nonstress testing and amniotic fluid index) and twice-weekly office visits. Antihypertensives are used for severe hypertension only. Frequently used drugs in pregnancy include methyldopa, labetalol, or hydralazine for outpatient oral therapy and intravenous labetalol or hydralazine for inpatient therapy. ACE inhibitors and angiotensin receptor blockers are contraindicated in pregnancy due to their teratogenic effects.

- If hospitalization is indicated, the patient is maintained on bed rest with frequent BP monitoring, daily weight examination, and observation for symptoms. CBC, platelet count, serum chemistries, and 24-hour urine collection for creatinine clearance and total protein are followed closely. Twice-weekly tests of fetal well-being (nonstress testing and amniotic fluid index) are done. Amniocentesis for fetal lung maturity may be indicated.
- If the diagnosis of severe preeclampsia/eclampsia is made, management should be directed toward delivery. The patient should be medically stabilized with control of blood pressure and seizures and reversal of hypoxia and acidosis, if present. Induction of delivery should be attempted if the cervix is favorable. Glucocorticoid therapy may be indicated to promote fetal lung maturity if the gestational age is less than 34 weeks.
- Magnesium sulfate is used in the peripartum period (labor/delivery/24 hours post partum) for prophylaxis and treatment of seizures. Therapeutic blood levels are 4 to 8 mEq/L. A magnesium level above 12 mEq/L is toxic. Phenobarbital may also be used.
- Hypertension and proteinuria usually resolve within the first week post partum. Liver function and platelet abnormalities begin to normalize by postpartum day 4 but may persist for up to 10 days. Hypertension remains a common medical complication of pregnancy. It accounts for a significant proportion of all maternal and neonatal morbidity and death.

XXI. Preterm Labor
  A. Basic science
- Preterm labor (PTL) is defined as labor beginning before the 37th week of gestation. PTL occurs in about 10% of pregnancies. Preterm delivery accounts for over 60% of perinatal morbidity and death.
- In most cases, the cause of preterm birth is unknown and spontaneous preterm labor occurs in 50% of cases of preterm delivery. Other conditions associated with preterm birth include preterm prelabor rupture of membranes (PPROM), multiple gestation, preeclampsia/eclampsia, antepartum bleeding, fetal growth restriction, and other causes (maternal infection, cervical incompetence, uterine abnormalities, etc.). The most important risk factor for preterm labor is a previous history of preterm birth, especially if it occurred before 28 weeks of gestation, or a history of more than one preterm delivery.
  B. History and physical examination
- The history should focus on known causes of PTL, particularly infectious etiologies. A history of PTL is a significant risk factor for recurrence. Smoking and cocaine abuse also increase the risk of PTL. Other risk factors include extremes of maternal age, poor socioeconomic and nutritional status, history of uterine fibroid or anomaly, prior uterine or cervical surgeries such as cone biopsy, lack of prenatal care, short interpregnancy intervals, anemia, genital infection, asymptomatic bacteriuria or urinary tract infection, and premature cervical dilatation (>2 cm) or effacement (>80%) detected on routine obstetric ultrasound. The assessment of the abovementioned risk

factors can help predict the small subgroup in which potential interventions may help.

- Common symptoms of PTL include change in cervical discharge, uterine cramps, lower back and pelvic pressure, and bloody show. Patients with PROM (premature rupture of membranes) often describe a sudden gush of fluid followed by continued leakage.
- If the membranes are not ruptured, and there is no history of placenta previa, a digital examination should be done to determine if the cervix is dilated or effaced.

C. Laboratory and diagnostic studies
- Cultures for bacterial vaginosis, gonorrhea, chlamydia, and group B streptococci (GBS) should be obtained. Urinalysis should be performed to detect asymptomatic urinary tract infections. If chorioamnionitis is suspected, amniotic fluid should be sent for Gram stain and culture.
- Amniocentesis may be indicated to determine fetal lung maturity. A lecithin : sphingomyelin ratio greater than 2 : 1 signifies fetal lung maturity. In cases of PROM, a sample of amniotic fluid from the vagina can be tested for phosphatidylglycerol. Its presence is an indicator of pulmonary maturity.
- The best indicator for PPROM is observing a pooling of amniotic fluid in the vagina. There are two rapid bedside tests that can confirm the diagnosis of PROM:
  1. Nitrazine test
     - Vaginal fluid that changes the color of nitrazine paper (from yellow-green to dark blue) indicates an amniotic fluid leak and suggests PROM.
  2. Fern test
     - Amniotic fluid is air-dried on a glass slide and then examined under the microscope. A characteristic ferning pattern is seen if amniotic fluid is present.
- Both these tests have a high false positive rate. Ultrasonography can be used to confirm a diagnosis of PPROM and may reveal anhydramnios or severe oligohydramnios. These findings combined with a characteristic history are highly suggestive, but not diagnostic, of rupture of membranes.
- Although the prediction and prevention of prematurity are major goals of obstetricians, effective tools for reducing preterm birth remain elusive. Many biochemical markers and ultrasonographic features have been evaluated for the prediction of preterm labor. The most clinically useful biochemical approach to differentiating women who are at high risk for impending PTD from those who are not at high risk is measurement of fetal fibronectin in the cervicovaginal secretions. It is a large-molecular-weight glycoprotein present in the amniotic fluid. Fetal fibronectin is currently used in women who present with signs and symptoms of preterm delivery and can be identified from vaginal swabs collected from the posterior fornix. Its presence has a high negative predictive value in the diagnosis of preterm labor; this means that if fibronectin is absent, there is a low likelihood for preterm labor.

D. Formulating the diagnosis
- True labor is characterized by regular uterine contractions (six to eight per hour, or four contractions within 20 minutes) associated with cervical change (either dilation or effacement). False labor is characterized by irregular uterine contractions without cervical change. Uterine contractions alone may suggest false labor or threatened PTL.

E. Evaluating the severity of problems
- Maternal temperature and fetal heart rate should be monitored. Elevation in either vital sign suggests chorioamnionitis. The presence of palpable contractions and uterine tenderness may indicate abruptio placentae.

F. Managing the patient
- Some preventive strategies are available in women who have a higher risk of preterm labor identified by history or by routine obstetric ultrasound showing cervical dilation or effacement. These strategies include smoking cessation, avoidance of illicit drugs and alcohol, appropriate nutrition, reduction of occupational fatigue, decreasing the rate of multiple pregnancies during ART, treatment of asymptomatic bacteriuria or UTI, treatment of genital infections, and cervical circlage surgery. Progesterone supplementation may help in some women; further studies are needed before this practice is adopted in clinical practice. Most of the cases of preterm labor, however, occur spontaneously, and there are limited effective interventions.
- Crucial determinants in the management of preterm labor include the gestational age and the integrity of membranes. The fetus is not viable at less than 24 weeks.
- Management modalities for preterm labor include the following:
  1. Bed rest and IV hydration
     - The goal of this therapy is to increase uterine blood flow and thereby "quiet" the uterus.
  2. Treatment of identified genital or urinary infections including bacterial vaginosis and asymptomatic bacteruria
     - In cases of chorioamnionitis, antibiotics (ampicillin and gentamicin) should be started and labor should ensue. Antibiotics have a role in preterm labor in three circumstances: if there is documented infection, as described above; in patients with associated PPROM to delay labor; and during labor to prevent neonatal GBS sepsis. Antibiotics are ineffective in prolonging labor if routinely used along with tocolysis in the absence of coexistent PPROM.
  3. Corticosteroids
     - Antenatal corticosteroid therapy (ACS) reduces the incidence of neonatal respiratory distress syndrome, intraventricular hemorrhage, and overall perinatal morbidity and mortality by approximately 50%. They should be given to any pregnant woman at 24 to 34 weeks of gestation at high risk for preterm delivery within 7 days of administration.
     - A single course of ACS consists of betamethasone 12 mg intramuscularly every 24 hours for two doses or four doses of 6 mg dexamethasone intramuscularly 12 hours apart.

- Corticosteroids are not recommended after 34 weeks of gestation because there are insufficient data regarding the risks and benefits of ACS at advanced gestational ages.

4. Pharmacologic tocolysis (i.e., delaying labor with medication)
   - Most studies show that the tocolytics are successful only in the short term by delaying labor up to 48 hours. Tocolysis is generally employed between 24 and 34 weeks of gestation. It is not routinely used in gestations above 35 weeks unless there is fetal lung immaturity, in which case tocolytics are used to delay labor until corticosteroids can be administered.
   - Contraindications to tocolysis include intrauterine fetal demise, lethal fetal anomaly, nonreassuring fetal heart tracing, severe intrauterine growth restriction, chorioamnionitis, severe preeclampsia or eclampsia, and maternal hemorrhage with hemodynamic instability.
   - Commonly used medications include magnesium sulfate and the β-mimetics: ritodrine and terbutaline. Magnesium acts as a calcium antagonist, competing with it for intracellular smooth muscle uptake. It is administered intravenously as a 4-g bolus.
   - Deep tendon reflexes should be tested frequently because they are a reliable index of high blood magnesium concentrations. Loss of the patellar reflex is the earliest sign of magnesium toxicity. Respiratory depression begins at 10 to 15 mg/dL, and cardiac arrest occurs at 30 mg/dL. Calcium gluconate is the antidote to magnesium toxicity. The β-mimetics act on $β_2$-receptors (of the myometrium) to cause relaxation.
   - Side effects (e.g., tachycardia, tremor, and hyperglycemia) occur because these agents have both $β_1$ and $β_2$ effects. They are contraindicated in patients with cardiac disease or hyperthyroidism.

5. Because of the devastating consequences of preterm neonatal group B streptococcal infection, women whose group B streptococcal carrier status is known to be positive or is unknown must be given antibiotic prophylaxis (with ampicillin or penicillin G) during labor.

6. General treatment for PTL is to delay delivery if the woman is less than 34 weeks pregnant so that antenatal corticosteroids can be administered to the mother. Labor may also be allowed to proceed if the mother is more than 34 weeks pregnant or tests show that the baby's lungs are fully developed. The management depending on the gestational age is outlined below:
   a. PPROM or PTL less than 32 weeks of gestation
      - In general, preterm delivery is the greatest risk to the fetus with PPROM and onset of labor at less than 32 weeks of gestation. Therefore, pregnancies at this gestational age should be managed expectantly in the absence of complications (e.g., infection, abruption, cord prolapse, nonreassuring fetal assessment). Monitoring for maternal or fetal infection and signs of fetal compromise should be initiated and consists of routine vital signs

(temperature, maternal and fetal heart rates, and subjective assessment of fetal activity) and can include serial nonstress testing or biophysical profile scoring.

- Antenatal corticosteroids should be given. Prophylactic antibiotics should be given for all cases with PPROM; they prolong the latent period between the time of membrane rupture and the onset of labor and significantly reduce the frequency of maternal and neonatal infection. Tocolytics are used to attempt to delay delivery 48 hours in women with preterm labor who are receiving steroids for fetal lung maturation.
- Antibiotic prophylaxis for possible GBS colonization should be given during labor in the absence of a documented, recent negative GBS culture.

b. PPROM or PTL between 32 and 34 weeks
- For patients admitted with PPROM at 32 to 34 weeks of gestation with fetal lung maturation confirmed via amniocentesis or collection of amniotic fluid from the vaginal pool, the risks of expectant management usually exceed those of delivery. Such women hospitalized at centers capable of providing intensive neonatal care are best managed by prompt induction of labor. However, if fetal lung maturity cannot be confirmed, then a course of corticosteroids is administered and the patient is delivered at 34 weeks.

c. PPROM or PTL after 34 weeks
- Patients admitted with PPROM at or after 34 weeks' gestation are begun on GBS prophylaxis and delivered.

XXII. Uterine Cancer
   A. Basic science
   - Uterine cancer is the fourth most common female malignancy in the United States. Most patients with endometrial cancer are older than 40 years. Risk factors for endometrial cancer include the following:
     1. Obesity (conversion of androstenedione to estrone in adipose tissue)
     2. Nulliparity
     3. Postmenopausal estrogen therapy (unopposed by progesterone)
     4. Early menarche or late menopause
     5. Diabetes mellitus
     6. Polycystic ovarian syndrome
     7. Extended use of tamoxifen
   - The most significant risk factor for the development of uterine adenocarcinoma is endometrial hyperplasia; this results from the excessive endometrial estrogen stimulation found in many of the aforementioned conditions.
   - Hormonal contraceptives (e.g., birth control pills and parenteral progesterones) are associated with up to a 50% reduction in endometrial cancer.

B. History and physical examination
   - The initial history should focus on age of menarche and menopause, number of pregnancies, and the use of steroid contraceptives or hormone replacement therapy. The most common symptom of uterine cancer is abnormal vaginal bleeding. Therefore, a complaint of postmenopausal bleeding warrants investigation.
   - Most cancers are discovered early; thus, manifestations of distant metastases to lung, brain, and bone are rare. Inguinal lymphadenopathy and an enlarged uterus are occasionally present. The adnexa must be examined for evidence of neoplasia.
C. Laboratory and diagnostic studies
   - Any bleeding following 6 months of postmenopausal amenorrhea deserves evaluation. This should include a speculum examination, Pap smear, and outpatient endometrial biopsy. An ultrasound of the pelvis can be obtained and the endometrial biopsy performed only if the lining is more than 4 to 5 mm thick.
   - The Pap smear is not a screening test for any neoplasm except squamous cell lesions of the cervix. Nevertheless, endometrial cells found on a postmenopausal woman's cytologic report should be investigated with a follow-up endometrial biopsy because many of these patients will have an endometrial cancer.
D. Formulating the diagnosis
   - Thirty percent of postmenopausal women with vaginal bleeding will have endometrial cancer. No therapy should be prescribed until a histologic diagnosis is obtained.
   - Approximately 95% of uterine neoplasms are adenocarcinomas. Up to 40% of patients will progress to cancer from hyperplasia with atypia if they remain untreated.
E. Evaluating the severity of problems
   - Once the diagnosis of endometrial cancer is confirmed, staging is performed. The only routinely indicated metastatic survey is a chest x-ray. Other tests including CT scan of the abdomen and pelvis; barium enema, sigmoidoscopy or colonoscopy, and IV urogram are performed based on symptoms.
F. Managing the patient
   - Endometrial hyperplasia (with or without atypia) can be managed in a premenopausal woman who desires to remain fertile with long-term progesterone (e.g., 12 weeks) and periodic endometrial biopsies.
   - Stage I cancer is confined to the uterus and should be adequately treated with hysterectomy and salpingo-oophorectomy. During the hysterectomy, lymph node biopsies should be obtained from the pelvis and periaortic areas to identify those patients who will benefit from postoperative adjuvant therapy. Patients at high risk for recurrence or those with extrauterine disease should receive radiation treatment to the pelvis and vaginal apex. Patients with evidence of cancer in the upper abdomen may be offered systemic chemotherapy or whole abdomen radiation treatment.

- Most patients with uterine cancer are cured. Therefore, long-term follow-up is needed to detect rare recurrences seen after treatment of early stage disease. Although patients with advanced disease are at high risk for recurrence, up to 50% may eventually be cured if the recurrence is detected early. A surveillance regimen should begin with a pelvic and speculum examination plus Pap smear every 3 to 4 months for the first 3 years following the completion of therapy.
- Endometrial cancer is a terminal disease if untreated. It can cause life-threatening vaginal bleeding and symptoms attributable to metastatic disease. Stage I disease has a 90% cure rate, but even the most advanced cases can benefit from palliative chemotherapy or radiation treatment. Besides stage, prognosis is related to histologic classification and grade.

Hematology and Oncology

I. Anemia
   A. Basic science
      - Anemia is a decrease in hemoglobin leading to a reduction in the oxygen-carrying capacity of blood. The finding of low hemoglobin should always prompt a workup.
      - Evaluation of anemia may be approached in two ways: (1) the mechanism which results in anemia; and (2) the morphologic approach, which is based on the mean corpuscular volume (MCV) and the red blood cell distribution width (RDW), a reflection of the variation in red blood cell (RBC) volume.
      1. Mechanism approach
         - The reticulocyte index is the percent of reticulocytes times the patient's hematocrit divided by 45. A reticulocyte index less than 1 is suggestive of inadequate RBC production, whereas a value greater than 2 suggests adequate RBC production but RBC loss from either bleeding or hemolysis. Anemia may result from underproduction, destruction or loss, or abnormal maturation of red blood cells. Often, more than one mechanism is involved.
      2. Morphologic approach
         - The morphology of the red blood cells as seen on a peripheral smear (microcytic, normocytic, or macrocytic) and the MCV help define the red blood cell morphology.
         - Microcytic anemia (low MCV) may be due to iron deficiency, thalassemia, lead poisoning, sideroblastic anemia, and chronic disease. Iron deficiency is suggested by a history of blood loss and the finding of a microcytic anemia.
         - Normocytic anemia (normal MCV) may be due to acute blood loss, secondary to chronic disease, renal insufficiency, hemolytic anemia, overwhelming involvement of the bone marrow with tumor or infection, multiple myeloma, or aplastic anemia.
         - Macrocytic anemia (high MCV) may be due to megaloblastic anemias that arise as the result of vitamin B_{12} or folate deficiency, liver disease, alcoholism, myelodysplastic syndrome, and hypothyroidism.
   B. History and physical examination
      - The symptoms due to anemia vary depending on how rapidly the anemia occurred.
      - Patients with mild anemia and those with hemoglobin as low as 6 g/dL in whom the anemia occurred over months are usually asymptomatic.

- Anemia may present with fatigue, weakness, palpitations, lightheadedness, decreased exercise tolerance, pica, dyspnea, chest pain suggestive of angina, syncope, dizziness, and headache. Physical examination may reveal pallor, tachycardia, bounding pulse, widened pulse pressure, orthostatic hypotension, hyperdynamic point of maximal impulse, and a systolic ejection murmur. Depending on the cause of anemia, the spleen may be enlarged; neurologic signs or jaundice may be present.
  1. Iron deficiency
     - Patients with severe iron deficiency may have a sore tongue due to glossitis, complain of dysphagia (Plummer-Vinson syndrome), and have koilonychia. Iron deficiency should never be attributed to poor dietary intake of iron alone.
  2. Thalassemia
     - A family history of anemia raises the possibility of thalassemia, particularly in those of Mediterranean or Asian descent.
  3. Hemolytic anemia
     - Patients with hemolytic anemia may be jaundiced but do not necessarily have dark urine because the indirect bilirubin released in excess from red blood cell lysis is insoluble in urine. Urinary hemosiderin, if present, may color the urine.
  4. Vitamin B_{12} and folate deficiency
     - Symptoms and signs of advanced vitamin B_{12} deficiency, which almost always occur because of pernicious anemia, include mental status changes (e.g., memory changes or dementia), ataxia, and peripheral neuropathy. Folate deficiency should be suspected in those with poor diets, malabsorption syndromes, or increased folate requirements (e.g., during pregnancy) or who are taking certain medications such as methotrexate.

C. Laboratory and diagnostic studies
  - The following tests are essential in evaluating the cause of anemia: MCV, the peripheral blood smear, the reticulocyte index, and the RDW. The RDW is typically elevated in iron deficiency, folate deficiency, vitamin B_{12} deficiency, sickle cell anemia, myelodysplasia, chronic liver disease, and immune hemolytic anemias.
  1. Microcytic anemias
     - The laboratory findings in iron deficiency anemic, anemia of chronic disease, the thalessemias, and sideroblastic anemia are listed in Table 14-1.
  2. Hemolytic anemias
     - Hemolysis may cause an elevation of the bilirubin and lactate dehydrogenase (LDH) and may lead to fragmentation (microangiopathic process) or spherocytosis (autoimmune process). If autoimmune hemolysis is suspected, a Coombs' test should be ordered.
  3. Anemia due to folate or vitamin B_{12} deficiency
     - Folate and vitamin B_{12} levels should be obtained in the patient with macrocytosis. The neutrophils are often hypersegmented in folate or

TABLE 14-1:

Laboratory Findings in Microcytic Anemias

Measurement	Iron Deficiency Anemia	Anemia of Chronic Disease	Thalassemia	Sideroblastic Anemia
Serum Fe	Low	Low	Normal	High
TIBC	High	Low	Normal	Normal
Ferritin	Low	High	Normal	High
Others	High RDW, Fe/TIBC < 18%	Fe/TIBC > 18%	Normal RDW, basophilic stippling, abnormal hemoglobin electrophoresis	Ringed sideroblasts in bone marrow

Fe, iron; RDW, red blood cell distribution width; TIBC, total iron binding capacity.

vitamin B_{12} deficiency states and the MCV is greater than 100 femoliters (fL). Other causes of macrocytosis include liver disease, alcoholism, hypothyroidism, hemolysis and aplastic anemia.

D. Formulating the diagnosis
- The cause of the patient's anemia can usually be determined with the evaluation described earlier. A bone marrow aspirate and biopsy may eventually need to be done in patients in whom the cause of anemia is not obvious. A bone marrow study is also indicated in patients suspected of having primary bone marrow failure, pancytopenia, or infiltrative disease of the marrow.

E. Evaluating the severity of problems
- Marked pallor, orthostasis, syncope, angina, and dyspnea all suggest severe anemia and should prompt immediate evaluation and treatment.

F. Managing the patient
- The cause of anemia should be aggressively sought in all patients. Transfusion of RBCs is generally indicated for severe anemia, significant acute and ongoing blood loss, and marrow failure.
  1. Iron deficiency
     - Iron deficiency can be treated with oral iron in most cases. The dose of elemental iron varies from 60 to 200 mg a day. The peak reticulocyte response occurs in 7 to 10 days and the hemoglobin should begin to increase in about 3 weeks. After the hemoglobin level has normalized oral iron should be continued for about 6 months to replete body iron stores. Parenteral iron therapy should be reserved for patients who cannot tolerate oral iron preparations (rare) or in those who have iron malabsorption.
  2. Folate and vitamin B_{12} deficiency
     - Intravenous folate is rarely required. Generally oral folic acid 1 mg daily or 5 mg daily in the presence of malabsorption is adequate. Patients

with vitamin B_{12} deficiency are treated with intramuscular or nasal vitamin B_{12}. In a folate or vitamin B_{12} deficient patient the patient begins to feel better even before a hematologic response can be detected. The reticulocyte count peaks by day 7 with progressive improvement in the hemoglobin in a matter of weeks. There may be an accompanying thrombocytosis.

3. Anemia in renal insufficiency
   - Patients with anemia due to chronic renal insufficiency respond to parenteral erythropoietin. Supplemental iron must be given to these patients.

4. Hemolytic anemias
   - Patients may present with symptoms of anemia previously described, pinkish urine (hemoglobinuria), fever, chills, and back and abdominal pain. On examination pallor, icterus, lymphadenopathy, and splenomegaly may be present. A peripheral smear may show polychromatophilia, spherocytes, nucleated red blood cells, an elevated serum LDH, low haptoglobin, and a positive Coombs' test.
   - Treatment: Any precipitating cause should be eliminated, if possible. This may involve stopping drugs known to cause hemolysis (methydopa, penicillin, cephalosporins, quinidine, INH, sulfonamides). Many autoimmune hemolytic anemias respond to prednisone. Splenectomy is indicated in patients unresponsive to prednisone. Patients who undergo splenectomy must receive pneumococcal, *Haemophilus influenzae* type B, and meningococcal vaccines.

II. Breast Cancer
   A. Basic science
   - Breast cancer is the neoplastic proliferation of cells in the lobules or ductules of the breast. It is the most common cancer in women in the United States and the second most common cause of cancer death in women. On average a woman has a 12% lifetime risk of developing breast cancer.
   - Median age of diagnosis is 60 years old. The risk of breast cancer starts to increase after the age of 35. Current data indicate that women who are taking contraceptives are not at increased risk for breast cancer, but women who are taking estrogen replacement therapy are at a higher risk for development of breast cancer. Important risk factors includes advanced age, family history (especially first-degree relatives), prolonged exposure to estrogen (nulliparity, early menarche before age 12, late menopause after the age of 55), previous history of breast cancer (subsequent breast cancers usually develop 4 years after first), the presence of proliferative nonmalignant breast conditions such as intraductal papilloma, and familial and socioeconomic factors, with women of higher socioeconomic status being at increased risk.
   - Male breast cancer accounts for about 1% of all new breast cancer.
   - The most common type of breast cancer is infiltrating ductal carcinoma (80% of all patients). About 10% is accounted for by lobular carcinoma and others like Paget's disease of the breast.

- Inflammatory breast cancer is a clinical, not a pathologic, diagnosis. It is characterized by the presence of an inflamed, erythematous, tender breast.
- Prognostic markers in breast cancer are axillary lymph node involvement, invasion, and tumor size. An estrogen- and progesterone–receptor-positive patient has approximately 10% improved survival rate compared to patients who are receptor negative. The presence of a tyrosine kinase receptor, HER2 neu, is a poor prognostic marker.

B. History and physical examination
- Most breast cancers are discovered when the patient or physician discovers a painless breast mass. The presence of bloody or nonmilky nipple discharge especially if unilateral, skin dimpling over the breast, palpable axillary nodes/supraclavicular nodes, excoriations over the nipple and areolar area otherwise unexplained by other causes should also alert one to the possibility of breast cancer.
- If a mass is felt, its size, consistency, and mobility should be noted. The skin overlying the breast should be examined for erythema and adema and the nipple for retraction or discharge.

C. Laboratory and diagnostic studies/formulating the diagnosis
- If a breast mass is found, a mammogram should be done to assess the characteristics of the mass and to assess for multicentricity and bilaterality. Further tests such as breast ultrasound and magnetic resonance imaging (MRI) can help delineate the characteristics of the mass. Pathologic examination of the mass is mandatory either by fine needle aspiration biopsy, a core biopsy, or excisional biopsy.
- Other ancillary procedures such as chest x-ray and liver enzymes may alert one to possible metastatic manifestations of the disease. Breast cancer metastasizes to the bones, brain, lungs, and liver.

D. Management of the patient
- The current management scheme is based on the American Joint Committee on Cancer (AJCC) staging system and the presence or absence of hormone receptors. Premalignant breast disorders and early stage breast cancers are usually treated with surgery. On the other hand, metastatic breast cancers are usually treated with chemotherapy or hormonal therapy.
  1. Surgical therapy
     a. Ductal carcinoma in situ
        - Breast conservation surgery (lumpectomy) + irradiation
     b. Early stage breast cancer
        - Breast conservation surgery (lumpectomy) + irradiation + axillary lymph node dissection
  2. Pharmacologic therapy
     - See Table 14-2 for recommended pharmacologic regimens.
     - Hormonal therapy may be in the form of antiestrogens such as tamoxifen or aromatase inhibitors such as anastrazole.
     - There are several chemotherapeutic regimens and they include cyclophosphamide + an anthracycline + 5 FU (fluorouracil) or taxanes + anthracycline compounds

TABLE 14-2:

Pharmacologic Therapy for Breast Cancer

	Premenopausal	Postmenopausal
Hormone receptor (+) Axillary LN (−)	Chemotherapy + tamoxifen	Tamoxifen
Hormone receptor (−) Axillary LN (+)	Chemotherapy	Chemotherapy
Hormone receptor (+) Axillary LN (+)	Chemotherapy + tamoxifen	Tamoxifen +/− chemotherapy
Hormone receptor (−) Axillary LN (−)	Chemotherapy	Chemotherapy

LN, lymph node.

III. Colon Cancer
- See Chapter 6, Gastroenterology, for a discussion of colon cancer.

IV. Hemophilia
  A. Basic science
   - The hemophilias are X-linked inherited defects that result in abnormal amounts of certain plasma clotting proteins. The two common hemophilias are hemophilia A (factor VIII deficiency) and hemophilia B (factor IX deficiency). The ratio of hemophilia A to B is about 4:1. Both hemophilias result in joint and soft tissue hemorrhage as well as exsanguinating hemorrhage after minor trauma.
   - Hemophilia is classified as follows:
     1. Severe: less than 1% coagulant activity
     2. Moderate: 1% to 5% coagulant activity
     3. Mild: more than 5% coagulant activity
  B. History and physical examination
   - The distinction between hemophilia A and B cannot be made clinically. In the typical family, male patients are affected and female patients are carriers. Severe hemophilia usually leads to spontaneous hemorrhage early in life. Milder forms of the disease may not be apparent until after trauma or surgical procedures.
   - Hemarthrosis is the most common spontaneous bleeding complication in the patient with hemophilia. Hemarthrosis is rare before the age of 9 months. Recurrent bleeding into the joints leads to pain and deformity and often requires fusion of the joint or total joint replacement. Muscle hematomas may occur, causing compartment syndrome. Ecchymoses, retroperitoneal hematomas, oral bleeding, and gastrointestinal bleeding are all common in severe hemophilia. Intracranial bleeding is the most common cause of hemorrhagic death.
   - Since the availability of recombinant factor VIII and factor IX the risk of hepatitis and HIV transmission is nonexistent. Patients who received blood

products in the mid-1980s have a high rate of transfusion-acquired HIV (human immunodeficiency virus), hepatitis B and hepatitis C infections. The resultant cirrhosis and complications of portal hypertension contribute significantly to morbidity and death.

C. Laboratory and diagnostic studies
- Most patients with hemophilia have an elevated partial thromboplastin time (PTT), whole blood clotting time, and prothrombin consumption test because of deficiencies in the intrinsic pathway coagulation proteins. The prothrombin time (PT), bleeding time, and fibrinogen level are all normal. Patients with mild hemophilia may have a normal PTT. Direct assays of both factor VIII and factor IX levels can be done to measure the coagulant activity in the patient's blood.

D. Formulating the diagnosis
- The diagnosis of hemophilia is usually made in a bleeding patient with a positive family history. The results of assays of specific factors will confirm the clinical suspicion. Patients with mild hemophilia may go undiagnosed until significant bleeding occurs at surgery.

E. Evaluating the severity of problems
- All bleeding in a patient with hemophilia must be considered life-threatening. Physical examination of the hemophiliac may not reflect the severity of the bleeding, especially when the bleeding is into the retroperitoneum or the thigh.

F. Managing the patient
- Symptomatic patients should be evaluated immediately. Consultation with a hematologist should be sought promptly. As many as 20% of patients with hemophilia A have antibodies to factor VIII, making their management challenging.
- Factor VIII and factor IX concentrates are the mainstays of treatment. The aim is to replace the diminished factor to 50% to 100% of normal coagulant activity.
- Hemarthroses should be managed with orthopedic consultation. The suspicion of compartment syndrome in a limb should lead to prompt surgical evaluation.
- Perioperative management involves replacing the abnormal factor until the levels are 50% to 100% of normal. Treatment with the factor should be continued for up to 7 days postoperatively.

V. Leukemias
A. Basic science
- Leukemias are a group of orders characterized by the presence of neoplastic white blood cells that may be present in the peripheral blood, bone marrow, or in other organs. Historically leukemias have been subdivided into acute and chronic, based on "duration of survival." Today the term "acute" refers more to presence of immature proliferating cells and "chronic" to the presence of more mature cells. Distinguishing between abnormal lymphocytic and myeloid proliferation is important because of differences in treatment and prognosis.

B. Acute leukemias
  1. Acute myelogenous leukemia (AML)
     - AML is a clonal proliferation of abnormal neoplastic immature myeloid cells. Two classification systems are in use in clinical practice: the French, American, and British Classification (FAB), which groups AML into seven categories, namely M1 to M7, and the World health Organization (WHO) Classification I through IV.
     - Of every 100,000 new patients, 3 are diagnosed with AML each year in the United States. The median age of diagnosis is about 60 years. Male-to-female ratio is 1.3:1. Risk factors include exposure to ionizing radiation, benzene, and chemotherapeutic agents such as topoisomerase inhibitors (i.e., etoposide) and alkylating agents (i.e., cyclophosphamide).
     a. History and physical examination
        - The clinical manifestations are generally nonspecific and are related to depression of the blood cell lines namely RBCs (symptoms associated with anemia such as fatigue and dyspnea), WBCs (infections), and platelets (bleeding diathesis).
        - M3 or the promyelocytic type may sometimes present with features of disseminated intravascular coagulation.
        - M5 or acute monoblastic type can present with gingival hyperplasia.
        - AML rarely presents with splenomegaly, which when discovered should alert one to the presence of a concomitant myeloproliferative disorder.
        - Other less common manifestations are skin infiltration and central nervous system involvement, which manifests itself with meningeal signs. Dysphagia may be a result of oropharyngeal candidiasis; symptoms of prostatism may be due to leukemic infiltration of the prostate.
        - Examination reveals an ill-appearing individual who is pale and febrile. The patient may be hemodynamically unstable if septic or has had gastrointestinal bleeding. There may be evidence of pneumonia and the skin often reveals petechiae and less commonly leukemic infiltrates. Meningism suggests cervical nervous system involvement.
     b. Laboratory and diagnostic studies
        - The white blood cell count may be elevated or depressed; hemoglobin, hematocrit, and platelets are usually low and blasts are usually present.
        - Flow cytometry will confirm either myeloid or lymphoid origin of blasts.
        - Myeloid cells morphologically show granules and Auer rods, cytochemistry may demostrate myeloperoxidase or nonspecific esterase positivity, and immunophenotyping may be positive for the myeloid antigens CD13 and CD33.
        - Abnormal prothrombin time and partial thromboplastin time may indicate the presence of disseminated intravascular coagulation which in turn suggests an M3 AML.

- A bone marrow biopsy will help ascertain the presence of blasts and will allow cytogenetic studies. Cytogenetics abnormalities are the single most important prognostic indicators in AML patients. The t(15,17) associated with M3 AML or promyelocytic leukemia has the most favorable outcome.
  c. Formulating the diagnosis
  - The diagnosis of acute leukemia is made by demonstrating blasts in the peripheral blood or the bone marrow. In approximately 10% of patients the peripheral blood shows no evidence of blasts. Acute leukemia is indicated by the presence of more than 20% myeloid blasts in the bone marrow or the presence of clonal recurrent cytogenetic abnormalities such as t(8,21) in acute myeloid leukemia with differentiation (M2), inv/del (16) in acute myelomonocytic leukemia (M4Eo), or t(15,17) in acute myelomonocytic leumemia (M3), regardless of blast percentage.
  d. Evaluating the severity of the problem
  - Infection, bleeding, hemodynamic stability, and leukostasis are the most important concerns initially. If the blast count is more than 100,000/μL, leukophoresis should be considered.
  e. Management of the patient
  - While the type of leukemia is being characterized, infections must be treated aggressively. Cefepime is effective in neutropenic patients; thrombocytopenia may require platelet transfusions and packed red blood cells for anemia. The treatment of leukemia consists of three phases: induction (generates remission), consolidation (strengthens the remission), and maintenance (endures a prolonged remission).
  - During induction chemotherapy, cytarabine and daunorubicin are generally used, except for M3 which responds to all-*trans*-retinoic acid (ATRA).
  - After induction chemotherapy, the next step of treatment depends on whether or not the patient falls in the good, poor, or intermediate prognostic group.
  - Consolidation chemotherapy (with high-dose cytarabine) is for those with good prognostic factors such as t(15,17), t(8,21), inv 16 cytogeneric abnormalities and under 60 years of age. Patients with poor prognostic factors such as AML secondary to myelodysplastic syndrome (MDS) or another hematologic disorder, 5q-, 7q-, trisomy 8, t(9,22) or Philadelphia chromosome, t(6,9), the patient is best treated with allogeneic bone marrow transplantation after remission with induction chemotherapy. Older patients usually have a poorer prognosis and are often not candidates for bone marrow transplant.

2. Acute lymphocytic leukemia (ALL)
  a. Basic science
  - ALL is a clonal proliferation of neoplastic immature lymphoid cells. It accounts for 80% of childhood leukemias and 20% of adult leukemias. Adults tend to do worse than children. The current classification

system uses the FAB system L1 to L3 and the immunotype system, which classifies ALL as pre-B cell, T cell, and B cell.
- The incidence is 1 to 1.5 per 100,000 persons in the United States. ALL has a bimodal age incidence (ages 2 to 4 and age above 50 years). It is more common among whites than African Americans. Risk factors are Down syndrome, HTLV-1 (human T-lymphotrophic virus) for adult T cell leukemia, and Epstein Barr virus for mature B cell ALL.
  b. History and physical examination
- History and physcial examination are similar to AML. Most of the early clinical manifestations are due to suppression of the blood cell lines. The most common presenting symptoms are pallor and petechiae or ecchymoses. Hepatosplenomegaly is uncommon.
  c. Laboratory and diagnostic studies
- As with AML, CBC with differential counts should be obtained to assess abnormalities of the cell counts (WBC count may be elevated or depressed), and a blood smear is taken to detect the presence of blasts.
- Flow cytometry determines the origin of the blasts (myeloid or lymphoid).
- Evidence of lymphoid blasts is supported by the absence of granules on morphologic examination, (+) TdT by cytochemistry, and presence of CD7, CD10, CD19, CD20 surface Ig by immunocytochemistry. T-cell ALL occasionally presents with a mediastinal mass that may be seen on chest x-ray
  d. Formulating the diagnosis
- The diagnosis is established by finding lymphoid blasts in the peripheral blood or bone marrow.
  e. Evaluating the severity of problems
- The presence of the Philadelphia chromosome in patients with ALL is a marker of poor prognosis. These patients are best treated with allogeneic bone marrow transplant after remission induction chemotherapy.
  f. Management
- As with AML infection, anemia and severe thrombocytopenia should be aggressively managed.
- Induction chemotherapy consists of vincristine, prednisone, and an anthracycline (e.g., daunorubicin, idarubicin) with or without asparaginase. CNS prophylaxis is paramount in ALL treatment because of the high risk of CNS relapse.
- Treatment of CNS involvement is with intrathecal methotrexate, systemic methotrexate, or cranial irradiation.
- Optimal consolidation and maintenance regimens are still under investigation. Most regimens used in adults are patterned after pediatric protocols. Relapse is common in adults in whom the cure ratio is 40% versus 80% in children.
- C. Chronic leukemias
  1. Chronic myelogenous leukemia (CML)
    a. Basic science

- CML is a myeloproliferative disorder. It is an abnormal clonal proliferation and accumulation of granulocytic cells, especially neurophils. Central to the pathogenesis of CML is the Philadelphia chromosome t(9,22), found in 90% of patients, which produces the *bcr-abl* chimeric gene coding for a protein with tyrosine kinase activity.
- CML invariably progresses to acute leukemia. The median age of diagnosis is between 50 and 60 years of age. There are 4000 new cases in the United States every year. It accounts for 15% of adult leukemias, with a slight male predominance.
- There are three clinical phases of CML: a chronic phase that may last for years, an accelerated phase, and a blast phase.

b. History and physical examination
- Most people are diagnosed during the chronic phase and about 30% to 50% are asymptomatic with a high WBC count (usually >50,000 cells/μL) detected on routine laboratory tests. Less commonly, patients may present in a blast crisis. Symptoms of anemia are common because of the high myeloid versus erythroid ratio in the bone marrow. The most common physical finding is the presence of splenomegaly, which correlates with the degree of leukocytosis.
- Lymphadenopathy and hepatomegaly are uncommon. Symptoms of acute leukemia may be seen during the blast phase. Because of the high WBC count, symptoms and signs of hyperviscosity syndrome (i.e., stupor, strokes, visual changes, and retinal hemorrhages) may be present.

c. Laboratory and diagnostic studies
- The WBC count is high with a predominance of neutrophils and metamyelocytes. The presence of basophilia should raise questions about the accuracy of the diagnosis. Eosinophilia may be present. Thrombocytosis is almost always present. Vitamin B_{12} levels are elevated secondary to increased production of transcobalamin I by high numbers of granulocytes. Uric acid and LDH levels are also elevated. Leukocyte alkaline phosphatase (LAP) is low, which may help differentiate CML from leukemoid reactions in which LAP is normal or elevated.
- Bone marrow biopsy confirms the presence of Philadelphia chromosome (usually done by fluorescent in situ hybridization, or FISH). Anemia is usually mild except in blast crisis.

d. Formulating the diagnosis
- The history, physical examination, demonstration of an elevated WBC count with an appropriate differential count, and the previously mentioned laboratory tests will help support the diagnosis of CML. Bone marrow biopsy should be pursued in the appropriate setting and if positive for Philadelphia chromosome will clinch the diagnosis. If the Philadelphia chromosome is negative, PCR (polymerase chain reaction) or FISH for *bcr-abl* if postive will also confirm the diagnosis. The chronic phase is characterized by WBC count greater than 50,000/μL with fewer than 5% blasts in peripheral blood.

- The accelerated phase has more than 5% but fewer than 30% blasts in the blood or bone marrow, and the blast phase is considered an acute leukemia with more than 30% blasts, which may be either myeloid or lymphoid.
  e. Evaluating the severity of the problem
  - Patients in an accelerated phase or blast crisis are severely ill and suffer from the same complications related to anemia and infection as patients with acute leukemias.
  f. Management
  - Imatinib mesylate (Gleevec) is the drug of choice for all phases of CML, chronic, accelerated, or blast crisis. Gleevec, an oral tyrosine kinase inhibitor, is unique in that it is able to induce both hematologic and cytogenetic remission in patients. Hydroxyurea can control leukocyte and platelet counts. Interferon-α has also been used to treat patients during the chronic phase but has limited use because of its side effects.
  - The best chance for cure is by allogeneic bone marrow transplant in those who fulfill the appropriate criteria
  - Hyperviscosity syndrome symptoms can be managed with hydroxyurea with or without leukopheresis.
2. Chronic lymphocytic leukemia (CLL)
   a. Basic science
   - CLL is the proliferation of neoplastic mature but functionally defective monoclonal B lymphoid cells. It is characterized by the accumulation of lymphocytes in the liver, spleen, bone marrow, and less commonly other organs.
   - CLL is the most common adult leukemia. It is the same disease as small lymphocytic lymphoma, but at a different stage. It may present as immune thrombocytopenic purpura (ITP) or Coombs-positive autoimmune hemolytic anemia (AIHA). The etiology is unknown. Median age of onset is 50 years old and it has a male predominance. There were 7300 new cases in the United States in 2003 alone.
   b. History and physical examination
   - Most patients are asymptomatic at presentation with an incidentally discovered lymphocytosis on a blood sample drawn for evaluation of a medical condition or as part of a "routine" medical evaluation.
   - If symptomatic, fatigue, malaise, weight loss, and decreased exercise tolerance are common presenting symptoms. Opportunistic infections with *Pneumocystis carinii* pneumonia and disseminated zoster may occur because of hypogammaglobulinemia. Symptoms of anemia and thrombocytopenia can also be present. Physical examination may be normal, or reveal lymphadenopathy or hepatosplenomegaly.
   - A sudden clinical deterioration can indicate the transformation to a diffuse large B cell lymphoma (Richter's transformation), which carries a poor prognosis.

   c. Laboratory and diagnostic studies
   - The presence of lymphocytosis (>5000 mature-appearing small lymphocytes) in the peripheral blood with no other apparent cause should alert one to the possibility of CLL. Hyperviscosity symptoms usually do not occur until the WBC count is above 500,000.
   - Immunocytochemistry may reveal the B cell markers CD19, CD20, and CD23 and a T cell marker CD5 along with weak surface immunoglobulins staining.
   - A bone marrow biopsy is not routinely necessary to make a diagnosis of CLL, but it helps in predicting prognosis.

   d. Formulating the diagnosis
   - Many diseases can cause a lymphocytosis. For example, cytomegalovirus, infectious mononucleosis, pertussis, chronic inflammatory states, and autoimmune symdromes. The lymphocytes are, however, polyclonal and the patients generally younger.

   e. Evaluating the severity of the problem
   - In the absence of hepatomegaly, splenomegaly, anemia, and thrombocytopenia treatment is unnecessary. The rationale for this approach is that current agents have not been shown to prolong life and may increase the risk of secondary malignancies.

   f. Management of the patient
   - Chemotherapy upon initial diagnosis is generally unnecessary. Most of the initial therapy should be focused on treating infections and other supportive management.
   - Indications for chemotherapy should include disease-related symptoms such as fevers, weight loss, sweats, progressive lymphadenopathy and hepatosplenomegaly, AIHA, ITP, rapidly progressive lymphocytosis, and recurrent infections. The regimen commonly used consists of fludarabine or chlorambucil +/− rituximab (anti-CD20) or alemtuzumab (anti-CD52). Prednisone is indicated for AIHA and ITP associated with CLL.

VI. Lung Cancer
   A. Basic science
   - This is the second most common cancer in the United States in both the female and male population. It accounts for more cancer deaths in the United States than any other neoplasm. Cigarette smoking is responsible for 80% to 90% of lung cancers. The risk of developing lung cancer increases with both the number of cigarettes smoked per day and the number of years of smoking. After a patient stops smoking, the risk of developing lung cancer declines over 2 to 15 years. Other potential carcinogens include asbestos, radon, radiation, chromates, nickel, arsenic, hydrocarbons, vinyl chloride, and mustard gas.
   - Although early localized lung cancer may be cured with surgical resection, more advanced disease is incurable, and the prognosis for affected patients is dismal.
   - It is commonly divided into two major categories:

1. Small cell lung cancer (SCLC)
   - SCLC is usually central in distribution, affects the proximal bronchi, is strongly associated with smoking, and has the most aggressive course compared to other histologic types.
2. Non–small cell lung cancer (NSCLC)
   a. Adenocarcinoma: lesions are usually peripheral in location. It is the most common subtype of lung cancer.
   b. Bronchoalveolar carcinoma: a subset of adenocarcinoma not associated with smoking. It involves the alveolar septa and may arise in scar tissue
   c. Squamous cell carcinoma: lesions are usually located centrally
   d. Large cell carcinoma
- The incidence of death due to lung cancer continues to increase in both men and women. There are about 172,000 new cases in the United States each year. Cigarette smoking continues to be the leading risk factor.

B. History and physical examination
   - The clinical presentation may be related to local effects, intrathoracic effects secondary to local invasion, paraneoplastic syndrome, and metastasis. Symptoms due to local effects include cough that is persistent or a change in the character of a chronic cough. Hemoptysis should prompt immediate evaluation. If there is bronchial obstruction, examination may reveal wheezing, or evidence of a pneumonia (postobstructive pneumonia). Local invasion can cause chest pain and pleural effusion as well as superior vena cava syndrome, Horner's syndrome (ptosis, miosis, and hemifacial anhidrosis), and Pancoast syndrome (apical sulcus tumor giving rise to shoulder pain and evidence of brachial plexus involvement, most often of the ulnar nerve with or without Horner's syndrome).
   - Symptoms related to metastasis or paraneoplastic syndromes are commonly seen in both NSCLC and SCLC. Lung cancers metastasize to the brain, bones (particularly the vertebra and ribs), liver, adrenal glands, skin, and lymph nodes.
   - Commonly seen paraneoplastic syndromes include syndrome of inappropriate antidiuretic hormone secretion (SIADH), the Eaton-Lambert syndrome secondary to SCLC, hypercalcemia because of ectopic parathyroid hormone secretion in squamous cell lung cancer, pulmonary hypertrophic osteoarthropathy in adenocarcinoma, and ectopic hCG (human chorionic gonadotropin) production from large cell lung cancer. Additionally, the patient may complain of weight loss, fatigue, anorexia, and fever.

C. Laboratory and diagnostic studies
   - Chest radiographs should be carefully reviewed in all patients suspected of having lung cancer. Reviews of serial chest x-rays is particularly useful. A lung lesion that has not changed in size over years or has heavy central calcification is unlikely to be malignant. Computed tomography (CT) scans will define the location, size, and nature of a parenchymal lung lesion and will aid in pursuing tissue. It should be noted that the mediastinum is more

readily evaluated with CT scan than with x-ray films. CT scans should include views of the liver and adrenals as part of the staging workup.

- In addition to chest and abdominal scans, staging usually includes a bone scan and if the patient has neurologic symptoms, a contrast CT scan of the head. Patients who have resectable NSCLC do not need bone scans in most situations.

- If the cancer is thought to be resectable, the patient needs to have an assessment of the expected postoperative pulmonary reserve. Workup may include spirometry, arterial blood gas, and ventilation-perfusion (V/Q) scans to establish that FEV_1 will be more than 1.2 L after resection and that the patient does not have hypercapnia or cor pulmonale. If such pulmonary requirements are not met, then surgical resection of the lesion is best not done.

D. Formulating the diagnosis
- As with all malignancies, a confident diagnosis requires a histologic or cytologic diagnosis. Transbronchial biopsy, transthoracic needle aspiration, thoracentesis, and thoracotomy/mediastinoscopy are techniques used to obtain tissue from primary lung lesions. Patients with metastatic disease often have lesions that are more easily sampled; examples include cervical lymph nodes, bone lesions, and liver metastases. Sputum cytologic examination may occasionally reveal malignant cells.

E. Evaluating the severity of the problem
- The prognosis is clearly correlated with the stage of the disease. In general, patients with significant weight loss, chest wall pain, large primary tumors, and metastatic disease have a poor prognosis. If the tumor is considered resectable, the patient's prognosis is markedly improved, and cure can be expected in a significant proportion of these patients.

F. Managing the patient
1. Non–small cell lung cancer (NSCLC)
- In NSCLC, potentially curative surgical resection is indicated when a complete resection is anticipated, even in those with more advanced disease. Patients with nonresectable disease are treated primarily with radiation therapy; chemotherapy has effected a modest improvement in survival in patients who are active and have minimal symptoms. The treatment of metastatic disease is aimed toward palliation of symptoms such as pain, dyspnea, and hemoptysis. Chemotherapy, in hope of obtaining a response, can be offered to patients with good performance status. The chemotherapy agents that are used for the treatment of NSCLC include docetaxel, gemcitabine, vinorelbine, and irinotecan. Table 14-3 provides a summary of the treatment strategies for NSCLC.

2. Small cell lung cancer (SCLC)
- Most SCLC is disseminated at presentation. Limited stage small cell lung cancer is treated with combination radiation and chemotherapy. Extensive disease is treated with chemotherapy. In contrast to NSCLC, SCLC does respond well to chemotherapy. Survival is increased from 2 to 3 months without chemotherapy to 8 to 14 months with chemotherapy. Despite

TABLE 14-3:
Treatment Strategies for Non–Small Cell Lung Cancer

Stage	Treatment Modality
Stage I	Surgical resection +/– chemotherapy
Stage II	Surgical resection +/– radiation +/– chemotherapy
Stage IIIa	Neoadjuvant chemotherapy +/– radiation → surgical resection
Stage IIIb	Combination of +/– radiation +/– chemotherapy
Stage IV	Chemotherapy +/– supportive care

this good response to chemotherapy, long-term survival remains dismal because of high rates of relapse. Long-term survival (>5 years) rate is less than 1%. Most commonly used chemotherapeutic regimens include platinum-based medications and etoposide.

VII. Lymphomas
  A. Non-Hodgkin's lymphoma (NHL)
    1. Basic science
      • NHLs are a heterogeneous group of B cell and T cell malignancies that usually originate from any lymph node but may also originate from any organ in the body either as a result of lymphatic spread or as a manifestation of a primary extranodal disease. It originates from a single clonal lymphocyte progenitor. By convention, any lymphoid neoplasm arising from the bone marrow is called lymphocytic leukemia, and those originating from any other lymphoid site are referred to as lymphomas.
      • Most lymphomas are B cell in origin. Epstein-Barr virus and human T cell leukemia virus have been linked to lymphoma development. Immunodeficient patients, such as those on immunosuppressive medications after organ transplantation or acquired immunodeficiency syndrome (AIDS) are at increased risk for the development of lymphomas.
      • There is a gradually increasing incidence of NHL in the United States. There are approximately 60,000 new cases per year, with a slight male predominance.
    2. History and physical examination
      • Most patients with lymphoma present with painless adenopathy in the neck, inguinal region, or axillae. Mediastinal involvement may cause a persistent nonproductive cough. Patients are generally diagnosed after failing antibiotic therapy for presumed bronchitis. Massive mediastinal disease may also present with superior vena cava syndrome (swollen face and arms, and a prominent venous pattern on the chest indicating venous engorgement and formation of collateral circulation) due to obstruction of the superior vena cava.

- Patients with intra-abdominal lymphoma may have abdominal or back pain, bowel obstruction, extrinsic compression of the urinary tract, or gastrointestinal bleeding.
- Lymphoma of the central nervous system (CNS) may present with headache, cranial nerve palsies, or symptoms of spinal cord compression. The diagnosis of CNS lymphoma should be considered in any AIDS patient with neurologic symptoms.
- The presence of B symptoms (fever, chills, night sweats, and weight loss) may be present at diagnosis and usually suggest advanced disease.
- Physical examination may reveal enlargement of the lymph nodes, liver, and spleen. Rapidly growing lymph nodes may be tender.

3. Laboratory and diagnostic studies
- Tissue biopsy is mandatory. Patients should undergo surgical biopsy of the most accessible lymph node. Because lymph node architecture is important in defining the type of lymphoma, needle aspiration and frozen section of the lymph node are considered inadequate in making a precise diagnosis of lymphoma.
- Cell marker studies may be helpful in confirming the diagnosis if they demonstrate monoclonality of the cell population.
- In order to rule out the diagnoses of tuberculosis and fungal infection, tissue should also be sent for microbiologic studies, including acid-fast bacillus and fungal stains.
- Staging involves imaging the neck, chest, abdomen, and pelvis by CT scanning.
- Other tests that should be done include CBC, liver function tests, LDH, β_2-microglobulin, erythrocyte sedimentation rate (ESR), and HIV serologic test.

4. Formulating the diagnosis
- The most important feature in determining outcome and treatment of the non-Hodgkin's lymphomas is the pathologic grade. The working formulation in Table 14-4 classifies the non-Hodgkin's lymphomas into three major groups based on microscopic appearance.

5. Evaluating the severity of problems
- Emergent medical care is indicated in only a few situations: severe pain, spinal cord compression, increased intracranial pressure or cranial nerve palsies, superior vena cava syndrome, ureteral obstruction or obstruction of another vital organ, and metabolic abnormalities such as tumor lysis syndrome. In most other circumstances, treatment and staging workups can be done on an outpatient basis.
- Tumor lysis syndrome is a condition characterized by rapid cell death, which causes release of intracellular potassium, phosphate, and nucleic acids. Irreversible renal failure may be the end result of severe tumor lysis.

6. Managing the patient
   a. Low-grade lymphoma
   - The low-grade lymphomas often present with advanced stage disease (for example, with bone marrow, splenic, or liver involvement). The

TABLE 14-4:
REAL/WHO Working Formulation for the Classification of Lymphomas

Grade	Cell Types
Low grade (indolent)	Small lymphocytic Follicular small cleaved cell Follicular mixed cells
Intermediate grade	Follicular large cell Diffuse small cleaved Diffuse mixed cells Diffuse large cell
High grade	Immunoblastic Lymphoblastic Small non-cleaved (including Burkitts' lymphoma)

median survival, however, is generally greater than 5 years. Low-grade lymphomas are treatable but are usually incurable with conventional therapy.
- Treatment of the indolent lymphomas is usually undertaken only when the patient develops symptomatic lymphadenopathy, cytopenia, or compression of a vital organ.
- Commonly used agents to treat low-grade lymphoma include chlorambucil and cyclophosphamide (used alone or with prednisone).
- Combination chemotherapy includes regimens such as cyclophosphamide, vincristine, and prednisone and the monoclonal antibody rituximab (anti-CD20).

b. Intermediate- and high-grade lymphoma
- The intermediate- and high-grade lymphomas are characterized by rapid disease progression but higher rates of remission and cure.
- Combination chemotherapeutic regimens such as CHOP (cyclophosphamide, doxorubicin, vincristine, and prednisone) commonly in combination with rituximab (CHOP-R) effect a complete remission in many patients. Multiple other regimens are also commonly used. Combination radiation therapy and chemotherapy are used and improve complete remission rates in patients with localized disease.

B. Hodgkin's disease
1. Basic science
- Hodgkin's lymphomas account for approximately 25% of all lymphomas and occur in about 8000 patients a year in the United States. Its incidence has remained unchanged over the past few decades. The malignant cell is thought to be the Reed-Sternberg cell.

TABLE 14-5:
Staging for Hodgkin's Disease

Stage/Modifier Stage	Description
I	Involvement in a single lymph node region or lymphoid structure
II	Disease in two or more lymph node regions on one side of the diaphragm
III	Involvement of lymph node structures on both sides of the diaphragm
IV	Involvement of one or more extranodal sites
Modifiers	
A	No symptoms
B	Presence of B symptoms
X	Bulky disease (nodal mass) > 10 cm or more than $\frac{1}{3}$ of the width of the thorax
E	Involvement of a single extranodal site contiguous or proximal to a known site

- Hodgkin's disease tends to spread along contiguous lymph node regions. Almost one third of patients will present with B symptoms (fever, night sweats, and 10% or more weight loss in 6 months).
- The staging of the disease, rather than the histopathologic picture, is the most important prognostic feature. The Ann Arbor system (also used for the non-Hodgkin's lymphomas) classifies the stage of the disease according to the number and distribution of lymph nodes involved (Table 14-5).
- Patients who have bulky mediastinal disease or modifier X (measuring greater than one third of the transthoracic diameter) are treated as stage IIB disease.
- Histologically, the Rye classification identifies four subtypes of Hodgkin's lymphoma: lymphocyte predominant, nodular sclerosing (most common), mixed cellularity, and lymphocyte depleted.
2. History and physical examination
   - The history and physical examination are the same as those described for non-Hodgkin's lymphomas.
3. Laboratory and diagnostic studies
   - The laboratory and radiographic workup for non-Hodgkin's lymphoma is the same as for the patient with Hodgkin's lymphoma.
4. Formulating the diagnosis
   - As in all malignancies, tissue is required to make the diagnosis of Hodgkin's disease.
5. Evaluating the severity of problems
   - The prognosis correlates with the stage of the disease at diagnosis. Another important prognostic feature is the responsiveness of the tumor to treatment.

6. Managing the patient
- All patients with Hodgkins lymphoma, irrespective of their stage or histologic features, should be treated with the intent to cure.
- Early stage disease carries a 75% to 90% cure rate and stages III and IV disease carry a 50% to 70% cure rate. Stages I and IIA disease may be treated with radiation therapy alone; stage IIB requires combination of radiotherapy with chemotherapy, and stages III and IV are treated with chemotherapy alone.
- Effective chemotherapy regimens:
  a. Mechlorethamine, vincristine, procarbazine, and prednisone (MOPP)
  b. Doxorubicin, bleomycin, vinblastine, and dacarbazine (ABVD)
- Stem cell transplantation for disease relapse or chemotherapy-refractory patients is an option.

VIII. Multiple Myeloma (MM)
A. Basic science
- Multiple myeloma is a clonal disorder of plasma cells characterized by the production of monoclonal protein, IgG. It commonly occurs about the age of 60 and is twice as common in African Americans. MM accounts for 10% of all hematologic malignancies in the United States.
B. History and physical examination
- MM should be suspected in individuals with normocytic normochromic anemia, renal insufficiency, hypercalcemia, and bone pains (particularly pain of the spine and ribs, accompanied by reduced height and pathologic fractures). Occasionally these individuals can also have recurrent bacterial infections, particularly pneumonia and pyelonephritis and bleeding.
C. Laboratory and diagnostic studies
- Laboratory investigations reveal a normocytic, normochormic anemia, an elevated creatinine and calcium.
- The incidental finding of lytic lesions on x-rays (taken for another reason) should raise the possibility of MM.
- A urine dipstick may miss the light chain or Bence Jones protein in the urine, so a sulfasalicylic acid test must be done to ascertain light chain proteinuria.
- Urine protein electrophoresis (UPEP), serum protein electrophoresis (SPEP), and immunofixation will identify the presence of monoclonal antibodies. The IgG M protein is found in approximately 50% of all patients followed by IgA in about 20%.
D. Formulating the diagnosis
- Hypercalcemia, renal insufficiency, anemia (usually normocytic normochromic), and back pain should alert one to the possibility of multiple myeloma. The presence of monoclonal proteins in the urine or serum, the presence of skeletal lytic lesions by skeletal x-ray, the presence of plasmacytomas, or more than 30% plasma cells in the bone marrow will help establish the diagnosis.

E. Evaluating the severity of the problem/management of the patient
  • Treatment is rarely curative.
  • If a patient has serum monoclonal protein of less than 3 g/dL, less than 10% plasma cells in the bone marrow and no anemia, renal failure, or lytic bone lesions, these patients have monoclonal gammopathy of undetermined significance. These patients should be followed at 6- to 12-month intervals. No treatment is indicated. M protein levels in the urine and blood should be monitored.
  • The melphalan and prednisone combination or vincristine, doxorubicin (adriamycin), and dexamethasone (VAD) are the most widely used chemotherapy regimens for MM. Most recently, thalidomide, which is an antiangiogenesis agent, has been used with success. Other novel treatments are autologous bone marrow transplant and borteozemib.
  • Radiation may help alleviate bone pain or localized plasmacytoma unresponsive to chemotherapy.

IX. Ocologic Emergencies
  A. Superior vena cava syndrome
    1. Basic science
      • This is no longer considered a true oncologic emergency. It is a result of obstruction to blood flow through the superior vena cava. This syndrome is most often the result of a bronchogenic carcinoma (70% to 80%) and less often due to a lymphoma, retrosternal goiter, thoracic aortic aneurysm, or fibrosing medasitinits due to histoplasmosis or tuberculosis.
    2. History and physical examination
      • The patient may be asymptomatic or complain of shortness of breath, cough, dysphagia, or headache. Examination may reveal evidence of weight loss, neck and chest wall distention, edema of the upper extremities, and facial swelling and discoloration. Hoarseness due to vocal cord paralysis and Horner's syndrome may also occur.
    3. Laboratory and diagnostic studies
      • Chest x-ray may reveal a widened mediastinum.
    4. Management of the patient
      • Low-salt diet, head elevation, and oxygen may be the initial symptom-alleviating maneuvers. Diuretics and steroids may be helpful at initial presentation. If compression is not life-threatening, then a tissue diagnosis must be sought first before proceeding with treatment. Radiation therapy is useful for non–small cell lung cancer and metastatic cancer. Chemotherapy is indicated for small cell lung cancer and lymphoma. If the obstruction is secondary to thrombosis of the superior vena cava, anticoagulation is indicated.
  B. Tumor lysis syndrome
    1. Basic science
      • This syndrome is caused by the lysis of a huge number of neoplastic and normal cells as a consequence of chemotherapy, radiation, or steroids. Rarely, it can occur spontaneously. It is most commonly seen in leukemias

especially ALL and non-Hodgkin's lymphoma. Patients with rapidly proliferating tumors, bulky tumors, underlying chronic kidney disease, and an elevated LDH are most susceptible to this syndrome.

- The presence of risk factors combined with metabolic abnormalities, commonly hyperuricemia, hyperphosphatemia, hyperkalemia, and hypocalcemia, helps establish the diagnosis. These patients are at risk of developing renal failure or worsening of underlying renal failure.

2. Management of the patient
   - Patients with the tumor lysis syndrome should be aggressively hydrated with hypotonic or isotonic saline, given allopurinol, and the urine alkalinized. Electrolyte abnormalities should be treated concomitantly.

C. Spinal cord compression due to malignancy

1. Basic science
   - Spinal cord compression is a common emergency and is a result of bony metastasis. The typical cancers that cause spinal cord compression are breast cancer, renal cell cancer, lung cancer, and prostate cancer. The most common site of involvement is the thoracic vertebra. Spinal cord compression occurs in 5% of cancer patients.

2. History and physical examination
   - The most common symptom is radicular pain secondary to nerve compression. Other symptoms include paresthesias, weakness and abnormalities suggestive of a cauda equina syndrome. Local pain may be a prominent symptom.

3. Laboratory and diagnostic studies/formulating the diagnosis
   - This is generally a clinical diagnosis. MRI of the spine is the imaging study of choice.

4. Management
   - Dexamethasone is initial treatment of choice. Emergent radiation and surgical decompression are generally indicated.

D. Neutropenic fever

1. Basic science
   - Neutropenic fever is fever (single oral temperature $\geq 38.3°C$ or $\geq 38.0°C$ lasting for longer than 1 hour) in the absence of an obvious cause, in a patient with an absolute neutrophil count of less than 500 cells/μL or less than 1000 cells/μL with a predicted nadir of less than 500 cells/μL.

2. History and physical examination
   - Indicators of infection may not be readily evident because of the presence of low numbers of neutrophils. A thorough history and physical examination must be done, though, to help exclude common sources of infection such as oral ulcers, pharyngeal infection, pneumonias, urinary tract infection, and intra-abdominal infections.

3. Laboratory and diagnostic studies
   - Tests should include CBC with differentials to confirm the presence of neutropenia by ANC. Blood cultures, urinalysis and urine culture, chest x-ray, and stool cultures are performed if indicated.

4. Management of the patient
- Risk stratification is most important in determining whether the patient should either be on oral or intravenous antibiotics. Criteria for low risk include individuals younger than 60 years old living in the community who have good performance statuses, serum creatinine of less than 2.0 mg/dL, and an anticipated duration of neutropenia less than 7 days. Patients who fall in the low risk category can be treated with oral antibiotics such as ciprofloxacin plus amoxicillin/clavulanate. Intravenous antibiotics are indicated in patients at high risk. If monotherapy is decided on a carbapenem (imipenem-cilastatin, meropenem) or an antipseudomonal cephalosporin (e.g., ceftazidine or cefepime) may be used. Therapy with two antibiotics should include an antipseudomonal penicillin with an aminoglycoside or ciprofloxacin.
- The duration of treatment is determined by the presence of an identifiable source for the neutropenic fever and the ANC. Generally if the cause of infection is found treatment should be continued for 14-day course (unless the patient has osteomyelitis or infective endocarditis). If no source is identified and the patient is low risk, afebrile for 48 hours, and ANC above 500 the antibiotic can be stopped.

X. Polycythemia Vera
  A. Basic science
- Polycythemia vera is a clonal expansion of multipotent progenitor cells in which there is accumulation of phenotypically normal red blood cells, and usually granulocytes and platelets in the absence of a recognizable physiologic stimulus. It is the most common of the myeloproliferative disorders and occurs in 2 in 100,000 persons. There is a slight male predominance.
  B. History and physical examination
- The signs and symptoms are protean but are commonly related to hyperviscosity, thrombosis, bleeding, or pruritus. Hyperviscosity symptoms are vertigo, visual disturbances, tinnitus, and headaches. Symptoms related to venous or arterial thrombosis may be the initial presenting symptom for some (erythromelalgia). Uncontrolled systolic hypertension may occur. Bleeding may result because of dysfunctional platelets.
  C. Laboratory and diagnostic studies
- The complete blood count confirms the presence of increased hemoglobin and hematocrit and, when present, an increase in WBC and platelets. Vitamin B_{12} levels, leukocyte alkaline phosphatase, and uric acid levels are usually elevated. The presence of a low erythropoietin level further supports the diagnosis.
  D. Formulating the diagnosis
- Diagnoses are based on a set of criteria established by the Polycythemia Vera Study Group (PVSG): 3 major and 1 minor or 2 major and 2 minor criteria (Box 14-1).

BOX 14-1

THE POLYCYTHEMIA VERA STUDY GROUP CRITERIA FOR DIAGNOSIS

Major Criteria
1. Increased red blood cell mass
2. Normal O_2 saturation
3. Splenomegaly

Minor Criteria
1. Thrombocytosis
2. Leukocytosis
3. Elevated leukocyte alkaline phosphatase
4. Elevated vitamin B_{12}

Secondary causes of erythrocytosis must be excluded, especially hypoxemia, renal disease, and neoplasms such as hepatoma and pheochromocytoma.

E. Management
- The goal of treatment is to reduce blood volume to normal level and to prevent complications such as thrombosis or bleeding.
- Phlebotomy is useful in decreasing the hematocrit level to about 45%. It is the mainstay of treatment. Chemotherapy and radioactive phosphorus are associated with acute myelogenous leukemia transformation. Use of cytoreductive agents such as hydroxyurea is helpful in reducing counts to acceptable levels. Aspirin may be useful and is indicated for patients with erythromelalgia (painful red extremities), cardiovascular disease, and microvascular disorders.

XI. Prostate Cancer
A. Basic science
- Prostate cancer is the most common noncutaneous cancer in males. It accounts for 36% of male cancers and 13% of all male cancer deaths. Most prostate cancers are adenocarcinomas.
- The cause of prostate cancer is not known. In the United States it is more common among African Americans. The lifetime male risk of developing prostate cancer is about 10%. Risk factors include age, race, and family history. Benign prostatic hypertrophy is not a risk factor for prostate cancer.
B. History and physical examination
- Since the widespread use of prostate specific antigen (PSA) and digital rectal examinations most patients are asymptomatic at diagnosis. The presence of asymmetric areas of induration or hard nodules on the prostate is suggestive of cancer. If symptomatic, the initial presenting symptoms are usually related to obstruction. Other concomitant or initial presenting symptoms include hematuria, dysuria, and back pain. New onset erectile dysfunction should also raise suspicion of prostate cancer. Evidence of metastatic disease as manifested by deep vein thrombosis and spinal cord compression may be the initial presentation.

C. Laboratory and diagnostic studies
- The most commonly used laboratory test is the PSA. A normal level is less than 4 ng/mL. It should be noted that a normal PSA value does not rule out prostate cancer.
- If the PSA is 4 to 10 ng/mL the positive predictive value (PPV) that there is cancer is 20% to 25%; if it is over 10 ng/mL the PPV is 50%; and if the PSA is over 4 ng/mL and the rectal examination is abnormal, the PPV is 60%.
- If the same assay is used, measurement of PSA velocity (>0.75 ng/mL/year) may also be a helpful indicator of prostatic malignancy.
- Diagnosis is established by transrectal biopsy under ultrasound guidance.

D. Formulating the diagnosis
- Tissue is essential for diagnosis. The histologic grade is the most important determinant of disease course and patient survival. The currently used system is the Gleason grading scheme. The higher the score, the less differentiated the tumor is, and the poorer the prognosis.

E. Management of the patient
- When the disease is confined to the prostate the options are radical prostatectomy, radiation therapy (external beam or interstitial radioactive implants referred to as brachytherapy), or watchful waiting. Androgen deprivation therapy is generally reserved for locally advanced or metastatic disease. Chemotherapeutic options are available for hormone therapy resistant patients.

XII. Renal Cell Cancer
A. Basic science
- Renal cell carcinoma (RCC) originates within the renal cortex and accounts for 80% of all neoplasms in the kidney. The predominant histologic type is the clear cell carcinoma, which accounts for 60% of all cases. Transitional cell carcinomas arise in the renal pelvis. RCCs are more common in males by a 2 : 1 ratio. Risk factors include advanced age, smoking, obesity, and the presence of hereditary abnormalities such as von Hippel-Lindau syndrome and polycystic kidney disease.

B. History and physical examination
- The classic triad of symptoms is hematuria, flank/abdominal mass, and abdominal pain or symptoms related to distant metastasis in the lung, lymph nodes, bones, or liver. Other symptoms include fever, weight loss, malaise, anemia, and a varicocele, particularly on the left.

C. Laboratory and diagnostic studies
- It is not uncommon for renal masses to be detected incidentally during imaging tests performed for some other reason. Local disease and vein invasion is best evaluated by CT scan. Once a mass has been discovered, further workup should include chest x-ray to assess for possible metastasis, urinalysis, and urine cytologic test. CBC may show evidence of erythrocytosis secondary to increased erythropoietin production by the tumor.

D. Management
- The current management scheme depends on the Robson Classification and American Joint Committee on Cancer (AJCC) staging system. It involves the use of radical nephrectomy for stage I (only kidney involved) or II (has extended beyond renal capsule but within the Gerota's fascia) and selected cases of Stage III localized tumors. Radical nephrectomy involves removal of the Gerotas' fascia, its content including the kidneys, the ipsilateral adrenal gland, and adjacent hilar lymph nodes. There is no proven role for adjuvant chemotherapy.
- Advanced or metastatic disease is poorly responsive to any type of therapy, including chemotherapy or immunotherapy.

XII. Sickle Cell Disease
A. Basic science
- Sickle cell disease is an autosomal recessive hemoglobinopathy that results from a single base mutation in DNA that leads to an amino acid substitution (valine for glutamic acid) in the hemoglobin molecule. The abnormal hemoglobin (Hb S) polymerizes in the deoxygenated state and causes red blood cell sickling. The sickled cells in the microvasculature cause vaso-occlusion. Hemolysis of the sickled cells leads to anemia.
- An individual must be homozygous to develop sickle cell disease. Heterozygosity leads to the carrier state; such patients are said to have sickle trait.
B. History and physical examination
- The clinical manifestations vary considerably.
- Patients with sickle cell anemia experience both acute crises and chronic medical problems. Most problems are due to vaso-occlusion rather than anemia. Dehydration, infection, pregnancy, and fever can precipitate vaso-occlusion. Vaso-occlusion affects the bones, joints, mesentery, and lungs. This causes painful crises, bone infarction, and cerebrovascular accidents. Acute pain is the reason patients most often seek medical care. Any part of the body can be affected, most commonly the chest, abdomen, back, and extremities.
- Acute chest syndrome is a vaso-occlusive process characterized by fever, chest pain, dyspnea, hypoxia, and pulmonary infiltrates. It can be life-threatening.
- Chronic sickling and splenic infarction lead to functional asplenia. Sickle cell patients are particularly susceptible to infection with encapsulated pathogens (e.g., pneumococcus) and *Salmonella*. Meningitis due to *S. pneumoniae* is seen in infants and young children. Osteomyelitis and pneumonia are other infections that can occur in these patients.
- Related medical problems also contribute to morbidity and death. Growth retardation, chronic bone disease, leg ulcers, cardiac disease due to chronic anemia and iron overload (from hemolysis and blood transfusions), renal disease, proliferative retinopathy, and chronic pulmonary disease develop in

the adolescent and adult patient. The chronic hemolysis leads to pigment gallstones, frequently requiring cholecystectomy.

C. Laboratory and diagnostic studies

- Widespread screening of infants in the United States detects both sickle trait and sickle cell disease. Early detection helps in management and decreases the chances for morbidity and death.
- Quantitative hemoglobin electrophoresis confirms the diagnosis by showing a predominance of hemoglobin S. Heterozygotes have both hemoglobin A and hemoglobin S. The patient with sickle cell disease who presents with a painful crisis should have a complete blood count, chemistry panel (including LDH and bilirubin as measures of hemolysis), and a reticulocyte count. Blood samples for cultures and for typing and crossmatching are usually obtained during the initial evaluation as well. MRI scans of bones may be helpful in differentiating between infarcts and osteomyelitis. In the patient with pulmonary symptoms, a chest radiograph and arterial blood gas should also be done.
- Abdominal ultrasound may be indicated in the patient with possible cholelithiasis or cholecystitis.

D. Formulating the diagnosis

- The screening of infants provides early diagnosis. In the rare patient who eludes diagnosis in infancy, a painful crisis coupled with sickled cells on the peripheral smear will lead to the diagnosis. The finding of osteomyelitis caused by *Salmonella* should also raise the suspicion of sickle cell disease.

E. Evaluating the severity of problems

- The patient's pain is the most important indicator of crisis severity. The degree of anemia often does not correlate with the severity of the painful crisis, particularly as dehydrated patients may have a falsely elevated hematocrit upon presentation. The reticulocyte count will correlate with the degree of hemolysis and can be followed during the crisis.

F. Management of the patient

- Pneumococcal and *Haemophilus influenzae* type b vaccination is indicated for all sickle cell patients. Any trigger for the crisis should be treated, if possible. Patients should avoid dehydration, cold, and high altitude to prevent vaso-occlusive crises.
- Early treatment with penicillin in the febrile pediatric patient reduces morbidity from meningitis. Treatment of a sickle cell crisis includes intravenous hydration, narcotic analgesics, folate supplements, antibiotics if an infection is suspected, and red blood cell transfusions as indicated. Acute chest syndrome is treated with oxygen, fluids, antibiotics, and exchange transfusion in the more severe cases.
- Patients with iron overload can be treated with deferoxamine, an iron chelator.
- Hydroxyurea increases hemoglobin F and reduces leukocyte and sickle cell counts. It has been shown to decrease acute pain episodes, transfusion requirements and increase life expectancy.

XIV. Thalassemia
  A. Basic science
   • The thalassemias are a group of genetic disorders that affect the globin protein of hemoglobin. Defects are due to mutations in the DNA that code for these globin chains. Each normal adult has four α-globin genes and two β-globin genes.
  B. History and physical examination
   • The clinical manifestations of thalassemia depend on the location of the DNA mutation and the number of involved genes.
  C. Laboratory and diagnostic studies
   1. α-Thalassemia
    • There are four α-thalassemia syndromes, most of which arise because of α-globin gene deletions:
     a. The silent carrier state
      • One of the four α-chain loci is absent; this syndrome has no clinical or laboratory implications for the carrier.
     b. α-Thalassemia trait
      • Two of the four loci are abnormal or absent.
      • This form will produce microcytosis, with or without mild anemia. Hemoglobin electrophoresis is normal. Patients are rarely symptomatic unless they have a second cause for anemia.
     c. Hemoglobin H disease
      • This syndrome arises from deletions of three of the four α-chain genes.
      • It causes moderate to severe microcytic anemia with red blood cell changes, including target cells, stippling, and hypochromia. Besides anemia, affected patients have jaundice and hepatosplenomegaly as early as 1 year of age.
     d. Hydrops fetalis
      • Caused by deletions of all four α-chain loci.
      • Incompatible with life, affected fetuses are stillborn.
   2. β-Thalassemia
    • The β-thalassemias are the result of mutations within the genes encoding the β-globin chains. There are two β-thalassemia syndromes:
     a. β-Thalassemia minor (β-thalassemia trait)
      • This type occurs in those who are heterozygous for the β-thalassemia gene. Laboratory findings include microcytosis, hypochromia, target cells, cigar-shaped cells, basophilic stippling, and hypochromia. Anemia, if present, is usually mild. Hemoglobin electrophoresis demonstrates increased amounts of hemoglobin A_2. Because of the microcytosis, many patients with β-thalassemia trait have been treated with iron for what was thought to be iron-deficiency anemia.
     b. β-Thalassemia major (Cooley's anemia)
      • This form arises from the homozygous state of the β-thalassemia gene. Affected patients are severely anemic and have signs of hemolysis, iron overload, and skeletal abnormalities (due to

expansion of the marrow). The peripheral smear demonstrates marked shape changes and often normoblasts. Hemoglobin electrophoresis reveals an increased amount of fetal hemoglobin (Hb F). Patients are transfusion dependent and have a decreased life expectancy. Folate supplementation is appropriate. Splenectomy may be helpful in increasing the red blood cell survival. Bone marrow transplantation is potentially curative in the patient with a human lymphocyte antigen-compatible sibling. Many patients require iron chelation therapy to avoid the complications of iron overload.

D. Formulating the diagnosis
   - The diagnosis of α-thalassemia trait or β-thalassemia minor is suspected in the patient with microcytosis (with or without anemia) whose iron studies are normal. A family history of mild anemia also suggests thalassemia. Hemoglobin electrophoresis will help distinguish these two syndromes, being normal in α-thalassemia trait and showing increased amounts of hemoglobin A_2 in β-thalassemia minor. Hemoglobin H disease and β-thalassemia major are generally diagnosed because of the unique clinical features described in the preceding paragraphs.

E. Evaluating the severity of problems
   - The degree of anemia, the transfusion requirement, and the severity of hemolysis are important factors in determining the severity of the disease.

F. Managing the patient
   - Transfusion support is often needed. Patients do not need to be transfused to a normal hematocrit; most are asymptomatic with hematocrits in the low 20%.
   - Because of the hazards of iron overload from chronic transfusion therapy, most patients should be considered for treatment with chelation therapy. The most common chelator is deferoxamine, a drug that can be given via subcutaneous injection through a home pump.

XV. Thrombocytopenia
   - Thrombocytopenia is a quantitative drop in platelets usually to below 150,000/μL. The risk of bleeding increases with the degree of thrombocytopenia (Table 14-6).
   - Thrombocytopenia can be due to (1) decreased production (e.g., aplastic anemia, marrow suppression due to medications, alcohol, infection, or ionized radiation); (2) replacement of marrow (e.g., leukemias, metastatic deposits, folate or vitamin B_{12} deficiency); or (3) increased destruction (e.g., idiopathic thrombocytopenia purpura, thrombotic thrombocytopenia purpura, hemolytic uremic syndrome, sepsis, disseminated intravascular coagulation and hypersplenism).

A. Disseminated intravascular coagulation (DIC)
   1. Basic science
      - DIC is an acquired disease characterized by a loss of equilibrium in the coagulation system resulting in consumption of the coagulation factors with widespread microthrombi formation and bleeding.
      - DIC may be the result of infection, neoplasms, burns, trauma, pancreatitis, obstetric complications, snake venom, cocaine use, and vasculitides.

TABLE 14-6:
Risk of Bleeding in Thrombocytopenia

Platelet Count	Risk of Bleeding
>100,000	No increased risk
50,000–100,000	Risk of bleeding only with major trauma but may proceed with general surgery
20,000–50,000	Risk with minor trauma or surgery
<20,000	Risk of spontaneous bleeding
<10,000	Risk of severe spontaneous bleeding, e.g., intracranial bleeding

2. History and physical examination
   - Patients are typically critically unwell. Bleeding from the gums, mucosal surfaces, gastrointestinal tract, or into the skin may occur.
3. Laboratory and diagnostic studies
   - The blood smear may show fragmented red blood cells. There is thrombocytopenia, low serum fibrinogen, elevated PT, INR, PTT, fibrin split products, and D-dimer levels.
4. Formulating the diagnosis
   - DIC should be suspected in a patient with bleeding in the presence of prolonged PT, INR, and PTT; thrombocytopenia; decreased serum fibrinogen; and elevated fibrin degradation products (FDPs) and D-dimer levels.
5. Management of the patient
   - The most important goal in treatment is to correct the underlying cause of the DIC such as antibiotics for infection, removal of products of conception if it's secondary to a retained fetus, etc. Supportive treatment includes platelet, red blood cell, fresh frozen plasma, and cryoprecipitate transfusions. Heparin may be administered in selected patients to help neutralize thrombin.
B. Heparin induced thrombocytopenia/thrombosis (HITT)
   1. Basic science
      - HITT is a heparin antibody medicated thrombocytopenia. Both unfractionated and low-molecular-weight heparin can cause thrombocytopenia.
      - Two types of this syndrome are recognized:
        a. HIT 1 (also known as nonimmune HIT)
           - This is a self-limited form that is not associated with thrombotic complications. It is associated with only a modest drop in the platelet counts.
        b. HIT 2 (immune-mediated HIT)
           - This is the more serious form. It results from antibodies formed against the heparin-platelet factor 4 complex and occurs 5 to 7 days after exposure to heparin if this is the initial exposure. It can still

occur within 100 days of treatment with heparin. It may occur immediately if the patient has been previously exposed to heparin. The drop in the platelet count is usually modest, rarely below 50,000/μL, but a drop by 50% (even if within normal limits) suggests the diagnosis.

- HITT occurs in 3% of people who received heparin. There is a 30% incidence of concomitant thrombosis in patients diagnosed with HIT.

2. History and physical examination
   - The finding of a thrombotic event within 10 days of starting heparin is suggestive. Thrombotic complications may be both venous and arterial (25% of cases). Evidence of leg swelling may suggest deep vein thrombosis (DVT) of the lower extremity, and shortness of breath with concomitant pleuritic chest pain suggests pulmonary embolism. Acute coronary syndromes and cerebrovascular accidents can also occur. Thrombosis of blood vessels at unusual sites should point to a diagnosis of HITT.

3. Laboratory and diagnostic studies
   - A complete blood count will document thrombocytopenia and exclude some of the other causes of thrombocytopenia. Heparin-induced platelet aggregation and demonstration of antiplatelet factor 4 antibody are sensitive tests. The serotonin release assay is confirmatory.

4. Formulating the diagnosis
   - HITT should be suspected in any individual who develops thrombocytopenia during heparin treatment. The diagnosis is made by demonstrating thrombocytopenia, thrombosis, and abnormal laboratory data as outlined above.

5. Evaluating the severity of the problem
   - Thrombosis can result in life-threatening ischemia to a limb, myocardial infarction, or a cerebrovascular accident.

6. Management of the patient
   - Heparin should be discontinued immediately. Low-molecular-weight heparin (LMWH) cannot be used in place of unfractionated heparin. If there is a concomitant thrombotic complication, the patient should be started on an alternative anticoagulant such as lepirudin or argatroban which are direct thrombin inhibitors, the patient should be maintained on warfarin. If there is no thrombosis, alternative anticoagulation in the form of direct thrombin inhibitors should still be used until the platelet count normalizes. There is still no clear consensus as to the duration of subsequent anticoagulation.

C. Idiopathic thrombocytopenic purpura (ITP)
   1. Basic science
      - ITP is an acquired quantitative platelet abnormality characterized by an isolated thrombocytopenia not accounted for by any other clinical condition. The red and white blood cell counts are normal.
      - Current evidence suggests that it is likely to be secondary to an antibody-mediated problem that causes an increased clearance of the platelets by the spleen.

- ITP has a bimodal distribution, one during childhood which is characterized by a self-limited disease and an adult variant that tends to run an indolent course. In adults, it is more common in females than in males and the age of onset is between 18 and 40 years old.
2. History and physical examination
   - Signs and symptoms are usually related to low platelet counts and include bruising, petechiae, and epistaxis. Despite increased clearance of platelets by the spleen, spelnomegaly is uncommon and is seen in only 3% of all patients. Therefore, a palpable spleen should make one consider an alternative diagnosis.
3. Laboratory and diagnostic studies
   - A complete blood count will demonstrate a low platelet count and the absence of quantitative abnormalities in the other cell lines. A peripheral smear will help exclude the other causes of thrombocytopenia such as TTP/HUS and DIC. A bone marrow biopsy is usually not indicated unless morphologic abnormalities are seen in the other cell lines, the patient is over 60 years old, and splenectomy is being considered.
4. Formulating the diagnosis
   - ITP is a diagnosis of exclusion: infections (e.g., HIV, infectious mononucleosis), medications (e.g., heparin, sulfonamides), liver disease, hypothyroidism, systemic lupus erythematosus, TTP, HUS, preeclampsia, and the rare congenital thrombocytopenias.
5. Management of the patient
   - Treatment depends on the degree of thrombocytopenia and patient's age.
   - Platelet transfusion is indicated if the platelet count is below 10,000/μL or if there is evidence of spontaneous bleeding.
   - Oral prednisone is given in noncritical cases and intravenous methylprednisolone in significant life-threatening bleeding. Intravenous immunoglobulin (IVIg) is first line treatment in pregnancy and in severe disease. Splenectomy should be considered in patients with persistent thrombocytopenia despite 6 weeks of medical treatment. Rituximab may be effective in patients who do not respond to conventional treatment.

D. Thrombotic thrombocytopenic purpura (TTP) and hemolytic uremic syndrome (HUS)
   1. Basic science
      - TTP and HUS result in platelet destruction and have clinical similarities characterized by the presence of microangiopathic hemolytic anemia and thrombocytopenia. The incidence of TTP is about 3.7 cases per 100,000.
   2. History and physical examination
      - Both TTP and HUS may have symptoms of hemolytic anemia and thrombocytopenia. A helpful way to differentiate them clinically is the predominance of neurologic findings in TTP and predominance of renal findings in HUS.
      - HUS is a disease primarily of infants and young children and is seen most often following bloody diarrhea caused by *E. coli* 0157:H7. Hypertension is common. The pentad of thrombocytopenia, fever, microangiopathic

hemolytic anemia, neurologic fndings, and renal failure should make one think of TTP and HUS. Purpura, mucosal bleeding (from thrombocytopenia), and jaundice (hemolysis) may also occur.

3. Laboratory and diagnostic studies
   - A white blood cell count will help determine the decrease in platelet count and anemia. A peripheral smear will show the presence of schistocytes. Low haptoglobin, elevated indirect bilirubin, elevated LDH, and the presence of hemosiderin in the urine support the diagnosis. Normal PT, INR, and PTT will help exclude DIC. ADAMTS13, a von Willebrand factor cleaving protein, has been associated with TTP. It is, however, not currently recommended as a test for TTP.

4. Formulating the diagnosis
   - TTP or HUS should be suspected in patients with low platelets, low hemoglobin and hematocrit, microangiopathy (schistocytes in peripheral blood smear), hemolytic anemia, and normal PT, INR, and PTT in the appropriate clinical setting.

5. Management
   - Plasmapheresis with plasma exchange is the treatment of choice. Response to the treatment can be monitored by following LDH and CBC. Prednisone alone may be effective in mild disease. Platelet transfusions are generally contraindicated because they promote platelet aggregation and further thrombus formation.
   - Drug-induced TTP secondary to mitomycin and cyclosporine are poorly responsive to plasmapheresis and carry a poor prognosis.

XVI. Thrombosis
   A. Basic science
      - Thrombosis is the formation of clots in the arterial and venous vascular system.
      - Hypercoagulable states, stasis, and endothelial injury (Virchow's triad) predispose to thrombosis.
      - Acquired predisposing causes include include surgery especially orthopedic, neoplasms, pregnancy, prolonged immobilization, presence of antiphospholipid antibodies, trauma, infections, and drugs. Acquired causes are more common than those that are inherited.
      - Inherited causes include factor V_{Leiden} mutation, prothrombin G20210A mutation, hyperhomocystinemia, protein C or S deficiency, and antithrombin deficiency.
   B. History and physical examination
      - Identifying patients at risk for thrombosis is essential to the diagnosis because the presenting signs and symptoms of deep venous thrombosis (DVT) may be minimal or absent. When present, the clinical signs of a DVT are nonspecific and include pain, warmth, tenderness, and swelling or color changes in the area of the thrombus, or a palpable "cord."
   C. Laboratory and diagnostic studies
      - The "gold standard" for evaluation of a lower extremity DVT is contrast venography. This is an invasive test and is painful. The hazards of giving IV

contrast agent also exist. Duplex ultrasonography is the procedure of choice for diagnosing DVT. Ultrasonography can be obtained quickly and has excellent sensitivity for detecting proximal thrombi. Impedance plethysmography has poor sensitivity for calf-vein thrombi and nonobstructive proximal thrombi. False positive results can occur in patients with peripheral vascular disease and postoperative lower extremity swelling.

D. Formulating the diagnosis
  • A high index of suspicion is required to make the diagnosis.

E. Evaluating the severity of problems
  • The most serious consequence of a DVT is a pulmonary embolus.

F. Managing the patient
  • DVT prophylaxis includes the use of low-dose heparin, (unfractionated or low molecular weight) pneumatic stockings with at least one compression per minute. A patient with a documented DVT requires anticoagulation. Initially, continuous IV heparin or low-molecular-weight heparin is used with the goal of bridging to warfarin. Warfarin dosing should be guided by the INR. Warfarin should generally not be started alone because it puts the patient at a transient risk for thrombosis because of initial depletion of protein C. Heparin is usually discontinued 1 to 2 days after patient achieves therapeutic INR on warfarin. The duration of therapy depends on the cause of the DVT and the number of previous episodes of DVT.
  • Those patients at risk for bleeding or contraindication to anticoagulation should have an inferior vena cava filter placed if the DVT is in the lower extremity.
  • If the patient develops a DVT for the first time with a clearly identifiable cause, anticoagulation should be given for 3 to 6 months. If the DVT is idiopathic, coagulation should be continued for 6 months. If the DVT is the patient's second episode, or if the patient has underlying malignancy or a nonmodifiable risk factor, anticoagulation should be continued for life.

XVII. von Willebrand's disease
  A. Basic science
    • von Willebrand's disease is an inherited coagulation disorder caused by abnormal synthesis or release of von Willebrand factor (vWF) from endothelial cells. von Willebrand factor is a large adhesive glycoprotein required for platelet adhesion to the vessel wall and for stabilization of factor VIII.
    • The most common form of the disease, type I (partial deficiency), or classic von Willebrand's disease, is inherited as an autosomal dominant trait. The trait is seen in both males and females. Type III is near-complete deficiency and type II is a qualitative abnormality.
  B. History and physical examination
    • The most common type of bleeding in von Willebrand's disease is mucocutaneous bleeding. Examples of such bleeding are epistaxis, gingival bleeding, menorrhagia, and easy bruising. Variability of bleeding is characteristic of the disease. Therefore, although bleeding after surgery,

childbirth, and dental extractions is common, the patient may not have a consistent bleeding history. The family history may be helpful.

C. Laboratory and diagnostic studies
- The bleeding time, a measure of platelet function, is often prolonged in patients with von Willebrand's disease. The PTT is often but not always elevated. The ristocetin cofactor assay is a sensitive test for von Willebrand's disease.

D. Formulating the diagnosis
- The history, physical examination, and the laboratory tests will help establish the diagnosis of von Willebrand's disease. Because of the variability of the disease, however, one set of normal blood results does not rule out the diagnosis.
- Mild hemophilia may simulate this disease.

E. Evaluating the severity of the problem
- The extent of bleeding in the past is not necessarily a reliable indicator of disease severity. The level of factor VIII and the bleeding time are probably accurate measures of the status of the disease at the time of evaluation. Fatal bleeding from von Willebrand's disease is rare.

F. Managing the patient
- von Willebrand's disease can be treated prophylactically (or during bleeding episodes) with cryoprecipitate or factor VIII preparations that are "contaminated" with von Willebrand factor. Both must be given approximately every 12 hours.
- Patients with type I von Willebrand's disease, in whom the vWF is synthesized normally but secreted abnormally, may respond to treatment with ddAVP (i.e., desmopressin, an analog of vasopressin). This hormone, given intravenously, stimulates release of vWF from endothelial cells.

XVIII. Waldenstrom's Macroglobulinemia
- Waldenstrom's macroglobulinemia is a plasma cell disorder characterized by IgM monoclonal macroglobulins. It is differentiated from IgM myeloma by the absence of bone lesions.
- Most patients present with hyperviscosity syndromes characterized by headaches dizziness, peripheral neuropathy, and visual disturbances. Hepatomegaly, lymphadenopathy, vascular segmentation, and dilatation of retinal veins (sausage links by ophthalmologic examination) may be found. Renal disease is uncommon because very little light chain is excreted.
- Diagnostic approach is similar to multiple myeloma. Patients with hyperviscosity syndrome symptoms are best treated with plasmaphoresis, chlorambucil, and prednisone or a combination of melphalan and cyclophosphamide. Patients who do not respond are treated with fludarabine, 2-CdA (2-chloro-deoxyadenosine), or retuximab.

XIX. Appendix: Cancer Screening Recommendations (Table 14-7)

TABLE 14-7:

Age-Appropriate Cancer Screening*

Disease	Date of Recommendation	Recommendation
Lung cancer	May 2004	The evidence is insufficient to recommend for or against screening asymptomatic persons for lung cancer with either low-dose computed tomography, chest x-ray, sputum cytologic test, or a combination of these tests.
Breast cancer	February 2002	Screening mammography, with or without clinical breast examination (CBE), every 1–2 years for women aged 40 and older.
		The evidence is insufficient to recommend for or against routine CBE alone to screen for breast cancer.
		The evidence is insufficient to recommend for or against teaching or performing routine breast self-examination (BSE).
		There is no data to support screening mammograms between ages 35 and 40 years.
		If there is a strong family history of breast cancer, then screening should be started 5 years earlier than the age when the youngest member of the family was first diagnosed with breast cancer.
Prostate cancer	December 2002	The evidence is insufficient to recommend for or against routine screening for prostate cancer using prostate-specific antigen (PSA) testing or digital rectal examination (DRE).
Colon cancer	February 2005	It is strongly recommended that clinicians screen men and women 50 years of age or older for colorectal cancer.
		A digital rectal examination at age 40.
		Three stool Hemoccult test and flexible sigmoidoscopy at age 50 and every 3–5 years thereafter.
		Colonoscopy every 10 years.
Cervical cancer	January 2003	It is strongly recommended to do screening for cervical cancer in women who have been sexually active and have a cervix.
		Recommends against routinely screening women older than age 65 for cervical cancer if they have had adequate recent screening with normal Pap smears and are not otherwise at high risk for cervical cancer.
		Recommends against routine Pap smear screening in women who have had a total hysterectomy for benign disease.
		Concludes that the evidence is insufficient to recommend for or against the routine use of new technologies to screen for cervical cancer.
Bladder cancer	June 2004	Recommends against routine screening for bladder cancer in adults.
Ovarian cancer	May 2004	Recommends against routine screening for ovarian cancer.

*Based on the recommendations of the U.S. Preventive Services Task Force (USPSTF).

Preventive Medicine and Miscellaneous Topics

I. Adult Vaccinations
  A. Influenza vaccine
   - The killed viral intramuscular vaccine contains three subtypes: two subtypes of influenza A and one of influenza B. The specific strains are determined each year based on the previous year's isolated strains.
   - The following people should be vaccinated annually during the fall:
     1. Those older than 50 years of age
     2. Nursing home residents
     3. Adults with chronic illnesses (chronic obstructive pulmonary disease, coronary artery disease, diabetes, renal disease, sickle cell disease)
     4. Women who will be pregnant during the influenza season.
     5. Immunocompromised adults (HIV positive, cancer)
     6. Health care personnel, home care providers, and household members in close contact with patients with the other groups listed here
     7. Caretakers of children 0 to 24 months of age
     8. Children 6 to 23 months old
     9. Children with any condition that can compromise respiratory function, e.g., seizure disorders
     10. Children older than 2 years with chronic pulmonary or cardiac disorders
   - Hypersensitivity to eggs is a contraindication for this vaccine.
   - Additionally, a live-attenuated intranasal vaccine has been approved in 2003 for use in for healthy individuals ages 5 to 49; it should not be used in the immunocompromised individual.
  B. Pneumococcal vaccine
   - A heptavalent vaccine (PCV7) is approved for use in children. The adult vaccine (PPV23) contains 23 purified capsular polysaccharide angtigens.
   - Most healthy adults respond well to this vaccine, and antibodies persist for at least 5 years after immunization.
   - The vaccine should be administered once to the following groups if they have not previously been vaccinated:
     1. Those older than 65 years of age
     2. Those ages 2 to 64 with any of the following:
       a. Chronic illnesses (chronic obstructive pulmonary disease, coronary artery disease, diabetes, renal disease)

b. Alcoholism or cirrhosis

c. Residents of nursing homes

d. Immunocompromised adults (HIV positive, cancer)

e. Asplenia, including those with sickle cell disease

- First trimester of pregnancy is the only relative contraindication to this vaccine.
- Additionally, revaccination every 5 years is indicated only for those older than age 65 and in the immunocompromised.

C. Tetanus toxoid vaccine

- Active immunization for children is accomplished by using the DTaP (diphtheria, tetanus acellular, pertussis) vaccine at 2, 4, 6, and 18 months, and again at 4 to 6 years of age with boosters.
- For previously unimmunized adults, IM tetanus toxoid is administered in two doses 4 to 6 weeks apart, followed by a third dose 6 to 12 months later.
- Booster doses (Td in adults or DT in children) should then be given every 10 years or after a major injury that occurs more than 5 years after a dose. Diptheria immunization is always given with a tetanus booster.

D. Hepatitis B vaccine

- Hepatitis B vaccine is a series of three injections and should be given to:
  1. All neonates
  2. Sexually active individuals with multiple sex partners or same-sex partners
  3. Household contacts of patients with hepatitis B
  4. Intravenous drug users
  5. Patients on dialysis
  6. Health care workers
- Pregnant women and immigrants from endemic areas (Asia and Africa) should be screened and vaccinated if needed.
- A combination of hepatitis A and B vaccine is now available. Indications for hepatitis A immunization include travelers to developing countries, men who have sex with men, drug users, those with chronic liver disease, and those who receive clotting factors

E. Varicella vaccine

- Varicella vaccine for adults is indicated for patients who have no varicella titer but risk exposure, such as the elderly, health care workers, college students, day care workers, and parents of young children.

II. Cancer screening

- The following guidelines are based on the recommendations of the U.S. Preventive Services Task Force (USPSTF):

A. Breast cancer

- Screening mammography, with or without clinical breast examination, every 1 to 2 years for women aged 40 and older.

B. Prostate cancer

- Insufficient evidence to recommend for or against routine screening for prostate cancer using prostate-specific antigen (PSA) testing or digital rectal examination (DRE).

C. Colon cancer
- Three stool guaiac tests or flexible sigmoidoscopy every 5 years starting at age 50 for both men and women
- Colonoscopy every 10 years

D. Cervical cancer
- Pap smear beginning 3 years after the onset of sexual activity or at age 21 years, whichever comes first, and then every 3 years afterward, provided that all previous Pap smears have been normal in women who have been sexually active and have a cervix.
- No routine screening for:
  1. Women older than age 65 if they have had adequate recent screening with normal Pap smears and are not at high risk for cervical cancer
  2. Women who have had a total hysterectomy for benign disease

E. Lung, ovarian, and bladder cancer
- Insufficient evidence to recommend for or against routine screening.

III. Medical Ethics
   A. For the physician to act ethically, he or she must adhere to the following principles:
   1. Patient autonomy
      - The patient ultimately has the right to choose his/her treatment plan.
      - The physician must explain, without coercion, the risks and benefits of all diagnostic and therapeutic options in terms the patient understands (informed consent).
   2. Nonmaleficence
      - Do no harm, including overtreatment
   3. Beneficence
      - Suggests mercy, kindness, and charity (doing good)
      - Asserts an obligation to help others
   4. Justice
      - Persons with similar circumstances and conditions should be treated alike.
   B. Recognize that the patient's religious and cultural beliefs are not always the same as the physician's; therefore, decisions about treatment options may differ.
      - For example, a patient who is a Jehovah's Witness may refuse a lifesaving blood transfusion. It is unethical for the physician to impose this treatment on the patient even if the physician is, in his or her mind, acting in the patient's best interest. The patient must, however, understand the consequences of the decision; otherwise, a surrogate decision maker should be involved, especially in treating pediatric, incompetent, or elderly patients.

IV. Statistics in Medicine
   A. Test characteristics and use
      - The ideal screening test should have four qualities:
      1. Inexpensive
      2. Highly sensitive and specific
      3. Noninvasive
      4. Able to detect disease before symptoms occur, and early enough to affect outcome

TABLE 15-1:

Sensitivity and Specificity for Test Results

Test Result	Disease Present	Disease Absent
Positive	True positive (TP)	False positive (FP)
Negative	False negative (FN)	True negative (TN)

B. Sensitivity and specificity (Table 15-1)
   1. False positive (FP) rate is the percentage of patients with a positive test result who do not have the disease.
   2. False negative (FN) rate is the percentage of patients with a negative test result who actually have the disease.
   3. True positive (TP) rate is the percentage of patients with a positive test result who have the disease.
   4. True negative (TN) rate is the percentage of patients with a negative test result who do not have the disease.
   5. Sensitivity is the percentage of patients with the disease in whom the test is positive.
      • A high **sen**sitivity rules **out** disease (**snout**)

$$\text{Sensitivity} = TP/(FN + TP)$$

   6. Specificity is the percentage of patients without the disease in whom the test is negative.
      • A high **sp**ecificity rules **in** disease (**spin**)

$$\text{Specificity} = TN/(FP + TN)$$

   7. Positive predictive value (PPV) is the percentage of patients with a positive test result who actually have the disease.

$$PPV = TP/(TP + FP)$$

   8. Negative predictive value (NPV) is the percentage of patients with a negative test result who really do not have the disease.

$$NPV = TN/(TN + FN)$$

   9. Prevalence = the number of patients with the disease divided by the number of patients tested.
   10. Incidence = the number of all new cases with the disease (over a certain period of time) divided by the number of all patients tested (over the same period of time).
   11. Sensitivity and specificity do not depend on prevalence but do depend on the patient population.
   12. PPV and NPV are dependent on the prevalence of the disease in the tested population.
      • A test with a particular sensitivity and specificity has different PPV when used in populations that have different prevalences.

C. Descriptive statistics
- Mean is the arithmetic average of a series of numbers (sum of the series/number in series).
- Median is the number in a group for which 50% of the numbers are above and 50% are below.
- Mode is the most frequently occurring number in a series.

D. Other statistical tests
  1. Student's t-test
     - Used to calculate the probability with which two sets of measurements would have come from normal distributions with the same mean.
     - Assumes that the standard distributions are identical
  2. Chi square (χ^2)
     - It is used to test for dependence of outcome on treatment when the outcomes to be measured are divided into discrete outcomes or variables.
     - This is a two-tailed hypothesis in that it checks for both negative and positive correlation; therefore, data must be inspected carefully.
  3. p value
     - It measures the effect of chance within a study.
     - Statistical significance is usually set at $p < 0.05$, meaning that there is a less than 5% probability that the observed difference occurred by chance alone.
  4. Correlation coefficient (r)
     - This number indicates the degree of correlation between two sets of data or random variables.
     - The value ranges between −1 and +1.
     - A value of zero indicates that there is no relationship between the variables.
     - Values closer to −1 suggest a negative or inverse relationship (exercising more causes lower blood sugars), and values closer to +1 suggest a positive or direct correlation (higher blood sugars are related to more complications).

E. Error types and power
  1. Null hypothesis
     - This is the assumption that any observed difference between two samples of a statistical population is purely accidental and not due to systematic causes.
     - In other words, it proposes that the variables being analyzed are not related.
  2. Type I error
     - This error occurs when a true null hypothesis is rejected (you conclude that there is a relationship when in fact there isn't one).
     - The α value is the probability of committing a type I error.
  3. Type II error
     - This error occurs when a false null hypothesis is rejected (you conclude that there is no relationship when in fact there is one).
     - The β value is the probability of committing a type II error.
  4. Power ($= 1 - \beta$)
     - It is the statistical probability of avoiding a type II error in a study (probability that a study will not erroneously accept the null hypothesis and conclude that there was no effect or difference when there really was one).

Emergency Medicine

I. Emergency Stabilization
   A. Basic life support and advanced cardiac life support (ACLS) principles
   - Cardiopulmonary resuscitation (CPR) is performed to support the circulatory and respiratory systems of the patient in cardiac arrest in effort to prevent anoxia and ischemic damage to vital organs. CPR should be initiated within 4 minutes of cardiac arrest, and ACLS should commence within 8 minutes of arrest. The approach to the patient in cardiopulmonary arrest should be systematic and include primary and secondary surveys.
   - In the primary survey:
     1. Assess responsiveness
     2. Activate EMS
     3. Call for a defibrillator/automatic external defibrillator (AED)
     4. Position the patient and open the airway, immobilizing the cervical spine (C-spine) if trauma is suspected
     5. Assess respiratory effort
     6. If no spontaneous breathing, give 2 slow rescue breaths
     7. Check for pulse
     8. If no pulse, begin chest compressions. Chest compressions should be 1.5 to 2 inches deep, 100 compressions/minute, and 15 compressions per 2 breaths. (For the intubated patient, give 100 compressions/minute without pausing for ventilations.) Once an AED is available, attach the pads, analyze the rhythm, and shock if indicated by the AED. If using a conventional (monophasic) defibrillator, cardiovert ventricular fibrillation or pulseless ventricular tachycardia up to 3 times consecutively at 200, 300, and 360 J (unsynchronized).
   - A detailed review of ACLS is beyond the scope of this chapter, but remember the following during the secondary survey:
     1. Place an advanced airway
     2. Check placement by examination and confirmation device such as an end-tidal carbon dioxide monitor, secure the airway, oxygenate and ventilate the patient
     3. Establish intravenous (IV) access
     4. Identify the rhythm
     5. Give appropriate drugs
     6. Identify reversible causes and treat them accordingly.

- In children, most arrests are due to respiratory insults. Rule out foreign body aspiration. Follow the same principles as for adults, with some distinctions. Calculate endotracheal tube size by the formula (age/4) + 4. Defibrillation, if needed, is based on the child's weight. Shocks of 2 J/kg, 2–4 J/kg, and 4 J/kg are applied consecutively. Drug doses and fluid requirements are weight-based, as well.

B. Trauma

1. The primary survey of the trauma patient proceeds in an orderly fashion. You, the treating physician, must do the following:
   a. Maintain the patient's *airway* (providing C-spine immobilization when necessary)
   b. Assess *breathing* and assure adequate ventilation
   c. Control bleeding and support *circulation*
   d. Assess neurologic *disability*
   e. Entirely *expose* the patient in search of wounds

   - Patients with head or neck injuries may need a surgical airway.
   - Paralytics may be necessary to maintain the airway in an agitated patient.
   - After the patient is adequately ventilated, check for tracheal deviation, wounds, fractures, pneumothorax, and flail chest.
   - Assume that hypotension in the trauma patient is due to hemorrhage until proven otherwise. Blood may be lost to the following areas: external (to body), intrathoracic, intra-abdominal, retroperitoneal, and intracranial. Infuse enough crystalloid solution (normal saline [NS] or Ringer's lactate [LR]) to nearly normalize vital signs through two large-bore IV lines or a trauma introducer catheter. If blood pressure response is inadequate, give type O Rh-negative blood.
   - Assess for pericardial tamponade (muffled heart sounds, distended neck veins, and hypotension) and tension pneumothorax (tracheal deviation, breath sounds). Perform a needle thoracostomy (midclavicular line) immediately if a pneumothorax is found without waiting for imaging if the examination is convincing.
   - Comatose patients with a history of head injury should have an urgent head computed tomography (CT) after cervical spine (C-spine) immobilization and intubation.
   - For a patient presenting with penetrating abdominal trauma, proceed directly to the operating room (OR). Do not remove embedded objects outside the OR.

2. During the secondary survey:
   - Check for hemotympanum and epistaxis (signs of basilar skull fracture), obtain x-rays (anteroposterior [AP] chest, lateral C-spine, and AP pelvis), and place a nasogastric (NG) tube (or orogastric tube if a basilar skull fracture is suspected) to suction.
   - Image the C-spine *unless* the patient denies C-spine tenderness, is not intoxicated, is without neurologic deficit, and has no painful injury, and the patient is alert.
   - Inspect the genitalia and rectum for signs of trauma. Do not place a urinary catheter if there is blood at the urethral meatus or if there is suspicion of a

pubic symphysis fracture because these injuries may herald a urethral disruption.

- Perform vascular and neurologic examinations. Examination findings guide further imaging. Focused abdominal sonographic examination for trauma (FAST) is a rapid ultrasound assessment for bleeding in the pericardium, hepatorenal recess of Morrison (peritoneum), pelvis, and perisplenic region. FAST is an alternative to diagnostic peritoneal lavage for detection of hemoperitoneum.

C. Foreign body ingestion
- Children account for 80% of foreign body ingestion cases.
- Patients may present with neck or throat pain (adults often complain of retrosternal pain), dysphagia, vomiting, stridor, or poor feeding.
- In children, the five areas where objects commonly lodge are C6 (cricopharyngeal narrowing), T1 (thoracic inlet), T4 (aortic arch), T6 (tracheal bifurcation), and T10-T11 (hiatal narrowing).
- In adults, the three major areas of foreign body obstruction are the cricopharyngeus, aortic arch, and gastroesophageal junction.
- If there is esophageal obstruction, insert a tube above the obstruction and suction to prevent aspiration.
- Obtain a plain radiograph as the initial imaging study. Circular coin shadows in the esophagus are visible on an AP radiograph. If the circular coin is seen on the lateral film, the object is in the trachea.
- Endoscopy can be used for diagnosis and therapy (extraction). Button battery ingestion requires emergency endoscopic removal.
- If esophageal perforation is suspected, a contrast (Gastrografin or barium) swallow study can be done. Endoscopic intervention is required in 10% to 20% of cases.
- The majority of ingested foreign bodies pass without difficulty. A follow-up x-ray is recommended at 48 hours to assess foreign body migration.

D. Shock
- Shock refers the physiologic state whereby circulation is insufficient to maintain adequate organ oxygenation and perfusion, resulting in end organ damage (reversible or irreversible). Without adequate oxygenation, anaerobic metabolism dominates energy production, causing metabolic acidosis. The major categories of shock include *hypovolemic, cardiogenic,* and *distributive* shock.
  1. Hypovolemic shock is caused by significant loss of blood or other body fluid. Causes include hemorrhage, dehydration (gastrointestinal losses or poor intake), fluid third spacing, and fluid losses through burns. If hemorrhage is suspected, assess for trauma, gastrointestinal (GI) bleeding, and reproductive tract sources of bleeding. Consider third spacing in patients with liver disease, bowel infarction, pancreatitis, or nephrotic syndrome.
  2. Cardiogenic shock occurs when cardiac output is insufficient to meet metabolic demands. Intrinsic cardiac causes include myocardial infarction (which can lead to wall rupture or an acute valvular abnormality), decompensated heart failure, myocarditis, dysrhythmias, cardiac contusion, and cardiomyopathy. Other causes include pericardial tamponade, mediastinal hemorrhage, pneumomediastinum, tension pneumothorax, and positive pressure ventilation.

3. Distributive shock occurs because of poor vasomotor response to hypotension. Though intravascular volume may be adequate, inappropriate vasodilatation increases the effective intravascular space resulting in hypotension. Both neurogenic and septic shock are in this category.

4. Neurogenic shock can occur from central nervous system (CNS) injury. Neurogenic shock presents with bradycardia, arterial and venous dilatation, and hypotension due to decreased sympathetic output.

5. Septic shock may follow a significant infection.

- In general, the patient in shock presents with hypotension, altered mental status, decreased urine output, tachycardia, and tachypnea. History and physical examination findings may provide clues to the cause of the shock. Using a Swan-Ganz catheter may help determine the category of shock, but placing a Swan-Ganz catheter is more appropriate after the patient has been stabilized and transferred to an intensive care unit (ICU) setting.

- Initial treatment in the emergency department (ED) focuses on the ABCs. Evaluate the patient's vital signs. Secure the patient's airway; intubate the patient if necessary. Ventilate the patient. Place either two large-bore IV lines or a central venous introducer, and begin volume resuscitation with NS or LR. Determine the need for blood products (red blood cells, platelets, fresh frozen plasma [FFP]), and give type O Rh-negative blood if emergency red blood cell transfusion is needed. For hemorrhage, replace three times the estimated blood loss with NS or LR (to account for third spacing). If hypotension persists despite an aggressive fluid challenge, inotropes may be needed. Dopamine (α- and β-agonists) given through a central line is a good first choice for distributive shock and cardiogenic shock. If inotropes are needed, an arterial line should be placed. Attempt to correct dysrhythmias and replace electrolytes.

- For the patient presenting with shock, the differential diagnosis is wide. As you stabilize the patient, consider ordering the following studies: complete blood count (CBC), complete metabolic panel (CMP), type and crossmatch, arterial blood gas (ABG) with lactate, coagulation parameters (PTT/INR), and electrocardiogram (ECG). Depending on the suspected cause for the shock, blood cultures, chest x-ray (CXR), cardiac enzymes, and transthoracic echocardiogram may be indicated.

E. Anaphylaxis

- Anaphylaxis is classically an IgE-mediated hypersensitivity reaction that occurs after a subsequent exposure to a particular sensitizing antigen or hapten-protein antigenic complex. Clinically indistinguishable, non-IgE-mediated reactions are better referred to as "anaphylactoid."

- Patients usually present with itching, flushing, and hives. Symptoms, if untreated, can progress to involve the respiratory system, cardiovascular system, or both, eventually leading to airway compromise and shock. Half of the fatalities from anaphylaxis occur within the first hour.

- For the patient suspected to have anaphylaxis, assess the ABCs. Secure the airway, and quickly administer epinephrine 0.1 mg IV bolus. If this is ineffective at improving the patient's symptoms, infuse epinephrine 1 to 4 µg/minute IV.

- For less severe symptoms and anaphylactoid reactions, consider giving epinephrine 0.3 to 0.5 mg IM every 5 to 10 minutes or other diphenhydramine (an H_1-blocker) 25 to 50 mg PO/IM/IV. (Consider giving an H_2-blocker for cases of refractory anaphylaxis). Adults should also be given methylprednisolone 125 mg IV or hydrocortisone 250 to 500 mg IV. For children, give methylprednisolone 2 mg/kg IV or hydrocortisone 5 to 10 mg/kg IV. Anaphylaxis recurrence rates are 10% to 20% for penicillin, 20% to 40% for radiopaque IV contrast material, and 40% to 60% for insect stings.

II. Cardiopulmonary Issues
  A. Chest pain
    - Patients presenting with chest pain (CP) to the ED should be triaged promptly. Place the patient on a cardiac monitor, establish IV access, give oxygen, and obtain an electrocardiogram (ECG). Address the ABCs. Perform focused cardiovascular and respiratory examinations. Discern whether pain appears to be visceral CP, respiratory pain, or musculoskeletal pain. Rule out the life-threatening causes of CP: myocardial infarction (MI), unstable angina, aortic dissection, pulmonary embolism, tension pneumothorax or esophageal rupture.
    - In general, approximately 15% of patients over the age of 30 presenting to the ED with visceral CP have an acute coronary syndrome (ACS). ACS encompasses unstable angina (USA) and acute myocardial infarction (AMI). An ECG should be interpreted as soon as possible, and cardiac markers should be measured. The positive predictive value for AMI with new ST segment elevation is 80%. For new ST segment depression or T wave inversion, the positive predictive value is 20% for AMI and 14 to 43% for USA. CK-MB becomes detectable 4 to 8 hours after symptom onset, and troponin (I and T) is detectable 6 hours after. Treatment of ACS (including AMI) is explained in Chapter 5, Cardiology. If AMI is excluded (by cardiac markers and ECG), and there is still suspicion of ischemic CP, a cardiac stress imaging study or an exercise stress test can be arranged.
    - A pulmonary embolism (PE) causes a pulmonary infarction and inflammation of the overlying parietal pleura that presents as CP. The classic symptoms of PE are pleuritic CP, dyspnea, hypoxemia, tachycardia, and tachypnea.
    - The pain from an aortic dissection is usually worse at onset and located between the scapulae.
    - The diagnosis of spontaneous pneumothorax can be made by physical examination and chest x-ray.
    - Patients with esophageal rupture usually present after forceful vomiting.
    - Once these causes of acute CP are excluded, one should consider other causes of CP including musculoskeletal pain, pericarditis, pneumonia, mitral valve prolapse, panic disorder, peptic ulcer disease (PUD), and other causes of GI pain.
  B. Heart failure
    - Fluid overload is the most common presentation of heart failure (HF) in the ED. Patients may present with acute pulmonary edema (hypertension [HTN], respiratory distress). Chest x-ray findings of left-sided HF include vascular

redistribution and engorged upper lobe vessels, an enlarged cardiac silhouette, interstitial edema, prominent pulmonary arteries, pleural effusions, alveolar edema, a prominent superior vena cava, and Kerley B lines. A brain natriuretic peptide (BNP) level greater than 100 pg/mL predicts the presence of HF, and the magnitude of elevation correlates with HF severity.
- Initiate cardiac monitoring and pulse oximetry, establish IV access, obtain an ECG, and repeat vital signs frequently. With acute pulmonary edema, decrease afterload with nitrates or nesiritide, and reduce volume with IV furosemide or bumetanide. Vasodilatation is contraindicated in hypertrophic cardiomyopathy, aortic stenosis, and right ventricle infarction, and with volume depletion. Evaluate for AMI as the precipitating event, and treat accordingly. In general, patients with decompensated HF or acute pulmonary edema will require hospitalization in an ICU or telemetry bed.

C. Syncope
- Each year, syncope accounts for approximately 3% of ED visits. Decreased blood flow to the brain, for any reason, causes loss of consciousness. The patient regains consciousness only after perfusion to the brain is restored, which is usually when the patient assumes a horizontal position, collapsing after the moment of syncope. Thus, syncope is often short-lived.
- In reflex-mediated syncope, physical or emotional stressors bring about a dulled autonomic response. Increased vagal tone causes inappropriate hypotension with or without bradycardia. Examples of reflex-mediated syncope are vasovagal syncope, carotid sinus hypersensitivity, and situational syncope (such as may occur during micturition or defecation). Orthostatic hypotension with systolic blood pressure dropping more than 20 mm Hg on assuming a more upright posture may also provoke syncope.
- Neurovascular syncope is the result of cerebrovascular disease such as a transient ischemic attack, subclavian steal, basilar artery migraine, or vertebrobasilar atherosclerosis. Usually there are other neurologic symptoms preceding syncope.
- Cardiac syncope occurs secondary to dysrhythmias or structural heart disease. Consider aortic stenosis in the elderly patient and hypertrophic cardiomyopathy in the young. Other causes of syncope include PE, medication effects, and psychiatric illnesses.
- Check bilateral arm blood pressures and orthostatic vital signs. Search for signs of trauma. Listen for murmurs or other extra cardiac sounds, and obtain an ECG. Obtain basic laboratory tests. Hospitalize patients who have acute neurologic disease or the suspicion of a cardiac reason of the syncope.

III. Environmental Emergencies
A. Burns
- Burns can be categorized as thermal burns or chemical burns. Thermal burns can cause both local and systemic injuries. Cellular damage occurs at temperatures greater than 45°C. The resulting wound has three zones: the zone of coagulation (central), the zone of stasis (surrounding the zone of coagulation), and the zone of hyperemia (the penumbra). The latter two zones have salvageable tissue.

- Burn size is measured in total body surface area (TBSA) that is estimated by the Rule of Nines [legs 18% TBSA, arms 9% TBSA, anterior trunk 18% TBSA, posterior trunk 18% TBSA, head 9% TBSA] or, alternatively, measured in hands (the back of a hand equals approximately 1% TBSA).
- Burn depth is described in degrees:
  1. First-degree burns are limited to the epidermis, are hyperemic without blistering, heal without scarring in about 7 days, and require only symptom management.
  2. Second-degree burns involve the dermis and are further characterized as superficial and deep partial thickness. In the former, injury involves the papillary layer of the dermis, and there is blistering (with a red base) and pain. Superficial second-degree burns heal in 2 to 3 weeks without scarring. Deep second-degree burns involve the reticular layer of the dermis where there is damage to hair follicles, sebaceous glands, and sweat glands. The burn may be insensate and have blistering (with a white-yellow base). Healing may take 3 weeks to 2 months and may require surgical intervention. Scarring is common.
  3. Third-degree burns involve the entire dermis, are leathery and painless, are without capillary refill, and require surgery.
  4. Fourth-degree burns extend beyond the skin to deeper structures.
- The most commonly used method to calculate IV fluid requirements is to multiply the percent TBSA by weight (kg) by 4 mL LR (Parkland Formula). Give half of this amount in the first 8 hours, and the remainder in the following 16 hours. Give this in addition to calculated hourly requirements. Aim for urine output of 0.5 to 1.0 mL/kg/hour. In children, aim for 1 mL/kg/hour. Cover large burns with dry sterile burn pads. Smaller burns may be covered by dressings soaked in normal saline. Treat pain and anxiety, preferably with IV agents. Patients with all but minor burns (i.e., those sparing the face, perineum, hands, and feet) should be admitted.
- Death in burn victims is primarily due to inhalation injury with bronchospasm and edema in the terminal bronchioles. If inhalation injury is suspected, administer humidified oxygen and determine the need for intubation. Establish IV access, insert a urinary catheter, and if there is greater than a 20% TBSA partial-thickness burn, place a nasogastric (NG) tube because ileus is common.
- In general, chemical burns produce damage by causing capillary and arterial vasodilatation. Superficial vessels are affected first, followed by deeper vessels. Tissue hyperemia, pain, burning, and itching occur. Acids tend to cause coagulation necrosis and produce a leathery eschar. Alkalis cause more damage by producing liquefaction necrosis of the skin that further compromises the skin's barrier to infection.
- Minimize the patient's contact with the chemical causing the burn. Remove the patient's clothing, brush off dry chemicals, and for most chemicals, irrigate copiously with water or saline (gentle continuous irrigation, avoid forceful irrigation). After normalizing the skin's pH (can use pH indicator paper), debride any necrotic tissue, apply a topical antimicrobial, and give a tetanus shot

if needed. Fluid resuscitation and pain control should be managed as with thermal burns.

B. Electrical injury

- Flowing electric current has variable predilection for conductive tissues depending on the resistance to electric current flow of that particular tissue. Bone provides greater resistance than muscle, which in turn has greater resistance than nerves or blood vessels. Electricity finds the path of least resistance; nervous tissue conducts electricity better than does blood vessels, and blood vessels conduct electricity better than bone. Therefore, nerves sustain significant damage because they have a high current density despite their smaller surface area.

- Electric current may cause delayed spinal cord injury. Heating of tissues from current flow is generally the mechanism of injury. Current can also induce dramatic muscle contraction, which can throw a patient from the source and cause other trauma. Hence, a person gripping an electrical source can experience hand flexor tetany that exceeds extensor contraction and causes the person to grip the source more tightly.

- Electrical skin burns can occur at high voltage in under a second, or at household voltage with prolonged exposure.

- Household electric alternating current can produce seizures, respiratory arrest, or dysrhythmias.

- In the ED, evaluate the ABCs, place the patient on telemetry if there are neurologic or cardiac signs or symptoms, and immobilize the spine until trauma is ruled out. Give isotonic crystalloid solution 20 to 40 mL/kg in the first hour, and reassess further needs for IV fluid. Patients who have electrical injuries may require more IV fluid than patients who have thermal injuries, because the extent of internal injury may be underestimated by minimal external signs of damage. As with other burns, escharotomy may be required to prevent compartment syndrome or airway compromise.

C. Heat illness

- Normal core body temperature is 36°C to 38°C. Below 35°C and above 40°C, thermal regulation is compromised.

- There are five types of heat illness:

  1. Heat edema
     - Heat edema is swelling of the distal extremities due to cutaneous vasodilatation in response to heat stress. It requires no specific treatment.

  2. Heat tetany
     - Heat tetany frequently affects the calves and occurs mainly in individuals who sweat and attempt to replace fluid losses with hypotonic fluids. The treatment is to replace fluid and salt orally or intravenously. Rhabdomyolysis is a rare complication of heat tetany because the muscle groups involved are usually small.

  3. Heat syncope
     - Heat syncope is the result of vasodilation in an effort to cool the body after exertion in hot weather. The treatment is rest in a cooler environment, elevation of the feet, and drinking salt-containing fluids.

4. Heat exhaustion
   - Heat exhaustion presents as hyperthermia, tachycardia, tachypnea, diaphoresis, orthostatic hypotension, and possibly syncope, with *normal* mentation.

5. Heat stroke
   - Heat stroke is characterized by body temperature greater than 40°C, alteration of consciousness, and anhidrosis. The patient with heat stroke may be significantly cooler than 40°C by the time he arrives at the ED because cooling measures may already have been implemented. Treatment general adds to augment evaporative cooling, e.g., mist of lukewarm water applied to skin with cooling fans and cold packs to neck, axillae, and groin areas.

D. Accidental hypothermia and cold injury

1. Accidental hypothermia (core body temperature below 35°C)
   - Accidental hypothermia can follow immersion and nonimmersion cold exposures.
   - Standard thermometers may not measure temperatures below 34.4°C. Therefore, core temperature should be taken with an esophageal probe, tympanic thermometer, or special urinary catheter thermometer.
   - Effects of hypothermia include CNS depression, cold diuresis (causing volume loss), intravascular thrombosis or bleeding, acute pancreatitis, liver dysfunction, dysrhythmias (such as recalcitrant atrial fibrillation, ventricular tachycardia, or ventricular fibrillation), and respiratory depression. Below 30°C to 32°C, shivering stops.
   - Passive rewarming involves removing the patient from the cold environment and providing clothing/linens.
   - With active external rewarming, heated blankets or other heat sources are applied to the body surface. Active core rewarming involves administering oxygen or fluids heated to 40°C. Alternatively, irrigation of the bladder, gastrointestinal tract, thoracic cavity, or peritoneal cavity with warmed fluid may be necessary. Measures beyond this generally involve cardiopulmonary bypass.

2. Cold injury
   - Cold injury is classified by degree of severity:
     a. In first-degree injury, there is erythema and partial skin freezing. Desquamation may occur several days later.
     b. With second-degree injury, there is full-thickness skin injury, edema, erythema, and blistering. Within days, the blisters desquamate and form eschars.
     c. In third-degree injury, subdermal damage causes hemorrhagic blisters and necrosis.
     d. With fourth-degree injury, subcutaneous tissues, muscle, tendon, and bone are damaged. The skin mottles, becomes cyanotic, and later forms a deep eschar. Prognosis is poor for third-and fourth-degree injury.
   - Rapid rewarming is critical. Do not rub affected tissue because rubbing may promote damage. Extremities should be rewarmed in 40°C to 42°C water for

10 to 30 minutes until the skin is erythematous. Separate digits by wrapping them in cotton and gauze. Treat blisters with topical aloe vera cream every 6 hours. Provide analgesics because the rewarming process can be very painful. Infection is a potential complication, but use of prophylactic antibiotics is controversial.

- Chilblains (pernio) is characterized by pruritic red or purple bumps, the result of localized vasculitis, caused by chronic intermittent exposure to damp, nonfreezing temperatures. Chilblains may occur on the digits several hours after acute exposure to cold. Treatment options are limited and include topical steroids and antibiotics.

E. Carbon monoxide poisoning
- Carbon monoxide (CO) competes with oxygen binding sites on various enzymes and pigments. Hemoglobin (Hgb) binds CO with 300 times the affinity it has for oxygen, and the COHgb complex prevents oxygen release to metabolically active tissue. CO binding to myocardial myoglobin and neuroglobin may depress cardiac and neurologic function, respectively.
- CO poisoning can cause many syndromes, including multiorgan failure, disseminated intravascular coagulation (DIC), rhabdomyolysis, circulatory shock, renal failure, and noncardiogenic pulmonary edema.
- Treat the patient with 100% oxygen by face mask. Monitoring oxyhemoglobin saturation with pulse oximetry is unreliable because it measures both oxyhemoglobin and COHgb. If mild symptoms do not improve within 4 hours and there is no other obvious cause for the symptoms, consider hyperbaric oxygen.
- Traditionally, major signs or symptoms (altered mental status, loss of consciousness, seizure, coma, hypotension, MI, prolonged exposure, and pregnancy with COHgb >15%) have warrant treatment with hyperbaric oxygen. Untreated pneumothorax is a contraindication to hyperbaric oxygen.

F. Poisonous plants
- Poisonous plant ingestions are best treated with GI decontamination and supportive care.
- The castor bean *(Ricinus communis)* and the jequirity bean *(Abrus precatorius)* are extremely poisonous. Either can cause delayed (potentially hemorrhagic) gastroenteritis, mental status change, seizures, and death.
- Foxglove *(Digitalis purpurea)* has effects similar to digitalis.
- Oleander *(Nerium oleander)* contains cardiac glycosides, which inhibit the Na^+K^+-ATPase pump, leading to hyperkalemia and dysrhythmias.
- Poison hemlock *(Conium maculatum)* can cause weakness, seizures, ascending paralysis, renal failure, rhabdomyolysis, coma, and death.
- Water hemlock *(Cicuta maculata)* inhibits gamma-aminobutyric acid (GABA) receptor antagonists and may cause death within 15 minutes.
- Yew (*Taxus* species) rarely causes seizures, arrhythmias, and coma. Many other common plants can cause a variety of lesser symptoms.
- In general, ingestion of or contact with suspicious plants should be reported to the regional poison control center for guidance in management.

G. Near-drowning
- Near-drowning defines survival beyond 24 hours after submersion.

- "Wet-drowning" refers to victims who aspirate water, resulting in washout of surfactant, atelectasis, and ventilation-perfusion mismatch. Hemolysis may occur with fresh water.
- "Dry-drowning" refers to those who lose consciousness (generally from laryngospasm-induced hypoxia) before aspiration can occur.
- In the ED, address ABCs, and rewarm the patient. If there is pulmonary edema, the patient should be kept for observation. If the patient recovers to baseline or is only minimally symptomatic in 4 to 6 hours, discharge from the ED may be feasible.

H. Envenomations
   1. Arthropods
      - The order Hymenoptera encompasses wasps, bees, and ants. Hymenoptera venom contains histamine and melittin (a membrane-active polypeptide that can cause the granulation of basophils and mast cells), and cross-sensitization can occur in humans allergic to any of the species.
      - Reactions can be local or systemic, ranging from mild rash to anaphylaxis, and can occur in response to a single sting (in sensitized individuals) or after multiple stings.
      - If a stinger is present, remove it promptly, provide symptomatic relief (ice, NSAIDs, antihistamines), and prepare to give epinephrine (0.3–0.5 mg IM in adults, 0.01 mg/kg to maximum 0.3 mg IM in children). If epinephrine is needed, also give antihistamines and consider H_2-blockers. Treat anaphylactic shock as described earlier in this chapter. Patients should be prescribed injectable epinephrine to carry and should be referred to an allergist.
      - The majority of spider bites lead to local reactions only. However, *Loxosceles* spiders (brown recluse, corner spider, Arizona brown spider) produce local necrosis and possibly systemic toxicity. The bite is often painless, and the onset of necrosis is delayed. For this reason, serial examination of the bite should be performed. The brown recluse has a characteristic violin shape on its body. The hobo spider *(Tegenaria agrestis)* bite may also produce a delayed necrotic lesion, often preceded by headache. There is no antivenom available for either of these envenomations.
      - A black widow spider (five species of *Latrodectus*) bite is typically felt as a prick on the hand or forearm, producing pain and erythema that rapidly involves the extremity. At the puncture site there may be a classic target lesion, and patients often experience severe generalized muscle spasms. The treatment is *Lactrodectus* antivenom, analgesics, and anxiolytics.
      - Of scorpions, only the bark scorpion *(Centruroides exilicauda)* produces severe systemic toxicity. Patients can present with paresthesias, cranial nerve findings, and somatic motor dysfunction. Treatment is supportive, and antivenom is reserved for severe cases. Any bite that causes necrosis may require excision.
   2. Reptiles
      - Pit viper bites may cause local injury, coagulopathy, or systemic effects. The treatment is supportive, and Crotalidae immune Fab should be given. Affected limbs should be examined repeatedly for compartment syndrome, which warrants additional antivenom.

- Coral snakes are characterized by red, yellow, and black rings, and in the United States, the red and yellow rings touch, signifying poisonous venom. Antivenom should be given, because the primarily neurologic effects can be fatal (respiratory muscle paralysis). Remember, "red next to yellow, kill a fellow; red next to black, venom lack." In general, all snakebites should be considered to be from poisonous species until proved otherwise, and the poison control center should be alerted.

IV. Gastrointestinal/Abdominal Emergencies
  A. Gastrointestinal bleeding (GIB)
   - A GI bleed (for purposes of emergency medicine) can present with hematemesis (frank blood or coffee-ground emesis), melena, or hematochezia. Upper GI bleeds originate from a source proximal to the ligament of Treitz, and lower GI bleeds originate distal to this. First and foremost, assess ABCs. Determine if the patient is in shock, and manage appropriately. The GI bleeding patient requires adequate IV access (two 16- to 18-gauge IV lines). Begin volume repletion, and determine the need for blood products. A nasogastric tube should be placed, and lavage should be performed gently with room temperature water. The purpose of the NG lavage is to look for "coffee grounds" or fresh blood. Such information can assist in the initial triage and management of the patient. A Foley catheter should be placed to assess response to volume resuscitation. Aim for urine output of 0.5 to 1.0 mL/kg/hour. Vital signs should be taken frequently.
   - When taking the history, inquire about NSAID, steroid, alcohol, and anticoagulant use. Depending on the presentation, assess the patient for nasopharynx and vaginal bleeding that may mimic GI bleeding. Obtain blood for type and cross, PTT/INR, CBC, and CMP. ECG should be done in the elderly patients with known coronary artery disease, and those with dyspnea or chest pain (to assess for anemia-induced ischemia). GI consultation should be obtained for any hemodynamically significant GI bleed. Determine the need for urgent (upper or lower) endoscopy, angiography, or surgery. Octreotide is effective in reducing GI bleeding from varices and peptic ulcer disease, and octreotide can be started while awaiting endoscopy.
   - Causes of life-threatening upper GI bleeds include peptic ulcer disease, esophageal varices, and Mallory-Weiss (partial-thickness esophageal) tears. Other causes of upper GI bleeding are gastritis, esophagitis, and Dieulafoy lesions. Diverticula, arteriovenous malformations, and aortoenteric fistulas cause life-threatening lower GI bleeding. Other sources of lower GI bleeding include malignancy, hemorrhoids, anal fissures, inflammatory bowel disease (IBD), ischemic bowel, and infectious diarrhea.
  B. Esophageal emergencies
   - Esophageal perforation typically presents with pain (neck, chest, or abdominal), fever, and subcutaneous emphysema. Patients may also present in shock. Be suspicious of underlying esophageal disease (esophagitis, malignancy, radiation, etc.), ingestions, trauma, recent procedures, and foreign bodies. Boerhaave's syndrome is spontaneous perforation occurring after prolonged vomiting, coughing, or other unusual strain. With perforation, secretions and acid are released into the mediastinum, and mediastinitis follows.

- The emergency workup should include chest x-ray and, possibly, chest CT. Evaluate for mediastinal widening, air/fluid levels, or abscess, as well as pneumomediastinum, subcutaneous emphysema, and pleural effusion. If these studies are nondiagnostic and the suspicion is still high, EGD or esophagoscopy may be done. The patient should be made NPO (nothing by mouth) and given broad-spectrum IV antibiotics, and surgical consultation should be obtained.

C. Abdominal pain
  - In patients presenting with abdominal pain, consider GI, genitourinary (GU), gynecologic (GYN), and vascular sources of pain. Further symptoms may help in distinguishing among these. (We will focus on GI emergencies here.) Attempt to localize tenderness to a quadrant on abdominal examination, and consider the structures in that area. A pelvic examination should be performed in women of childbearing age. Yield of laboratory and radiographic tests is variable.
  - Consider the following diagnoses, which may warrant a surgical consultation.
    1. Appendicitis
       - With appendicitis, the five features with positive predictive value are right lower quadrant (RLQ) pain, movement of pain from periumbilicus to RLQ, rigidity, pain before vomiting, and a psoas sign. Ultrasound and CT scan are, both, reasonable imaging studies, and positive findings on either favors surgery.
    2. Small bowel obstruction
       - With suspected small bowel obstruction (SBO), only a few features have predictive value: colicky pain, prior abdominal surgery, abnormal bowel sounds, and distention. Plain radiographs may be sufficient to detect SBO, but CT scan is better for diagnosis of bowel strangulation or ischemia.
    3. Large bowel obstruction
       - Large bowel obstruction (LBO) generally affects the elderly. The leading causes are malignancy, volvulus, and diverticulitis. Look for clues such as constipation (less commonly diarrhea), emesis, and distention. Start with a plain radiograph.
    4. Ogilvie syndrome
       - Ogilvie syndrome is similar to LBO and looks similar radiographically, but it is due to colonic gaseous distention without a physical obstruction. The abdomen on physical examination should be nontender in Ogilvie syndrome.
    5. Diverticulitis
       - Diverticulitis may be diagnosed by ultrasound, but CT (with colonic contrast) is better for detecting complications such as abscess or perforation.
    6. Acute pancreatitis
       - The diagnosis of acute pancreatitis is difficult to make by physical examination alone. Lipase should be at least twice the upper limit of normal. Ultrasound may be useful in diagnosing biliary pancreatitis, whereas CT scan with PO/IV contrast is superior in identifying complications such as fluid collections, hemorrhage, or necrosis.
    7. Abdominal aortic aneurysm
       - Abdominal aortic aneurysms (AAA) present with a pulsatile abdominal mass, abdominal or back pain, and hypotension less than 50% of the time. Physical examination is likely to reveal abdominal tenderness. Attempt to

determine the size of the aorta by palpation. Surgery is warranted for AAAs 5 cm or larger and considered for rapidly progressing smaller AAAs. Ultrasound may be done to confirm the diagnosis. CT, however, is used to determine if there is leak or rupture, both of which are indications for prompt surgery.

8. Mesenteric ischemia
   - Mesenteric ischemia usually presents with nonfocal abdominal pain without tenderness. It can be caused by thrombosis, embolism, or a low-flow state affecting either the arterial or venous supply to the bowel. There is no reliable laboratory test to make this diagnosis, although CT scan may pick up, among other diagnoses in the differential, mesenteric venous thrombosis. Treatment depends on the cause of the ischemia.

9. Ischemic colitis
   - Ischemic colitis presents as abdominal pain with or without diarrhea (possibly bloody). Diagnosis is typically made by colonoscopy. Bowel necrosis may occur and cause peritonitis, in which case colectomy is required.

10. Incarcerated hernia
    - Patients presenting with an incarcerated or strangulated hernia often have a history of the hernia with new, sudden onset of pain. If it is clear that incarceration occurred very recently, an attempt may be made to gently reduce it. Strangulation may progress to abscess, perforation, peritonitis, or shock.

11. Ruptured ectopic pregnancy
    - Ruptured ectopic pregnancy must be evaluated in any women of childbearing age presenting with abdominal/pelvic pain or abnormal vaginal bleeding. Order a qualitative urine human chorionic gonadotropin (hCG) (if positive, then a quantitative serum hCG). If indicated (such as in cases with an hCG elevated but incompatible with dates, adnexal tenderness, or mass), proceed to transvaginal ultrasound. If an intrauterine pregnancy is not seen and the hCG is positive (in a woman not under treatment for infertility), the differential includes ectopic pregnancy, blighted pregnancy, and threatened abortion. Patients with a rupture, hemorrhage, infection, or torsion of an ovarian cyst can present similarly to a patient with a ruptured ectopic pregnancy.

12. Ovarian torsion
    - Ovarian torsion is a surgical emergency as it can lead to loss of ovarian function.

13. Pelvic inflammatory disease
    - For diagnosis of pelvic inflammatory disease, transvaginal ultrasound (with doppler flow) is superior to physical examination findings and laboratory studies. Screening for pregnancy is particularly important for choice of medications and diagnostic procedures.
    - The causes of vaginal bleeding in the nonpregnant patient that need to be established in the ED are trauma, foreign bodies, infection, and bleeding disorders.

V. Toxicology
- Nearly all substances have the potential for toxicity in sufficient quantities. In addition to a careful, focused history and physical examination, patients should be checked for hidden substances or clues (needles, packets, notes, etc.).
- In the unresponsive patient, four toxic etiologies can be quickly treated with antidotes contained in the "coma cocktail." This contains oxygen (hypoxia), thiamine (Wernicke's encephalopathy, dose 100 mg IV), naloxone (opiates, dose 0.1–2.0 mg IV/IM in adults; 0.01 mg/kg in children), and $D_{50}W$ (hypoglycemia, glucose 50 mL in adults, 1 g/kg in kids). Toxicology screens may be done, but bear in mind that positive results may not fully explain a patient's presentation, and intervention is often needed before the results are available.
   A. General principles
   - Patients should be undressed and washed.
   - For eye exposures, irrigate the affected area with 2 L NS (alkalis require 1- to 2-hour irrigation, stop when pH less than 8.00), and consult ophthalmology.
   - For GI exposures, treatment depends upon the time after ingestion. Inducing vomiting is contraindicated in patients with caustic ingestions or at risk for aspiration and is not recommended, in general.
   - For GI exposures within the hour, orogastric (OG) lavage may be done. Place the patient in the left lateral decubitus position and in slight Trendelenburg; place an OG tube (36–40 F for adults, 22–24 F for kids), and lavage with room temperature water until the effluent is clear. Finish by instilling 1 g/kg activated charcoal. Activated charcoal adsorbs toxin in the gut, creating a relatively toxin-free gradient in the lumen. Thus, other tissues take up fewer toxins. It can be given alone or with 1 dose of a cathartic such as sorbitol. Although the initial dose is 1 g/kg, repeated dosing is 0.25 to 0.5 g/kg every 1 to 4 hours for large or slow-release ingestions. Whole bowel irrigation is done with 2 L/hour polyethylene glycol PO/NG (for children, 50–250 mL/kg/hour). This may be helpful for ingestion of heavy metals, lithium, sustained-release formulations, or substances with potential for bezoar formation. Stop when rectal effluent is clear.
   - Alkalinizing the urine with IV sodium bicarbonate enhances the elimination of acidic toxins. The goal for urine pH is 7.50 to 8.00, whereas serum pH should remain less than 7.50 to 7.55. Monitor the patient for hypokalemia, and correct it as needed. This method can aid elimination of chlorpropamide, herbicides, methanol, phenobarbital, and salicylates.
   - Hemodialysis should be reserved for substances not amenable to correction by the aforementioned methods or for remote ingestions of dangerous substances. Isopropanol, salicylates, theophylline, uremia, methanol, barbiturates, lithium, and ethylene glycol (I STUMBLE) may be dialyzed.
   B. Alcohols
   - Patients with alcohol intoxication can present with disinhibition, CNS depression, slurred speech, nystagmus, and incoordination. Exclude hypoglycemia and give thiamine. If there are signs of volume depletion, give $D_{5}\frac{1}{2}$ NS IV. Without intervention, alcoholics eliminate ethanol from the bloodstream at the rate of 25 to 35 mg/dL/hour, and others eliminate ethanol at a rate of 15 to 20 mg/dL/hour.

- Ethanol causes an osmolar gap, but if there is also an anion-gap metabolic acidosis, it may indicate methanol or ethylene glycol ingestion.
- Isopropanol (rubbing alcohol) has twice the CNS toxicity of ethanol but is less toxic than methanol or ethylene glycol. Ketonemia and ketonuria without hyperglycemia or glycosuria is classic for isopropanol ingestion. In addition to prolonged CNS toxicity, hemorrhagic gastritis may be a complication. Treatment is supportive with consideration for hemodialysis.
- Methanol is found in commercial and industrial solvents and can cause CNS depression, visual disturbance (including blindness!), abdominal pain, and vomiting. Treatment involves supportive care, correction of acidosis, fomepizole or ethanol, and hemodialysis.
- Ethylene glycol (antifreeze, polishes, detergent) has three phases of clinical features: (1) CNS toxicity (hallucinations and seizures), (2) cardiopulmonary phase (tachycardia, tachypnea, hypertension, sometimes heart failure, adult respiratory distress syndrome [ARDS], and shock), and (3) nephrotoxicity (oliguria, acute tubular necrosis [ATN]). Half of these patients have calcium oxalate crystalluria. Treatment includes correcting hypocalcemia and hypomagnesemia, giving parenteral pyridoxine and thiamine, fomepizole or ethanol, and performing hemodialysis.

C. Opioids

- The opioid toxidrome includes CNS depression, respiratory depression, and miosis. (Exceptions are meperidine and hydromorphone, which do not cause miosis.) Treat overdose with naloxone and respiratory support. Activated charcoal can also be given.
- Meperidine overdose may cause seizures, which may be treated with benzodiazepines.
- Propoxyphene has cardiotoxic effects, which may be reversed with IV bicarbonate.
- For ingested packets of drug, use whole bowel irrigation and multiple doses of activated charcoal.
- It is important to be aware that clonidine, pilocarpine, sedative-hypnotics, and pontine hemorrhage also cause miosis with mental status change!

D. Cocaine/amphetamines

- Cocaine and amphetamine intoxication can present with mydriasis, adrenergic stimulation, arrhythmias, MI or ischemia, aortic or coronary rupture or dissection, seizures, stroke, barotrauma, rhabdomyolysis, and renal failure. Examining vital signs (e.g., tachycardic and hypertensive) and mental status in the right clinical setting can help aid in making the diagnosis. Treatment is activated charcoal, oxygen, and sedation with benzodiazepines. Blood pressure may be controlled with nitroprusside, calcium channel blockers, or phentolamine (*not* β-blockers) if benzodiazepines are insufficient.

E. Hallucinogens

- Hallucinogens include lysergic acid diethylamide (LSD), psilocybin (mushrooms), mescaline, MDMA (Ecstasy), phencyclidine (PCP), and marijuana.
- LSD toxicity is typically limited to mild sympathomimetic symptoms and psychological effects. Treatment of a "bad trip" includes reassurance, and perhaps benzodiazepines or haloperidol.

- A recognized constellation of MDMA intoxication symptoms includes hyperthermia, DIC, rhabdomyolysis, renal failure, and seizures. Treatment is with activated charcoal and supportive care.
- Distinct features of PCP intoxication include bidirectional nystagmus and dulled perception. Because PCP is often a contaminant in other street drugs, it can present with a wide array of symptoms and may be difficult to diagnose.
- Acute medical complications of marijuana are rare.

F. Salicylate
- Salicylate toxicity causes a mixed respiratory alkalosis, metabolic alkalosis, and anion-gap metabolic acidosis. Symptoms range from nausea, vomiting, and abdominal discomfort (mild toxicity), to vomiting, hyperpnea, diaphoresis, tinnitus, and metabolic disturbances. Concentrate on the ABCs, elimination (charcoal, bowel irrigation, urinary alkalinization), volume repletion (NS), and hypoglycemia prevention. Check serum salicylate levels every 1 to 2 hours until they are declining. Hemodialysis can also be provided for patients with acute renal failure, hemodynamic instability, or refractory acidosis.

G. Acetaminophen
- Anorexia, nausea, vomiting, and malaise mark the first 24 hours of acetaminophen toxicity. On days 2 to 3, right upper quadrant pain and elevation of lever enzymes occur. On days 3 to 4 fulminant liver failure ensues. The final stage (in survivors) is recovery.
- The Rumack-Matthew nomogram is helpful in guiding treatment 4 to 24 hours after ingestion. Treatment is with activated charcoal, N-acetylcysteine (140 mg/kg PO load and 70 mg/kg every 4 hours for 17 doses), and supportive care. Use of IV N-acetylcysteine is not yet standard of care in the United States (it is used in Europe). Patients progressing to fulminant hepatic failure should be referred to a liver transplant center.

H. Tricyclic antidepressants
- Tricyclic antidepressants (TCAs) bind to and inhibit fast sodium channels in myocytes. This impairs conduction (prolonging QRS) and contractility, and can also create ventricular dysrhythmias. TCAs block potassium channels in phase 3 repolarization of His-Purkinje myocytes, causing QT prolongation. TCAs also produce negative inotropic effects by blocking calcium channels. Peripheral vasodilation and hypotension result from inhibition of α_1-adrenergic receptors. TCAs block norepinephrine reuptake in the CNS and peripheral nervous system (PNS), causing early tachycardia and hypertension, and later, bradycardia and hypotension. TCAs are competitive antagonists at muscarinic acetylcholine receptors (central and peripheral), producing anticholinergic effects. Furthermore, there is blockade of H_1-histamine, GABA, and NDMA–glutamate receptors.
- Neurologic effects can include mental status change, seizures, and myoclonus. Cardiovascular effects include hypertension, hypotension, dysrhythmias, and conduction blocks. Potential ECG findings are numerous: sinus tachycardia, long QRS, RBBB (right bundle branch block), VT, VF, long QT, negative R wave in lead aV_R, and negative S wave in leads I and aV_L. Patients present with anticholinergic symptoms. Hypoventilation and acute respiratory distress syndrome (ARDS) can occur.

- Gastric lavage may be done in patients presenting within an hour of a life-threatening TCA ingestion. Activated charcoal is indicated, though multiple dose charcoal is controversial. Manage hypotension with isotonic IV fluid, Trendelenberg position, and inotropic support if needed (norepinephrine or dopamine). If the QRS is 110 milliseconds or longer, give sodium barcarbonate IV to achieve a goal pH of 7.45 to 7.55. Treat seizures with benzodiazepines and phenobarbital.

I. Organophosphates
- Organophosphates (pesticides) inhibit acetylcholinesterase. Thus, muscarinic, nicotinic, and CNS effects ensue. Muscarinic effects include "DUMBELS" (diaphoresis and diarrhea; urination; miosis; bradycardia, bronchospasm, and bronchorrhea; emesis; lacrimation excess; salivation excess) and "SLUDGE" (salivation, lacrimation, urination, diarrhea, GI upset, emesis). Nicotinic effects consist of mydriasis, tachycardia, hypertension, cramps, weakness, fasciculations, and diaphragmatic failure. CNS effects include tremors, seizures, anxiety, insomnia, ataxia, dysarthria, paralysis, and coma.
- Decontaminate the patient (bathe, charcoal). Maintain the airway. Pharmacologic treatment consists of atropine (1–2 mg IV, then 2 mg every 5–15 minutes prn) or glycopyrrolate (0.1 mg IV every 3–4 hours prn), 2-PAM (pralidoxime; 1–2 g IV over 15–30 minutes, may repeat prn in 1 hour and then every 3–8 hours), and diazepam (for seizures; 5–15 mg IV every 5 minutes prn).

J. Other medications
- Theophylline toxicity can occur at therapeutic doses and can cause dysrhythmias, seizures and milder neurologic symptoms, and GI symptoms. Treatment is gastric lavage or activated charcoal, supportive care, and if needed, appropriate antiarrhythmics.
- Digitalis toxicity may present with dysrhythmias (particularly bradyarrhythmias) in a patient with a detectable serum digoxin level. Patients with hypokalemia, hypomagnesemia, or hypercalcemia are predisposed to toxicity. Give activated charcoal, digoxin-specific Fab antibody fragments (antidote, multiple doses may be needed), and supportive care.
- β-Blocker toxicity leads to bradycardia and hypotension. Drug levels are not particularly helpful, aside from confirming exposure. Give activated charcoal, IV fluid, and glucagon (1 mg IV every 5 minutes). Atenolol, nadolol, and sotalol can be dialyzed.
- Calcium channel blockers can cause similar effects with varying degrees of atrioventricular (AV) block. Lactic acidosis and hypercalcemia are common. Give IV fluid, calcium chloride or calcium gluconate, adrenergic agents (for those not responding to calcium salts), glucagon, and insulin.
- Hydrocarbons may be ingested on inhaled. Patients should be decontaminated, and treatment should focus on the ABCs. Hypotension should be treated with IV fluid. Avoid catecholamines because they can precipitate dysrhythmias.

Pediatrics

I. Bronchiolitis
   A. Basic science
   - Bronchiolitis is an acute infectious illness of the small airways occurring most commonly in infants 2 to 12 months of age. Respiratory syncytial virus (RSV) is the most common agent causing bronchiolitis and encompasses nearly 75% of all cases. However, several other viruses have been implicated, including parainfluenza, influenza, rhino-, and adenoviruses.
   B. History and physical examination
   - Bronchiolitis usually begins as an upper respiratory infection with clear nasal discharge, cough, and variable degrees of fever. However, apnea may be the presenting symptom in some infants, especially those infants born prematurely and younger than 2 months of age.
   - Over 3 to 7 days there is a progression to lower respiratory tract infection that manifests as tachypnea, wheezing, rhonchi, or crackles. Some infants can present with significant respiratory distress including grunting, nasal flaring, and retractions (subcostal, intercostal, and supraclavicular) as well as hypoxemia. Findings on chest x-ray are variable and nonspecific and may include patchy atelectasis, hyperinflation, and peribronchial thickening.
   C. Laboratory and diagnostic studies
   - Pulse oximetry is useful to assess oxygen saturation in infants with bronchiolitis. More severe cases may require serial arterial blood gas monitoring. Chest x-ray may be useful in patients who present with significant respiratory distress and hypoxemia. A fluorescent antibody test and an ELISA (enzyme-linked immunosorbent assay) are available for the rapid diagnosis of RSV.
   D. Formulating the diagnosis
   - The diagnosis is usually clear from the history and physical examination. Recurrent episodes of wheezing in a young child may suggest foreign body aspiration, reactive airway disease, vascular rings, or cystic fibrosis.
   E. Evaluating the severity of problems
   - Infants with significant respiratory distress manifested by increased work of breathing, tachypnea, and cyanosis have severe disease. Infants with persistently increasing oxygen requirements or rising P_{CO_2} levels may require intubation.

F. Managing the patient
   • Otherwise healthy infants with mild symptoms can be managed at home. Hospitalization is required for children with moderate to severe respiratory distress or hypoxemia, those who have underlying cardiopulmonary disease and immunodeficiencies, and infants born prematurely (less than 34 weeks' gestation). Hospital management is mostly supportive, as most patients require some type of supplemental oxygen or respiratory support (mostly nasal suctioning) as well as fluid therapy to prevent dehydration. Initial and subsequent monitoring of oxygenation by pulse oximetry facilitates the appropriate management of hypoxia.
   • Treatments with racemic epinephrine, albuterol, and corticosteroids have not been proven to make a significant difference in the management of infants and young children with bronchiolitis. Other therapies including ribavirin (an antiviral agent that is active against RSV), heliox, and surfactant have been used in the past for critically ill infants, although there are no specific recommendations for their use.
   • Passive immunization with a monoclonal antibody to RSV once each month during RSV season is now available for specific high-risk groups of infants and children as recommended by the American Academy of Pediatrics.

II. Child Physical Abuse
   A. Basic science
      • Child abuse often presents to the physician with a chief complaint of "accidental injury." The key aspect to managing this problem is to identify and differentiate accidental versus deliberate injury patterns and to identify the factors that put families at risk for child physical or sexual abuse. The broader term "child maltreatment" includes acts of commission (abuse) and acts of omission (neglect) that adversely affects a child. These encompass physical, psychological, and sexual abuse as well as neglect.
   B. History and physical examination
      1. Child abuse must be suspected when:
         • The history of an injury is vague.
         • History is incompatible with physical signs.
         • History changes when the story is retold.
         • Parents and other caregivers give different histories.
         • History is incompatible with the child's developmental stage.
         • Child gives a different history from the parent. Note that often the child will not reveal that he or she was deliberately injured.
      2. Other red flags include the following:
         • Significant delays in seeking medical care
         • A detached or inattentive parent
         • Unrealistic parental expectations (e.g., demanding a 1-year-old to sit still)
      3. The physical examination includes checking for the following:
         • Head and neck injury
         • Ophthalmologic injury
         • Abdominal injury

- Genital trauma
- Skin bruising
- Skeletal injury
4. Classification of injuries:
    a. Bruises
        - Bruises are the commonest manifestation of child abuse and can be found anywhere on the body.
        - Accidental bruises tend to occur over bony prominences, such as the forehead, chin, elbows, and shins. Inflicted bruises are usually found on soft tissue areas such as the cheeks, buttocks, trunk, and upper arms.
        - The human hand which is the most common "instrument" of child abuse may leave parallel linear stress petechiae representing the spaces between the fingers. It is important to remember that petechiae of the face and shoulders can be the result of intense stretching, crying, or ongoing coughing and can be mistake for abuse. Objects used to inflict injury such as belts and cords often leave marks conforming to the shape of the object used.
    b. Head injury
        - Abusive head injuries are responsible for more fatalities and long-term morbidities than any other form of physical abuse. Children rarely sustain significant head injury or skull fractures due to falling from a couch or bed, or running and falling onto the ground. Evidence of head trauma includes vomiting, irritability, altered mental status, scalp injuries, and skull fractures.
    c. Shaken baby syndrome
        - Shaken baby syndrome occurs when a perpetrator holds the infant by the chest, arms, or back and then shakes the infant causing rupture of bridging veins, diffuse axonal injury, and hypoxia. The infant usually presents with signs of increased intracranial pressure. These signs include apnea, alternating lethargy and irritability, altered level of consciousness, a full fontanel, retinal hemorrhage(s), and poor or increased muscle tone. Retinal hemorrhages occur in approximately 85% of shaken infants. They are rarely seen in coagulopathies, blood dyscrasias, accidental head injury, or meningitis. These children often suffer severe neurologic injury with permanent deficits.
    d. Thoracic injuries
        - Thoracic and abdominal injuries result from the child's being hit, kicked, thrown, or struck with an object. Often these battered children present with no history of trauma and delayed medical care. Symptoms of thoracic trauma include hematemesis, respiratory distress, poor feeding, and fever.
    e. Abdominal injuries
        - Abdominal injuries are the second most common cause of death. Abdominal injury often presents with abdominal pain, sometimes accompanied by distention and signs of obstruction (e.g., vomiting),

and areas of localized tenderness. The major injuries include duodenal hematoma, mesenteric injury, pancreatic and renal contusions, liver and splenic laceration/hematoma, and small bowel lacerations.

  f. Skeletal injuries

  - About 80% of abuse fractures are seen in children younger than 18 months of age. The four most common sites of abuse fractures (excluding skull fractures) are the femur, humerus, tibia, and posterior arc of the ribs. The classic metaphyseal lesion of long bones ("corner fracture," "bucket handle fracture") is considered pathognomonic for abuse. Old fractures in various stages of healing also suggest child abuse.

    - Factors that increase the likelihood of fractures being due to abuse:

      - Fractures in children younger than 2 years of age
      - Presence of developmental handicaps in the child
      - Premature birth of the child
      - Presence of other associated injuries in addition to the fractures
      - Absence of a history explaining the fracture

  g. Burns

  - Burns represent approximately 10% of all physical abuse cases. The peak age of burn victims is 13 to 24 months. Tap water scalds, contact burns, and hot grease burns are the most prevalent. Cigarette burns account for up to 5% of burns.

  - Accidental burns are rarely full thickness because the child quickly withdraws from pain. Inflicted burns are often full thickness and can imprint the source of the burn. Inflicted burns are often caused by immersing the child in hot water. Immersion burns often leave a sharp line of demarcation between the normal and the burned skin. Often immersion burns of the buttock leave a doughnut lesion and immersion burns of the hands and feet leave a stocking-glove pattern.

C. Laboratory and diagnostic studies

  1. Bruising

  - A complete blood count (CBC), platelet count, and coagulation screen should be performed to rule out medical causes of abnormal bruising such as leukemia or idiopathic thrombocytopenia.

  2. Shaken baby syndrome

  - The child should have an eye examination to look for retinal hemorrhages and a head computed tomographic (CT) scan to look for intracranial hemorrhage. Cerebrospinal fluid (CSF) examination may reveal blood and xanthochromia.

  3. Thoracic injuries

  - Diagnosis of the injuries is by plain radiographs or chest CT scan.

  4. Abdominal injuries

  - Plain radiographs may show dilated loops of bowel. An abdominal CT scan may be required for definitive diagnosis. Hematuria may indicate renal trauma.

5. Fractures
- Medical causes of unusual fractures, such as osteogenesis imperfecta, should be ruled out. Children younger than 5 with any unusual fracture warrant an entire skeletal survey performed by a trained pediatric radiologist to detect old fractures.

D. Formulating the diagnosis
- If the physician suspects child abuse a comprehensive investigation is necessary. All medical personnel are mandated by law to report suspicious cases to child protective services. A social worker generally examines the psychosocial factors that place families at risk for child abuse. Some of these factors include financial problems, unemployment, social isolation, domestic violence, young or single parents, use of corporal punishment, poor impulse control, depression, and substance abuse. However, child abuse is seen in all ethnic, religious, educational, and socioeconomic backgrounds. Spouse abuse increases the likelihood of child abuse.
- After the history, physical examination, x-ray films, and social work analyses are complete, a determination is made regarding whether child abuse has occurred.

E. Evaluating the severity of symptoms
- The psychological sequelae of abuse and neglect are often the most permanent and devastating injury suffered by the child.

F. Managing the patient
- If child abuse is highly suspected:
  1. The child should not be allowed to return home until any risk of injury is ruled out.
  2. The physician must report findings immediately to the proper child protective agency.
  3. All medical problems should be treated.

III. Child Sexual Abuse
A. Basic science
- The annual number of cases of child sexual abuse reported in the United States is approximately 250,000 to 350,000. Perpetrators are most often male, relatives, or are well known to the victim.

B. History and physical examination
- Often the victim does not reveal a history of any sexual abuse. When a child does disclose sexual abuse, a history should be taken by someone skilled in interviewing children.
- Children may have symptoms that suggest sexual abuse. These include difficulty walking or sitting; abdominal pain; constipation; dysuria; vaginal, urethral, or rectal discharge or bleeding; change in behavior; and depression. Children may also have recurrent urinary tract infections (UTIs) or may present with a sexually transmitted disease.
- The majority of sexually abused children have no physical findings.
- Examination with a forensic evidence kit ("rape kit") should be performed for acute assaults occurring within 72 hours of presentation.

C. Laboratory and diagnostic studies
- Sexually transmitted disease testing should be done. This includes appropriate specimens for gonorrhea, chlamydia, syphilis, hepatitis, and human immunodeficiency virus (HIV).

D. Formulating the diagnosis
- The diagnosis is made when there is adequate suspicion, despite the absence of physical findings.

E. Evaluating the severity of problems
- Even without significant physical injury, sexual abuse victims develop severe emotional problems.

F. Managing the patient
- Once it has been determined that a child has been sexually abused, management includes treatment of medical problems, protection from the perpetrator, and counseling for the child and family.

IV. Colic

A. Basic science
- Colic is defined as excessive, unexplained crying, lasting more than 3 hours per day, more than 3 days per week, and persists for more than 3 weeks in an otherwise healthy and well-fed infant.
- At 2 weeks of age, infants normally cry about 2 hours per day. Crying tends to increase to an average of 3 hours per day at 6 weeks and then decreases to 1 hour per day by 3 months of age.
- Ten percent of all infants have colic. Crying episodes typically begin in the first 3 weeks of life. Persistent crying episodes often start abruptly and may last for several hours. Most often, crying occurs in the evening hours. Infants often draw their knees up and pass flatus. The infant with colic is difficult to console with usual measures.
- The etiology of colic is poorly understood and is probably multifactorial. Proposed theories have included immaturity of the infant's gastrointestinal tract, trapped intestinal gas, hyperperistalsis, allergy, and maternal anxiety.

B. History and physical examination
- The history and physical examination should rule out other causes of excessive infant crying. The history should review the timing, duration, and character of the crying, as well as the parent's responses. Vomiting, diarrhea, or blood in the stools may indicate a sensitivity to cow milk protein or other gastrointestinal problem. A detailed social history is helpful and the physician must consider the potential for child abuse.
- Physical examination must include a complete neurologic examination looking for evidence of infection, increased intracranial pressure, and shaken baby syndrome. Otitis media should be ruled out. Abdominal and genitourinary examination should look for evidence of trauma, intussusception, incarcerated hernia, or testicular torsion. The extremities should be examined for trauma and digits examined for strangulation by an encircling hair. A fluorescein eye examination will rule out corneal abrasion as the cause.

C. Laboratory and diagnostic studies
- Laboratory studies are not indicated unless the history or physical examination suggests an etiology other than colic.

D. Formulating the diagnosis
- The diagnosis of colic is one of exclusion.

E. Evaluating the severity of problems
- Colic is benign. The infant is generally healthy and will outgrow the behavior.

F. Managing the patient
- The natural history of colic is improvement over time, with resolution by 3 to 4 months of age, regardless of the management strategy used. Reassurance, support, and a review of behavioral tactics should be the mainstays of management. Parents should be reassured that their infant is healthy and the crying will not hurt the baby but will improve with time. The physician should acknowledge parental feelings of frustration toward their baby.
- Behavioral tactics that may be beneficial include swaddling, walking, rocking, and other comforting measures. To avoid overstimulation, parents should not use more than one or two comforting methods per 20-minute period.
- There is no drug proved effective and safe for colic. Parents should be discouraged from switching formulas unless there is evidence of dietary intolerance such as diarrhea, vomiting, or blood in stools.

V. Croup
   A. Basic science
   - Croup, or laryngotracheobronchitis, is an acute, viral upper respiratory infection of the larynx and surrounding areas. The vocal cords become inflamed and edematous, leading to stridor, hoarseness, and a barking cough. Croup is usually a mild, self-limited process; severe cases with significant upper airway obstruction may be life-threatening. The major site of obstruction is the subglottic area.
   - Parainfluenza virus is the most common pathogen; influenza A, adenovirus, respiratory syncytial virus (RSV), and other viruses have also been implicated. Croup occurs most frequently in the winter months. Allergies and psychological factors can also be causative.

   B. History and physical examination
   - Croup most commonly affects children ages 6 months to 3 years. Fever and upper respiratory symptoms are usually present for 1 to 3 days before the onset of hoarseness, stridor, and a characteristic, barking cough. Wheezing and chest retractions may be present. Symptoms are typically worse at night. Agitation and crying may aggravate the signs and symptoms. Severe cases may result in tachypnea, nasal flaring, and retractions. The child who is hypoxic, cyanotic, or obtunded needs urgent airway management.

   C. Laboratory and diagnostic studies
   - There is little role for laboratory testing in croup. Airway radiographs, if obtained, show subglottic narrowing ("steeple sign") and are most useful to rule out retropharyngeal abscess or airway foreign bodies. Radiographs do not

correlate well with disease severity. Direct fluorescent antibody testing is available for the common viruses that cause croup.

D. Formulating the diagnosis
- Croup is diagnosed clinically. Bacterial tracheitis, diphtheritic croup, epiglottitis, foreign body aspiration, and retropharyngeal abscess must be excluded in all patients who present with croup.
- Spasmodic croup is a variant consisting of the precipitous, nighttime onset of barking cough, stridor, and dyspnea in an otherwise apparently well child. Symptoms resolve quickly with mist or cool air but often recur on several successive nights.

E. Evaluating the severity of problems
- Children with severe chest retractions, stridor at rest, tachypnea, hypoxia, cyanosis, agitation, or lethargy may progress to respiratory failure and require close observation. Respiratory difficulty may interfere with drinking, leading to dehydration.

F. Managing the patient
- Home management, consisting of the use of a humidifier and placing the child in a steamy bathroom. Exposure to cool night air is often effective.
- In the hospital, humidified air or nebulized saline is helpful. As with epiglottitis, invasive procedures should be kept to a minimum. Children with moderate to severe disease usually benefit from parenteral corticosteroids, often given as a single dose of dexamethasone. Administration of nebulized racemic epinephrine is an effective way to rapidly reduce airway inflammation in children with severe croup. Because rebound airway edema may occur, children should be observed for several hours before being discharged home.
- Children with croup should be hospitalized if they demonstrate progressive stridor, severe stridor at rest, hypoxia, obtundation, or the need for reliable observation. Antibiotics are not indicated in croup.

VI. Dehydration
- Dehydration is a decrease in total body water and can be associated with loss of sodium and potassium.

A. Basic science
- The water deficit is the percent dehydration multiplied by the patient's body weight. Maintenance fluid requirements for children can be calculated based on their body weight according to Table 17-1.

B. History and physical examination
- The history may reveal sources of increased fluid loss (e.g., fever, vomiting, diarrhea, increased respiratory rate) or decreased intake.
- Mild dehydration (3% to 5%) is present when the pulse is normal or increased, urine output decreased, the child is thirsty, and physical examination is normal.
- Moderate dehydration (7% to 10%) is present when the patient is tachycardic, irritable or lethargic, eyes and fontanel sucken, tears decreased,

TABLE 17-1:

Maintenance Fluid Requirements for Children

Body Weight	Fluid Requirements
First 10 kg	100 mL/kg/24 hours
Second 10 kg	50 mL/kg/24 hours
Remaining body weight	20 mL/kg/24 hours

mucous membranes dry, mild loss in skin turgor, delayed capillary refill, cool and pale skin, and little or no urine output.

- Severe dehydration (10% to 15%) is diagnosed when all the above symptoms and signs are more pronounced. Additionally, the patient is hypotensive, the skin may be mottled, and there is no urine output. Severe dehydration is a medical emergency.

C. Laboratory and diagnostic studies
- The hematocrit may be falsely elevated owing to hemoconcentration. Electrolytes are usually abnormal and vary based on the amount and source of fluid loss(es). Of note, the serum sodium provides one with information about the type of dehydration (i.e., hypernatremic, isotonic, or hyponatremic).
- Urinalysis shows an elevated specific gravity, often accompanied by the presence of ketones. Volume loss alone will result in a disproportionate increase in the blood urea nitrogen (BUN) without a concomitant increase in serum creatinine.
- Other studies may be necessary depending on the underlying cause of the dehydration.

D. Formulating the diagnosis
- The diagnosis is based on the patient's history. Particular attention should be paid to oral intake and urine output. Parents should also be questioned on how they prepare the formula, and on what fluids they have used to try to rehydrate the child.

E. Evaluating the severity of problems
- Children with decreased urine output, dry skin, dry mucous membranes, mild tachycardia, and a normal mental status are mildly to moderately dehydrated and can often be orally rehydrated. Children with no urine output for 24 hours, delayed capillary refill, decreased blood pressure, or altered mental status require aggressive intravenous fluid resuscitation.

F. Managing the patient
- Children with mild to moderate dehydration can be orally rehydrated with electrolyte solutions such as the WHO/UNICEF rehydration solution and Pedialyte.
- Children with severe dehydration (or those with persistent vomiting) require intravenous fluid resuscitation. This consists of an initial 20 mL/kg bolus of isotonic fluid without glucose, such as lactated Ringer's solution or normal

saline. This bolus can be repeated multiple times as long as the patient's clinical status is reassessed. Patients may need up to 60 mL/kg in bolus solutions. Consider blood or plasma (10 mL/kg) if there is no response after two boluses of isotonic fluid or if there is acute blood loss.

- The estimated fluid deficit should be replaced over 24 hours in the following manner:
  1. Hours 1 to 8: maintenance + one-half deficit
  2. Hours 16 to 24: maintenance + one-half deficit
- Patients with electrolyte abnormalities such as hypernatremia require special management.

VII. Enuresis

A. Basic science

- Enuresis is defined as the voluntary or involuntary passage of urine after an age when bladder control should have been established. It usually refers to bedwetting at night, although it can also occur during the day. Approximately 20% of children with nighttime enuresis also have daytime symptoms as well. Enuresis is a common occurrence in children, although boys are twice as likely than girls to have symptoms. Most children develop bladder control between the ages of 3 and 6 years, but as many as 7% of 5-year-old boys and 3% of 5-year-old girls still wet the bed.

- Enuresis is primary or secondary. Primary enuresis refers to a situation in which the child has never achieved an adequate period of nighttime dryness and this accounts for the majority of children with nocturnal enuresis. Secondary enuresis refers to wetting in a child who had been dry for at least the previous 6 months. Secondary enuresis is often attributed to various stressors at home including an illness, family move, or birth of a new sibling.

- Although the cause of enuresis is still unclear, it is believed that some children experience persistent bedwetting because of a small bladder capacity or the inability to control their urge to urinate. Others drink too much before bed and do not wake up to empty their bladder. Some may make large amounts of urine because they do not have a nighttime rise in antidiuretic hormone.

- Only a small percentage of children have enuresis as a symptom of an underlying condition, most commonly a urinary tract infection or diabetes mellitus. Other neurologic or genitourinary tract abnormalities should be considered.

B. History and physical examination

- Most children with enuresis not caused by an underlying condition will have a normal history and physical examination. Important details in the history include birth history, growth, development, previous urinary tract infections, urinary symptoms, and quality of stream. The family history often reveals childhood enuresis in one or both parents.

- The physical examination is usually normal. The examiner should, however, check closely for elevated blood pressure and abdominal, genital, and neurologic abnormalities.

C. Laboratory and diagnostic studies
- In general, all patients should have a urinalysis and urine culture. The decision to obtain other studies should be based on findings in the history and physical examination.

D. Formulating the diagnosis
- A normal history, physical examination, urinalysis, and urine culture rules out most medical and surgical causes of enuresis of concern.

E. Evaluating the severity of problems
- Successful treatment of underlying disorders that cause enuresis will usually result in resolution of the enuresis.

F. Managing the patient
- Once a pathologic etiology has been excluded, treatment should include behavior modification. Bladder-stretching exercises and pharmacologic intervention are second-line treatment modalities. Parents should be reassured that enuresis is common among school-age children and that spontaneous resolution occurs in 15% of children each year. Children usually do not wet the bed purposefully and should not be punished. Instead, they should be encouraged to take responsibility when bedwetting does occur; for example, they should be involved in changing sheets and doing laundry. They should be actively involved in their treatment plan and receive positive reinforcement, such as gold stars on dry days.
- Initial attempts to manage enuresis should begin around 4 years of age with establishing a day and night toileting routine. Daytime urination should be postponed to increase bladder capacity. Daytime fluid intake should be encouraged and nighttime fluids discouraged. Children who have secondary nocturnal enuresis as a symptom of stress or regressive behavior can be managed with time and patience.
- If enuresis persists, children can use bedwetting alarms at night that sense moisture and waken them before fully voiding. Alternatively, a bedside alarm can be set as a reminder to urinate in the middle of the night.
- Older children who continue to have enuresis may benefit from intranasal desmopressin (an analog of antidiuretic hormone) or imipramine (a tricyclic antidepressant). Both drugs have been demonstrated to be effective, but when stopped the enuresis often recurs. It may be helpful to use these drugs with other therapies such as the alarm and bladder-stretching exercises.

VIII. Epiglottitis
A. Basic science
- Epiglottitis is a life-threatening acute infection of the supraglottic region of the upper airway. As the arytenoids, aryepiglottic folds, and the epiglottis swell, the upper airway becomes obstructed.
- *Haemophilus influenzae* type b (Hib) is the most common identified etiologic agent. The incidence of epiglottitis has decreased considerably since the introduction of Hib vaccination. *Streptococcus pneumoniae* and other bacteria have also been implicated and should be considered in a fully immunized child.

B. History and physical examination
  • The affected child is usually 1 to 5 years of age, although adult and infant cases have been reported. The child will have had a sudden onset of fever, severe sore throat, dysphagia, and drooling. Fever between 38.8°C and 40°C is typical. Children assume a characteristic posture: sitting quietly while leaning forward with the neck extended, mouth open, and an anxious expression. This position is in an effort to maximize the airway diameter. Children with advanced airway obstruction may have decreased air exchange, altered level of consciousness, and gray color. Stridor generally indicates near-complete airway obstruction. Because agitation of the child may lead to laryngospasm, no attempt should be made to separate a conscious child from the parents, to force the patient to lie down, or to view the child's pharynx with a tongue blade.

C. Laboratory and diagnostic studies
  • Laryngoscopy should only be performed in a controlled environment such as an intensive care unit or operating room. It will show a swollen "cherry red" epiglottis. Although an enlarged epiglottis seen on a lateral neck radiograph will confirm the diagnosis, this is not advisable given the tenuous nature of the patient's airway. The etiologic diagnosis is made by blood culture or by culture of the surface of the epiglottis.

D. Formulating the diagnosis
  • Epiglottitis is a clinical diagnosis made on the basis of the history and physical examination. The differential diagnosis consists of: croup or spasmodic croup, bacterial tracheitis, uvulitis, foreign body, peritonsillar or retropharyngeal abscesses, and chemical or thermal upper airway injury.

E. Evaluating the severity of problems
  • Epiglottitis is a medical emergency. Complete airway obstruction is the most important complication.

F. Managing the patient
  • Every emergency department should have a plan for management of the epiglottitis patient. Oxygen should be administered and monitors applied as tolerated. Equipment and medications for intubation and resuscitation should be at the child's bedside, an operating room rapidly prepared, and a team skilled at endotracheal intubation and tracheostomy assembled. In the operating room, the trachea is intubated, intravenous access obtained, and broad-spectrum antibiotics administered. Should endotracheal intubation fail, a tracheostomy should be performed.
  • Once the airway is secured, the patient is admitted to an intensive care unit. Intubation is usually necessary for 48 hours; as bacteremia is often present, intravenous antibiotics are usually administered for 7 to 10 days.

IX. Fever without Localizing Signs
  A. Basic science
    • Acute febrile illnesses constitute the majority of pediatric visits to a pediatric office or emergency room. Although many pediatric infectious diseases present with classic features that make the diagnosis obvious for the

BOX 17-1

COMMONLY ISOLATED BACTERIAL AGENTS IN THE PEDIATRIC POPULATION

Newborn (0–6 Weeks)	**6–8 Weeks to 4–5 Years**	**Over 5 Years**
Group B streptococcus (*Streptococcus agalactiae*)	*Haemophilus influenzae* type B	*Streptococcus pneumoniae*
Gram-negative enterics, mostly *Escherichia coli*	*Streptococcus pneumoniae*	*Neisseria meningitidis*
Listeria	*Neisseria meningitidis*	*Staphylococcus aureus*

physician, occasionally, infectious agents may cause fever without localizing signs, presenting the physician with a diagnostic challenge. Although most infectious illnesses are benign and self-limited, high fever in a child (particularly a child under 2 years of age) should prompt an investigation for more serious bacterial disease.

- At different ages, children have different exposure and susceptibility to bacterial agents (Box 17-1). In general, newborns usually become infected with organisms acquired by passage through the birth canal or by ascending infection of the lower female genital tract. Older infants and children are exposed to pathogens through close contact by caregivers, pets, day care, and school attendance.

- Although the majority of infant and childhood illnesses are viral infections, physicians always must be aware of the potential for an underlying serious bacterial illness (SBI). Important sources of bacterial infections causing serious bacterial illnesses in young infants and children include bacteremia, meningitis, pneumonia, urinary tract infections, gastroenteritis, septic arthritis, and osteomyelitis. Some of these illnesses present with classic clinical features; however, sometimes infants and young children will only present with a history of fever and not a clear source.

B. History, physical examination, laboratory evaluation, and management

- Several subjective features are often cited to distinguish those infants who are more ill from those who have a benign, self-limited febrile disease. Among large studies of febrile infants, the degree of playfulness, alertness, consolability, use of eye contact, and other age-appropriate behaviors are all favorable clinical observations. However, proper interpretation of these features requires the experience of the examiner as well as the realization that some infants who initially look well can clinically worsen over time. A thorough physical examination should be performed in an attempt to identify the source of the fever. Young infants are unable to localize infection and may rapidly disseminate bacteria. Clinical and laboratory evaluations should be thorough but selective, with an emphasis on attempting to identify those infants who are at high risk of bacterial disease. This is one of the most critical and difficult decisions in the care of children.

- Neonates do not have reliable findings on physical examination, so any fever (38.0°C or greater) in neonates 28 days old and younger is considered serious and requires a full sepsis evaluation including the following laboratory investigations: CBC with differential, blood culture, and urine culture, and CSF for cells, biochemistry, and culture. These infants should be admitted to the hospital for intravenous (IV) antibiotic therapy and close observation.

- In general, fever in infants 30 to 90 days of age also requires a detailed history and physical examination as well as blood and urine cultures so that a serious bacterial illness is not missed. However, any infant or young child who is ill-appearing, regardless of age, will require a full "sepsis workup" as well as hospital admission and treatment with IV antibiotics. A white blood cell count greater than 15,000 in infants and young children with a fever of 38.0°C or greater, combined with a bandemia and a suggestive clinical picture, identified a significant number of infants who subsequently were found to have bacteremia.

- In the past, many infants under the age of 3 months with fever were automatically admitted to the hospital for several days of empiric antibiotic therapy pending the results of blood, urine, and spinal fluid cultures. With the advent of broad-spectrum antibiotics that can be administered by the intramuscular route, some physicians now favor the outpatient use of IM antibiotics if a febrile infant older than 28 days is at low risk for bacterial infection. However, this decision should be made only by an experienced clinician who can evaluate the child and ensure appropriate follow-up. The infant must have parents willing and capable of assessing their child for changes in status. If all these criteria are not met, the child should be hospitalized pending results of cultures.

C. Managing the patient

- Because the bacterial agent causing sepsis are different in different pediatric age groups, empiric antibiotic therapy will vary with the age of the child. Ampicillin and gentamicin or ampicillin and cefotaxime are often used in the newborn period and can be useful until about 2 or 3 months of age. These two regimens will cover group B streptococci, gram-negative enterics, and *Listeria monocytogenes*. Third-generation cephalosporins alone are not appropriate for this age group because listeria are resistent to third-generation cephalosporins. Third-generation cephalosporins alone are used at many centers for infants greater than 2 to 3 months of age.

- The emergence of penicillin-resistant pneumococci and other resistant organisms may alter the recommendations for empiric antibiotic therapy in the near future.

- At all ages, antibiotics should be directed at the most likely pathogen(s); if an organism is isolated, therapy should be modified to cover only the isolated

TABLE 17-2:

Common Bacterial and Viral Pathogens in Diarrhea and Their Treatment

Pathogen	Pathogenesis	In Blood	In Mucus	Treatment
Bacterial Pathogens				
Campylobacter	Invasion and enterotoxin	Yes	Variable	Supportive; erythromycin if severe
Vibriocholerae	Invasion and enterotoxin	No	No	Bactrim
Escherichia coli	Invasion and enterotoxin; cytotoxin	Variable	Variable	Supportive, or Bactrim or ampicillin
Salmonella	Invasion and enterotoxin	Variable	Moderate	None unless severe, ampicillin, chloramphenicol, Bactrim
Shigella	Invasion and enterotoxin	Yes	Yes	Bactrim
Yersinia	Invasion and enterotoxin	Yes	Yes	None or Bactrim
Viral Pathogen				
Rotavirus	Mucosal destruction	No	No	Supportive

organism. If bacterial cultures are negative within 48 to 72 hours and the child is clinically well without any development of new signs or symptoms suggesting bacterial disease, antibiotics can often be stopped.

X. Gastroenteritis
  A. Basic science
    • Gastroenteritis is a syndrome of diarrhea (≥5 loose stools/day) usually accompanied by emesis. It is generally self-limited. In children, it is most often of viral cause. During the summer months enteroviruses are the most common agents, whereas in the late winter and early spring, rotavirus is the usual culprit. However, many other viruses can cause gastroenteritis.
    • The most common bacterial causes of gastroenteritis include *Salmonella, Shigella, Yersinia, Campylobacter,* and enteroinvasive *Escherichia coli.* Less common are *Staphylococcus, Clostridium difficile,* and the parasites *Giardia lamblia, Entamoeba histolytica, Cryptosporidium,* and *Trichuris trichiura.* Viral causes include rotavirus, enteric adenovirus, norovirus, and calcivirus. The specific characteristics of selected pathogens are listed in Table 17-2.
  B. History and physical examination
    • In general, viral disorders of the gastrointestinal tract produce gastroenteritis with vomiting preceding or concurrent with the diarrhea. In contrast, most (but not all) bacterial pathogens produce enteritis with little or no emesis.

The exception to this is staphylococcal food poisoning, which produces both vomiting and diarrhea. In addition, bacterial diarrhea when due to invasive organisms can produce bloody and mucus diarrhea. There may be history of contact with ill persons, animals, contaminated water, undercooked food, or travel outside the area of residence.

- On physical examination, the presence of fever should be sought. The examination may be normal but is often remarkable for hyperactive bowel sounds, a scaphoid abdomen, and the clinical signs of dehydration (see Section VI, Dehydration).
- Occasionally extraintestinal complications of gastrointestinal infections may be seen, depending on the causative organism (e.g., osteomyelitis, endocarditis, and septic thrombophlebitis).

C. Laboratory and diagnostic studies

- Examination of a freshly voided stool is the mainstay of diagnosis for both viral and bacterial pathogens. The presence of occult blood and fecal leukocytes as detected by Wright's stain, often in sheets, are characteristic of stools due to an invasive bacterial pathogen. Viral diarrhea usually does not contain blood but may produce blood-streaked stool if the child develops an anal fissure; an irritated, bleeding hemorrhoid; or a severe diaper rash secondary to the passage of copious stools.
- If the history and stool examination suggests a bacterial pathogen, a stool culture and sensitivity should be done. If the child's age and season of the year suggest viral diarrhea, a rotazyme (an ELISA specific for rotavirus), an ELISA for enteric adenovirus, or a stool culture for enterovirus may be appropriate. Depending on the severity of illness, ancillary tests including electrolytes, complete blood count with differential, and blood cultures may be warranted.

D. Formulating the diagnosis

- Appropriate history and examination of the stool will aid in the identification of most cases of gastroenteritis. Occasionally an acute abdominal process or a urinary tract infection may present with similar gastroenteritis. Examination of the urine or abdominal films may be warranted in children who do not have a clearly identified case of gastroenteritis, particularly if the child is acutely ill.

E. Evaluating the severity of problems

- Questions regarding the quantity of stool passed, ability of the child to retain oral fluids, and assessment of the child's hydration status by physical examination and electrolyte measurements will allow the clinician to determine the severity of the child's condition. Any child unable to retain oral fluids or with severe GI fluid losses should be admitted for rehydration and observation. In addition, any child with a toxic appearance should be admitted and given antibiotics pending the results of cultures.

F. Managing the patient

- Viral gastroenteritis requires only supportive therapy. Correcting dehydration and electrolyte imbalance, if present, and maintaining hydration are the mainstay of therapy. There is no specific antiviral therapy. The illness usually starts within 12 hours to 4 days after exposure and lasts 3 to 7 days. Most infants and children can be managed with oral rehydration consisting of a balanced salt solution with a simple sugar (Pedialyte, Lytren, or the WHO oral rehydration solution). Fruit juices, tea, and similar fluids are inappropriate because they lack the appropriate carbohydrate concentration and electrolyte content. Bland meals such as the BRAT diet (bananas, rice, applesauce, and toast) are often well tolerated. Breastfeeding should continue through the course of the illness. If emesis is protracted or severe, an infant or young child can become dehydrated, necessitating intravenous rehydration.

- Bacterial diarrhea is also often treated symptomatically, without the use of antimicrobial agents. The exceptions to this are *Shigella* (treated to prevent spread of infection) and other bacterial diarrhea that is particularly severe and not resolving spontaneously. The choice of antibiotic for each pathogen is listed in Table 17-2. In general, the use of Lomotil (diphenoxylate) or Imodium (loperamide) to decrease gastrointestinal motility is not recommended for children.

XI. Gastroesophageal Reflux
   A. Basic science
   - Gastroesophageal reflux can be seen normally in all age groups ranging from infancy to adulthood. Gastroesophageal reflux occurs secondary to decreased lower esophageal sphincter tone and increased transient lower esophageal sphincter relaxation. The peak age group affected is around 4 months of age.
   - The majority of episodes of gastroesophageal reflux are brief and do not cause any distress to the patient. Clinically significant gastroesophageal reflux is referred to gastroesophageal reflux disease (GERD). Infants and children with gastroesophageal reflux disease usually present with a history of symptoms such as poor weight gain, irritability, feeding refusal, and recurrent vomiting.
   B. History and physical examination
   - In most infants with mild gastroesophageal reflux, there is usually a history of nonprojectile, nonbilious vomiting after feeding. The infant is afebrile, with normal appetite and activity. The infant should be vigorous and nontoxic appearing, with a normal physical examination. When the gastroesophageal reflux is significant, some infants may present with apparent life-threatening events. Respiratory symptoms such as stridor, chronic cough, wheezing, and recurrent pneumonia can be seen. Sandifer syndrome (anemia and hematemesis) has also been described in infants and young children with significant gastroesophageal reflux disease. Severe gastroesophageal reflux disease may also cause failure to thrive in infants and young children. Cow milk protein allergy can also present with symptoms of gastroesophageal reflux in this age group.
   - Preschool-aged children can present with respiratory symptoms and abdominal pain, as well as a decreased amount of food intake. Older children and adolescents present with similar symptoms as adult patients, including heartburn or regurgitation symptoms.

C. Laboratory and diagnostic studies
- Laboratory studies such as CBC and electrolyte analyses are usually not required but should be normal. Esophageal pH probe studies can confirm the diagnosis of acid reflux. Other studies such as barium contrast radiography can help identify problems associated with severe reflux such as strictures, however the sensitivity and specificity for GERD itself is low. Nuclear scintigraphy is another study which can be used to help identify delayed gastric emptying as well as reflux of nonacid stomach contents. If symptoms are severe, some infants and children undergo endoscopic evaluation.

D. Formulating the diagnosis
- The diagnosis can usually be made based on a detailed history and physical examination.
- The diagnosis may be confirmed by one of the previously mentioned studies.

E. Evaluating the severity of problems
- Gastroesophageal reflux rarely causes dehydration or failure to thrive. However, the infant must be assessed for these conditions. The presence of these, or an ill-appearing infant, warrants consideration of other possible diagnoses.

F. Managing the patient
- For infants, treatment consists of giving the infant thickened feeds and placing him or her in an upright posture after feeding. On occasion, metoclopramide is given to enhance gastric emptying. Some infants and young children are also placed on a histamine blockers or proton pump inhibitors to help reduce acid production in the gut. Gastroesophageal reflux usually resolves by the time the infant reaches 12 months of age.
- In older children and adolescents, recommendations to avoid certain foods may be helpful. Some food and beverages that have been found to decrease the lower esophageal pressure and exacerbate reflux include peppermint, alcohol, caffeine, and chocolate. Avoidance of acidic beverages including orange juice and colas may also be helpful. Proton pump inhibitors as well as H_2 blockers are also used for this age group.
- Patients with severe gastroesophageal reflux that is refractory to medical treatment may need to be referred to a pediatric surgeon for possible fundoplication procedure

XII. Immunizations
A. Basic science
- In "active" immunization, a form of the infectious agent is introduced via injection or ingestion, which in turn stimulates the immune system to develop antibodies. Most routine childhood immunizations, such as DTP (diphtheria, tetanus, and pertussis), MMR (measles, mumps, and rubella), and IPV (inactivated poliovirus vaccine), are forms of active immunization.
- Passive immunization involves using antibodies produced by other animals to treat a patient already exposed to a disease. Examples include hepatitis B immune globulin (HBIG) and tetanus immune globulin. Although passive

immunization takes effect immediately, it is short-lived. It is often combined with active immunization to result in long-term disease prevention.

B. Specific immunizations

1. MMR (measles, mumps, and rubella) vaccine
   - MMR is a live attenuated virus vaccine and should be only given to immunocompetent children. The first dose of MMR is given at 12 to 15 months. The second dose of MMR should be given at school entry (between 4 and 6 years of age). Adverse reactions include low-grade fever, rash, hypersensitivity reactions, the development of idiopathic thrombocytopenic purpura, and febrile seizure. Egg allergy is not a contraindication to receiving the vaccine. Large prospective studies have shown that there is no causal link between the MMR vaccine and autism.

2. Poliovirus vaccine
   - Inactivated poliovirus vaccine (IPV) is the standard of care in the United States. In other countries, the oral poliovirus vaccine is utilized. The vaccine is administered at 2, 4, and 6 to 18 months of age and prior to entering school (4 to 6 years). Adverse reactions include fever and rash. The only contraindication to the vaccine is anaphylaxis to a previous dose.

3. Hepatitis B vaccine (HBV)
   - HBV is given at birth, 1 to 2 months, and 6 months, although the vaccine series may be started at any age. Because of the risk from vertical transmission, infants born to mothers who are hepatitis B positive should receive hepatitis B immunoglobulin and HBV immediately after birth. This provides both passive and active protection. Infants born to mothers whose hepatitis status is unknown should receive the vaccine immediately after birth, and the mother should be tested at the time of delivery for the hepatitis B antigen to determine further treatment. Hepatitis B vaccines are now free of thimerosal.

4. DTaP (diphtheria, tetanus, and acellular pertussis) vaccine
   a. The immunization series consists of five doses of vaccine given at 2, 4, 6, and 15 to 18 months, and before school. Adverse reactions include swelling and tenderness at the injection site, low-grade fever, and fussiness.
   b. Contraindications
      - Anaphylaxis to a prior dose or to any vaccine component
      - Encephalopathy without a known cause within 7 days of a dose of pertussis vaccine
   c. Relative contraindications
      - Inconsolable crying for 3 or more hours within 48 hours of the vaccination
      - Collapse or shock within 48 hours of vaccination
      - High fever within 48 hours of vaccination
   d. DTaP vaccine should be postponed for infants with an evolving neurologic disorder or unevaluated seizures, or who have a neurologic event between vaccinations. For children over 7, diphtheria

immunization consists of Td (the tetanus and diphtheria toxoids without pertussis). This vaccine is less likely to produce adverse reactions in adults and older children.

    5. *Haemophilus influenzae* type b (Hib)

- Now rarely seen because of immunization, this organism was the most common cause of bacterial meningitis in infants and young children and the most frequent cause of epiglottitis and septic arthritis in young children. Generally, it is administered at 2, 4, and 6 months.

    6. Varicella vaccine

- A single subcutaneous dose of this live attenuated vaccine is recommended for all healthy children between 1 and 12 years of age. Children 13 years of age and older require two doses of the vaccine at least 4 weeks apart. The vaccine is also effective in preventing or modifying varicella infection if given within 3 days of exposure to chickenpox. Adverse reactions include fever and localized rash. It is contraindicated in immunocompromised children and pregnant patients.

C. Site and route of immunization

- Injectable vaccines should be administered in the anterolateral aspect of the upper thigh or the deltoid area of the upper arm. The upper, outer aspect of the buttocks in infants should not be used for injections because these injections can damage the sciatic nerve.

D. Lapsed immunizations

- A lapse in an immunization schedule does not require one to repeat the entire schedule. If a dose of DTP, IVP, Hib, or HBV is missed, immunization should occur on the next visit as if the usual interval had elapsed.
- In a patient who is lacking at least three doses of tetanus vaccine and has a wound that requires tetanus prophylaxis, both active and passive immunization are necessary. Such a patient would initially receive tetanus immune globulin (TIG) and Td or DTaP at the time of injury, and then he or she would be scheduled to complete the Td or DTP series in 2-month intervals.
- If the patient has previously received the series of four tetanus vaccinations, he or she would require Td if it has been over 5 years since the last vaccination.

E. Misconceptions regarding vaccine contraindications

- Some physicians inappropriately defer or delay immunizations. In the following cases immunizations should be given:
    1. Mild acute illness with low-grade fever or mild diarrhea in an otherwise well child
    2. Child taking antibiotics
    3. Reaction to previous DTaP involving only soreness, redness, or swelling at vaccination site or mild temperature
    4. Prematurity: the appropriate age for initiating immunizations in a preemie is the chronologic age. Vaccine doses should not be reduced for preterm infants.
    5. Pregnant household contacts

6. Recent exposure to infectious disease
7. Allergies to penicillin or any other antibiotic except anaphylactic reactions to neomycin or streptomycin (IPV contains trace amounts of streptomycin and neomycin).
8. Family history of sudden infant death syndrome (SIDS)
9. Family history of seizures
10. Malnutrition

XIII. Infantile Hypertrophic Pyloric Stenosis
  A. Basic science
  - Pyloric stenosis is hypertrophy of the pyloric sphincter that prevents passage of gastric contents into the duodenum. It occurs in 3 in 1000 live births, often in males, and in 30% of cases the children are the firstborn. The age range typically is 3 to 6 weeks of age. The cause is unknown, but there is an association between pyloric stenosis and the administration of erythromycin.
  B. History and physical examination
  - The history consists of projectile, nonbilious vomiting directly after feeding usually about week 3 of age. The infant does not have fever, diarrhea, or loss of appetite. The hypertrophied pylorus may be palpated as an "olive"-sized mass in the epigastric area.
  C. Laboratory and diagnostic studies
  - Electrolytes are remarkable for a hypochloremic metabolic alkalosis if vomiting has been persistent. Ultrasound should be performed by a pediatric radiologist, and the pyloric muscle thickness, length, and diameter should all be assessed. Barium swallow will show delayed gastric emptying and a positive "string sign" caused by the narrow lumen of the pylorus.
  D. Formulating the diagnosis
  - The diagnosis can be made based on the history and physical examination. If no mass is palpable, ultrasound or barium studies can confirm the diagnosis in patients in whom this diagnosis is suspected.
  E. Evaluating the severity of problems
  - Initially infants with pyloric stenosis are vigorous with a normal to increased appetite; however, they may become dehydrated over time and should be assessed for this (see Section VI, Dehydration).
  F. Managing the patient
  - Once the diagnosis has been made, treatment consists of correction of dehydration and electrolyte abnormalities with intravenous fluids in preparation for definitive treatment, which is pyloromyotomy. The operation involves surgical incision of the hypertrophied pylorus and is curative.

XIV. Intussusception
  A. Basic science
  - Intussusception is the telescoping of a proximal segment of the bowel into the lumen of a distal segment. The ileocecal junction is the most commonly affected region. When the proximal segment of the bowel starts telescoping into the more distal segment, its associated mesentery follows and

subsequently venous and lymphatic congestion result. The edema from the compression of these vessels eventually results in ischemia and possible perforation of the bowel.

- Intussusception is the most common cause of bowel obstruction in the 3 to 12 month age group and it is also the most common abdominal emergency in early childhood.

B. History and physical examination

- Intussusception usually occurs in previously healthy children. A gastrointestinal infection or introduction of new food may precede an intussusception. There is usually a sudden onset of intermittent abdominal pain (manifesting as crying episodes in the preverbal child). Anorexia, lethargy, and vomiting are common associated symptoms. Microscopic blood in the stool is common. Currant jelly stool is a late finding. Physical examination demonstrates lethargy or irritability and the abdomen may be tender. Sometimes the intussusception can be palpated as a sausage-like mass, most often in the child's right upper quadrant.

C. Laboratory and diagnostic studies

- The barium contrast enema is the best study for diagnosing and reducing the intussusception. The less common ileoileal intussusception is not visualized on barum enema. Plain film findings are variable. The radiograph may be normal or may demonstrate signs of bowel obstruction, such as distention and air-fluid levels. Abdominal ultrasound has an excellent sensitivity and specificity in making the diagnosis, as well as evaluating the blood flow to the involved segment of bowel with Doppler imaging.
- Laboratory studies, such as a CBC, may reflect a stress response or, in the case of perforation, may be markedly elevated with a left shift. Electrolytes are usually are normal at presentation, although they will show evidence of a metabolic alkalosis if vomiting has been prolonged or pronounced.

D. Formulating the diagnosis

- The diagnosis is based on the history, physical examination, and contrast enema (when appropriate, see below) findings.

E. Evaluating the severity of problems

- Protracted intussusception can lead to gangrenous bowel or perforation, which are surgical emergencies. Any child with suspected intussusception, who is ill-appearing with altered mental status (i.e., lethargy to the point of not responding to parents) and signs consistent with shock, such as delayed capillary refill or low blood pressure, peritonitis, or perforation (free air on plain film) requires immediate surgical consultation and surgical repair. A contrast enema is contraindicated in such a patient.

F. Managing the patient

- Contrast enema is the procedure of choice to reverse intussusception when there are no features to suggest shock, ischemia, or perforation. Any child with suspected intussusception should be made NPO (nothing by mouth) and given intravenous fluids. Abdominal films should be done to look for features of obstruction and perforation. Surgical consultation should be obtained when perforation or ischemia are suspected.

- Even in cases of successful reduction of the intussusception with contrast enema, there is a small recurrence rate. If the contrast enema reduces the intussusception, the child should remain in the hospital for 24 hours to observe for signs of recurrence. If the enema is not successful in reducing the intussusception, surgical repair is indicated.

XV. Measles
  A. Basic science
- Measles, or rubeola, is a RNA virus belonging to the Paramyxoviridae family and is transmitted by contact with respiratory secretions. Patients are contagious from 24 to 48 hours before the onset of symptoms and remain so for 4 days after the appearance of the rash. The incubation period is from 8 to 12 days.
  B. History and physical examination
- Measles is characterized by the three Cs—cough, conjunctivitis, and coryza—as well as fever and morbilliform rash. Koplik spots (small gray-white spots that appear inside the buccal and labial mucosa early in the disease) are the pathognomonic enanthem of measles. Koplik spots disappear in 12 to 18 hours. The rash usually appears 3 to 5 days after the initial symptoms. Red maculopapular lesions begin on the head and neck and progress to cover the trunk and extremities, becoming confluent. During the next 6 to 7 days, the rash turns a brownish color and then fades. Uncommonly hemorrhage into the rash may occur (black measles). Fever is common in the first 3 to 4 days of illness and can be as high as 40°C. Lymphadenopathy and splenomegaly may be present.
  C. Laboratory and diagnostic studies
- Measles virus infection can be diagnosed by a positive serologic test for measles IgM antibody. Measles IgM is detectable for 1 month after rash onset. All patients suspected to have measles should be reported to the state or local health department prior.
  D. Formulating the diagnosis
- The diagnosis is made based on the clinical findings, history, and exposure to measles in an unvaccinated child.
  E. Evaluating the severity of problems
- Most children with measles experience fever, pharyngitis, and rash. Lymphadenopathy, splenomegaly, vomiting, and diarrhea are also common symptoms but can usually be managed on an outpatient basis. Other complications include pneumonia, both viral and bacterial, which may require hospitalization for oxygen and parenteral antibiotics.
- Neurologic complications include encephalitis, which occurs in 1 per 1000 cases of typical measles. The mortality rate from respiratory and neurologic complications is 3 per 1000 patients. Subacute sclerosing panencephalitis (SSPE) occurs in about 1 per 100,000 cases. SSPE is a degenerative nervous system disease caused by persistent measles infection of the central nervous system. It causes intellectual deterioration progressing to dementia, myoclonic jerks, and cerebellar signs. The disease is usually fatal.

F. Managing the patient
- Typical measles in a normal host is managed at home with antipyretics, fluids, and rest. Complications from measles infection as discussed above often require hospitalization. Ribavirin and vitamin A have been used for some patients. Hospitalized patients should also be placed on respiratory precautions for 4 days after the onset of rash. Also, live-virus measles vaccine if given within 72 hours of exposure may provide protection from the illness. Immunoglobulin given within 6 days of exposure may decrease disease severity and possibly prevent it.

XVI. Mumps
A. Basic science
- Mumps is a paramyxovirus infection of the salivary glands (predominantly the parotid glands). It is transmitted by exposure via respiratory droplets, fomites, or direct contact with the infected patient. The incubation period from exposure to glandular swelling is approximately 18 days. Patients with mumps are infectious from 1 to 2 days before the onset of glandular swelling and remain so for 8 to 10 days.
- MMR vaccine given at 1 year of age and prior to the start of kindergarten prevents the disease and has resulted in a marked decrease in the incidence of this disease.
B. History and physical examination
- The presentation of mumps may range from an asymptomatic infection (up to 20%) to mild upper respiratory symptoms (up to 50%) to the classic illness, which is characterized by fever, malaise, headache, abdominal pain, and glandular swelling.
C. Laboratory and diagnostic studies
- Although laboratory studies are usually not necessary to make the diagnosis, the serum amylase, if measured, may be elevated. The diagnosis can be confirmed by an ELISA demonstrating IgM antibodies.
D. Formulating the diagnosis
- The diagnosis of mumps is based on the clinical presentation of generalized symptoms in combination with parotid swelling in unimmunized, previously uninfected individuals. Usually the parotid swelling begins in one gland and then becomes bilateral, although some patients have only unilateral involvement. Before vaccination, the most common age of infection was 5 to 9 years.
E. Evaluating the severity of problems
- Mumps is usually a mild, self-limited disease that requires no specific treatment, but it can be complicated by orchitis in males, which occurs in approximately 40% of postpubertal males who contract mumps. Far less frequent complications include meningoencephalitis; pancreatitis; thyroiditis; oophoritis; mastitis; neuritis, especially of the facial and auditory nerves; myelitis; arthritis; and myocarditis.

- Other viruses and some bacteria, such as *Staphylococcus aureus,* can also cause parotitis. In these cases, there is usually erythema and tenderness of the skin overlying the involved gland, and antibiotic therapy is indicated.
 F. Managing the patient
- Most patients with mumps require only symptomatic treatment, such as acetaminophen, fluids, and rest until symptoms resolve (in 7 to 10 days). Orchitis is also treated with rest and avoidance of contact sports until it has completely resolved. Meningoencephalitis needs to be considered in a patient with mumps who presents with high fever and headache. Pancreatitis should be suspected in a patient with mumps who has high fever and severe abdominal pain.

XVII. Pharyngitis
 A. Basic science
- Many viruses can cause pharyngitis, particularly the group of viruses that cause other respiratory symptoms such as influenza viruses, parainfluenza viruses, adenoviruses and rhinoviruses, and HIV. Streptococci, usually group A (but also group C and group G), may cause bacterial pharyngitis. Epstein-Barr virus can cause pharyngitis as part of the clinical picture of infectious mononucleosis. Diphtheria, although rare in this country, can cause membranous pharyngitis and should be considered in an unimmunized patient.
- For convenience one can classify the appearance of the tonsils or pharynx into one of three classifications: exudative, ulcerative, or membranous.
 1. Exudative pharyngitis
- Exudative pharyngitis is defined by the presence of white or gray spots on the surface of the tonsils or pharynx that resembles skim milk and could be readily wiped off without bleeding. White, hard material occasionally seen in the tonsillar crypts is more appropriately called crypt debris and is not an exudate.
- Exudative pharyngitis is the most common manifestation of group A streptococcal pharyngitis.
 2. Ulcerative pharyngitis
- Ulcerative pharyngitis is characterized by the presence of circular or shallow ulcers on the soft palate, tonsillar area, or posterior pharynx. Herpangina is sometimes used to describe ulcerative pharyngitis (usually caused by coxsackieviruses) associated with fever and often dysphagia. Herpes simplex viruses may also cause an ulcerative pharyngitis.
 3. Membranous pharyngitis
- Membranous pharyngitis is the presence of a grayish white membrane adherent to the surface of the pharynx and tonsils. When removed, there is bleeding from the surface underneath.
- In the United States, most cases of membranous pharyngitis are caused by Epstein-Barr virus (EBV) mononucleosis, particularly in teenagers and young adults. Pharyngitis coupled with fever, fatigue, generalized

nontender adenopathy, and enlarged liver or spleen should make one consider the possibility of EBV mononucleosis.

- In unimmunized children, diphtheria is a more common cause of membranous pharyngitis.
- Primary HIV infection can also cause an acute retroviral syndrome consisting of pharyngitis, fever, weight loss, adenopathy, rash, and splenomegaly.

B. History and physical examination
   - Pharyngitis may occur alone or in combination with other symptoms in many pediatric infectious diseases. Fever, headache, and abdominal pain may accompany the sore throat.
   - When evaluating complaints of a sore throat it is important to get a thorough look at the pharynx with adequate illumination. One should closely examine the oral and buccal mucosa for associated redness or lesions, examine the cervical lymph nodes for lymphadenopathy or adenitis, and palpate the abdomen for the presence of an enlarged liver or spleen.

C. Laboratory and diagnostic studies
   - The most useful adjunct to the diagnosis of pharyngitis is the throat culture for identification of group A streptococcus. The throat culture remains the gold standard, but rapid antigen detection methods are now frequently used in practioners' offices. Not every patient with a complaint of sore throat should have a throat culture. This should be reserved for those patients with a history of exposure to streptococcal infections or clinical features that suggest streptococcal pharyngitis, including exudative or membranous pharyngitis, enlarged tonsils with tender cervical adenopathy, and fever. The recovery of β-hemolytic colonies on throat culture does not prove the presence of a streptococcal infection (due to the possibility of a carrier state), but in the presence of suggestive clinical features, a positive throat swab for group A streptococcus is sufficient to warrant therapy. Culturing for other agents of pharyngitis is possible but usually unnecessary.
   - Patients who have features suggesting EBV infection should undergo a complete blood count, differential, and a monospot test. Often one will find an elevation of the total white blood cell count with a predominance of atypical lymphocytes and monocytes in the peripheral blood smear. Eighty percent of patients with EBV mononucleosis can be diagnosed by a monospot test. However, in children under 5 years of age, a monospot test will not necessarily be positive, even in cases of proven EBV infection. The preferred method of diagnosis in a young child is the evaluation of IgG and IgM antibody titers against EBV viral capsid antigen (EBV-VCA). The IgM antibody is positive during the acute phase of illness, whereas IgG antibodies develop during convalescence. These may also be useful in monospot-negative EBV infections to clarify the diagnosis.
   - If there is concern for a primary HIV infection illness, the appropriate diagnostic test would be a detection of HIV RNA by reverse transcriptase polymerase chain reaction. Antibody assays may be negative in the initial stage of HIV infection.

D. Formulating the diagnosis
- The diagnosis of pharyngitis is based on the clinical presentation and physical findings. Laboratory tests for group A streptococcus, viruses, or Epstein-Barr virus (mononucleosis) are not always necessary but help confirm the specific diagnosis.

E. Evaluating the severity of problems
- Pharyngitis is rarely a serious problem. Occasionally a patient with severe infectious mononucleosis or diphtheria will have obstructive symptoms requiring medical intervention.

F. Managing the patient
- Most viral infections causing pharyngitis are managed with symptomatic therapy. The treatment for group A streptococcal pharyngitis is a 10-day course of oral penicillin. Children are considered noninfectious after 24 hours of therapy and can return to school if they feel well. For the penicillin-allergic patient, erythromycin may be used. The rationale for treating patients with group A β-hemolytic streptococci is to prevent rheumatic heart disease. In contrast, the incidence and severity of glomerulonephritis are not altered by treatment of streptococcal pharyngitis.
- Treatment of EBV infection is mostly supportive. Children with splenomegaly should not be allowed to participate in contact sports until their spleen has returned to normal to prevent splenic rupture. Rarely, steroids may be necessary for cases of EBV infection where the tonsillar enlargement is severe enough to cause compromise of the airway, but the routine use of steroids for uncomplicated EBV infection is unwarranted and may prolong the course of infection.

XVIII. Pneumonia
A. Basic science
- In all ages of pediatric patients, pneumonia is most commonly caused by *Streptococcus pneumoniae, Mycoplasma pneumoniae,* and respiratory syncytial virus. Respiratory syncytial virus, influenza virus, parainfluenza virus, and adenoviruses are the majority of viral agents responsible for pediatric viral pneumonia.
- Primary bacterial pneumonia is less common in pediatric patients but still occurs. Children with poor control of their oral secretions are particularly prone to pneumonia secondary to frequent aspiration.
- Newborn infants may develop group B streptococcal pneumonia (*Streptococcus agalactiae)* or, less commonly, gram-negative pneumonia due to aspiration of secretions contaminated by maternal vaginal flora at the time of delivery. *Chlamydia trachomatis* pneumonia usually occurs in the first few weeks of life in infants exposed to maternal genital tract chlamydia.
- Older infants and children are more likely to develop pneumococcal pneumonia. *Streptococcus pyogenes* or *Staphyloccus aureus* may also cause pneumonia in children, particularly following a viral illness such as measles or influenza.

- *Mycoplasma pneumoniae* and *Chlamydia pneumoniae* may cause an atypical pneumonia syndrome in school-aged children and young adults.

B. History and physical examination
- In the newborn or young infant, pneumonia may present with extreme respiratory distress, hypoxia, hypercapnia, and cyanosis. Many infants will be tachypneic and have varying degrees of respiratory difficulties manifested by nasal flaring, substernal, intercostal, or supraclavicular retractions, and occasionally abdominal breathing patterns. Some infants may even be apneic, particularly those infants with respiratory syncytial virus. Cough and audible wheezing may also be clinical findings in infants with pneumonia. Posttussive emesis may make feeding difficult for the infant and predispose to dehydration. During physical examination, an examiner may have difficulty hearing crackles or wheezes in a young infant with pneumonia.
- In older children, decreased breath sounds, crackles, and rhonchi are all characteristics of pneumonia.
- *Chlamydia trachomatis* pneumonia is usually an afebrile pneumonia and may be preceded by conjunctivitis in affected infants.

C. Laboratory and diagnostic studies
- Arterial blood gas sampling is suggested for children with severe respiratory distress, but measurement of pulse oximetry may be sufficient for less severe cases. A CBC and differential may reveal an elevated white blood cell count with a left shift in cases of bacterial pneumonia. For infants with *Chlamydia pneumonia*, a peripheral eosinophilia may be a clue to the diagnosis. Viral pneumonia can often be diagnosed by obtaining a viral culture of respiratory secretions obtained through an endotracheal tube, by a throat swab, or by a nasopharyngeal wash. Rapid diagnostic tests for RSV, parainfluenza virus, and influenza virus can also be performed. Nasal secretions can also be obtained for culture or for ELISA to detect *Chlamydia*. In general, a febrile child with pneumonia should also have a blood culture because there may be an associated bacteremia.
- A chest x-ray is a useful adjunct to the physical examination of a patient with suspected pneumonia. Viral pneumonia often shows patchy alveolar infiltrates or interstitial disease. *Mycoplasma pneumoniae* and *Chlamydia pneumoniae* pneumonia may have mild chest symptoms but, when viewed by radiography, may demonstrate a fairly extensive interstitial pneumonia. Bacterial pneumonia is much more likely to produce a consolidation that appears on chest x-ray as an opacified area of lung. Chest x-rays are also useful when a pleural effusion is present. If there is sufficient pleural fluid, a pleural tap should be performed for diagnostic and therapeutic purposes. The fluid should be analyzed for protein, LDH, cell count, and Gram stain, and sent for bacterial cultures.

D. Formulating the diagnosis
- The presence of rales, rhonchi, and absent or decreased breath sounds in a febrile child suggests pneumonia. A chest x-ray confirms the diagnosis and is helpful in assessing the extent of the pneumonia as well as the presence of effusions present.

E. Evaluating the severity of problems
- Significant respiratory distress, cyanosis, and labored breathing signify extensive lung involvement and warrant prompt medical intervention. The physician should always start by assessing the ABCs (airway, breathing, circulation) in any infant or child presenting as critically ill.

F. Managing the patient
- Most mild viral pneumonias can be managed with symptomatic support. Supplemental oxygen should be administered to any child with pneumonia who has respiratory distress and hypoxemia. Any infant or child with significant respiratory distress secondary to pneumonia needs to be admitted and given IV antibiotics. Intubation and assisted ventilation may be necessary for some severe cases of pneumonia.
- Neonates with pneumonia are usually started empirically on ampicillin and gentamicin or ampicillin and cefotaxime. If *Chlamydia trachomatis* pneumonia is suspected in young infants, oral erythromycin therapy can be used.
- After age 3 months, antimicrobial therapy should be directed more toward coverage of pneumococcal pneumonia, and a third-generation cephalosporin such as ceftriaxone can be used. Sometimes higher doses of penicillin are needed to overcome pneumococcal resistance. The mechanism of resistance with pneumococcal infections is related to changes in penicillin-binding proteins and high doses of penicillin will usually overcome this resistance.
- Older infants and young children with severe respiratory distress requiring admission into the intensive care unit may need to be started on vancomycin along with a third-generation cephalosporin. For complicated cases of community-acquired pneumonia, the addition of clindamycin may also be helpful when considering susceptible strains of MRSA. For older infants and young children who are clinically stable and do not require hospital admission, treatment with oral antibiotics such as amoxicillin, amoxicillin plus clavulanate, or cefuroxime is generally adequate. Aspiration pneumonia is usually treated with a combination of a penicillin and another antibiotic that has good anaerobic coverage. Azithromycin is usually used for treatment of atypical community acquired pneumonia caused by either *Mycoplasma* or *Chlamydia*.
- Pleural effusions will often resolve spontaneously, but pleural empyemas associated with pneumonia may require longer courses of antibiotics before resolution (up to 3 weeks). Early removal of a pleural empyema with serial taps or a chest tube may hasten clinical improvement. Open thoracotomy to remove empyema fluid is rarely necessary in pediatric patients. Follow-up chest x-rays in children with empyema demonstrate complete or nearly complete resolution within 6 months.

XIX. Retropharyngeal Abscess
A. Basic science
- Infection can fill the potential space between the deep layers of the cervical fascia, which abuts the esophagus anteriorly and the cervical vertebrae posteriorly, leading to symptoms of dysphagia, drooling, stridor, and airway

compromise. Group A streptococci, anaerobes, and *Staphylococcus aureus* are the most common pathogens.

B. History and physical examination
   - These infrequent infections occur most commonly before age 6 years. A history of trauma to the neck or pharynx or recent infection should be sought. A child with a retropharyngeal abscess usually is unwilling to move the neck and often complains of a stiff neck as well. History may be significant for a preceding upper respiratory infection or sore throat. High fever and toxic appearance are common. Drooling and stridor are often present. A midline mass may be visible on inspection of the posterior pharynx.

C. Laboratory and diagnostic studies
   - A lateral radiograph of the soft tissues of the neck usually demonstrates enlargement of the retropharyngeal space. Blood cultures may identify the infecting organism. As fever and stiff neck may simulate meningitis, lumbar puncture for CSF collection may be necessary. Gram stain and culture should be performed on abscess material.

D. Formulating the diagnosis
   - The diagnosis is made both clinically and via radiologic studies. Lateral neck radiograph is helpful, but CT scan of the neck provides more information about whether there is abscess formation versus cellulitis in the retropharyngeal space, as well as whether there is extension of the infection to other vital structures. Other common causes of upper airway obstruction include peritonsillar abscess, epiglottitis, croup, and infected foreign bodies.

E. Evaluating the severity of problems
   - Major complications include complete airway obstruction and aspiration. The abscess may spontaneously rupture or erode into other major structures, such as the mediastinum or lung.

F. Managing the patient
   - All children with retropharyngeal abscess require hospitalization and surgical drainage of the abscess. Broad-spectrum intravenous antibiotics and fluids should be administered. Endotracheal intubation or, rarely, tracheostomy may be necessary to secure the airway.

XX. Reye Syndrome
A. Basic science
   - Reye syndrome is characterized by a rapidly progressive encephalopathy and fatty degeneration of the liver. The pathophysiology involves generalized loss of mitochondrial function leading to disordered carnitine and fatty acid metabolism. There are many mitochondrial hepatopathies that create a similar clinical picture.
   - The syndrome is preceded by a viral illness, especially influenza B and varicella. A 35-fold increase in the incidence of Reye syndrome has been reported when aspirin or other salicylate products are used during an acute viral illness. Because of this, the use of aspirin in children is contraindicated during "flu" season or chickenpox infection.

B. History and physical examination
- Patients most commonly present with a history of an upper respiratory tract viral infection. The patient may also report aspirin usage during the illness. About a week after the start of symptoms severe vomiting begins, followed by mental status changes. Mental status changes range in severity from a mild amnesia to irritability, confusion, disorientation, delirium, and coma.
- Children are usually not febrile and not jaundiced (although hepatomegaly does occur in about half of the patients). Meningeal signs and focal neurologic signs are absent. As the illness worsens the patient may manifest decorticate or decerebrate posturing. Seizure and respiratory arrest may also occur.

C. Laboratory and diagnostic studies
- The diagnosis is made by liver biopsy showing changes of microvesicular steatosis and by mitochondrial function studies. Laboratory abnormalities include elevated liver and muscle enzymes and elevated ammonia levels. Hypoglycemia is an early laboratory finding in more severe cases.

D. Formulating the diagnosis
- Reye syndrome should be suspected in any child with a history of viral illness and aspirin usage in combination with mental status change and vomiting. Consideration should be given to metabolic disorders that resemble Reye syndrome. Serum chemistry tests that demonstrate high levels of ammonia and liver dysfunction support the diagnosis.

E. Evaluating the severity of problems
- The prognosis is related to the degree of neurologic deficit. The overall mortality rate is 21%; it is higher in patients who develop seizures and respiratory arrest.
- Neurologic deficits (mental retardation, epilepsy, and the like) are commonplace among those patients who develop decerebrate and decorticate posturing or seizures while ill.
- Recurrence is uncommon, and most survivors have a good prognosis.

F. Managing the patient
- The brain is the principal organ affected in Reye syndrome. Cerebral edema is the major factor contributing to morbidity and death. Therefore, intracranial monitoring and reduction of increased intracranial pressure is essential. Hypoglycemia must also be corrected.
- Vitamin K and fresh frozen plasma may help to reverse the patient's coagulopathy. Serum electrolytes should be monitored frequently.

XXI. Rubella
A. Basic science
- Rubella, also known as "German measles," is a viral infection that has its greatest clinical impact on fetal development during the first and second trimesters of pregnancy (see Chapter 13, Section XIII, Infections during Pregnancy). The virus is a RNA virus belonging to the Tongaviridae family and is acquired by exposure to oral droplets or via the placenta in the fetus.

- The peak incidence of infection is during late winter and early spring. The incubation period is 14 to 23 days, with a 1- to 5-day prodrome of cough, conjunctivitis, coryza, lymphadenopathy, and low-grade fever. An erythematous maculopapular rash follows and lasts about 3 days. The patient is contagious the week before and the week after onset of this rash.

B. History and physical examination
- The history is one of low-grade fever, respiratory symptoms, and lymphadenopathy for about 5 days before the onset of the rash. Pale red spots on the soft palate may be seen just before the appearance of a rash. The most commonly affected lymph nodes are the cervical, posterior auricular, and suboccipital. Adolescents and adults (females more than males) may also have arthritis and arthralgia of multiple joints, both small and large. This usually begins during or after the rash. As in rubeola (measles), the rash of rubella begins as discrete, red, maculopapular lesions, first on the head, progressing down to the trunk and extremities. However, it does not coalesce or turn brown and has a shorter duration than the rubeola rash. The symptoms usually resolve within 2 weeks.

C. Laboratory and diagnostic studies
- The diagnosis can be obtained by confirming a fourfold or greater acute and convalescent titers 10 to 14 days apart.

D. Formulating the diagnosis
- Rubella's symptoms and rash are nonspecific and difficult to distinguish from those associated with enterovirus, scarlet fever, mycoplasma, or human papovavirus 19 infection. The history of missed MMR immunization is important in making the diagnosis, as is serologic testing.

E. Evaluating the severity of problems
- Rubella ranges from an asymptomatic illness (25% of patients) to arthritis requiring aspirin or nonsteroidal anti-inflammatory drug (NSAID) therapy, but it is usually a mild, self-limited infection, managed at home with supportive care. Severe and rare complications such as encephalitis and thrombocytopenia can also occur.
- Congenital rubella causes anomalies in 30% to 60% of infants infected during the first month of pregnancy. These anomalies include intrauterine growth retardation, hepatosplenomegaly, lymphadenopathy, anemia, thrombocytopenia, meningoencephalitis, myocarditis, nephritis, cataracts, glaucoma, microphthalmia, sensory neural deafness, patent ductus arteriosus, and peripheral pulmonary artery stenosis. Patients also may have a "blueberry muffin" appearance of their skin due to dermal erythropoiesis.

F. Managing the patient
- Preventing exposure of a nonimmunized pregnant women to infected patients is paramount. The infection in the nonpregnant patient is usually mild and requires only rest and analgesics. In pregnant women, the infection during the first or second trimesters is managed by counseling women about the risk to the fetus. Immunization after exposure is not helpful and is actually contraindicated during pregnancy (see Section XII, Immunizations). However, immunization of the postpartum woman is essential.

XXII. Urinary Tract Infection
A. Basic science
- Urinary tract infections (UTIs) are common in pediatrics. The incidence of UTI in the neonatal period is approximately 1%. UTI is up to 1.5 to 5 times more common in male neonates than female neonates and uncircumcised male infants are also at higher risk. The incidence of UTI in male infants then decreases during the first 6 months of life while there is a concomitant increase in the incidence of UTI in female infants such that by 1 year of age, females are three times as likely to have a UTI than males. The prevalence of UTI in white children is also two- to fourfold higher than in African American children.
- The organism most frequently implicated in causing UTIs in infants and young children is *Escherichia coli*. However, sexually active adolescent females may have a higher incidence of *Staphylococcus saprophyticus,* in addition to gram-negative bacteria such as *Escherichia coli*. Viruses can also cause cystitis.
B. History and physical examination
- History suggestive of UTI in an infant may include foul-smelling urine, poor feeding or growth, and recurrent episodes of unexplained fever. Older children may complain of increased frequency of urination, urgency, or dysuria. Some children may present with nighttime wetting or the reappearance of frequent accidents following successful toilet training.
- Physical examination is often unhelpful in an infant, but in an older child suprapubic tenderness or flank tenderness are useful physical findings. Asymptomatic bacteriuria occurs almost exclusively in females.
C. Laboratory and diagnostic studies
- Urine culture is the only way to accurately diagnose UTI in infants and young children. Although a urine analysis (UA) may be helpful, up to 20% of infants and young children with a UTI will have normal results on their UA. Some findings on the UA are more sensitive and specific than others in terms of predicting the probability of UTI. For example, nitrite is a very specific marker for UTI when it is found on UA as well as bacteria noted on Gram stain of a fresh urine sample. White blood cells in the urine should be interpreted cautiously because they may arise from other structures, such as the vagina. Fever, glomerulonephritis, renal stones, appendicitis, or any extrinsic ureteral irritation also may produce white blood cells in the urine without bacterial infection.
- In general, suprapubic aspiration is the considered the gold standard for obtaining a urine culture; however, most parents find this procedure unacceptable and many physicians are also very uncomfortable performing the procedure. Any growth of organisms from a suprapubic aspiration is considered positive for a UTI. Catheterized urinary specimens are preferred and they provide both a high sensitivity and specificity. Collection of urine via a perineal bag collection is not recommended secondary to the high false positive cultures rate of approximately 85%. For all collection methods, there is an increased rate of false positive cultures if the sample is not quickly processed. In catheterized specimens, infection is highly likely if there are

greater than 100,000 colony-forming units (CFU)/mL of one pathogen or 10,000 CFU/mL of a single type isolated.

- Many studies have been conducted in an attempt to differentiate upper tract infection from lower tract infection (i.e., to differentiate pyelonephritis from cystitis). However, in most acutely ill patients, the clinical symptoms and signs of infection will be the most important source of information. The use of radionuclide studies such as technetium glucoheptinate or technetium dimercaptosuccinic acid (^{99m}Tc-DMSA) are helpful in cases of severe pyelonephritis to identify areas of scarring due to infection.

D. Formulating the diagnosis
- The definitive diagnosis of urinary tract infection is based on the finding of significant bacteria in the urine obtained by catheterization, suprapubic aspiration, or clean voided specimen in a patient with an age appropriate constellation of symptoms.

E. Evaluating the severity of problems
- In general, the febrile infant, particularly if younger than 3 months of age, should be admitted to the hospital for intravenous antibiotic therapy.

F. Managing the patient
- The management of urinary tract infections is influenced by several factors, particularly the age of the child.
- In the febrile infant younger than 3 months of age, the initial choice of antibiotics should include a synthetic penicillin such as ampicillin for gram-positive coverage and an aminoglycoside or second- or third-generation cephalosporin for gram-negative coverage. A repeat urine culture is recommended after 2 or 3 days to ensure clearance of the organism and at the completion of antibiotic treatment. Intravenous antibiotics may be continued for at least 5 days or until the patient has resolution of fever and other symptoms followed by a 10- to 14-day course of an oral antibotics.
- In children older than 6 months of age who have symptoms and signs of a UTI, outpatient treatment with oral antibiotics for 7 to 10 days is recommended unless patients have high fever, any concerning findings on physical examination, or other symptoms that imply upper tract disease. Although successful in adults, there are little data currently to support the use of short-course antibiotic therapy for uncomplicated UTIs in children. Useful oral antibiotics in this age group include ampicillin, amoxicillin, or trimethoprim/sulfamethoxazole. Antibiotic therapy should be modified according to the antibiotic susceptibility pattern of the isolated bacteria.
- Routine imaging including renal ultrasound and VCUG (voiding cystourethrogram) is recommended for children younger than 5 years of age with a febrile UTI, females under the age of 3 with a UTI, males of any age with a UTI, and any child with a history of recurrent UTI as well as children who do not respond promptly to antimicrobial therapy. Routine imaging is extremely important in infants and young children with UTI in order to identify any underlying anatomic abnormalities such as vesicoureteral reflux, which can lead to renal scarring, hypertension, and end-stage renal disease if not diagnosed early in life.

XXIII. Varicella (Chickenpox)
  A. Basic science
   - Chickenpox represents primary infection with the varicella-zoster virus, a herpesvirus. It is a highly contagious virus and prior to immunization, the virus infected up to 90% of the population at some point during the first 2 decades of life.
   - Herpes zoster or shingles results from the latent form of this virus, which becomes reactivated later in life, usually during illness or stress. At this stage, the infection consists of burning pain, followed by a vesicular eruption in areas usually limited to one sensory dermatome.
  B. History and physical examination
   - Even prior to immunization, chickenpox was generally a mild, self-limited disease in previously healthy children. The clinical manifestations of chickenpox in healthy children usually develop within 15 days of the exposure. The primary infection often starts within a day or two of fever and mild systemic symptoms (e.g., malaise and headache) followed by the characteristic rash, consisting of groups of vesicles, usually beginning on the trunk or face and spreading distally. The rash has the initial appearance of "dewdrops on a rose petal" (i.e., small, clear vesicles on an erythematous base), which may spread over a 5- to 7-day course. In 48 hours the clear vesicles become cloudy and become umbilicated followed by crusting and healing. Immunized children may still develop a mild version of clinical varicella, and develop only a few skin lesions.
  C. Laboratory and diagnostic studies
   - The diagnosis is largely clinical, but it can be confirmed by two methods: the Tzanck preparation and immunofluorescent assays.
  D. Formulating the diagnosis
   - The diagnosis is commonly based on recognition of the rash, especially in a patient who has recently been exposed to varicella. The diagnosis can be confirmed by the Tzanck preparation or immunofluorescent assays; however, this is usually not necessary.
  E. Managing the patient
   - In previously healthy children, chickenpox is usually treated with rest and medications to control itching (diphenhydramine, Aveeno baths) and fever (acetaminophen). Aspirin is contraindicated because of the increased risk of Reye syndrome.
   - A complication afflicting healthy children is cerebellar ataxia, which occurs approximately 7 to 21 days after the development of the varicella rash. Encephalitis and Reye syndrome are rare, serious sequelae of varicella infection. Adolescents and adults are often more seriously afflicted with varicella infection than younger children. The elderly and immunocompromised patients are at increased risk for severe varicella infection, including complications such as pneumonia, pancreatitis, hepatitis, central nervous system problems (transverse myelitis, encephalitis, aseptic meningitis, and peripheral neuritis), and invasive group A streptococcal skin infections leading to possible myositis or necrotizing fasciitis.

- A single varicella infection generally gives lifelong immunity. However, immunocompromised persons who have been exposed to varicella should receive VZIG (varicella-zoster immune globulin) to prevent infection because they are very susceptible to disseminated varicella and its associated complications.
- Routine administration of acyclovir is generally not recommended for otherwise healthy children. However, immunocompromised patients with varicella should be treated with acyclovir because studies have demonstrated a significant reduction in visceral dissemination and other varicella-related complications in these patients.
- Neonatal varicella is another serious illness in which the mortality rate can reach up to 25%. Newborns born to mothers who are exposed to VZV or have clinical manifestations of the disease within 2 weeks of delivery are at highest risk for acquiring infection, especially those infants of mothers who develop symptoms less than 5 days prior to delivery as well as 2 days after delivery. These infants are treated with VZIG as well as acyclovir to help modify their clinical course and reduce the risk of death.

18

Surgery

I. Abdominal Aortic Aneurysms
  A. Basic science
   • Abdominal aortic aneurysms (AAAs) are the most common true aneurysms.
   • It is defined as a localized dilation of the abdominal aorta to a 50% increase in diameter compared with the normal expected diameter. A diameter of 3 cm or more is considered an aneurysm.
   • AAAs are predominantly located between the renal and inferior mesenteric arteries. They are four to five times more common in men than in women and their prevalence increases dramatically after age 60.
   • Other major risk factors include atherosclerosis, smoking, hypertension, and family history.
   • The etiology of AAA in most patients remains unclear. Familial clustering suggests a multifactorial, nonatherosclerotic causal hypothesis, such as a defect in vascular structural proteins with atherosclerosis playing a secondary role.
   • Less frequently, AAA can result from cystic medial necrosis, infections (salmonella and syphilis), Marfan syndrome, or Ehlers-Danlos syndrome.
   • Aneurysms less than 5 cm are unlikely to rupture; AAA greater than 6 cm are at significant risk for rupture.
  B. History and physical examination
   • AAAs present in three general ways:
    1. Asymptomatic AAA
      • The most common presentation
      • Usually discovered incidentally by physical examination or radiographically by ultrasound (US), abdominal computed tomography (CT), or magnetic resonance imaging (MRI) done for other purpose
    2. Symptomatic AAA
      • Abdominal or low back pain which is generally vague and hard for the patient to describe
      • Pain can be severe, deep, and boring and may be confused with renal colic or musculoskeletal low back pain. This happens when there is an acute enlargement of the aneurysm.
    3. Ruptured AAA
      • Acute onset of severe abdominal or low back pain
      • Usually accompanied by profound hypotension. If blood pressure (BP) is relatively stable, the aneurysm rupture usually has been contained in the retroperitoneum.

- Symptoms may be confused with renal colic, acute pancreatitis, acute diverticulitis, inferior wall myocardial ischemia, perforated viscus, or mesenteric ischemia.
- In thin individuals an aneurysm may reveal an expansile pulsation in the midline. This is in contrast to the normal pulsations that may be felt. The physical examination may not detect an aneurysm in up to 70% of patients, particularly those who are obese. Auscultation over the pulsatile mass may reveal the presence of a bruit. Unstable aneurysms are frequently tender.

C. Laboratory and diagnostic studies
- Plain x-rays may identify AAA incidentally because of the "egg shell" pattern of calcification in the aortic wall. This imaging technique is not a reliable means of detecting AAA.
- Abdominal ultrasound is the screening test of choice; it is used to define the size and can reveal the presence of wall thrombus. This modality is also used for monitoring change in the size of the aneurysm.
- CT angiography and MR angiography are useful for defining the size, anatomy, relationship to adjacent structures, and the presence or absence of rupture in the acute setting.
- Aortograms may be done in planning operative management, but with the advent of high-resolution CT scanning, they are being used less frequently.

D. Evaluating the severity of problems
- Rupture or potential rupture is a surgical emergency. Vascular surgical consultation should be sought immediately and the patient prepared for surgery. About 50% of patients with an AAA rupture die before they reach a hospital.
- If paraplegia is noted, one must suspect involvement of a low artery of Adamkiewicz, a major collateral of the anterior spinal artery. This complication may rarely be seen after elective repair.

E. Management of the patient
1. Elective surgical repair is indicated if:
   - AAA expands more than 0.5 cm per year.
   - AAA grows to more than 5.5 cm.
   - AAA becomes symptomatic.
   - AAA expands rapidly regardless of its size.
2. Traditional surgical approach is open repair. Endovascular stent grafts are a less morbid option for select patients, particularly those at high risk for an open procedure, and are being increasingly done.
3. For medium-sized asymptomatic AAA surveillance with serial imaging (US or CT) is recommended:
   - AAA 3 to 4 cm—should be imaged yearly
   - AAA 4 to 4.5 cm—should be imaged every 6 months
   - AAA greater than 4.5 cm—referral to a vascular surgeon
4. Medical management:
   - Risk factor modification including cessation of smoking is essential in all AAA patients. Therapy with β-blockers is also recommended.

II. Acute Appendicitis
   A. Basic science
      - The appendix, generally 6 inches long, originates from and lies directly behind the cecum. It is fixed retrocecally in approximately 15% of adults and freely mobile in the remainder.
      - Acute appendicitis results from obstruction of the appendiceal lumen, usually from fecaliths, fibrous bands, foreign bodies, parasites, or lymphoid hyperplasia. Appendiceal inflammation and edema cause increased wall tension, eventually disrupting blood flow leading to ischemia and ultimately to appendiceal perforation. The time from obstruction to perforation may be as little as 24 hours.
   B. History and physical examination
      - There are four classic symptoms of appendicitis:
         1. Right lower quadrant (RLQ) abdominal pain
         2. Anorexia
         3. Nausea and vomiting
         4. Fever
      - Less than one half of patients have typical signs and symptoms of appendicitis.
      - Appendicitis usually begins as periumbilical abdominal discomfort, followed by anorexia, nausea, and often vomiting.
      - After several hours, the pain usually moves to the RLQ due to regional peritoneal irritation.
      - The pain is worsened by movement or change in the intra-abdominal pressure (e.g., sneezing or coughing). In the case of a retrocecal or pelvic location of the appendix, the pain may remain poorly localized, making the diagnosis difficult.
      - The patient may experience low-grade fevers with RLQ tenderness, most commonly over McBurney's point.
      - Peritoneal signs (guarding and rebound tenderness) appear with peritoneal irritation.
      - Other helpful signs of appendicitis include the following:
         1. Psoas sign: pain from passive extension of the right hip
         2. Internal obturator sign: pain on passive internal rotation of flexed thigh
         3. Rovsing's sign: RLQ pain during palpation of the left lower quadrant
      - There is a great deal of variation in the signs and symptoms of acute appendicitis. A few patients with acute appendicitis may report pain with rectal examination, particularly in children; however, if present, rectal pain more often points to an alternative cause for the symptoms.
      - A pelvic examination is required in all women with abdominal pain; pelvic inflammatory disease may mimic the symptoms of appendicitis.
   C. Laboratory and diagnostic studies
      - There is often a leukocytosis with left shift (bandemia), but many patients, particularly the elderly, those who are immunosuppressed (HIV, steroids), and patients already on antibiotics, may have a normal white blood cell (WBC) count.

- A urinalysis is usually normal.
- Imaging:
  1. Plain x-ray (KUB): Findings are usually nonspecific and rarely help in the diagnosis.
  2. Ultrasound: may show appendiceal inflammation and help rule out other pelvic pathologies (ovarian masses, ruptured ectopic pregnancy, etc.) but is heavily operator-dependent
  3. CT scan of the abdomen: considered the best imaging modality. CT may show an enlarged appendix with wall thickening and periappendiceal fat stranding. The value of a CT scan is greatest in atypical presentations. However, in the setting of a classical presentation a CT scan is often superfluous and can even be misleading if it is negative.

D. Formulating the diagnosis
- In the classic case, the history should be diagnostic and readily supported by the physical examination and ancillary tests. The rate of false positive diagnosis in this group is around 10%.
- In equivocal cases, the best approach is to observe the patient for a period of about 6 hours (patient with appendicitis usually have progression of inflammatory signs and symptoms) and consider imaging with a CT scan of the abdomen.
- The diagnosis is usually more difficult in the very young and in the elderly. In these groups the diagnosis is often delayed and the incidence of perforation is most common.
- The highest rate of false positive diagnosis (~20%) occurs in young females (ages 20 to 40), in which the differential diagnosis includes gynecologic causes of abdominal pain.

E. Evaluating the severity of problems
- Appendicitis is a life-threatening disease, with possible progression from obstruction to perforation in 24 hours. A ruptured appendix may result in peritonitis and death.
- Additional complications include appendiceal abscess and pyelophlebitis (suppurative thrombophlebitis of the portal venous system).

F. Management of the patient
- Emergent surgery (open or laparoscopic) and initiation of antibiotics (covering aerobic and anaerobic enteric pathogens) is the standard of care. Patients often require fluids in preparation for surgery or for hypotension due to sepsis from a perforated appendix.

III. Anal Fissure
A. Basic science
- An anal fissure is a tear or ulcer in the anal canal distal to the dentate line (most commonly in the posterior midline). Most anal fissures result from local trauma due to passage of large, hard stool.
- Other less common reasons for an anal fissure include anatomic abnormalities, infections (sexually transmitted diseases, tuberculosis), inflammatory bowel disease (IBD), and leukemia.

- If the fissure rests on the internal sphincter, it may cause it to spasm. This results in pain leading to avoidance of defecation and development of hard, constipated stools.

B. History and physical examination
- Symptoms include tearing pain during defecation and bleeding upon wiping. Pain may persist for hours after defecation.
- On examination, the best way to diagnose an anal fissure is to spread the buttocks apart gently and look carefully in the posterior midline. Digital rectal examination or anoscopy are often too uncomfortable in this condition.
- Chronic fissures may be associated with a skin tag protruding from the anus and hypertrophied anal papillae proximally.

C. Laboratory and diagnostic studies
- No specific studies have been proved useful.

D. Formulating the diagnosis
- The diagnosis should be apparent after history and physical examination.
- For nonhealing fissures, alternative diagnoses need to be considered including Crohn's disease, cytomegalovirus (CMV), herpes simplex virus (HSV), human immunodeficiency virus (HIV), syphilis, and tuberculosis. Biopsy should also be considered to rule out malignancy.

E. Evaluating severity of problems
- As above, nonhealing fissures may be associated with alternative diagnoses.

F. Management of the patient
- Primary therapy includes stool softeners, bulking agents (psyllium), high-fiber diet, and frequent sitz baths. This approach will heal 90% of fissures. Even after a second event, 70% respond to medical management.
- Additional nonsurgical therapies include botulinum toxin infiltration (reversible paralysis of the internal sphincter) and nitroglycerin or nifedipine ointment (relaxation of the internal sphincter).
- Chronic fissures (>1 month) or fissures refractory to 3 to 4 weeks of conservative therapy should be considered for surgical correction.

IV. Complications of Anesthesia
- Anesthesia complications usually occur during or immediately after operation. The most common or serious complications are as follows:

A. Nausea and vomiting
- Nausea and vomiting are the most common complications of anesthesia.
- Narcotic analgesics are a frequent cause of postoperative nausea (40% of patients experience nausea with meperidine or morphine). Postoperative nausea is also attributable to induction and inhalational anesthetics. Induction agents implicated include propofol (the least), barbiturates (intermediate), ketamine, and etomidate (the worst).
- Other causes of nausea and vomiting include hypotension, hypoxemia, hypoglycemia, increased intracranial pressure, gastrointestinal bleeding, gastric distention, and ileus.
- Postoperative nausea can be prevented by administering antiemetics. Droperidol, metoclopramide, transdermal scopolamine, prochlorperazine,

promethazine, and newer agents, such as 5-HT$_3$ receptor antagonist ondansetron, are all effective.

B. Persistent sedation
- Persistent sedation most commonly results from overuse of sedatives (pentobarbital, droperidol, lorazepam, and diazepam).
- Sedation linked to inhalational agents is characterized by shallow respirations. Persistent inhalational anesthetic sedation is most likely to occur after relatively long periods of use of the inhalational agent and is worse in obese patients because of the high lipid solubility of the agents.
- Oversedation secondary to narcotic overdose is characterized by pinpoint pupils and slow respiratory rates. If narcotic sedation is deep enough to interfere with respiratory drive, it may be reversed with the use of naloxone.
- In the cases of persistent sedation secondary to benzodiazepine overdosage, reversal with flumazenil (a benzodiazepine antagonist) is appropriate.
- Persistent paralysis may be mistaken for oversedation and should be excluded by observing the patient's ventilation, active movements, and reflex activity.
- Metabolic derangements such as hypercapnia, hypoxia, hypoglycemia, hyperglycemia/hyperosmotic coma, and hyponatremia must be excluded. Hypothermia must also be considered.

C. Bronchospasm
- Patients with asthma are six times more likely to develop bronchoconstriction in response to intubation.
- Bronchoconstriction is treated with β_2-agonists (fast-acting) such as albuterol nebulizers or metered dose inhalers. Administration of intravenous corticosteroids will help decrease bronchospasm (delayed action).

D. Hypothermia
- Perioperative hypothermia is an extremely common problem. Trauma and burn patients, patients with a large blood loss, and patients at the extremes of age are all at risk for hypothermia.
- Temperatures less than 33°C cause platelet and coagulation abnormalities, dysrhythmias, and increased blood viscosity. Intraoperative normothermia has been proved to reduce the postoperative infection rate and length of hospital stay.
- Warmed air heating blankets and warmed intravenous solutions are commonly used to raise the patient's core body temperature. Additionally, low doses of meperidine are used to control excessive shivering and decrease oxygen consumption.

E. Malignant hyperthermia
- Malignant hyperthermia is an autosomal dominant genetic trait. The condition is characterized by often fatal hyperthermia with rigidity of muscles occurring in affected patients exposed to certain anesthetic agents, particularly halothane, succinylcholine, and methoxyflurane. It is thought that the triggering agent causes the patient's cells to lose the ability to control intracellular levels of calcium, resulting in high intracellular calcium levels.
- Signs of malignant hyperthermia include tachypnea, tachycardia, unstable blood pressure, hypoxemia, rigidity, sweating, and fever. Laboratory

abnormalities include respiratory and metabolic acidosis, electrolyte abnormalities (especially hyperkalemia), rhabdomyolysis, and myoglobinuria.
- Treatment of malignant hyperthermia involves the following:
  1. Discontinuing all possible agents that could have triggered the attack and concluding surgery as quickly as possible
  2. Hyperventilation with 100% oxygen
  3. Dantrolene (IV)
  4. Aggressive IV fluid resuscitation
  5. Cooling measures
  6. Correction of acidosis and hyperkalemia
  7. Transfer to ICU
- Patients with known malignant hyperthermia should be pretreated with dantrolene for 1 to 3 days, and triggering agents should be avoided. These patients are able to undergo future anesthesia as long as triggering agents that caused the previous attack are completely avoided. However, no anesthetic approach is completely safe

V. Decubitus Ulcer
  A. Basic science
  - A decubitus ulcer is also known as a bed or pressure sore. It is defined as the necrosis of tissue and subsequent ulceration in areas with bony prominences.
  - Decubitus ulcers are a complication of prolonged immobilization. They are a direct result of localized pressure. Decubitus ulcers most frequently occur in debilitated patients that are either bedridden, wheelchair bound, or left in the same position for prolonged periods of time. Many of the affected patients have decreased or absent sensation and are unable to feel pain associated with ischemia. Tissues overlying the occiput, scapulae, sacrum, ischia, greater trochanters, calcanei, and lateral malleoli are the most frequent sites of pressure necrosis.
  - Prolonged pressure over a period longer than 2 hours will lead to tissue ischemia that results in tissue necrosis. The necrosis can involve any tissue that is located between the external pressure source and the bony prominence. Skin, subcutaneous tissue, and muscle can be involved.
  - Factors that increase a patient's predisposition to the development of a decubitus ulcer include contact with perspiration, urine, and feces. Poor nutritional status of the patient, anemia, as well as infection predispose the patient to formation of decubitus ulcers.
  B. History and physical examination
  - The history is of a patient who is paralyzed, insensate, or debilitated in some other way, and who spends prolonged periods of time in the same position. Most of the patients are either bedridden or wheelchair bound. Additional factors can include poor nutritional status, anemia, diabetes, incontinence, or concomitant infection.
  - Physical examination will demonstrate an ulcer in one of the areas just mentioned. The depth of the ulcer determines its severity.

C. Laboratory and diagnostic studies
- None are needed.

D. Formulating the diagnosis
- Diagnosis is evident from history and physical examination.

E. Evaluating the severity of problems
- Stage 1 consists of an area of reddened skin. There is no underlying tissue involvement.
- Stage 2 is characterized by reddened, edematous skin with induration and dermal necrosis.
- Stage 3 involves exposed fat or muscle tissue.
- Stage 4 involves destruction of soft tissue and the involvement of bone, which may lead to osteomyelitis.

F. Management of the patient
- The best treatment for decubitus ulcer is its prevention. This entails relief of pressure over the areas of bony prominence. Special devices are available that distribute the patient's weight evenly and alleviate increased pressure over the points of prominence. Additional padding should be placed over areas that are prone to the development of decubiti. It is also imperative that the patient's position be changed every 2 hours in order to prevent the development of ischemic changes that will ultimately lead to necrosis. Patients who are wheelchair bound are at risk for the same complications and should be able to change their position frequently. In the case of braces or casts, windows may have to be cut at potential pressure sites in order to decrease the risk.
- Patients at risk must be carefully monitored for any cutaneous changes. This entails careful inspection of pressure points, at least on a daily basis. Patients have to be kept clean and dry. Especially in cases of incontinence it is imperative that the patient be checked frequently in order to avoid prolonged exposure to moisture and soilage.
- Patients' nutritional status must be optimized, and any deficits, such as anemia, corrected in order to facilitate the healing process.
- The early stage of the decubitus requires aggressive measures of prevention and optimization of the patient nutritional status. All pressure should be relieved from the area of the potential decubitus, and it should be kept dry and exposed to air. Unless progression or infection occurs at this site, the early stage of a decubitus ulcer should heal spontaneously.
- The later stages of a decubitus ulcer are manifested by the presence of tissue necrosis. On the discovery of such changes an aggressive approach must be instituted in order to minimize its progression. Surgical treatment is required for any area that is full thickness and greater than 2 cm in diameter. Any necrotic tissue must be debrided, and the underlying tissues protected from desiccation with, for example, wet to dry dressings.
- The likelihood of infection of the open wound is high. Uncontrolled local infection may lead to bacteremia and death. For bacterial counts greater than 10^3 organisms, topical antibiotics should be instituted. Once the progression of necrosis has been stopped and healing has started, closure of the defect may be undertaken. In the case of small defects, less than 2 cm in diameter, they may

heal spontaneously once granulation tissue develops. Larger defects may have to be closed surgically, either by simple closure, split-thickness skin grafts, or by the utilization of flaps.
- In the case of chronically debilitated patients or in the case of significant bone involvement, removal of the affected bone may be necessary.

VI. Hemorrhoids
   A. Basic science
      - Hemorrhoids are varicosities of the hemorrhoidal venous plexus in the anorectal area.
      - Hemorrhoids originate from arteriovenous communications between the superior rectal arteries and the superior, inferior, and middle rectal veins.
      - They function as protective cushions that become engorged with blood during the act of defecation, protecting the anal canal from direct trauma due to passage of stool.
      - External hemorrhoids are located below the dentate line and are covered by squamous epithelium.
      - Internal hemorrhoids are found above the dentate line and are lined with rectal and transitional mucosa.
      - Hemorrhoidal tissues become engorged when intra-abdominal pressure is increased, which occurs with obesity, pregnancy, lifting, and straining with defecation.
      - Hemorrhoids are infrequent in patients with portal hypertension. There is no direct communication with the portal system, although hemorrhoids may be in the proximity of rectal varices in patients with portal hypertension
   B. History
      1. Internal hemorrhoids
         - Bright rectal bleeding, usually painless
         - Rectal fullness or discomfort when very large
         - Prolapse into the anal canal (infrequent). Rarely, they can become incarcerated, thrombosed, and necrotic, causing pain.
         - Mucous discharge due to prolapsed hemorrhoids
      2. External hemorrhoids
         - Severe pain, usually caused by thrombosis (anal fissure and perianal abscess have a similar presentation)
         - Pruritus
         - Perianal mass
   C. Physical examination
      - Examination of the rectum may demonstrate various findings including normal-appearing perineum, edema, prolapse, or a gangrenous and incarcerated hemorrhoid.
      - Maceration from chronic mucosal discharge can be seen.
      - Acutely thrombosed external hemorrhoids are tender, tense, purple, swollen perianal masses.
      - Internal hemorrhoids are classified as follows:

      1. First-degree: bleeding, no prolapse

      2. Second-degree: prolapse out of the anal canal with spontaneous reduction (with or without bleeding)

      3. Third-degree: prolapse, requires manual reduction

      4. Fourth-degree: irreducible and may strangulate

  D. Laboratory and diagnostic studies

- Anoscopy is the initial tool in the evaluation of painless rectal bleeding.
- Anemia may be found in patients with hemorrhoids. However, its cause should be further investigated by colonoscopy to rule out colonic neoplasias and other causes of bleeding

  E. Formulating the diagnosis

- A detailed history and physical examination are essential for an accurate diagnosis.
- The decision to pursue further evaluation after anoscopy or flexible sigmoidoscopy depends on the patient's risk factors and medical condition.
- Hemorrhoids alone do not typically cause a positive guaiac stool test, so fecal occult blood should warrant adequate colonic examination.
- Differential diagnoses include anal fissures, rectal prolapse, rectal ulcers, polyps, vascular malformations, colorectal cancer, and inflammatory bowel disease. Thus, these diagnoses should be excluded, particularly if conservative treatment for hemorrhoids has not been successful.

  F. Evaluating the severity of problems

- As above, other more serious conditions should be ruled out before rectal bleeding is attributed to hemorrhoids.

  G. Management of the patient

- Asymptomatic hemorrhoids need no treatment.
- Initial medical management for symptomatic hemorrhoids consists of dietary changes and to avoid straining with defecation. Dietary changes include increasing dietary fiber, stool softeners (psyllium), bran, and fluid intake and decreasing constipating foodstuffs. Therapy includes sitz baths and topical pain and itching preparations (witch hazel, hydrocortisone cream).
- Surgical therapy should be considered if there is no response to 1 to 2 weeks of conservative measures. Options include the following:

      1. Injection sclerotherapy

- Commonly used for first- and second-degree hemorrhoids. Sclerosing agent is injected at the base of the hemorrhoidal complex. Complications include pain, abscess, impotence, and urinary retention.

      2. Rubber band ligation

- Commonly used for first-, second-, third-, and selected fourth-degree hemorrhoids. The protruding internal hemorrhoid is ligated with rubber band, causing necrosis and sloughing. The most common complication is pain, but abscess, urinary retention, band slippage, prolapse and thrombosis of adjacent hemorrhoids, and minor bleeding from the ulcer occur in less than 5% of patients.

3. Hemorrhoidectomy or stapled hemorrhoidopexy
   - Rarely performed, hemorrhoidectomy is reserved for larger third- and fourth-degree hemorrhoids, acutely incarcerated and thrombosed hemorrhoids, hemorrhoids with an extensive and symptomatic external component, and patients who have undergone less aggressive therapy with poor results.

VII. Hernias
   A. Basic science
   - A hernia is a protrusion of intra-abdominal tissue through a fascial defect in the abdominal wall.
   - The majority of hernias are groin hernias (indirect/direct inguinal and femoral hernias). Other less common hernias include incisional, epigastric, and umbilical hernias.
   - Indirect inguinal hernias are the most common type groin hernia (in both men and women). They develop at the internal ring, where the spermatic cord in males and the round ligament in females exit the abdomen. Indirect inguinal hernias arise lateral to the inferior epigastric artery (direct hernias arise medially). The cause is thought to be the defective obliteration of the fetal processus vaginalis.
   - Direct inguinal hernias occur through Hesselbach's triangle, formed by the inguinal ligament, the inferior epigastric artery, and the lateral border of the rectus muscle. The cause is thought to be a weakness in the floor of the canal. The relationship between direct inguinal hernias and straining or heavy lifting is not clear.
   - Femoral hernias account for less than 10% of all groin hernias, but they have the highest risk for incarceration and strangulation. These develop in a small empty space at the medial aspect of the femoral canal, medial to the femoral nerve, artery, and vein.
   - Causes of increased in intra-abdominal pressure are cited as risk factors for developing hernias. These include marked obesity, pregnancy, peritoneal dialysis, excess straining (prostatism and constipation), chronic cough, and ascites.
   B. History and physical examination
   - Most inguinal hernias are asymptomatic and are found on routine physical examination. On occasion a patient may present with a bulge in the groin that causes aching on exertion.
   - Commonly, direct inguinal hernias produce fewer symptoms and are less prone to incarceration and strangulation than indirect hernias.
   - Palpation of an inguinal hernia is performed by placing one's finger at the superior border of the scrotum in men and invaginating the skin into the inguinal canal toward the superficial ring. It is usually easier to demonstrate the presence of a hernia while examining the patient standing.
   - A mass or bulge structure can be felt when the patient coughs or strains. Differentiating between indirect versus direct hernia is of limited clinical significance and often very difficult to achieve on physical examination.

C. Laboratory and diagnostic studies
- In the majority of cases the diagnosis of a hernia can be made based on history and physical examination.
- Various imaging techniques have been used when the clinical diagnosis is unclear including herniography, ultrasound, and MRI. However, the optimal diagnostic tool is unclear.

D. Evaluating the severity of problems
- Occasionally a hernia may become incarcerated. This is a more serious presentation, as the hernia contents can become strangulated and eventually infarct. The patient will complain of a mass that does not reduce and is tender to palpation.
- Often with gentle pressure and occasionally with sedation the mass can be reduced into its proper place. If this is not possible, emergent surgery is required.

E. Management of the patient
- Patients with hernias should be referred to a surgeon. The majority of hernias will require surgical repair because the defect will only increase in size over time, resulting in the possibility of bowel incarceration.
- However, watchful waiting can be considered for asymptomatic hernias. Education as far as symptoms of incarceration and strangulation should be provided to the patient.
- Umbilical hernias often regress during adolescence but if still present during adulthood they should generally be repaired.
- For inguinal hernias, various repairs of the hernia have been proposed (including open and laparoscopic approaches), but they all have one goal in common, which is to fortify the inguinal floor and tighten the internal ring. Similar principles are used for the other types of hernia when closure of the defect is the desired result.

VIII. Intestinal Obstruction
A. Basic science
- Intestinal (or bowel) obstruction is a failure or interruption of the normal transit of intestinal contents.
- Obstruction of the small intestine can be complete or partial.
- The most common causes of bowel obstruction:
  1. Extrinsic causes
     a. Postoperative adhesions (overall most common cause)
     b. Hernias and wound dehiscence
     c. Masses (i.e., anomalous vasculature, abscess, hematomas, neoplasms)
     d. Volvulus
     e. Aganglionic megacolon (Hirschsprung's disease)
  2. Intrinsic causes:
     a. Congenital: atresia or stenosis, imperforate anus, Meckel's diverticulum
     b. Trauma
     c. Inflammatory: inflammatory bowel disease (Crohn's disease, ulcerative colitis), diverticulitis, radiation, toxic megacolon

      d. Neoplastic (most common cause of colon obstruction)

      e. Luminal lesions: meconium in newborns, intussusception in infants, gallstones, fecal impaction, foreign bodies

- Swallowed air is the major source of the gaseous abdominal distention early in the course of the disease. In later stages bacterial fermentation becomes a significant contributor.
- Large quantities of extracellular fluids are lost into the gut and into the peritoneal cavity (third spacing of fluid), leading to intravascular volume depletion, which can progress to shock and multiorgan system failure if not recognized and treated.
- As the disease progresses the vomitus becomes feculent due to bacterial fermentation, and translocation of bacteria may occur.
- Strangulation almost always occurs in the setting of complete obstruction (one notable exception is a Richter's hernia, in which only part of the circumference of a segment of intestine passes through a hernia orifice).

B. History and physical examination

- The most common symptoms are abdominal distention (more common with distal obstruction), abdominal pain (diffuse, poorly localized, crampy with paroxysms occurring every 5 to 15 minutes, more common with midlevel small bowel obstruction), nausea and emesis (more common in proximal obstruction), and obstipation.
- A history of prior abdominal surgeries must be sought because postoperative adhesions are the most common cause for bowel obstruction.
- Findings on examination include abdominal distention (particularly with distal obstructions), tympany, peristaltic rushes (early) followed by absence of bowel sounds (late), inability to pass flatus. Localized tenderness and presence of peritoneal signs suggest the presence of strangulation, which typically has systemic signs such as fever, tachycardia, hypotension, dry mucosa, and oliguria (all indicative of hypovolemia from third spacing of fluid in the abdominal cavity).
- Rectal examination should be performed in search of masses and gross blood (which can be found in intestinal neoplasms, ischemia, and intussusception), but most commonly reveals an empty rectal vault.

C. Laboratory and diagnostic studies

- In early stages all laboratory tests may be normal. As the disease progresses leukocytosis, hemoconcentration, electrolyte abnormalities, prerenal acute renal failure, and metabolic (lactic) acidosis develop owing to progressive hypovolemia and strangulation. Serum amylase is often elevated (nonspecific).
- Imaging:

    1. Plain x-ray (KUB)

- X-ray may show distention of small bowel or colon, ladder-like pattern of dilated small bowel loops with air-fluid levels, lack of air in the colon (except in partial obstruction or after an enema or sigmoidoscopy).

    2. Contrast studies

- Barium enema is useful for the diagnosis of colonic obstruction and can be therapeutic for intussusception; oral barium or Gastrografin studies (small bowel series or enteroclysis) can confirm the presence of mechanical obstruction and rule out ileus.

3. CT scan of the abdomen
   - CT is highly accurate in diagnosing and determining the level of bowel obstruction. It is also useful in documenting thickening, edema, or intramural air of the bowel wall—all highly suspicious for intestinal ischemia.

D. Formulating the diagnosis
   - The diagnosis of bowel obstruction is generally made based upon clinical and radiographic features and must be distinguished from nonmechanical causes of bowel dilatation (adynamic ileus, intestinal pseudo-obstruction—a chronic condition characterized by symptoms of recurrent abdominal distention).

E. Evaluating the severity of problems
   - Once a diagnosis of bowel obstruction is established, the approach will vary depending on whether the obstruction is partial or complete and whether strangulation is present or not.
   - The objectives of the initial evaluations are to establish the following:
     1. The degree of volume depletion and metabolic derangement
     2. The need for and timing of operative intervention

F. Management of the patient
   - Initial measures for all patients with bowel obstruction include nasogastric suction to relieve vomiting, reduce further swallowed air, and avoid aspiration of gastric contents. This, however, is not an effective means to decompress the bowel.
   - Fluid and electrolyte resuscitation are initiated after adequate intravenous access is obtained. Crystalloids (normal saline or lactated Ringer's solution) are the preferred solutions. Central hemodynamic monitoring may be required especially in patients with a history of congestive heart failure.
   - Urine output should be monitored by means of a Foley catheter.
   - Impending or ongoing strangulation requires urgent surgical intervention ("never let the sun rise or set on a small bowel obstruction"). For other situations a period of close observation may be warranted.
   - The surgical approach for most types of small bowel obstruction requires exploratory laparotomy, usually via a midline incision. For incarcerated inguinal hernias an inguinal approached may be used.
   - The extent of surgery is dictated by the assessment of bowel viability. Gangrenous intestine must be resected, but the difficulty lies in determining viability in the remainder of the obstructed bowel. The traditional approach is to wrap questionably viable bowel in warm saline-soaked pads and then look for signs of viability: return of motility, normal color, and the presence of mesenteric pulses.
   - Better approaches include the use of intraoperative doppler ultrasound to assess blood flow or the qualitative fluorescein test (1000 mg intravenous fluorescein injected into a peripheral vein) followed by inspection of the intestine using ultraviolet (UV) light. Areas of nonfluorescence or patchy fluorescence are indicative of nonviable bowel, which should be resected.

IX. Peripheral Arterial Disease
  A. Basic science
  - Atherosclerosis is the most common cause of peripheral arterial disease (PAD). Other causes include thrombosis, embolism, and trauma. Other less common causes include vaculitis and thromboangiitis obliterans.
  - Intermittent claudication is pain that occurs in affected muscle groups during exercise, especially walking, and resolves with rest. Gluteal claudication indicates obstruction of the aorta or iliac arteries, whereas calf claudication is suggestive of femoral or popliteal artery obstruction. Subclavian artery obstruction can cause claudication in the upper extremity. If the obstruction worsens, flow becomes insufficient even at rest, and pain is present at all times (rest pain). The end stage of arterial insufficiency to the extremity is tissue loss due to insufficient flow. Claudication due to vascular compromise should be distinguished from neuropathic pain due to lumbosacral radiculopathy (neurogenic pseudoclaudication).
  B. History and physical examination
  - Patients are often older men with risk factors for atherosclerosis such as smoking, hypertension, diabetes, lack of exercise, and hyperlipidemia. They will often give a history of atherosclerotic disease in other areas such as the carotid or coronary circulation. Patients will give a history of claudication and can often describe how many feet they walk before pain ensues. Rest pain and tissue loss signify advanced disease.
  - Physical findings are classically described by the six Ps:
    1. Pain
    2. Pallor
    3. Pulseless
    4. Paresthesia
    5. Paralysis
    6. Poikilolthermy or coolness
  - The physical examination may also reveal cool skin and hair loss, as well as some muscle wasting in the area that is hypoperfused. Bruits may be heard over the stenosed arterial segments. Pulses may be decreased or absent in the affected limb. Patients with severe disease have lower extremity blood flow that is dependent on gravity. They may complain of symptoms that are present when lying flat but are relieved by hanging their legs over the side of the bed.
  C. Laboratory and diagnostic studies
  - The ankle-brachial index (ABI) is defined as the ratio of systolic BP at the ankle to SBP in the arm (normal ABI $\geq$ 1). In peripheral vascular disease the ABI will be decreased to less than 1 (abnormal). Patients with an ABI is less than 0.5 generally have critical limb ischemia.
  - Doppler ultrasound studies may demonstrate a dampened flow pattern caused by the obstruction proximal to the measured point. MRA may also be useful.
  - The gold standard for evaluating the peripheral vasculature is angiography. This will demonstrate areas of stenosis, collateral circulation, adequacy of vessels distal to obstruction, and the presence of anomalies or aneurysms.

D. Formulating the diagnosis
  - Diagnosis is made by history and physical examination and from the results of the diagnostic tests just listed.
E. Evaluating the severity of problems
  - Severity of problems can be measured clinically (i.e., rest pain in the involved extremity) or with the use of diagnostic studies as outlined earlier.
  - PAD is more a marker of early death (from cardiovascular cause) than an indicator of imminent limb loss.
F. Management the patient
  - Most patients who present with claudication will improve with cessation of smoking, a graduated exercise program, improved diet, and aggressive management of comorbid medical conditions such as diabetes or hyperlipidemia.
  - Those patients with rest pain or tissue loss often require revascularization. This is done with autologous grafts (the patient's own saphenous vein). Other materials that may be used for bypass include prosthetic materials such as polytetrafluoroethylene (PTFE). In the appropriate patient balloon angioplasty and stenting is an alternative to surgical bypass.
  - Patients whose limbs are not salvageable with bypass require amputation.

X. Surgical Complications
  - Any postoperative occurrence that adversely affects a patient's health or survival is termed a complication. Complications may be specifically related to the operation performed. Others are more general and can occur after any surgical procedure.
  - A very important aspect of surgical care is to anticipate potential problems and take preventive measures to minimize their incidence. This is usually done during the preoperative consultation in order to do the appropriate patient evaluation, which involves the detection of both medical risk factors and psychiatric conditions that may interfere with a desirable outcome. Recognized early, problems may be treated so as to lessen the severity and prevent more serious outcomes. This ultimately has an impact on decreasing a patient's morbidity and mortality rates.
  - Important aspects of prevention of complications in the postoperative period include early mobilization, adequate respiratory care, and careful management of fluids and electrolytes.
  - The most common nonspecific postoperative complications are discussed in Sections B through D in this section.
A. History and physical examination
  1. Often the risk of any given patient suffering postoperative complications is directly related to that patient's general health. A thorough history and physical examination, including neurologic examination and assessment of peripheral arterial pulses, will alert the physician to an individual patient's risk for complications. Preventive measures and surgical care can be tailored to minimize postoperative problems.
  2. Specific helpful information that can be obtained by preoperative evaluation includes the following:

- Allergies to medications, anesthetics, topical antibiotics, latex, and bandage adhesives
- Medications (e.g., NSAIDs, antiplatelet agents, anticoagulants)
- Smoking and alcohol consumption
- Chronic medical conditions (hypertension, coronary artery disease, chronic obstructive pulmonary disease, diabetes mellitus, etc.)
- Past surgical history, including history of complications
- Presence of pacemaker/defibrillator, prosthesis, or other foreign body.
- Review of indicated preoperative tests (e.g., ECG, chest x-rays, hemoglobin level)

3. Specific factors affecting operative risk are found in patients with:
- Immunocompromised states (e.g., HIV positive, uncontrolled diabetes, use of immunosuppressive agents or steroids or prolonged use of antibiotics, renal failure, and neutropenia)
- Pulmonary dysfunction
- High risk of venous thromboembolism
- Elderly and obese patients

B. Respiratory complications
- Respiratory complications of surgery are extremely common. Patients with underlying lung disease and smokers are at significantly increased risk of postsurgical respiratory complications, as well as patients undergoing chest and upper abdominal surgeries, emergency operations and elderly patients.
- The major postoperative pulmonary complications:
1. Atelectasis
- Atelectasis is the collapse and failure to reexpand of small airways and alveoli. It is responsible for over 90% of febrile episodes during the first 48 hours after surgery.
- Clinical signs include fever, tachypnea, and tachycardia. Physical examination is often normal but may elicit rales, decreased breath sounds, and diaphragm elevation. Chest x-ray demonstrates platelike opacities.
- Atelectasis may be prevented by early use of incentive spirometry devices, early mobilization, and frequent position changes.
- Untreated atelectasis may lead to pneumonia.
2. Pulmonary aspiration
- Inhalation of oropharyngeal or gastric contents can cause aspiration pneumonitis.
- Predisposing factors are insertion of nasogastric or endotracheal tubes, depression of central nervous system in trauma victims and by drugs, pregnant women, and patients with intestinal obstruction, thoracic or abdominal surgeries.
- Aspiration can be prevented by preoperative fasting, careful endotracheal intubation, and proper positioning of the patient.
3. Postoperative pneumonia
4. Postoperative pleural effusion and pneumothorax

C. Infection
   1. Factors increasing the risk for infection include presence of necrotic and devitalized tissue, hematomas or seromas, foreign bodies, immunosuppressed states, existence of underlying chronic disease, and malnourishment.
   2. Preventive measures include meticulous attention to operative detail, hemostasis, maintaining sterile technique, and occasionally preoperative antibiotics. Early recognition of infection is important so that serious complications (e.g., dehiscence and/or incisional hernia) can be minimized.
   3. The cardinal signs of an inflammatory response are as follows:
      • Calor (fever, warmth)
      • Dolor (pain)
      • Rubor (erythema)
      • Tumor (edema and swelling)
   4. The four Ws represent the most common sites of infection during the postoperative period.
      • Wind (respiratory)
      • Walk (phlebitis)
      • Wound (wound infection)
      • Water (urinary tract infection, which is the most frequent acquired nosocomial infection)
   5. Other infections include *Clostridium difficile* colitis, cholecystitis, and parotitis.
D. Venous thromboembolism
   • Risk factors for the development venous thromboembolism (VTE) are advanced age, previous history of VTE, obesity, birth control pills, hypercoagulable state, underlying malignancy, orthopedic and pelvic surgeries, pregnancy, and postpartum status.
   • Risk for VTE in the perioperative period can be classified as low, moderate, or high:
      1. Low risk: age younger than 40, general anesthesia time less than 30 minutes, and patients who are undergoing minor elective, abdominal, or thoracic surgery. Preventive measures include early ambulation, and pharmacological measures are optional.
      2. Moderate risk: age older than 40, general anesthesia time longer than 30 minutes, and have one or more risk factors for VTE. Preventive measures include use of subcutaneous unfractionated or low-molecular-weight heparin (LMWH). Use of intermittent pneumatic compression devices is optional.
      3. High risk: age older than 40, patients having surgery for malignancy or an orthopedic procedure of the lower extremity lasting longer than 30 minutes, hypercoagulable state, or other risk factors. These patients are usually treated with subcutaneous LMWH or low-dose oral anticoagulants and additionally with intermittent pneumatic compression devices in select cases. Specific guidelines for knee and hip surgeries should be followed.
   • Classic findings of deep vein thrombosis (DVT) include a swollen, tender calf, fever, and Homan's sign (calf pain with dorsiflexion of the foot). However, 50% of patients are asymptomatic.

- Diagnostic studies to confirm DVT include Duplex ultrasound, plethysmography, and venography. Treatment for DVT includes systemic anticoagulation which reduces the risk of pulmonary embolism (PE) and extension of the DVT.
- PE results from migration of a DVT to the lungs. Signs and symptoms of PE include tachypnea, tachycardia, decreased O_2 saturation, and an A-a gradient that does not improve with O_2 administration.
- Diagnostic tests include helical CT scan (CT angiography), ventilation/perfusion scan, and pulmonary angiography (gold standard, rarely used).
- Treatment for PE is systemic anticoagulation typically with unfractionated heparin (bolus and then at a constant infusion rate) or LMWH, with eventual transition to oral therapy, typically with warfarin. If anticoagulation is contraindicated, placement of an inferior vena cava filter should be considered. Thrombolytic agents and thrombectomy are options in hemodynamically unstable patients.

Radiology

It is important to realize that the USMLE does not expect you to be a radiologist. In some cases, you might be able to select the correct answer based solely on the clinical information without even looking at the images. However, the images are there to help you and you should take full advantage of them. This chapter is designed to show common radiologic appearances of different diseases and injuries. Each image is accompanied by a concise history and pertinent description followed by a brief discussion including clinical information, differential diagnosis, and in many cases tips or "buzzwords" that usually go hand in hand with the described abnormality.

I. Head CT (Fig. 19-1)
  A. History
    • Sudden onset of severe headache and effortless vomiting that has progressed to obtundation
  B. Description
    • Noncontrast axial computed tomography (CT) image at the level of the pons. Blood is present throughout the basal cisterns, even outlining the basilar artery. The blood extends into the sylvian fissures bilaterally and is present in the fourth ventricle. No mass effect is demonstrated.
  C. Discussion
    • Blood within the subarachnoid space and sometimes within the ventricles is a classic presentation of a subarachnoid hemorrhage (SAH). The most common causes are a ruptured aneurysm (90%), arteriovenous malformation, trauma, and hypertension. Complications include obstructive or communicating hydrocephalus, cerebral infarction due to vasospasm (maximal at 48 to 72 hours), and cerebral herniation.
    • The initial radiologic study for a patient with suspected SAH is a noncontrast head CT scan. The hemorrhagic cerebrospinal fluid is hyperdense (bright) secondary to fresh blood, and progressively falls to below the attenuation of the brain over the next 2 weeks. Blood in the subarachnoid space classically fills the basilar cisterns and sulci. An intraventricular component may be present. The blood is often distributed asymmetrically. Cerebral angiography may be performed on an urgent basis to identify the bleeding source prior to surgery.
    • *Buzzwords: "Worst headache of my life"*

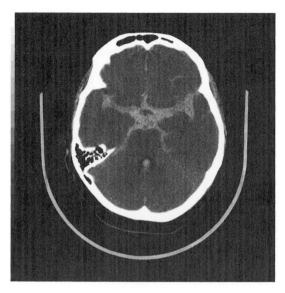

19-1

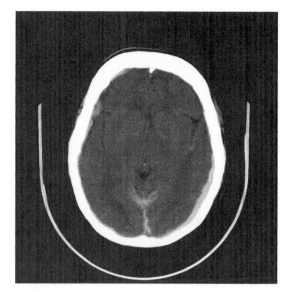

19-2

II. Head CT (Fig. 19-2)
   A. History
      • Motor vehicle accident with head trauma
      • Patient is unconscious.
   B. Description
      • Axial CT image at the level of the thalami. Blood is present in an extra-axial crescentic distribution in the left frontal and right parietal regions as well as the posterior interhemispheric fissure. No mass effect is demonstrated at this level. Foci of calcification are present in the choroid plexus.
   C. Discussion
      • This patient has bilateral acute subdural hematomas (SDHs). This is a neurosurgical emergency requiring immediate evacuation. Despite appropriate care, acute SDH carries a poor long-term prognosis due to underlying brain injury. The most common location for SDH is overlying the cerebral convexities. They also occur over the occipital poles, adjacent to the tentorium, and in the interhemispheric region. The latter is very characteristic of child abuse (shaken baby syndrome). Owing to the distribution in the subdural space, these hemorrhages can cross the suture lines but not the dural reflextions (falx, tentorium). They are crescent-shaped and high in attenuation (bright). These are venous bleeds, but if large enough, they can produce a mass effect and midline shift.
      • Chronic subdural hematomas (not shown) are often due to minor or forgotten trauma at a time remote from the clinical presentation. Although the shape seen on CT scan is the same as for acute SDH, they are often of low or mixed attenuation due to blood breakdown or rebleeding from a

neovascular membrane. Internal septations, calcifications, and fluid-fluid levels may be seen. Clinical signs and symptoms of chronic SDH are vague and unreliable. They are not a surgical emergency.

- *Tip: Question mentions child or elder abuse, or an acute deceleration injury.*

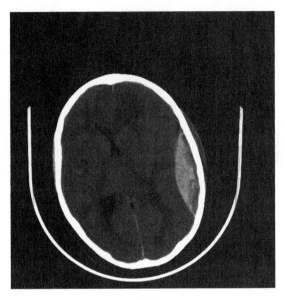

19-3

III. Head CT (Fig. 19-3)
   A. History
      - Head trauma with transient loss of consciousness
   B. Description
      - Axial image from a head CT scan at the level of the cerebral hemispheres. Blood in the left frontoparietal region exerts mass effect (convex surface) on the underlying brain. The ipsilateral lateral ventricle is effaced, and subfalcine herniation is demonstrated by a shift of the midline structures to the right.
   C. Discussion
      - This patient has an acute epidural hematoma, a neurosurgical emergency. They are much less common than subdural hematomas, accounting for about 10% of all head trauma. They are usually caused by laceration of a meningeal artery or vein, commonly with associated skull fracture (90%). The vast majority occur in the temporoparietal region. The latter is differentiated from a subdural hematoma by crossing of the falx and tentorium, but not the sutures. They are biconvex (lenticular) in shape and unilateral.
      - *Tip: Question mentions the presence of a skull fracture. Remember that you might not see it if only an axial CT of the brain is done, and not windowed to image the cranial bones.*

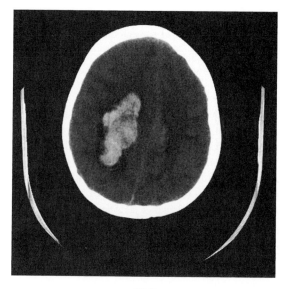

19-4

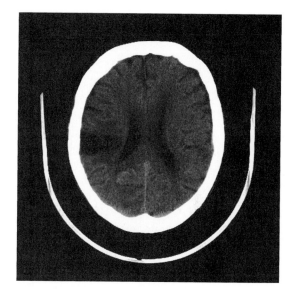

19-5

IV. Head CT (Fig. 19-4)
   A. History
      • Child with a new onset generalized seizure and now unresponsive
   B. Description
      • Axial image from a noncontrast head CT scan at the level of the cerebral hemispheres. A lobulated mass (hematoma) fills the lateral ventricle and exerts significant mass effect on surrounding structures. A low attenuation halo indicates brain edema.
   C. Discussion
      • This patient has a large intraparenchymal hematoma. Patients are invariably symptomatic with altered mental status, headache, and effortless vomiting. Neurologic signs are present as well. Parenchymal bleeds have an initial higher mortality rate than infarcts, but on recovery fewer deficits remain. Common causes include hypertension (most common), ruptured aneurysms, arteriovenous malformations, trauma, tumors, bleeding diathesis, and hemorrhagic infarction. The distribution and associated findings will often give clues as to the cause. Hypertensive hemorrhages classically occur in the basal ganglia (80%), brain stem, or cerebellum. Trauma will often have associated extra-axial blood or skull fractures. Complications and sequelae include encephalomalacia, rebleed, and abscess formation.
      • *Tip: Question mentions uncontrolled hypertension.*

V. Head CT (Fig. 19-5)
   A. History
      • Left-sided weakness

B. Description
   • Axial CT image without contrast at the level of the cerebral hemispheres demonstrates low attenuation in the right frontoparietal region involving the cortex and subcortical white matter.
C. Discussion
   • This patient has a right hemispheric stroke in the distribution of the middle cerebral artery. CT is the initial study of choice in acute stroke to exclude underlying mass or intracranial hemorrhage. Most CT examinations will appear normal in early stroke. Early signs of stroke in CT include loss of the gray-white matter junction interface, effacement of the sulci, or a hyperdense thrombus within the location of the affected vessel. Stroke syndromes are named for the vascular territory they involve. Each has a characteristic constellation of clinical findings. Strokes are further classified as bland (i.e., ischemic), such as this one, or hemorrhagic. Secondary hemorrhage into a bland stroke may occur. Risk factors include all those for atherosclerotic vascular disease, atrial fibrillation, and collagen vascular diseases. Treatment consists of supportive care as well as anticoagulation for bland strokes.

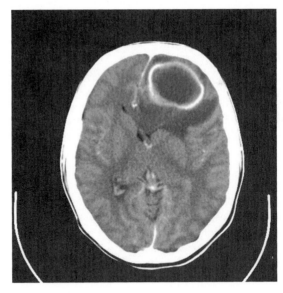

19-6

VI. Head CT (Fig. 19-6)
   A. History
      • IV drug user, septic and obtunded
   B. Description
      • Axial contrast-enhanced CT of the head demonstrates a large round lesion with ring enhancement involving the left frontal lobe with a moderate surrounding edema. Effacement of the anterior horn of the left lateral ventricle and midline shift is present as well.

C. Discussion
- Cerebral abscesses can occur via hematogenous dissemination (commonly in IV drug users), direct extension (trauma, sinusitis), or idiopathically. They can be single or multiple. They usually appear as parenchymal masses with surrounding edema. Over 90% of them will demonstrate peripheral ring enhancement after the administration of contrast agent. The most common differential considerations include metastatic lesions and a glioma. The clinical presentation will narrow the options to the appropriate diagnosis.

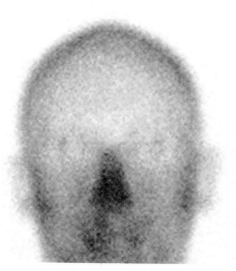

19-7

19-8

VII. Head HMPAO nuclear scan (Fig. 19-7)
   A. History
   - Brain death study
   B. Description
   - No tracer activity is identified in the supratentorial region. Blush of activity in the region of the nose is present ("hot nose" sign).
   C. Discussion
   - In cases in which brain death needs to be documented in patients who maintain cardiac and respiratory function, the study of choice is a ^{99m}Tc HMPAO nuclear scan to demonstrate the absence of blood flow into the cerebrum.

VIII. Waters' View of Facial Radiograph (Fig. 19-8)
   A. History
   - Facial pain and fever

B. Description
  • Waters' radiograph of the paranasal sinuses shows air-fluid levels in both maxillary and frontal sinuses (arrows).
C. Discussion
  • This patient has acute sinusitis. Differential diagnosis includes facial fractures with bloody effusions and barotrauma. Totally opacified sinuses have a wider differential diagnosis and are nonspecific. CT of the sinuses is now being used more commonly to assess bone detail and sinus anatomy. Treatment is with antibiotics if the sinusitis is due to bacteria. Involvement of the frontal and sphenoid sinuses is a concern because of the proximity of the brain and meninges and preformed pathways that may allow spread of infection intracranially. Intraorbital spread may occur from ethmoid sinusitis.

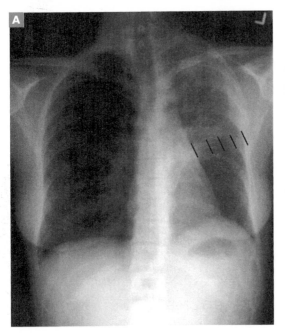
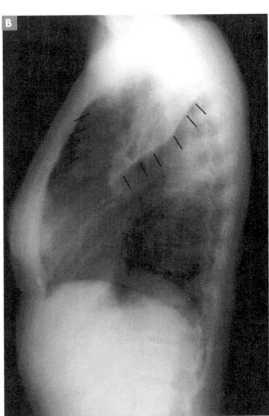

19-9

IX. Chest Radiograph (Fig. 19-9)
  A. History
    • Fever and productive cough

B. Description
   - Posteroanterior (see Fig. 19-9A) and lateral (see Fig. 19-9B) radiographs of the chest demonstrate confluent density and volume loss of the left upper lobe with air bronchograms throughout (markings). A portion of the aortic knob is obscured.

C. Discussion
   - This patient has left upper lobe pneumonia. Bacterial pneumonias tend to involve contiguous segments of a lung rather than the diffuse disease of viral pneumonia. Etiologic division into community- and hospital-acquired disease directs treatment plan.
   - The differential diagnosis of the radiographic pattern includes atelectasis (due to mucus plugging or endobronchial tumor), localized pulmonary hemorrhage, and pulmonary infarction. Rarely a bronchoalveolar cell carcinoma will present this way.
   - Up to 90% of pneumonias will resolve in 4 weeks. Subsequent films are indicated to demonstrate resolution.

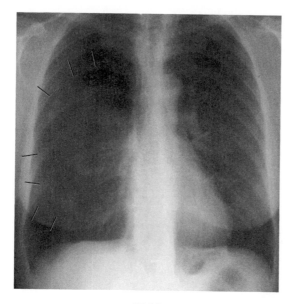

19-10

X. Chest Radiograph (Fig. 19-10)
   A. History
      - Shortness of breath
   B. Description
      - Posteroanterior radiograph of the chest demonstrates a shrunken right lung with absence of pulmonary vessels (lung markings) beyond a thin white pleural line.

C. Discussion
- This patient has a large right pneumothorax. The thin white line is the visceral pleura. An upright expiration film is usually the study of choice. In patients who cannot maintain the upright position, a lateral decubitus film is indicated. Symptomatic pneumothoraces are treated with chest tube drainage. The causes for pneumothorax are myriad. Primary pneumothoraces have no definable cause. Secondary pneumothoraces may be seen in asthmatics, in those with interstitial lung diseases or barotrauma, in patients on positive-pressure ventilation, and following invasive procedures such as thoracentesis. Traumatic pneumothoraces are due to pulmonary parenchymal damage or central airway damage.
- A tension pneumothorax (not shown) compresses the systemic venous return to the heart and results in rapid death if not treated immediately. The radiologic appearance includes an overexpanded chest with depression of the hemidiaphragm and shift of the mediastinum away from the pneumothorax.
- *Tip: Clinical presentation for a tension pneumothorax is not very specific but it can be dramatic and includes "tachypnea, tachycardia, cyanosis, sweating, and hypotension." A chest tube should be placed immediately.*

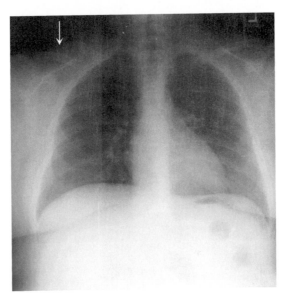

19-11

XI. Chest Radiograph (Fig. 19-11)
- A. History
  - Trauma
- B. Description
  - Chest radiograph shows a displaced midshaft fracture of the clavicle (arrow).

C. Discussion
- The clavicle is very commonly fractured (especially in children) and heals without surgical intervention in over 95% of patients. Fractures at the extreme ends of the bone may need surgical repair because of associated ligamentous injury.
- *Tip: Remember to look at the corners of the films, i.e., the clavicles, humeral heads, lower ribs.*

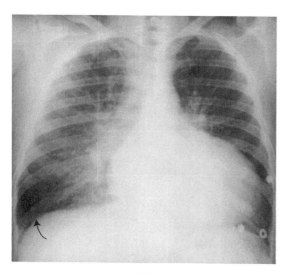

19-12

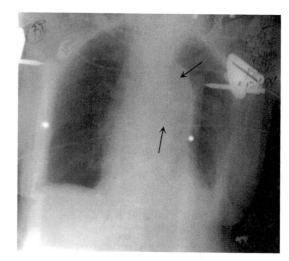

19-13

XII. Chest Radiograph (Fig. 19-12)
  A. History
    - Shortness of breath
  B. Description
    - A single frontal radiograph of the chest demonstrates a globally enlarged heart, engorged pulmonary vasculature with predominance in the upper lobes (redistribution or cephalization), perihilar haze, blunt right costophrenic angle, and Kerley B lines. The azygous vein is engorged as well.
  C. Discussion
    - This patient is in congestive heart failure. The majority of the radiographic signs just mentioned indicate left-sided heart failure. Two important signs of right-sided heart failure are noted: distended systemic veins and an enlarged right side of the heart (remember that the most common cause of right-sided heart failure is left-sided heart failure).

XIII. Chest Radiograph (Fig. 19-13)
  A. History
    - Trauma

B. Description
  - This portable radiograph of the chest was obtained with the patient on a backboard. There is a widened mediastinum with abnormal contours. The aortic arch is too large and a mural calcification does not project at the periphery (arrows). A left apical cap is present as well as depression of the left mainstem bronchus. The right paratracheal stripe is widened. Bilateral rib fractures, including the left first rib, are noted.

C. Discussion
  - This patient has many of the signs of a mediastinal hematoma. The main concern is that of an aortic transection, which was proved angiographically in this case (not shown). This sort of injury is caused by deceleration and tension on the aorta at its fixed points: the root, the great vessels, the ligamentum arteriosum, and the diaphragmatic crura. It is estimated that only 10% of the patients with traumatic aortic transections survive long enough to obtain definitive care. Other clues to the diagnosis in plain films are deviation of the trachea and nasogastric tube, if present, to the right. The differential diagnosis includes other major vascular injuries. Currently, contrast-enhanced CT is preferred over aortography as screening evaluation to exclude aortic injury because it is faster to obtain and useful to evaluate other intrathoracic structures.

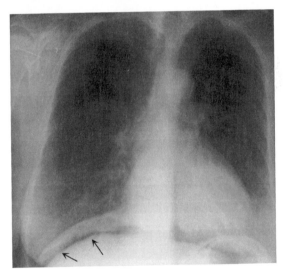

19-14

XIV. Chest Radiograph (Fig. 19-14)
  A. History
    - Acute onset abdominal pain
  B. Description
    - Air is present between the right hemidiaphragm and the liver (arrows). A smaller amount of gas lies between the left hemidiaphragm and the air-filled stomach.

C. Discussion
   • This patient has free intraperitoneal air, indicating a perforated hollow
     viscus. Common causes include peptic ulcer disease (most common),
     carcinoma, penetrating trauma, and postlaparotomy state. Treatment is
     surgical repair of the perforation and débridement of the peritoneum.
     Antibiotics are given for peritonitis.

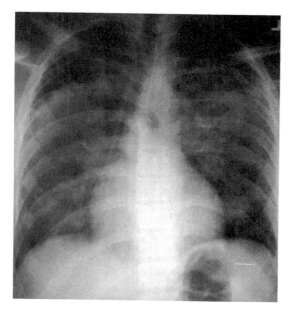

19-15

XV. Chest Radiograph (Fig. 19-15)
   A. History
      • Shortness of breath
   B. Description
      • Frontal radiograph of the chest demonstrates diffuse bilateral interstitial
        disease with foci of airspace consolidation. Apical cystic changes are present.
   C. Discussion
      • This patient has *Pneumocystis carinii* pneumonia (PCP). The radiograph
        shows all the classic findings for AIDS-associated PCP except a
        pneumothorax. The diagnosis is made by demonstrating the organism in
        sputum or bronchial washings.
      • Other pulmonary diseases seen in AIDS patients include tuberculosis,
        atypical mycobacterial infections, fungal pneumonia, and viral pneumonia.
        Kaposi sarcoma and lymphoma may involve the lung as well.
      • *Tip: Most common in AIDS patients; look for chest x-ray with a diffuse or
        bilateral perihilar interstital infiltrates.*

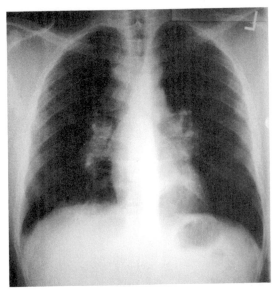

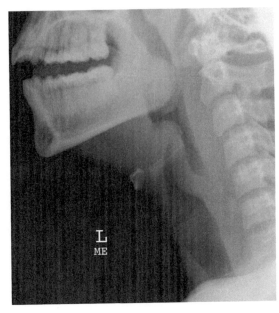

19-16

19-17

XVI. Chest Radiograph (Fig. 19-16)
   A. History
      • Young black female with cough and fever
   B. Description
      • Posteroanterior view of the chest shows marked symmetric hilar adenopathy.
   C. Discussion
      • Sarcoidosis is a systemic granulomatous disease that affects the lungs in over 90% of patients. Most often it presents as symmetric hilar adenopathy, but it can progress to frank pulmonary fibrosis in up to 20% of patients. The adenopathy usually regresses in 2 to 3 years. Most patients are asymptomatic, but some have dyspnea, nonproductive cough, or systemic symptoms such as fever or malaise.

XVII. Lateral Soft Tissues Neck (Fig. 19-17)
   A. History
      • Four-year-old boy with dysphagia, stridor, fever, and sore throat
   B. Description
      • Lateral image of the soft tissues of the neck demonstrates thickened aryoepiglottic folds and epiglottis.
   C. Discussion
      • These findings are characteristic of epiglottitis. This is a life-threatening disease that needs to be diagnosed and treated immediately. Examination of the child should be done in an intensive care unit or in an operating room

because it can induce complete occlusion of the airway, which requires intubation. *Haemophilus influenzae* is the most common etiologic agent.
- *Tip: This is one of the few cases in which a lateral soft tissues image of the neck would be shown. Make sure they are not trying to show you the spine.*

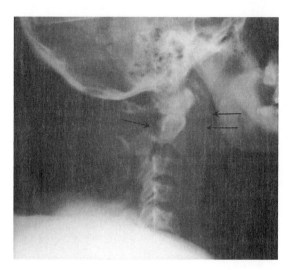

19-18

XVIII. Cervical Spine Radiograph (Fig. 19-18)
-   A. History
    - Trauma
-   B. Description
    - Cross-table lateral radiograph of the cervical spine shows a displaced and angulated fracture through the pars interarticularis of C2 bilaterally (arrow). Retropharyngeal soft tissue swelling is noted (double arrows).
-   C. Discussion
    - This patient has a "hangman's" fracture, which is a hyperextension and traction injury usually secondary to a motor vehicle accident. This fracture is unstable and requires immobilization (a halo device) to protect from further neurologic injury. Evaluation of the amount and level of neurologic deficit is also important.
    - Note that the entire cervical spine is not visualized on this radiograph. If the cervical spine from the skull base through top of T1 cannot be seen on cross-table lateral radiographs, CT scan is the study of choice.

XIX. Leg Radiograph (Fig. 19-19)
-   A. History
    - Trauma
-   B. Description
    - Anteroposterior radiograph of the lower leg of a child shows buckling of the distal tibial cortex (arrow).

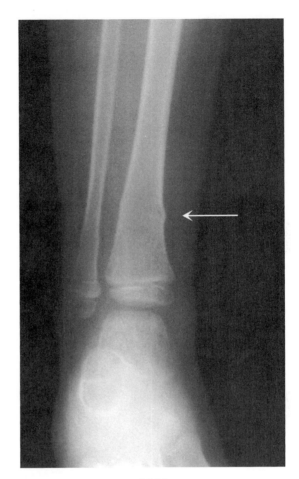

19-19

C. Discussion
- This patient has a torus fracture. These fractures occur only in young children and are due to relative plasticity of their immature skeleton. Characteristic locations include the radius and tibia. Treatment is conservative.
- Another fracture peculiar to children is the greenstick fracture (not shown), usually seen in children of elementary school age, in which a single bony cortex fractures (convex side) with bowing of the opposite side (concave side). Depending on the angulation, treatment might require casting only, reduction and casting, or completing the fracture under anesthesia followed by closed reduction.

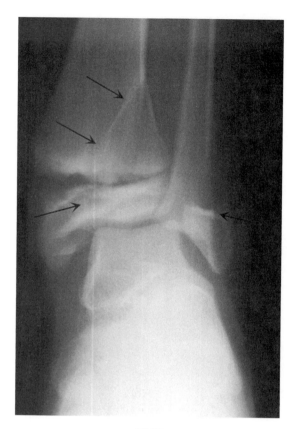

19-20

XX. Ankle Radiograph (Fig. 19-20)
   A. History
      • Trauma
   B. Description
      • A single radiograph of the ankle shows a fracture line (arrows) extending
        from the lateral portion of the tibial metaphysis through the central portion
        of the epiphysis. A fracture through the fibular physis has occurred with
        associated widening of the mortise.
   C. Discussion
      • This skeletally immature (pediatric) patient has a Salter-Harris IV fracture
        of the tibia and a Salter-Harris I fracture of the fibula. The ligaments
        stabilizing the ankle and the interosseous membrane are disrupted, too. The
        most common sites of this injury are the wrist and ankle. Reduction may be
        either closed or open. However, the patient must be monitored for
        abnormal growth patterns after clinical union (adequate weight bearing) has

been achieved. Premature physeal closure may cause limb shortening. Partial closure will lead to angulation deformity. Hyperemia to the entire limb may cause overgrowth at the other physes, leading to overall lengthening. Classified in 5 grades (types), the greater the grade, the greater is the likelihood of deformity.

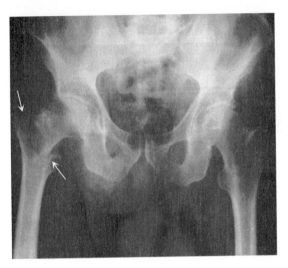

19-21

XXI. Pelvis Radiograph (Fig. 19-21)
   A. History
      • Elderly male found on the floor at home
   B. Description
      • There is a simple extra-articular fracture through the greater trochanter (arrows) extending to the basicervical region medially. Varus angulation is present.
   C. Discussion
      • Hip fractures are actually fractures through the femoral neck or trochanteric region. They occur most commonly in elderly or debilitated patients. Osteoporosis is a risk factor, and incidence increases with age. In the elderly hip fracture is associated with a high mortality rate. Females are affected three to six times more often than males.
      • The prime concern is that fractures may compromise the blood supply to the femoral head and cause osteonecrosis. Treatment is with pins or screws for fractures less likely to lead to osteonecrosis. More severe fractures are treated by femoral head resection and replacement. When inconclusive, MRI or bone scintigraphy is indicated.
      • Did you notice the large right inguinal hernia containing stool-filled colon? A smaller hernia is present on the left.

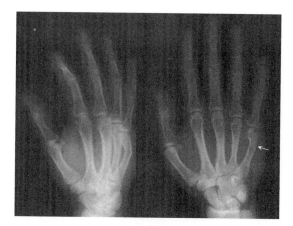

19-22

XXII. Hand Radiograph (Fig. 19-22)
    A. History
        • Pain in hand after a fight
    B. Description
        • Two views of the hand show a simple transverse fracture (arrow) of the distal fifth metacarpal shaft with volar angulation of the distal fragment (or dorsal angulation of the fracture site).
    C. Discussion
        • This is a form of a boxer's fracture. It is caused primarily by longitudinal forces on the metacarpal head and it is most commonly seen in the fifth metacarpal. Key concerns are rotation and excessive angulation causing protrusion of the metacarpal head through the palm pad, and associated lacerations caused by human teeth. If the rotation is mild, external reduction is sufficient. If markedly angulated or comminuted, then open reduction and internal fixation become necessary.

XXIII. Elbow Radiograph (Fig. 19-23)
    A. History
        • Fell on outstretched arm; pain upon pronation and supination
    B. Description
        • Anteroposterior (see Fig. 19-23A) and lateral (see Fig. 19-23B) radiographs of the elbow demonstrate prominent anterior and posterior fat pads ("sail sign") (markings).
        • A nondisplaced fracture of the radial head is present (arrow).
    C. Discussion
        • Radial head fractures are common and are usually treated conservatively by casting. If comminuted, the fracture fragment is excised. At times the fracture may not be seen on the initial radiographs. Alternative views (radial head, oblique view) can help in those cases.
        • *Tip: Look for the posterior fat pad on every elbow film.*

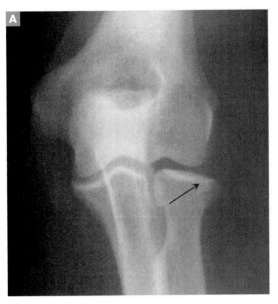

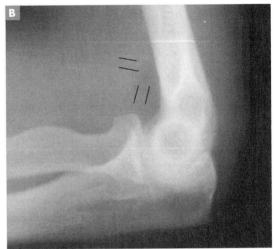

19-23

XXIV. Barium Enema (Fig. 19-24)
  A. History
    • Weight loss and guaiac positive stools
  B. Description
    • Lateral rectal view from an air contrast barium enema. An apple-core lesion is present at the rectosigmoid junction (markings). The presacral space is widened.
  C. Discussion
    • This patient has a colonic adenocarcinoma. Colon cancer is the third most common cancer in the United States and is the second most common cause of cancer deaths. Presentation usually includes symptoms related to anemia due to chronic occult blood loss, change in bowel habits, or weight loss. Risk factors include family history, low fiber/high fat diet, inflammatory bowel disease, and various polyposis syndromes. Diagnosis is made by barium enema, CT colonography, or colonoscopy. Staging is based on depth of penetration of the bowel wall and involvement of lymph nodes and distant organs. Metastases are primarily to the liver and can be seen by CT scan or ultrasound.
    • Current ACS screening recommendations include fecal occult blood test annually starting at age 50 combined with either flexible sigmoidoscopy every 5 years, double contrast barium enema every 5 years, or colonoscopy every 10 years.

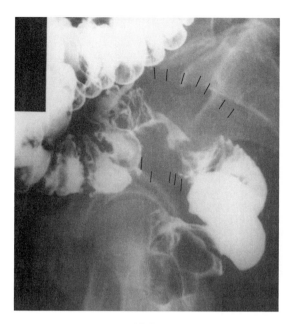

19-24

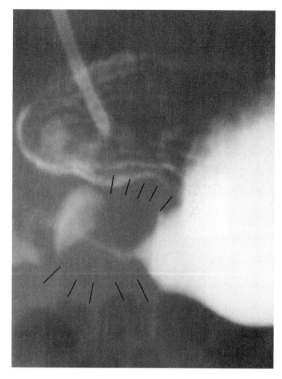

19-25

XXV. Upper Gastrointestinal Study (UGI) (Fig. 19-25)

   A. History

      • Infant with projectile vomiting

   B. Description

      • Image from an upper gastrointestinal series shows barium in the stomach and proximal duodenum. The pyloric channel is long and narrow with shoulders of mucosa at each end (markings).

   C. Discussion

      • This patient has hypertrophic pyloric stenosis. It is most commonly seen in firstborn males, often with a prior family history. Siblings may be affected, too. The clinical and radiologic manifestations are due to hypertrophy of the circular muscle layers surrounding the pylorus. Ineffective hyperperistalsis in the proximal stomach causes nonbilious projectile vomiting. (Bile in the vomitus would indicate obstruction beyond the ampulla of Vater.) Often the pylorus is palpable as an upper abdominal "olive" size mass. Ultrasound is useful as the first imaging modality, followed by barium study. Treatment consists of rehydration and pyloromyotomy.

      • *Buzzwords: "Olive" size mass palpated in the upper abdomen and projectile nonbilious vomiting. If the findings are seen only intermittently, pylorospasm should be considered.*

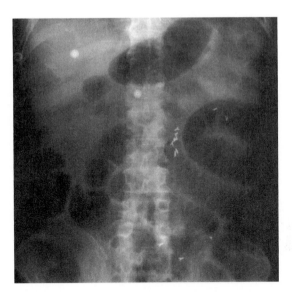

19-26

XXVI. Abdominal Radiograph (Fig. 19-26)
  A. History
    • Vomiting and abdominal pain
  B. Description
    • Supine radiograph of the abdomen shows dilated loops of small bowel with a small amount of air in the stomach and proximal colon. Surgical clips are present as well.
  C. Discussion
    • This patient has a small bowel obstruction. The majority of air in the bowel is swallowed. The small bowel normally has minimal air. Therefore dilated bowel containing easily seen air is abnormal. Dilated small bowel has the appearance of a "stack of coins." The presence of air in the colon in this case indicates either early or partial obstruction.
    • Small bowel obstruction in adults is usually caused by adhesions from prior surgery. Other causes include incarcerated hernias, intraluminal mass/foreign bodies, inflammatory processes, and intussusception. CT can help define the specific cause. Treatment consists of nasogastric tube decompression and rehydration. When the obstruction does not resolve with conservative treatment surgery is indicated.
    • *Buzzwords: The key to the diagnosis is the disproportionate amount of gas between the small bowel and colon, and between the proximal and distal small bowel. Retention of fluid also follows the distribution of gas, and air-fluid levels can be seen.*

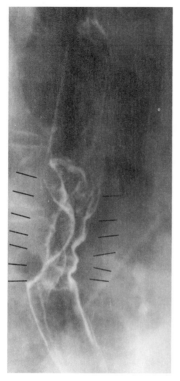

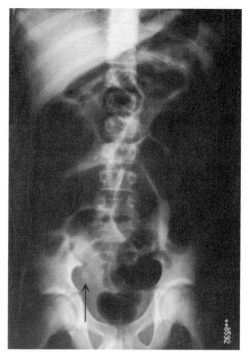

19-28

19-27

XXVII. Upper Gastrointestinal Study (UGI) (Fig. 19-27)
  A. History
    • Dysphagia
  B. Description
    • Single and double contrast esophagogram demonstrates a well-marginated, irregularly contoured, and ulcerated mass in the midesophagus (markings).
  C. Discussion
    • A mass with this appearance is almost pathognomonic for esophageal carcinoma. The majority are squamous cell carcinomas. The esophagus has no serosa to limit the spread of tumor; lymphatic dissemination occurs early. CT is used for staging. The prognosis is poor. Surgical treatment consists of resection with gastric mobilization or bypass. Chemotherapy and radiation are used as well.
    • *Tip: Consider adenocarcinoma if located in the lower esophagus at the gastroesophageal junction, where Barrett's esophagus occurs.*

XXVIII. Abdominal Radiograph (Fig. 19-28)
  A. History
    • Abdominal pain and fever

B. Description
  • Supine radiograph of the abdomen shows air throughout a redundant colon. Projecting over the right greater sciatic foramen is a well-marginated calcific density (arrow).

C. Discussion
  • This patient has acute appendicitis. Diagnosis is usually made purely on the basis of history and physical examination findings. Difficulty arises in the very young, women of childbearing age, and older patients. Plain films may be helpful, as in this case, but are generally nonspecific. The presence of an appendicolith in a patient with appendicitis is indicative of more severe disease. However, many normal appendices contain appendicoliths, making this sign less useful.
  • CT scan has the highest sensitivity and specificity of all the possible radiologic tests. Ultrasound can be very specific if the appendix is visualized, and is the study of choice in pregnant patients and the pediatric population.

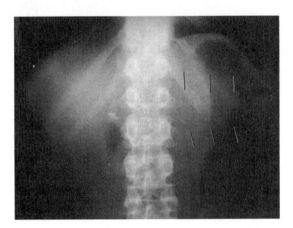

19-29

XXIX. Abdominal Radiograph (Fig. 19-29)
  A. History
    • Epigastric pain and vomiting
  B. Description
    • Supine radiograph of the abdomen demonstrates punctate calcifications projecting in the expected position of the pancreas (markings). Surgical clips are seen in the right upper quadrant. A nonspecific bowel gas pattern is present.
  C. Discussion
    • This patient has acute pancreatitis superimposed on chronic pancreatitis. No plain radiographic findings are specific for pancreatitis, which remains a clinical and laboratory diagnosis. The calcifications,

however, are very specific for chronic pancreatitis. CT scan is the modality of choice for assessing the extent of disease and to detect complications (e.g., pseudocyst, abscess, hemorrhage, or areas of necrosis). Common causes of pancreatitis include alcoholism, cholelithiasis (these two causes account for 70% of patients), hypercalcemia, certain medications, and trauma.

- *Tip: Calcifications in the pancreas = chronic pancreatitis.*

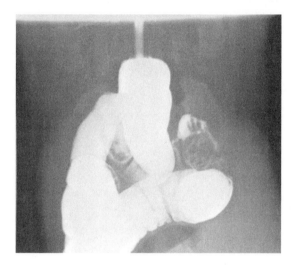

19-30

XXX. Barium Enema (Fig. 19-30)
- A. History
  - Child with intermittent abdominal pain
- B. Description
  - A single radiograph from a barium enema shows nearly complete filling of the colon. A filling defect is present in the proximal ascending colon and has a characteristic surrounding "coiled spring."
- C. Discussion
  - This child has an intussusception. This happens when one segment of bowel telescopes into another, causing intermittent obstruction. Eventually, vascular compromise of the intussusceptum may occur. Therefore, expeditious reduction should be carried out. Most intussusceptions can be reduced by enema, air, or barium. No underlying lead point is found in the majority of cases. The age group most often affected is between 3 months and 3 years. In adults a pathologic lead point (usually a tumor) is often found, and reduction requires surgery.

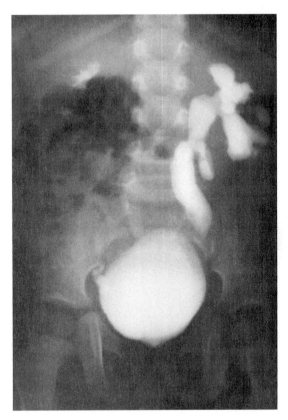

19-31

XXXI. Voiding Cystourethrogram (Fig. 19-31)
    A. History
        • Urinary tract infections
    B. Description
        • Image from a retrograde cystogram prior to voiding shows a normal
          bladder. The right ureter is filled with contrast material and is markedly
          dilated and tortuous. The right collecting system is dilated as well and its
          papillae are effaced. The left side is less severely involved.
    C. Discussion
        • This child has chronic severe vesicoureteral reflux (VUR). VUR is graded
          on a scale of 1 to 5 based on the level reflux reaches and anatomic changes
          in the ureter and collecting system. This patient has grade 5 reflux on the
          right and grade 4–5 on the left.
        • VUR is thought to be caused by maldevelopment of the ureterovesical
          junction (lack of the normal valve mechanism). Sterile, colonized, or
          infected urine ascends to the upper tracts, causing a focal tubulointerstitial
          nephritis most prominent in the polar regions. Patients may or may not be

symptomatic. Mild cases are treated with antibiotics and severe cases with ureteral reimplantation. More severe sequelae are renal failure and hypertension.

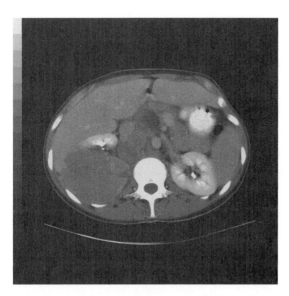

19-32

XXXII. Abdominal CT (Fig. 19-32)
  A. History
    • Right flank pain and microhematuria
  B. Description
    • Axial CT image of the abdomen at the level of the kidneys is shown. The patient received oral and intravenous contrast material. A large mixed attenuation mass arises from the right kidney, filling the perinephric space. The pararenal space is compressed but not invaded. Bulky adenopathy displaces the inferior vena cava anteriorly.
  C. Discussion
    • This patient has a large renal cell carcinoma with associated retroperitoneal adenopathy. These tumors occur later in life, especially in smokers, dialysis patients, and those with von Hippel-Lindau disease. Hematuria is the most common presenting sign. Staging is based on spread into contiguous structures and metastasis to distant structures. This patient's tumor is limited to the perinephric space, and there is no invasion of the renal vein (not shown). This is an aggressive tumor with a poor survival rate; therefore, therapy still consists of a radical nephrectomy, although some centers are pursuing radiofrequency ablations and partial nephrectomies as alternatives.

- *Tip: Hematuria plus a strongly enhancing solid lesion of the kidney. (Note that an enhanced CT scan is shown in this case by looking at the bright aorta. If there was no intravenous contrast agent administered with the same presenting history, the study they are showing you is probably one of renal stones.)*

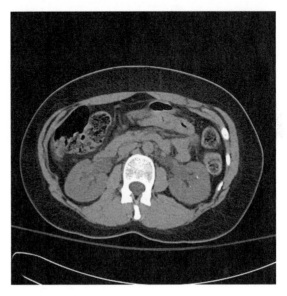

19-33

XXXIII. Abdominal CT (Fig. 19-33)
- A. History
  - Flank pain and hematuria
- B. Description
  - Noncontrast CT image through the level of the kidneys demonstrates a few calcifications within the renal collecting system.
- C. Discussion
  - Nephrolithiasis is a common disease occurring in up to 10% of the population. Although most stones can be seen on plain films, excretory urography is more sensitive in demonstrating filling defects within the opacified system, dilated collecting system and ureter, and aberrations in function. Complications include obstruction, infection, strictures, and even loss of renal function. CT is now commonly used to better detect the number and location of the stones and the presence of complications associated with them. Treatment varies, depending on the size and location of the stones.
  - *Tip: Most common causes of a filling defect in a urography are stones, blood clots, or tumor. If a noncontrast CT through the kidneys is shown, look for the calcifications.*

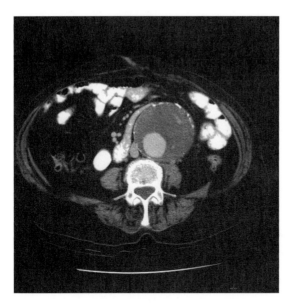

19-34

XXXIV. Abdominal CT (Fig. 19-34)
  A. History
    • Pulsatile abdominal mass
  B. Description
    • Single axial CT image of the abdomen is taken at the level of the transverse
      duodenum. The patient received oral and intravenous contrast material.
      The aorta is grossly enlarged with a peripheral rim of calcification. A large
      eccentric mural thrombus is present with a near-normal diameter true
      lumen. A high attenuation slit at 1 o'clock in the aortic cross section may
      be a normal vascular structure or intramural dissection.
  C. Discussion
    • This patient has an abdominal aortic aneurysm (AAA). Atherosclerotic
      aneurysms are a manifestation of generalized vascular disease. Risk
      factors include smoking, diabetes mellitus, high cholesterol, and
      sedentary lifestyle. The major risk of aneurysms is that they may rupture,
      showering emboli to the periphery, leading to infection and the creation of
      aortocaval or aortoenteric fistulas. Signs of rupture are usually clinically
      apparent and include acute onset of abdominal or back pain and
      hypotension.
    • Contrast-enhanced CT scan is the most precise study to determine the
      aneurysmal size and extent as well as involved branches. Angiography may
      play a preoperative role. AAA is diagnosed with aortic diameter greater than
      3 cm. The risk of rupture increases greatly at 6 cm or more in size.
    • *Buzzwords: "Pulsatile mass"*

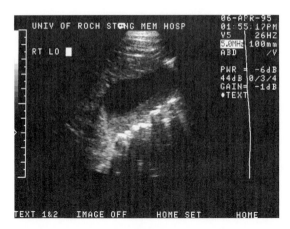

19-35

XXXV. Ultrasound (Fig. 19-35)
- A. History
  - Intermittent right upper quadrant pain
- B. Description
  - A longitudinal ultrasound image of the gallbladder demonstrates hyperechoic material layering dependently with shadowing (foci of obstruction of the sound beam).
- C. Discussion
  - This patient has multiple gallstones lying in "sludge" (inspissated bile). Stones present a strong echo with acoustic shadowing. Gallstones can be seen to move during a real-time examination. Ultrasound has a sensitivity of 95% in detecting gallstones.
  - Acute cholecystitis is diagnosed when stones are present, the gallbladder wall is thickened, and a sonographic Murphy sign is present. The latter consists of maximal pain elicited by pressing the transducer directly over the gallbladder. Associated findings may be biliary dilatation and ductal stones, or pericholecystic fluid.
  - *Tip: A positive Murphy sign plus the presence of gallstones.*

XXXVI. Transvaginal Ultrasound (US) (Fig. 19-36)
- A. History
  - Vaginal bleeding
- B. Description
  - Sagittal transvaginal ultrasound image shows a 1.5-cm complex cystic structure with a hyperechoic rim in the uterine fundus. An echogenic region is present eccentrically in the cystic structure.

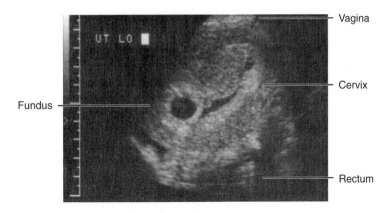

Vagina

Cervix

Fundus

Rectum

19-36

C. Discussion
- This patient has an intrauterine pregnancy of early gestational age. One fourth of all pregnant women will have bleeding in the first trimester. The differential diagnosis is based in the correlation with the last menstrual period, the quantitative β-hCG (human chorionic gonadotropin), and ultrasound.
- *Tip: A fetal pole should be seen by 6 weeks of gestation; if not present, differential considerations are early IUP, ectopic, or missed abortion. Don't forget to correlate with dates and β-hCG.*

20

Infectious Diseases

This chapter is divided into two parts: diseases by organ systems and specific diseases that are testable. Of the organ systems, infectious diseases of the ear, nose, and throat are covered in Chapter 3, Otorhinolaryngology. Infections during pregnancy and childhood are addressed in Chapters 13 (Obstetrics and Gynecology) and 17 (Pediatrics).

PART 1: DISEASES BY ORGAN SYSTEMS

I. Cardiovascular Infections
   A. Infectious endocarditis
      1. Basic science
         - Infectious endocarditis can involve the heart valves and other portions of the endocardium. The characteristic lesion of endocarditis is a vegetation, typically valvular; this represents deposition of fibrin and platelets at the infected site, often with ulceration and significant tissue damage. Risk factors include intravenous drug use (predominantly affecting the tricuspid valve) and abnormal valves due to disease (rheumatic fever), surgery (prosthetic valve), or congenital malformation (biscuspid aortic valve).
         - Endocarditis can present acutely or subacutely; both forms are fatal unless treated. Infection with *Staphylococcus aureus* usually results in acute endocarditis with rapid tissue destruction and progression of symptoms, while endocarditis due to streptococci often present subacutely. These two are the most common organisms; other bacteria and fungi occasionally cause endocarditis.
      2. History and physical examination
         - Individuals with preexisting cardiac lesions can develop subacute endocarditis after undergoing manipulation of the oropharynx (dental work), the genitourinary tract (catheterization), or the gastrointestinal system (colonoscopy).
         - Manifestations of endocarditis vary, but almost all patients will have fever. Arthritis and arthralgias are common, as are weight loss, fatigue, and malaise. Classically, there is either a new murmur or a change an existing murmur. Other physical findings include splenomegaly, petechiae, and clubbing. Found less commonly are Roth's spots (retinal hemorrhages with a clear center), Janeway's lesions (small nodular hemorrhages found on the palms and soles), splinter hemorrhages (small linear hemorrhages found in the nail bed), and Osler's nodes (tender subcutaneous fingertip nodules).

3. Laboratory and diagnostic studies
   - A typical feature of endocarditis is continuous bacteremia, as evidenced by blood cultures, due to the endovascular infection. Usually several sets of anaerobic and aerobic blood cultures are obtained from different venipuncture sites over time to improve sensitivity. Erythrocyte sedimentation rate is elevated and there is often a normochromic normocytic anemia with or without leukocytosis.
   - Chest x-ray often reveals cardiomegaly, and the echocardiogram will reveal vegetations in most patients.
4. Formulating the diagnosis
   - The diagnosis of endocarditis is dependent on the presence of positive blood cultures, without evidence of an obvious source of infection. Endocarditis may be present with other diseases, including cellulitis or pneumonia. Fever, echocardiographic findings and positive blood cultures with a history and risk factors consistent with endocarditis are essential to making the diagnosis.
5. Evaluating the severity of problems
   - The major complications of endocarditis are significant valvular damage and embolic events. Damage to the heart valves can result in congestive heart failure. Septic emboli and infarcts can occur in the lungs, brain (stroke), and kidneys (renal failure). New blocks on an electrocardiogram (ECG) may signify extension of the disease into the conduction system.
6. Managing the patient
   - Empiric intravenous antibiotics should be started after cultures are done. Initial combination therapy with a β-lactamase-resistant penicillin and an aminoglycoside (i.e., oxacillin and gentamicin) is an acceptable choice; if MRSA (methicillin-resistant *Staphylococcus aureus*) is suspected, vancomycin should be used instead of oxacillin. When culture and sensitivity results are available, therapy should be adjusted accordingly. All patients are at risk for recurrence and prophylaxis is suggested for many procedures, including those noted previously.

II. Central Nervous System Infections
   A. Meningitis
      1. Basic science
         - Meningitis is an inflammatory reaction of the meninges and subarachnoid space, including the cerebrospinal fluid (CSF) surrounding brain tissue. The two major types of meningitis are bacterial and nonbacterial (or aseptic), which is predominantly viral.
         a. Bacterial meningitis
            - Mechanisms of infection:
               - Blood-borne pathogens (systemic infection or respiratory infection)
               - Local extension from adjacent infected tissue (sinusitis, mastoiditis, otitis)
               - Direct invasion of pathogens (postsurgical or trauma)
            - Infecting organisms vary with the age of the patient and the mode of entry.

- The most common agents are *Streptococcus pneumoniae* (pneumococcus), Neisseria meningitidis, and *Haemophilus influenzae.*
- Important other agents in specific populations:
  - Neonates (group B streptococci, *Escherichia coli, Listeria monocytogenes*)
  - Infants and young children (*H. influenzae* if unvaccinated)
  - Elderly and the immunocompromised *(Listeria)*
  - Postneurosurgical patients *(Staphylococcus epidermidis)*

b. Other causes of meningitis
- Aseptic meningitis is an inflammatory reaction without an apparent infectious cause. Infectious agents include viruses (most common), bacteria, mycobacteria, and fungi. The enteroviruses constitute most cases of viral meningitis.
- In fungal meningitis, the host is usually immunocompromised (chemotherapy, chronic steroid use, or HIV) and has chronic, often low-grade, symptoms; these infections are often due to *Cryptococcus* (especially with HIV) or *Coccidioides* (prevalent in Arizona and the southwestern United States).
- Noninfectious causes:
  - Parameningeal process (such as a tumor or abscess) producing irritation
  - Presence of a foreign substance (such as air, drugs, or blood) in the CSF
  - Sulfa-containing agents, including TMP-SMZ (trimethoprim-sulfamethoxazole) and NSAIDs (nonsteroidal anti-inflammatory drugs)

2. History and physical examination
- The classic triad is headache, fever, and meningismus, but immunocompromised patients, including those at the extremes of age, may not develop these symptoms. Other symptoms may include photophobia, altered sensorium, seizures, and rash. The prodrome period for bacterial meningitis is short; for viral meningitis the prodrome may be characterized by an upper respiratory tract infection. Fungal meningitis causes an indolent infection, often with subtle signs and symptoms, often with only a headache and focal cranial neuropathy.
- Physical examination may reveal the source of infection (for example, otitis or pneumonia). Characteristic signs of meningeal irritation include Kernig's sign (neck pain with knee extension while the hip is flexed; **k**nee = **K**ernig) and Brudzinski's sign (hip flexion with passive neck flexion). Focal cranial nerve palsies may be present and are more common with bacterial meningitis. Fundoscopic examination may show papilledema, a sign of increased intracranial pressure, which is a contraindication to lumbar puncture (LP) because it may precipitate cerebral herniation.

3. Laboratory and diagnostic studies
- Once meningitis is suspected, a LP must be performed and opening pressure should be evaluated. A computed tomographic (CT) scan or funduscopic examination should be done prior to LP if mass lesion is suspected. CSF should be sent for cell count, protein, glucose, and Gram stain, and culture. Viral or fungal cultures may be sent if nonbacterial meningitis is suspected.

TABLE 20-1:

Characteristics of Meninigitis by Etiologic Agent

Etiologic Agent	CSF Opening Pressure	White Blood Cell Count (per μL)	Glucose (mg/dL)	Protein (mg/dL)	Microbiologic Findings
Bacterial	Normal to high	100–5000; >80% neutrophils	Very low	Very high	>75% culture positive
Viral	Normal	10–300; lymphocytes	Normal	Normal to slightly elevated	Viral isolation
Tuberculous	Normal to high	100–500; lymphocytes	Very low to low	Very high	Acid-fast bacillus stain and culture
Cryptococcal	Normal to high	10–200; lymphocytes	Low	Normal to slightly elevated	India ink or CSF antigen
Aseptic (including fungal)	Normal	10–300; lymphocytes	Normal	Normal to slightly elevated	Negative workup
Normal values	80–200 cm H_2O	0–5; lymphocytes	50–75	15–40	Negative workup

These studies can help differentiate bacterial, viral, fungal, and aseptic meningitis (Table 20-1). CSF monocyte predominance should prompt consideration of *Listeria monocytogenes*.

4. Formulating the diagnosis
   - Diagnosis is often clinical and confirmed by LP. Other important studies include chest x-ray, blood counts, urinalysis, and culture studies to identify the source of infection. Mimics of meningitis should be ruled out, including brain or epidural abscess (see Chapter 1, Neurology), post-ictal state, and stroke. The two latter conditions can also cause a mild CSF pleocytosis.
5. Evaluating the severity of problems
   - Without treatment of bacterial meningitis, the patient can develop brain edema, focal infarction, or die. Long-term sequelae include seizures, mental retardation, focal neurologic deficits, and chronic hydrocephalus. Hearing loss in children with *H. influenzae* meningitis is not uncommon. Complications with viral meningitis are less common.
6. Managing the patient
   - Supportive measures (airway protection, seizure precautions and electrolyte management) should be begun immediately.
   - If bacterial meningitis is suspected, immediately start empiric coverage with broad-spectrum antibiotics (i.e., vancomycin and ceftriaxone); vancomycin covers resistant pneumococccus.
   - Ampicillin can be added if *Listeria* is suspected. Narrow antibiotic coverage as culture results become available.
   - Dexamethasone should be given in all cases of suspected bacterial meningitis because, with pneumococcal meningitis, it has been shown to reduce the risk of death in adults and the risk of sensorineural hearing loss in children.

- Viral meningitis is usually a self-limited process and carries lower mortality and morbidity rates. If herpes simplex virus is suspected (many CSF red blood cells), start acyclovir. Mannitol or, if needed, ventriculostomy can be used to treat cerebral edema. Seizures are treated with benzodiazapenes and phenytoin.

III. Gastrointestinal Infections
  A. Toxin-mediated and infectious diarrhea
    1. Basic science
      - Food poisoning or infection can cause diarrhea of infectious etiology, as listed in Box 20-1.
      - Causative agents include enterotoxic (noninvasive) bacteria, invasive bacteria, viruses, and some parasites. Enterotoxins cause illness by producing a secretory diarrhea; traveler's diarrhea is most commonly caused by enterotoxic *E. coli* (E**TEC** = **t**ravel). The invasive organisms, with the exception of *Salmonella,* cause mucosal ulcerations of the bowel wall.
    2. History and physical examination
      - Signs and symptoms are based on the etiology of the gastroenteritis, but usually involve fever, abdominal pain, and diarrhea with nausea and vomiting.
      a. Enterotoxic bacteria
        - Patients with enterotoxic gastroenteritis complain of diarrhea, usually occurring within 24 to 48 hours of ingestion. *Bacillus cereus* (reheated rice) poisoning typically causes more nausea/vomiting than diarrhea; *Vibrio* species are associated with shellfish consumption. Most toxin-

---

BOX 20-1

DIARRHEAL PATHOGENS BY CLASS

Enterotoxic Bacteria	Invasive Bacteria	Parasites	Other
Enterotoxic *Escherichia coli*	*Salmonella*	*Giardia lamblia*	Enteroviruses
Bacillus cereus	*Shigella*	*Entamoeba histolytica*	Rotavirus
Vibrio vulnificus	*Campylobacter jejuni*		Norovirus (Norwalk virus)
Clostridium difficile	*Yersinia enterocolitica*		
	Enterohemorrhagic *E. coli* (O157:H7)		*Cryptosporidium* (immunocompromised)
			Cytomegalovirus (immunocompromised)

mediated food poisoning is self-limited and treatment is supportive. Stool is usually not bloody, and fecal leukocytes are rarely found. *Clostridium difficile* is associated with prior antibiotic use.

b. Invasive organisms
- Fecal leukocytes are common, and stools are occasionally bloody.
- Salmonella is an invasive organism and typically causes low-grade fevers, crampy abdominal pain, and diarrhea. Symptoms usually resolve in 3 to 5 days, unless the patient develops typhoid fever; this is characterized by persistent fever, rash, abdominal distention and rarely abdominal bleeding or perforation. Antibiotic treatment should be initiated with typhoid fever due to *Salmonella,* but should be withheld in self-limited gastroenteritis, as treatment may enhance the carrier state.
- *Shigella,* a highly infectious organism, presents much like *Salmonella* gastroenteritis and is also self-limited. Antibiotics should be used when patients appear toxic, are relatively immunocompromised (elderly, HIV), or work in health care or food service. *Campylobacter* causes symptoms similar to *Shigella* and *Salmonella.*
- *Yersinia enterocolitica,* in addition to causing gastroenteritis, may cause mesenteric adenitis, which can mimic acute appendicitis.
- Enterohemorrhagic *E. coli* (O157:H7) is associated with the hemolytic-uremic syndrome (HUS), in which the syndrome of renal failure, hemolytic anemia, fever, and thrombocytopenia follows an acute infection; use of antibiotics may increase the risk of HUS and should not be used. This strain of *E. coli* is associated with undercooked meat (EHEC = **h**amburgers).

c. Other organisms
- Viral gastroenteritis presents similar to a toxin-mediated process, though nausea/vomiting and diarrhea are often equally prominent.
- *Giardia* is a parasite found in contaminated water throughout the United States; it classically presents with profuse watery diarrhea starting 1 to 2 weeks after drinking from a mountain stream.
- *Entamoeba* is transmitted through contaminated water or fecal-oral contact and may cause nausea, abdominal pain, and bloody diarrhea. Liver abscesses may occur and are manifested by fever and abdominal pain for 1 to 2 weeks.

3. Laboratory and diagnostic studies
- Initial evaluation should include assessment of volume status and the need for hospitalization; further evaluation may be deferred for several days in those who do not have severe illness.
- Stool examination can guide therapy. The absence of occult blood and fecal leukocytes suggests either an enterotoxic bacteria or virus. The presence of fecal leukocytes strongly implies that an invasive organism is present and may require empiric antibiotic therapy while awaiting stool cultures. A complete blood count, serum electrolytes, and liver function studies may be appropriate.

4. Formulating the diagnosis
   - Gastroenteritis is a common illness; much of the diagnosis and treatment relies on clinical grounds. Testing for ova and parasites is indicated in those with HIV, persistent diarrhea, and bloody diarrhea without fecal leukocytes (amebiasis). Stool cultures can identity the pathogen. Endoscopy may be indicated if inflammatory bowel disease, ischemic colitis, or pseudomembranous *(C. difficile)* colitis is suspected. A cellophane tape or transparent adhesive tape test may be helpful to isolate pinworms in children.

5. Evaluating the severity of problems
   - Most enterotoxic diarrhea is self-limited, and severity is based on volume loss. Clinical deterioration tends to be more dramatic in patients with an invasive process. Radiologic studies to diagnose perforation or bowel obstruction may be indicated.

6. Managing the patient
   - Supportive therapy is the mainstay: aggressive hydration, with antiemetics and antimotility agents as needed. Antimotility agents such as loperamide (Imodium) or diphenoxylate (Lomotil) may be used when fevers are mild and stools are not bloody. Bismuth subsalicylate (Pepto-Bismol) may be useful when vomiting is prominent.
   - Antibiotic therapy, usually with TMP-SMZ or FQ (fluoroquinolone), is indicated for febrile illness with invasive features. Antimicrobials should *not* be used with enterohemorrhagic *E. coli* or self-limited *Salmonella* infection. Fluoroquinolones shorten the duration of traveler's diarrhea. Oral metronidazole is the treatment of choice for *C. difficile* infection and some parasitic infections such as amebiasis or giardiasis.

IV. HIV Infection
   A. HIV and AIDS
      1. Basic science
         - Human immunodeficiency virus (HIV), a retrovirus that infects the body's immune system, causes a spectrum of disease that ranges from asymptomatic to the acquired immunodeficiency syndrome (AIDS). With the advent of highly active antiretroviral treatment (HAART), HIV has become a treatable though not curable disease.
         - HIV is transmitted by body fluids, either through sexual contact, blood exposure (IV drug use, needle sticks in health care workers), or from mother to infant (either intrapartum or through breast milk). Homosexual men represent the largest percentage of patients, but currently the most common mode of transmission is between heterosexual partners.
         - HIV binds to the gp120 protein of the CD4 molecule on the surface of T helper lymphocytes. The virus is integrated into the T cell's DNA, leading to dysfunction and destruction of the T helper cells. B lymphocytes and macrophages are affected to a lesser extent. Acute infection may cause an acute syndrome or may be relatively asymptomatic; latency for a variable duration follows. AIDS is the end stage of HIV infection.

2. History and physical examination
   - Acute HIV infection can be characterized by the acute retroviral syndrome (fever, lymphadenopathy, pharyngitis, anorexia similar to mononucleosis). During clinical latency, persistent generalized adenopathy may be present. In advanced disease, temporal wasting and signs of opportunistic infections (thrush) may be evident.
3. Laboratory and diagnostic studies
   - Most laboratories use the enzyme-linked immunosorbent assay (ELISA); a positive finding is confirmed by a second ELISA and then with a Western blot. Newer rapid testing is available for both blood and saliva. Acute retroviral syndrome is diagnosed with a polymerase chain reaction (PCR) showing a high viral load (>100,000 copies/mL) with a negative ELISA because there has not been time to develop an antibody response.
4. Formulating the diagnosis
   - AIDS is defined by a CD4 less than 200 or HIV with an "AIDS-defining opportunistic illness." These illnesses include *Pneumocystis carinii* pneumonia (PCP, see next section), Kaposi sarcoma, non-Hodgkin's lymphoma, thrush, tuberculosis, cytomegalovirus (CMV), *Mycobacterium avium* complex (MAC), and toxoplasmosis. All patients with an STD, zoster (in the young), extensive psoriasis, or seborrheic dermatitis should be offered HIV testing.
5. Evaluating the severity of problems
   - HIV and AIDS predisposes patients to a host of opportunistic infection and malignancies, especially as the CD4 falls below 200; more types of infections are possible with a lower CD4 count. HIV infection invariably leads to death, though therapy can markedly slow the progression of disease and prevent infections.
6. Managing the patient
   - HAART is the mainstay of therapy, using three or four drugs in combination, and requires strict patient compliance. Initiation of therapy occurs when CD4 counts drop below 200, though this remains an area of controversy. CD4 counts should be initially monitored every 3 months to assess the efficacy of therapy. Use of AZT, the prototypical antiretroviral agent, by HIV-infected pregnant women decreases the chance of transmission to their child.
   - Once the CD4 is less than 200, prophylactic antibiotics for *Pneumocystis carinii* should be started, usually TMP-SMZ, but atovaquone and dapsone can be used in sulfa-allergic patients. When the CD4 falls below 50, azithromycin or another macrolide should be started for *Mycobacterium avium* complex prophylaxis. HIV patients should receive the pneumococcal, hepatitis B, and influenza vaccines because they are at high risk, and should be screened for tuberculosis (TB) with a purified protein derivative (PPD).
   - The treatment of common opportunistic infections is beyond the scope of this text; however, PCP is discussed below.

B. *Pneumocystis carinii* pneumonia

1. Basic science
   - *Pneumocystis carinii* is an organism that asymptomatically infects most individuals but often becomes symptomatic in immunosuppressed patients, most commonly those with AIDS. Unless patients with AIDS (CD4 < 200) receive PCP prophylaxis, the majority will become infected; in this population it is a major cause of death and can often be the first presentation of HIV.

2. History and physical examination
   - Early symptoms may be mild but usually include a nonproductive cough, fever, and progressive dyspnea. Patients should be questioned about the use of prophylactic measures and recent CD4 counts; fatigue, chest pain, and weight loss are associated symptoms.
   - Patients are often febrile and tachypneic on physical examination; if severe, they may be tachypneic or use accessory muscles. Up to 50% of patients will have clear lungs on initial presentation.

3. Laboratory and diagnostic studies
   - At minimum, resting pulse oximetry should be obtained, which often demonstrates significant hypoxia; in ill-appearing patients, an arterial blood gas (ABG) is preferred. An elevated lactate dehydrogenase (LDH) is characteristic. The CD4 is usually less than 200.
   - Chest x-ray typically reveals a diffuse bilateral interstitial pattern, though a minority has an unremarkable chest x-ray. Other less common radiologic findings include pneumothorax, nodules, cavitations, and cystic changes. PCP can be demonstrated from sputum, induced if needed, using the silver or Giemsa stain. If the sputum is negative for PCP, bronchoscopy can confirm the diagnosis.

4. Evaluating the severity of problems
   - Patients with this infection may progress to respiratory distress despite aggressive treatment. Persistent hypoxia and respiratory failure may require intubation and mechanical ventilation. Severe hypoxia (PaO_2 < 70 mm Hg on ABG) is an indication for steroids.

5. Formulating the diagnosis
   - The combination of fever, dyspnea, a nonproductive cough, and a bilateral interstitial infiltrate in a patient with HIV suggests PCP. The diagnosis is confirmed by finding the organism on specimens from either sputum or bronchoscopy.

6. Managing the patient
   - Mild to moderate PCP can be treated with oral TMP-SMZ or atovaquone. Severely ill patients should be hospitalized and started on IV TMP-SMZ or pentamidine along with steroids if indicated. The patient should be monitored closely, because they may develop respiratory failure requiring intubation or spontaneous pneumothorax. On discharge, patients should be placed on PCP prophylaxis with TMP-SMZ or dapsone.

V. Musculoskeletal and Soft Infections
  A. Osteomyelitis
    1. Basic science
      • Osteomyelitis is infection of bone, usually from one of two mechanisms.
      • In children, hematogenous seeding from a distant source is more common, and often occurs at the metaphysis of long bones, with more systemic signs.
      • In adults, the infection is usually from direct extension or penetration (diabetic foot ulcer or open fracture) but can occur with bacteremia; typically signs and symptoms are more localized. Typical pathogens are *S. aureus* and streptococci followed by the enteric pathogens; some have certain associations: *Pseudomonas* (penetrating wounds) and *Salmonella* (sickle cell). Infection due to TB or bacteremia in adults is often in the spine.
    2. History and physical examination
      • Hematogenous disease often presents with subacute symptoms, but direct osteomyelitis is more acute and localized. Systemic symptoms, including malaise and fever are often present. Tenderness, swelling, and erythema are usually present in the acute setting; chronic disease may present as draining wounds or cellulitis. Most patients with hematogenous seeding often have another identifiable recent or current source of infection.
    3. Laboratory and diagnostic studies
      • Acute phase reactants (erythrocyte sedimentation rate, C-reactive protein, platelets) are elevated. The white blood cell (WBC) count is usually elevated and may show a left shift. Blood cultures may be positive.
      • Plain radiographs of the affected area are the initial study; destruction of the normal bony architecture, evidence of soft tissue swelling, and periosteal reaction may be evident. Further investigation may require utilize bone scanning, CT, or magnetic resonance imaging (MRI).
      • A biopsy of the infected bone is recommended for organism identification, either percutaneously or surgically. If possible, the biopsy should be performed prior to initiation of antibiotics.
    4. Formulating the diagnosis
      • Osteomyelitis can sometimes present as cellulitis or a nonhealing ulcer overlying the affected bone. Diagnosis depends on the clinical presentation coupled with radiographic and microbiologic findings.
    5. Evaluating the severity of problems
      • Acute osteomyelitis may be a secondary process, so potential primary sources should be evaluated. If initial treatment is unsuccessful, chronic osteomyelitis may develop and eventually lead to amputation.
    6. Managing the patient
      • Acute osteomyelitis requires medical and surgical management. Intravenous antibiotics, such as vancomycin and FQ (depending on the causative organisms) are given for at least 4 weeks. Surgical irrigation and debridement is usually required for cure. Laboratory and radiographic follow-up are utilized to monitor progress.
      • Chronic osteomyelitis requires extensive surgery and long-term (6–12 months) antibiotics.

B. Septic arthritis
  1. Basic science
     - Infectious (septic) arthritis refers to infection of a joint, typically acute and suppurative. The etiology of the infection is usually bacterial and less commonly due to mycobacteria or fungi; the most common pathogen is *Staphylococcus aureus.* Other pathogens include streptococci, *Neisseria gonorrhoeae* (sexually active young adults), enteric pathogens, and Borrelia disease. Immunocompromised patients may be susceptible to any organisms, especially those uncommon to normal individuals. IV drug users provide direct access for the microorganisms to the circulatory system. Joint inflammation from other causes (e.g., rheumatoid arthritis) increases susceptibility to bacterial arthritis.
     - Polyarticular arthritis may be due to nonbacterial infections of the joint such as rheumatologic disease (rheumatoid arthritis) or viral arthritis (hepatitis A/B/C, mumps); the latter may be preceded by a viral prodrome.
  2. History and physical examination
     - Common complaints include pain, swelling, warmth, and erythema of the affected joint; bacterial arthritis can present as acute monoarticular joint pain and must be differentiated from gout. Range of motion will be markedly limited by pain with a septic joint. Patients may limp or may not use the affected extremity. The most common joint involved in bacterial arthritis is the knee.
     - Systemic symptoms, including malaise and fever, are often present, in addition to local warmth, swelling, and tenderness at the affected site. An effusion is usually present in the joint except with gonococcal arthritis, in which small joints (fingers) are often involved without effusion.
  3. Laboratory and diagnostic studies
     - The erythrocyte sedimentation rate, C-reactive protein, platelets, and other acute phase reactant tests are elevated. The WBC count is usually elevated and may show a left shift. Blood cultures may be positive if the infection has spread systemically.
     - Radiographic evidence of joint effusion is often present in septic arthritis. Aspiration of any effusion is recommended for diagnosis and organism identification, either percutaneously or surgically. Synovial fluid from an infected joint has a high WBC count (often >100,000 with >90% neutrophils). Fluid should also be evaluated for crystals.
  4. Formulating the diagnosis
     - A septic joint should be considered in any patient presenting with monoarticular arthritis; gout is also important to consider and demonstrates crystals in the fluid. Synovial fluid examination and culture are not always diagnostic, but often narrow the differential diagnosis considerably. Multiple joint involvement suggests a systemic process as noted above.
     - Diagnosis of viral arthritis may be difficult because it usually occurs in the postinfectious setting and acute phase viral serologic testing is negative.

5. Evaluating the severity of problems
   - Septic arthritis is severe and must be recognized promptly. Emergent referral to an orthopedic surgeon is necessary, for most cases require surgical intervention. Untreated bacterial arthritis can lead to joint destruction.
6. Managing the patient
   - Septic arthritis mandates drainage, usually with emergent surgical irrigation and debridement of the joint. Postoperative antibiotics are usually continued intravenously for several days and then orally for several weeks.
   - The choice of antibiotic should be made on the basis of Gram stain and, later, culture and sensitivity of the organism; usually vancomycin or a first-generation cephalosporin is used. If gonococcal arthritis is suspected, ceftriaxone is usually used.
   - Weight bearing should be minimized until pain and inflammation are resolved

C. Cellulitis and erysipelas
   1. Basic science
      - Cellulitis is an acute cutaneous bacterial infection often accompanied by systemic symptoms. Erysipelas is a very characteristic type of superficial cellulitis, involving only superficial dermal tissue and lymphatic vessels more extensively than cellulitis.
      - The causative agents of cellulitis are usually *S. aureus* and streptococci; with erysipelas, it is group A β-hemolytic streptococci. Diabetics tend to have a polymicrobial cellulitis with a greater potential for a septic presentation. Minor trauma or an existing skin dermatosis provide a portal of entry; predisposing conditions include diabetes, malnutrition, immunocompromised state, and lymphatic or venous obstruction.
   2. History and physical examination
      - Patients present with the abrupt onset of fever, chills, and malaise. Within 1 to 2 days of these symptoms an area of red, warm, and tender skin appears and begins to grow in size. A history of trauma to the affected area may be elicited from the patient.
      - Cellulitis is a hot, red, skin lesion with an indistinct border. Erysipelas causes a hot, bright red skin lesion with a sharply demarcated border, typically on the face or lower extremities. Involved areas may develop purpura, blisters, and even small areas of necrosis. Lymphangitis and painful, enlarged lymph nodes may occur. Cellulitis occurs most commonly on the lower extremities, although it may occur in any site after trauma (animal bites) and in chronically edematous skin (leg venous stasis).
   3. Laboratory and diagnostic studies
      - Culture or biopsy is usually negative and not typically done. Blood cultures also are usually negative but should be obtained if sepsis is suspected. WBC count is typically mildly elevated.
   4. Formulating the diagnosis
      - The diagnosis of cellulitis and erysipelas can be made clinically. The differential diagnosis includes osteomyelitis, contact dermatitis, venous thrombosis, and lymphatic obstruction by tumor.

5. Evaluating the severity of problems
  • Involved skin should be marked daily with a pen to ensure that patients are responding to antibiotics.
  • Systemic infection needs to be recognized when present; sepsis and death may occur in untreated patients. Local extension (osteomyelitis) or systemic infection with bacteremia can result without appropriate treatment.
  • Postinfectious glomerulonephritis is a potential complication of streptococcal cellulitis.

6. Managing the patient
  • Elevation of the involved site and cold compresses provide symptomatic relief. Antibiotic therapy with a β-lactamase-resistant penicillin (e.g., oxacillin) or cephalosporin is the mainstay of treatment. With the emergence of community-acquired methicillin-resistant *S. aureus* (MRSA), vancomycin and TMP-SMZ are rapidly becoming the IV and oral treatments of choice for soft tissue infections.

VI. Pulmonary Infections
  A. Pneumonia
    1. Basic science
      • Pneumonia is an infection of the lung parenchyma. Pneumonia can be caused by bacteria or viruses, and rarely by parasites or fungi. The environment in which the patient acquired the infection and the patient's health may predict the infectious agent (Table 20-2).
      • Morbidity and mortality rates from pneumonia can be high, especially in the elderly and those with chronic diseases; these populations should be vaccinated.
    2. History and physical examination
      • The presenting symptoms vary with the infecting agent. The "typical" pneumonia has an acute onset with fever, chills, productive cough, and pleuritic chest pain. The organisms involved are usually *S. pneumoniae, H. influenzae, Moraxella catarrhalis, S. aureus,* anaerobes, and gram-negative bacilli *(Klebsiella pneumoniae).*
      • The "atypical" pneumonia (*Legionella, Mycoplasma,* viruses) is insidious in onset. Lower fevers, nonproductive cough, headaches, myalgias, and the absence of organisms on Gram stain of sputum characterize these infections. *Legionella* often has extrapulmonary symptoms (confusion and diarrhea).
      • Viral pneumonia can be caused by adenovirus, parainfluenza virus, and respiratory syncytial virus; influenza can cause a primary pneumonia or lead to a secondary bacterial pneumonia.
    3. Laboratory and diagnostic studies
      • A chest x-ray reveals a lobar infiltrate with the "typical" pneumonias; patients with an "atypical" pneumonia more commonly present with a diffuse interstitial pattern.
      • In patients ill enough to be hospitalized, blood cultures and sputum should be sent for Gram stain and culture and sensitivity; patients with suspected tuberculosis or *Pneumocystis* should have appropriate special stains made. To

TABLE 20-2:

Important Pathogens and Their Associations with Pneumonia

Association	Organisms*
Community-acquired, otherwise healthy	**Streptococcus pneumoniae** Haemophilus influenzae Chlamydia Mycoplasma Viruses
Hospitalized	Enteric gram-negative bacilli, Pseudomonas Staphylococcus aureus
Winter (post-influenza pneumonia)	**S. aureus** S. pneumoniae H. influenzae
Age < 6 months	**Respiratory syncytial virus (RSV)** Chlamydia
Young adults (walking pneumonia) Elderly patients with chronic lung disease	Mycoplasma and Chlamydia S. pneumoniae H. influenzae Legionella pneumophila Moraxella catarrhalis
Alcoholism (aspiration) Asplenia (encapsulated organisms)	**Anaerobes** S. pneumoniae H. influenzae
Cystic fibrosis	**Pseudomonas**

*Organisms in boldface type are those most commonly encountered.

be interpretable, the Gram stain should have more than 25 polymorphonuclear cells (PMNs) and fewer than 10 epithelial cells per high-power field.
- *Legionella* is associated with a high LDH and low sodium and can be diagnosed with a urinary antigen test.
4. Formulating the diagnosis
    - Patients with typical symptoms and diagnostic findings are sufficient. Pneumonia should be distinguished from acute bronchitis (productive cough with simultaneous upper respiratory infection and normal chest x-ray); the latter is often viral and does not require treatment with antibiotics.
5. Evaluating the severity of problems
    - Patients with underlying pulmonary or cardiac disorders may become dyspneic with even a mild pneumonia. Arterial blood gas measurement may identify those patients in need of supplemental oxygen or more aggressive support (mechanical ventilation) during treatment.
6. Managing the patient
    - The keys to determine appropriate therapy are clinical suspicion, patient comorbidities (i.e., immunocompromised, diabetic), and Gram stain. Empiric therapy to cover both typical and atypical organisms generally employs a macrolide as an outpatient; a third-generation cephalosporin

should be added for patients requiring hospitalization. Alternative therapy uses a FQ. *Legionella* can be treated with a macrolide (azithromycin) or FQ (levofloxacin). Duration of therapy is 7 to 10 days.

B. Tuberculosis (pulmonary)

- Tuberculosis is common throughout most of the world; for USMLE Step 3, most questions focus on pulmonary manifestations, although the disease can affect any organ system. This section mainly addresses pulmonary disease.

1. Basic science

- *Mycobacterium tuberculosis* is carried through the air in infectious droplets produced when infected individuals cough, sneeze, or speak. The pathogenesis of tuberculosis (TB) occurs in two phases: acquisition and subsequent development of the active disease. Active tuberculosis may develop immediately following infection, later, or not at all. Certain populations, generally those with HIV, diabetes, or other immunocompromised states, are predisposed to the development of active TB once primary infection occurs.
- If the organism burden at exposure is high, a localized tuberculous pneumonia results, generally in the lower lobes, which heals spontaneously; it can leave a calcified parenchymal focus and hilar node that may be detected on a later x-ray. During this initial phase of infection, a tuberculous bacillemia occurs, and the organism settles in the lung apices chronically. The subsequent development of disease usually begins there.

2. History and physical examination

- Pulmonary tuberculosis should be suspected in patients with a persistent cough with or without hemoptysis, fever, weight loss, night sweats, malaise, and loss of appetite. Rales may be heard in the area of involvement, along with dullness and bronchial breath sounds if there is lung consolidation.
- Extrapulmonary disease (e.g., skeletal, gastrointestinal, meningeal, miliary) occurs in about 1% of all patients, but in the majority of patients with AIDS. Miliary TB represents widespread hematogenous dissemination and is difficult to diagnose because the clinical manifestations are protean.

3. Laboratory and diagnostic studies

a. Sputum

- Patients should have at least three sputum specimens examined by smear and culture. Cultures appear between 2 and 6 weeks. Sputum examination is considered the gold standard for pulmonary TB.

b. Tuberculin skin testing

- Dermal reactivity to purified protein derivative (PPD) is the hallmark of a cell-mediated response to tuberculosis. The test consists of the subcutaneous injection of tuberculin antigen with a subsequent reading in 48 to 72 hours. The reaction size is determined by the diameter of induration, not erythema. Definition of a positive reaction is population dependent (Box 20-2) and varies from 5 mm (in high-risk individuals) to 15 mm (in low-risk individuals) to minimize the number of false positives. False negatives can be cause by overwhelming tuberculosis,

BOX 20-2

**POSITIVE PURIFIED PROTEIN DERIVATIVE (PPD) TESTS
STRATIFIED BY INDURATION**

Considered positive with induration of 5 mm or more
(high-risk populations)
  HIV-positive individuals
  Recent contacts of tuberculosis case patients
  Patients with a chest x-ray consistent with prior tuberculosis (i.e., calcified hilar
    node)
  Patients with chronic immunosuppression (transplants, chronic steroid use)
Considered positive with induration of 10 mm or more
(increased probability of recent infection)
  Recent immigrants from high prevalence countries
  Intravenous drug users
  Residents and employees of high-risk settings (hospitals, jails, homeless, nursing
    homes)
  Those exposed to adults at high risk for active tuberculosis
Considered positive with induration of 15 mm or more
(routine tuberculin testing not recommended)
  All others undergoing screening

depressed cell-mediated immunity from HIV infection, lymphoma, malnutrition, and sarcoidosis.
  - Skin testing should *not* be used to assess for active pulmonary TB; sputum should be tested in this setting.
  c. Chest x-ray
  - Pulmonary TB nearly always causes detectable abnormalities on the chest film. Primary TB infection usually manifests as a middle or lower lung infiltrate, often with ipsilateral adenopathy. Reactivated TB usually causes cavitary lesions in the upper lobes of one or both lungs. In immunocompromised patients, particularly those with HIV, radiographic presentations are often "atypical" with diffuse lung disease instead of cavitations.
  d. Other tests
  - Rapid diagnostic tests are currently considered adjunctive because the sensitivity is variable. Diagnosis of extrapulmonary TB requires a high level of suspicion and usually tissue must be obtained.
5. Evaluating the severity of problems
  - Multidrug-resistant TB is rebounding, and patients require therapy individualized depending on sensitivities. As noted previously, TB can present outside the lungs.

6. Managing the patient
   a. Preventive therapy
      - Prophylaxis for patients with a positive PPD (more correctly termed treatment of latent tuberculosis) has been shown to decrease the incidence of conversion to active tuberculosis.
      - A positive PPD as defined in Box 20-2 should be treated with 9 months of prophylaxis; generally monotherapy with isoniazid is recommended for patients with a positive PPD. Isoniazid should always be given with vitamin B_6 (pyridoxine) to prevent peripheral neuropathy.
   b. Treatment of disease
      - The mainstay of treatment for tuberculosis is prolonged multiple drug therapy with directly observed therapy to reduce the incidence of resistance and treatment failure. Initiate a regimen including rifampin, isoniazid, pyrazinamide, and ethambutol (RIPE). Duration of total therapy is 6 months.
      - Important side effects of the major drugs to treat TB include hepatitis with rifampin, pyrazinamide, and isoniazid (no alcohol on treatment!), peripheral neuropathy with isoniazid (prevented with vitamin B_6) and red-green color blindness with ethambutol.

VII. Urologic and Reproductive Diseases
   A. Cystitis
      1. Basic science
         - Cystitis is an infection of the bladder. Isolated acute cystitis in a healthy adult nongravid female is considered uncomplicated; all other cases can generally be considered complicated. The most common cause is *E. coli; Proteus* and *Klebsiella* are less common. *S. saprophyticus* is common in young women.
      2. History and physical examination
         - The primary symptom is dysuria, often associated with frequency, urgency, suprapubic pain, and occasionally hematuria. Fever or systemic symptoms are unusual unless pyelonephritis is coexistent. Physical examination is often nonrevealing other than suprapubic discomfort.
      3. Laboratory and diagnostic studies
         - Urinalysis (UA) shows pyuria and occasionally hematuria; leukocyte esterase and nitrites are frequently positive. Urine cultures are not routinely needed in uncomplicated cases because the pathogens are predictable.
      4. Formulating the diagnosis
         - Dysuria and typical symptoms with pyuria on dipstick, in the absence of any vaginal discharge or systemic features, is sufficient to make the diagnosis. If the diagnosis is unclear, further evaluation is required; for example, vaginal discharge mandates a pelvic examination to rule out a sexually transmitted disease. Colicky pain should be evaluated with an abdominal CT to rule out nephrolithiasis.

5. Evaluating the severity of problems
   - Uncomplicated cystitis generally resolves quickly if treated; otherwise, it can progress to pyelonephritis. Complicated cystitis generally requires a longer, tailored treatment regimen.
6. Managing the patient
   - Treatment is generally with 3 days of either oral TMP-SMZ (preferred) or a FQ.

B. Pyelonephritis
1. Basic science
   - Pyelonephritis is a renal parenchymal infection; it is usually the result of a bacterial infection ascending from the lower urinary tract. Infection may also be caused by seeding from bacteremia or emboli. *E. coli* is the most common cause, along with the other organisms that cause cystitis.
2. History and physical examination
   - Patients complain of rapid onset of fever, chills, nausea, vomiting, and flank pain. Additionally, up to one third of patients complain of dysuria and frequency. Physical examination often demonstrates unilateral costovertebral tenderness.
3. Laboratory and diagnostic studies
   - UA shows the following characteristics:
     a. Detectable levels of leukocyte esterase (a WBC enzyme)
     b. Increased levels of nitrites (a bacterial metabolite)
     c. Increased pH with urea-splitting organisms (i.e., *Proteus,* associated with stones)
     d. Pyuria with or without RBCs, bacteria; WBC casts are nearly diagnostic
   - If the UA is positive, a urine culture and sensitivity should be obtained; cultures usually yield greater than 100,000 colony-forming units of a pathogen.
4. Formulating the diagnosis
   - History, physical examination, and laboratory studies suggest the diagnosis of pyelonephritis. Imaging studies are usually not needed unless there is concern for obstruction (stone or stricture) or abscess.
5. Evaluating the severity of problems
   - Patients who appear severely ill or cannot tolerate oral medications should be admitted (vomiting is common) and given parenteral antibiotics. Chronic pyelonephritis develops after repeated bacterial infection of the kidney and may progress to renal failure.
6. Managing the patient
   - Antibiotic treatment should be instituted immediately after blood and urine have been collected for culture. Patients requiring hospitalization are started on a regimen of intravenous antibiotics (ceftriaxone or FQ) and switched to oral medications once afebrile, for a total of 2 weeks. A few selected patients may be treated initially with oral agents (FQ or TMP-SMZ) under close supervision. Antibiotics should be modified once sensitivities are known.

C. Prostatitis

1. Basic science
   - Bacterial prostatitis is usually caused by the same gram-negative pathogens, such as *E. coli,* found in other urinary infections. Prostatitis generally occurs in older men and can be categorized as acute or chronic.
   - Less common pathogens in chronic prostatitis include tuberculosis and fungus. Nonbacterial prostatitis, which occurs in younger men, is a chronic prostatitis without an apparent causative organism.

2. History and physical examination
   a. Acute bacterial prostatitis
      - There is rapid onset of high fever, chills, dysuria, frequency, hesitancy, low back pain, and perineal discomfort. Fever is common and the patient may appear septic. Rectal examination shows a swollen, tender prostate; epididymitis may also be present.
   b. Chronic bacterial prostatitis/nonbacterial prostatitis
      - Recurrent urinary tract infections with the same organism, low back pain, urgency, frequency, and dysuria are typical. Fever is usually not present and the prostate is usually not tender or inflamed.

3. Laboratory and diagnostic studies
   a. Acute bacterial prostatitis
      - UA and a urine culture should be collected. Prostatic massage is contraindicated with acute bacterial prostatitis because of the risk of bacteremia. Cystitis often accompanies prostatitis, and a urine culture and sensitivity will usually reveal the offending organism.
   b. Chronic bacterial prostatitis/nonbacterial prostatitis
      - Urinalysis should be performed and a staged urine culture collected before, during, and after prostatic massage. Microscopic examination of the expressed prostatic secretions will usually show an increased number of WBCs. More than 20 WBCs per high-power field in the final sample with a identifiable pathogen is diagnostic for chronic bacterial prostatitis; with nonbacterial prostatitis, no organism is identified by culture.

4. Formulating the diagnosis
   - Age, prostate examination, analysis of prostatic fluid, UA, and culture guide diagnosis.

5. Evaluating the severity of problems
   - Acute bacterial prostatitis can lead to sepsis. Patients with acute bacterial prostatitis require hospitalization if septic or unable to tolerate oral medications.

6. Managing the patient
   a. Acute bacterial prostatitis
      - Marked bladder outlet obstruction may occur; in this setting, suprapubic drainage should be done. Oral TMP-SMZ or FQ should be started empirically. If the patient appears septic, an IV with FQ and gentamicin should be started. Antibiotic therapy should be tailored to the sensitivities from the culture and continued for 4 weeks.

b. Chronic bacterial prostatitis
- Treatment is based on urine culture and sensitivity results and is usually offered on an outpatient basis for at least 4 weeks. Ciprofloxacin is the drug of choice; TMP-SMZ is an alternative.

c. Nonbacterial prostatitis
- Nonbacterial prostatitis is difficult to treat owing to the lack of a definite cause. Treatment, usually as an outpatient, uses a trial of antibiotics for 4 weeks, α-blocking agents (terazosin), NSAIDs and sitz baths (if pain is predominant).

D. Sexually transmitted diseases (STDs)
- STDs can be divided into several syndromes: vaginitis/cervicitis, urethritis, nonulcerative genital lesions, and ulcerative genital lesions. Syphilis and HIV are discussed separately. All patients with an STD are offered HIV testing, and should be tested for *Chlamydia* and *Neisseria gonorrhoeae* (a gram-negative intracellular diplococcus). Table 20-3 summarizes the STDs.

1. Complications of STDs
- Pelvic inflammatory disease may develop in women with *Chlamydia* or gonococcal infection. Infection involving the fallopian tube may lead to scarring and ectopic pregnancy, infertility, or tubo-ovarian abscess.
- Disseminated gonococcal infection may occur by hematogenous spread of the organism. Fever, polyarthralgias, and skin lesions may occur. In young adults gonococcal infection is the most common cause of septic arthritis.

PART 2: TESTABLE DISEASE SYNDROMES

I. Infectious Mononucleosis
A. Basic science
- Infectious mononucleosis is a clinical syndrome consisting of the triad of pharyngitis, fever, and lymphadenopathy usually caused by the Epstein-Barr virus. The virus replicates in epithelial cells and B lymphocytes in the draining lymph nodes of the head and neck; it is secreted in the saliva (the "kissing disease"). The incubation period is approximately 4 to 8 weeks, but the virus can persist for up to 18 months.

B. History and physical examination
- Often, there is a prodrome of malaise, anorexia, and headaches 1 week before the onset of pharyngitis, fever, and lymphadenopathy; the acute symptoms last for 1 to 2 weeks. Severe sore throat is accompanied by pharyngeal exudate with occasional petechiae. Lymph nodes are most prominent in the posterior cervical region but can involve the axilla. The fever can be up to 40°C. Malaise and fatigue can be severe and persist for months after acute infection. Up to 50% of patients have splenomegaly. Rash may be present, especially if antibiotics were given for suspected streptococcal pharyngitis.

C. Laboratory and diagnostic tests
- Heterophil antibody testing is negative in 10% in the first week of illness; the monospot test is more specific and sensitive. Lymphocytosis is present in 75% of patients, and atypical or reactive lymphocytes are present. The patient may

TABLE 20-3:
Summary of the Sexually Transmitted Diseases

Syndrome	History	Examination	Physical Diagnostics	Causes	Treatment
Vaginitis/ cervicitis	Change in amount, odor, or color of vaginal discharge, vaginal/vulvar itching and irritation	Strawberry cervix (petechiae), gray frothy discharge	Motile trichomonads on wet prep	*Trichomonas*	Metronidazole × 7 days
		Fishy odor, thin homogenous coat on vaginal wall	Clue cells (epithelial cells with adherent bacteria) on wet prep	Bacterial vaginosis	
		Thick curdlike adherent discharge	Budding yeast on wet prep	*Candida*	Fluconazole PO × 1 dose or topical agents
		Mucopurulent cervical discharge	DNA probe	*Neisseria gonorrhoeae* (most common), *Chlamydia*	Ceftriaxone IM × 1 dose + Azithromycin PO × 1 dose
Urethritis (differentiate from UTI)	Dysuria, itching, and discharge	Mucopurulent discharge, if not evident, milk the urethra	WBCs on Gram stain from urethral swab	*N. gonorrhoeae, Chlamydia ureaplasma*	If penicillin allergic: fluoroquinolone
Nonulcerative genital lesions (asymptomatic)	Genital warts	Multiple rough papules, flat plaques, or soft exophytic lesions (condylomata accuminata)	Clinical diagnosis	Human papillomavirus (HPV)	Cryotherapy Surgery Biopsy needed for cervical warts (associated with malignancy)
	Molloscum contagiosum	Umblicated dome-shaped papules	Clinical diagnosis	Poxvirus	Surgery if symptomatic
	Syphilis (secondary)	Large elevated plaques (condylomata lata)	RPR/FTAB (see Section VI, Syphilis)	*Treponema pallidum*	Penicillin IM × 1 dose
Ulcerative genital lesions	Syphilis (primary)	Single painless indurated, clean-based ulcer (chancre)	Darkfield microscopy (for primary syphilis only)		If penicillin allergic, doxycycline × 14 days
	Herpes (may be recurrent)	Multiple painful ulcers or vesicles	PCR, culture, or Tzanck smear (multinucleated giant cells)	Herpes simplex virus (HSV)	Acyclovir for 7 days
	Chancroid	Multiple/single painful deep purulent ulcers	Gram-negative rod on Gram stain	*Haemophilus ducreyi*	Azithromycin or ceftriaxone × 1 dose

FTAB, fluorescent treponemal antibody test; PCR, polymerase chain reaction; RPR, rapid plasma reagin; UTI, urinary tract infection; WBCs, white blood cells.

also develop hematologic complications including neutropenia and thrombocytopenia.

D. Formulating the diagnosis
- Infectious mononucleosis is diagnosed clinically based on the preceding findings. A macular rash developing after use of antibiotics, typically amoxicillin for presumed strep throat, is classic with mononucleosis.

E. Evaluating the severity of problems
- Rare complications include autoimmune hemolytic anemia, splenic rupture, thrombocytopenia, and airway obstruction from pharyngeal edema (usually in younger patients). Typically patients recover spontaneously from the acute illness.

F. Managing the patient
- Supportive care and rest are the mainstays of treatment. Contact sports should be avoided for several weeks because of risk of splenic rupture. Airway obstruction can occur and should be treated with glucocorticoids.

II. Influenza

A. Basic science
- Influenza refers to the acute respiratory illness caused by influenza viruses A and B. It usually occurs in local outbreaks or worldwide epidemics. Local outbreaks occur annually during winter and are caused by antigenic drifts; pandemics are due to antigenic shifts (a rapid and marked change) of the influenza A genome. Generally, influenza B causes less severe disease than influenza A. The virus is transmitted by aerosolized respiratory secretions or direct hand-to-hand contact. Viral replication is rapid with an incubation period of less than 72 hours.

B. History and physical examination
- Most patients with influenza describe an abrupt onset of symptoms: fever, cough, sore throat, myalgias, arthralgias, and headache. There is a wide spectrum of disease severity. Most patients have fever, ranging from 38°C to 40°C for the first 3 to 4 days; diffuse myalgias and fatigue are prominent symptoms. Despite the severity of subjective symptoms, the physical findings are minimal if present in uncomplicated disease: mild erythema of the oropharynx and mild cervical lymphadenopathy. Lungs are usually clear except with underlying lung disease or primary influenza pneumonia.

C. Laboratory and diagnostic studies
- Nasal swab should be done and sent for viral culture is the diagnosis is unclear. Other studies are nonspecific are usually not indicated or helpful.

D. Formulating the diagnosis
- The diagnosis is made on clinical grounds; viral culture is especially indicated at the beginning of the influenza season or if there is no known outbreak. Aytpical pneumonia *(Mycoplasma)* or streptococcal pharyngitis can present similarly to influenza. Findings such as a markedly elevated leukocyte count, purulent sputum, or exudative pharyngitis suggest a bacterial cause. In a known outbreak, however, the diagnosis of influenza is more certain if the characteristic symptoms are present.

E. Evaluating the severity of problems
- The complications are more common in the immunocompromised, particularly at the extremes of age; pneumonia (either primary viral or secondary bacterial), Reye syndrome in children, myositis, myocarditis, encephalitis, and aseptic meningitis have all known complications.

F. Managing the patient
- Rimantadine and amantadine are two antiviral agents with activity against influenza A; they can be used prophylactically or to reduce the severity and duration of symptoms when given to patients with influenza A infection within 48 hours after the onset of disease. Zanamivir and oseltamivir (Tamiflu) are newer agents with activity against both influenza A and B and are rapidly replacing the older agents. Acetaminophen is the preferred analgesic and antipyretic because of the risk of Reye syndrome with aspirin. Antiviral therapy is not a substitute for vaccination, which is the best prevention (see Chapter 15, Preventative Medicine and Miscellaneous Topics).

III. Lyme Disease
A. Basic science
- Lyme disease is a tick-borne illness caused by the spirochete *Borrelia burgdorferi*. Lyme disease is prevalent in the Northeast, the northern Midwest, and in the Pacific Northwest, mostly in the late spring or early summer.

B. History and physical examination
- Recent travel or residence in an endemic area with a reported tick bite is the most important part of the initial history. Shortly after a tick bite, a characteristic skin lesion called erythema migrans develops at the bite site; it is a demarcated, circular, expanding, erythematous rash with central clearing ("bull's eye"). Accompanying symptoms of early Lyme disease are similar to those for influenza (myalgias, headache, arthralgias, and general malaise), but can progress within weeks to include the heart (conduction defects) and neurologic syndromes (meningitis or cranial nerve palsies such as Bell's palsy) as well as multiple sites of erythema migrans.

C. Laboratory and diagnostic studies
- Testing is problematic and diagnosis must use the combination of clinical findings and diagnostic studies. Typically an enzyme-linked immunosorbent assay (ELISA) is the screening test, but there is a high rate of false positive results and the diagnosis must be confirmed with a Western blot.

D. Formulating the diagnosis
- The diagnosis of early Lyme disease is simplest when a patient living in an endemic area presents with a tick bite followed by the typical rash; this situation, while classic, is unusual. Notably, early Lyme disease may cause disease before an antibody response is generated and may have false negative ELISA results. Diagnosis of late Lyme disease generally requires a compatible clinical syndrome with a positive ELISA and Western blot.

E. Evaluating the severity of problems
- Untreated Lyme disease can lead to meningitis, cranial neuropathies (e.g., Bell's palsy), cardiac conduction abnormalities, and significant arthritis, usually

involving the knee. Occasionally, late Lyme disease can manifest months to years later with central nervous system symptoms of cognitive dysfunction and neuropathy.

F. Managing the patient
- Treatment for most cases of Lyme disease is oral amoxicillin or doxycycline for at least 3 weeks. CNS involvement or conduction blocks require IV therapy with ceftriaxone or penicillin G for at least 4 weeks. The most frequent reason for treatment failure is an incorrect diagnosis. Patients should be advised to use insect repellents and to cover their arms and legs with clothing to avoid further tick bites.

IV. Rabies
A. Basic science
- Rabies is an encephalitis caused by a rhabdovirus following a bite from an infected animal. Animal vectors vary geographically in the United States and include bats, skunks, raccoons, coyotes, and foxes. Dogs are uncommon vector in the United States since animal vaccination was introduced, but remain common in developing countries.
- After inoculation, the virus travels in an antegrade fashion along the nerves toward the central nervous system, where it replicates and disseminates. The incubation period is dependent in part on the distance the virus must travel to reach the brain but averages 1 to 3 months.

B. History and physical examination
- Pain is followed by paresthesias at the site of the bite; hydrophobia results as attempting to drink causes extremely painful laryngeal spasms. Restlessness and changes in behavior are common. Extreme excitability and eventually convulsions and paralysis occur. The production of thick tenacious saliva is characteristic (think of a rabid animal "foaming at the mouth").

C. Laboratory and diagnostic studies
- No single simple diagnostic test is available. Saliva, serum, and CSF samples and neck biopsy (cutaneous nerve) tissue should be sent for testing after consultation with the state laboratory. Brain tissue from the animal should be tested, if available.

D. Formulating the diagnosis
- To decide whether to provide prophylaxis after a bite, the animal should be kept under observation for 10 days; if there is no evidence of disease in the animal, the patient does not need further treatment. If the animal cannot be found or examined, it should be assumed to be rabid and treatment initiated.
- In unimmunized individuals, presence of antibody in the CSF is diagnostic. If the individual has received postexposure prophylaxis, antibody titers should be repeated in several days to see if they are increasing. The pathognomonic lesion on brain histologic examination is the Negri body, although this is not present in all cases.
- The involvement of the brain stem distinguishes rabies from other viral encephalitides, though in practice this distinction is difficult. The history of

exposure is the most important clue. It is difficult to distinguish rabies from Guillain-Barré syndrome; other viral encephalitis syndromes may mimic rabies.

E. Evaluating the severity of problems
- Untreated rabies infection invariably results in death within a week after onset of clinical symptoms, usually from respiratory failure. Bites from a potentially infected animal must be assessed for the need for prophylaxis as noted previously.

F. Managing the patient
- Because the disease is almost always fatal, supportive care should be provided. After a bite, the wound should be thoroughly cleaned and repeatedly rinsed with soap and water. Both vaccine and human rabies immunoglobulin (divided between the wound site and the deltoid area) are recommended for exposures.
- Local reactions to the vaccine occur in up to 25% with mild systemic reactions (e.g., headaches, myalgias, and nausea) in 20% of recipients; true allergic reactions are rare.

V. Tetanus

A. Basic science
- Tetanus is caused by the toxin elaborated by *Clostridium tetani,* a sporulating gram-positive rod ubiquitous in soil. Although the bacteria are sensitive to several antibiotics, the spores are resistant to some disinfectants and can survive for long periods in the environment. The toxin disinhibits neurons that modulate excitatory impulses from the motor cortex, leading to increased muscle tone and spasm.
- In the United States most cases occur in unvaccinated individuals. Groups at risk include the elderly, newborns, migrant workers, and IV drug users. The incubation period is between 5 days and 15 weeks, averaging 8 to 12 days.

B. History and physical examination
- Patients may present with a history of an acute injury with soil contamination, such as a puncture wound, laceration, or abrasion; the injury can be trivial. *C. tetani* does not grow well in normal tissue and may also occur in patients with devitalized tissue (burns, frostbite, diabetic infections, dental infections, necrotic bowel, septic abortion, umbilical stumps of neonates, and injection sites of IV drug users).
- The first signs may be pain and swelling at the site of inoculation or spasticity of nearby muscles. More commonly the patient presents with stiffness of the jaw and neck, dysphagia, and irritability. The disease progresses to hyperreflexia and spasms of the jaw (trismus or lockjaw) and facial muscles. Rigidity and spasms can also involve the abdomen, neck, and back; acute asphyxia may result from spasms in the respiratory muscles and glottis. The patient is normally awake and alert throughout the illness, and the temperature is normal or only slightly elevated.

C. Laboratory and diagnostic studies
- Wound cultures may be done, though there are frequent false negatives and false positives. The WBC count may be elevated; however, the CSF is normal. An electromyogram may show continuous discharge of motor units and shortening or absence of the normal silent period after the action potential.

D. Formulating the diagnosis
- The diagnosis is made clinically and is usually obvious. The differential diagnosis includes various acute central nervous system infections such as meningitis, encephalitis, or rabies, as well as acute intra-abdominal processes that produce a rigid abdomen. Trismus may occur with acute local processes such a dental abscess, phenothiazine, metoclopramide, strychnine poisoning, and hypocalcemia. A marked increase in the tone of central musculature with superimposed generalized spasms involving the neck and face (sparing the hands and feet) strongly suggests tetanus.

E. Evaluating the severity of problems
- With the development of disease, the prognosis is worst in the elderly, neonates, and those with a short incubation period, a short period of onset, or rapid progression.

F. Managing the patient
- Management should be conducted in an intensive care unit with minimal environmental stimulation. The goals are to eliminate the source of the toxin, neutralize unbound toxin, prevent muscle spasm, and provide supportive measures (particularly respiratory) until recovery.
- Initially, it is important to adequately clean and debride the wound. Intravenous penicillin G or metronidazole should be started. Tetanus immune globulin is given to neutralize unbound toxin and should be given before manipulating the wound. The tetanus vaccine should also be given, as natural disease does not induce immunity.
- Muscle spasms may be controlled with benzodiazepenes or, in severe cases, with a neuromuscular blocking agent such as vecuronium. Mechanical ventilation and tracheostomy are often needed, especially if a paralytic agent is used. Labetalol may be used to control autonomic dysregulation.
- The course of the illness generally extends over 4 to 6 weeks. Increased tone and minor spasms can last for months, but recovery is usually complete. The overall mortality rate in the United States has been reported as 2%.
- Wound prophylaxis consists of combined adult absorbed tetanus and diphtheria toxoid (Td) and should be considered in those who are nonimmunized or incompletely immunized (less than three doses of vaccine greater than 10 years after a booster), or in those with uncertain status whenever a wound may contain contaminated material or devitalized tissue. Tetanus immune globulin is indicated for wounds (other than clean or minor wounds) if the patient is not fully immunized. Active immunization with tetanus toxoid should be started concurrently, using separate syringes and sites.
- The disease is completely preventable by active immunization—please see Chapter 15, Section I, Adult Vaccination.

VI. Syphilis
A. Basic science
- Syphilis is caused by the spirochete *Treponema pallidum*. Acquisition occurs via sexual contact, maternal transmission, or blood transfusions with an incubation period of 3 weeks. The organism penetrates through nonintact skin or

mucous membranes; it then enters lymphatic vessels and disseminates hematogenously.

- Four stages are recognized: primary, secondary, latent, and tertiary.

B. History and physical examination

1. Primary syphilis
   - A chancre, at the inoculation site, is a clean based, firm ulcer often accompanied by adenopathy; unlike chancroid and herpes, it is painless.
   - The chancre heals in 2 to 8 weeks without treatment.

2. Secondary syphilis
   - This stage occurs 2 to 12 weeks after contact.
   - It manifests with fever, headache, malaise, diffuse adenopathy, and copper-colored macular or papular rash involving the palms and soles.
   - The rash is primarily on the patient's trunk, but can involve any part of the skin or mucous membranes; papules in the groin folds can enlarge to form condylomata lata (broad, moist, gray-white plaques).

3. Latent syphilis
   - This stage follows secondary syphilis and represents a period of infection without clinical manifestations.
   - This stage may persist indefinitely.

4. Tertiary syphilis
   - This stage occurs in approximately one third of untreated patients.
   - It presents with gummas (nodular lesions of the skin or viscera), ascending aortic aneursysm, or neurosyphilis (meningitis or tabes dorsalis).

C. Laboratory and diagnostic studies

- Darkfield microscopy is the test of choice for primary syphilis. For secondary, latent, and tertiary syphilis, a rapid plasma reagin (RPR) or venereal disease research laboratory test (VDRL) should be performed; a positive result indicates that the patient has or has had syphilis. False positive results may occur in many disease states, so a confirmatory test (FTAB, the fluorescent treponemal antibody-absorption test) must be performed.

D. Formulating the diagnosis

- Primary syphilis is suggested by the chancre and lymphadenopathy. Secondary syphilis is "the great imitator" and should be considered in all patients with a suggestive rash, especially if there is palm and sole involvement, unexplained adenopathy, or flulike illness. The diagnosis requires a high level of clinical suspicion.

E. Evaluating the severity of problems

- Central nervous system, ocular, renal, splenic, or hepatic involvement may occur. Screening for other STDs is necessary, especially for HIV. Local laws may require notification of public health officials and all sexual partners.

F. Managing the patient

- The treatment for all stages of syphilis is penicillin. The recommended regimen for primary or secondary syphilis is IM penicillin (i.e., one dose of benzathine penicillin G; an alternative is doxycycline for 2 weeks). For latent syphilis, 3 weekly doses of IM penicillin or 4 weeks of doxycycline is sufficient. For

tertiary syphilis, IV penicillin must be given for 2 weeks. Pregnant women with any stage should be desensitized and treated with penicillin if allergic.
- Approximately two thirds of treated patients with secondary syphilis have an acute self-limited febrile reaction (Jarisch-Herxheimer reaction) caused by the rapid destruction of spirochetes; it is marked by the abrupt onset of headache, fever, chills, diaphoresis, gastrointestinal irritation, and exacerbation of cutaneous features. This is treated symptomatically with rest and aspirin or acetaminophen and usually resolves within 6 hours.

VII. Miscellaneous Infectious Disease Information (Box 20-3)

BOX 20-3

MISCELLANEOUS INFECTIOUS DISEASE PEARLS FOR STEP 3

West Nile virus, a mosquito-borne encephalitis (infection of the brain parenchyma), should be considered in any patient with fever and a neurologic deficit during the summer months.

Rash involving the palms and soles = syphilis or Rocky Mountain spotted fever (a rickettsial disease with fever, travel to the Rockies, low platelets, +/− tick bite).

Most rickettsia can be treated with doxycycline.

Travelers to malaria-endemic areas should receive prophyaxis; atovaquone-proguanil, doxycycline, mefloquine cover all species of malaria, including those resistant to chloroquine.

Fever in a returning traveler—think malaria, then everything else.

Neutropenic fever (absolute neutrophil count < 500 + temperature > 38°C) should be treated with double coverage for *Pseudomonas* (i.e., ceftazidime or pipercillin/tazobactam plus gentamicin); after 5 days of persistent fever, add amphotericin for fungal infections.

Palpable violaceous skin lesions in high-risk individual = Kaposi sarcoma—may be initial presentation of HIV.

H. pylori infections should be diagnosed by symptoms and cultures of ulcers and treated with a three-drug combination including agents such as bismuth, metronidazole, amoxicillin, and proton pump inhibitor (i.e., omeprazole).

Vesicular rash in dermatomal distribution = shingles (varicella zoster virus reactivation).

Descending paralysis after eating home-canned food or honey = botulism.

Common Laboratory Values

Test	Conventional Units	SI Units
Blood, Plasma, Serum		
Alanine aminotransferase (ALT, GPT at 30°C)	8–20 U/L	8–20 U/L
Amylase, serum	25–125 U/L	25–125 U/L
Aspartate aminotransferase (AST, GOT at 30°C)	8–20 U/L	8–20 U/L
Bilirubin, serum (adult): total; direct	0.1–1.0 mg/dL; 0.0–0.3 mg/dL	2–17 μmol/L; 0–5 μmol/L
Calcium, serum (Ca^{2+})	8.4–10.2 mg/dL	2.1–2.8 mmol/L
Cholesterol, serum	Rec: <200 mg/dL	<5.2 mmol/L
Cortisol, serum	8:00 AM: 6–23 μg/dL; 4:00 PM: 3–15 μg/dL 8:00 PM: ≤50% of 8:00 AM	170–630 nmol/L; 80–410 nmol/L Fraction of 8:00 AM: ≤0.50
Creatine kinase, serum	Male: 25–90 U/L Female: 10–70 U/L	25–90 U/L 10–70 U/L
Creatinine, serum	0.6–1.2 mg/dL	53–106 μmol/L
Electrolytes, serum		
Sodium (Na^+)	136–145 mEq/L	135–145 mmol/L
Chloride (Cl^-)	95–105 mEq/L	95–105 mmol/L
Potassium (K^+)	3.5–5.0 mEq/L	3.5–5.0 mmol/L
Bicarbonate (HCO_3^-)	22–28 mEq/L	22–28 mmol/L
Magnesium (Mg^{2+})	1.5–2.0 mEq/L	1.5–2.0 mmol/L
Estriol, total, serum (in pregnancy)		
24–28 wk; 32–36 wk	30–170 ng/mL; 60–280 ng/mL	104–590 nmol/L; 208–970 nmol/L
28–32 wk; 36–40 wk	40–220 ng/mL; 80–350 ng/mL	140–760 nmol/L; 280–1210 nmol/L
Ferritin, serum	Male: 15–200 ng/mL Female: 12–150 ng/mL	15–200 μg/L 12–150 μg/L
Follicle-stimulating hormone, serum/plasma (FSH)	Male: 4–25 mIU/mL Female: Premenopause, 4–30 mIU/mL Midcycle peak, 10–90 mIU/mL Postmenopause, 40–250 mIU/mL	4–25 U/L 4–30 U/L 10–90 U/L 40–250 U/L
Gases, arterial blood (room air)		
pH	7.35–7.45	[H^+] 36–44 nmol/L
P_{CO_2}	33–45 mm Hg	4.4–5.9 kPa
P_{O_2}	75–105 mm Hg	10.0–14.0 kPa
Glucose, serum	Fasting: 70–110 mg/dL 2 hr postprandial: <120 mg/dL	3.8–6.1 mmol/L <6.6 mmol/L
Growth hormone–arginine stimulation	Fasting: <5 ng/mL Provocative stimuli: >7 ng/mL	<5 μg/L >7 μg/L

Test	Conventional Units	SI Units
Blood, Plasma, Serum—cont'd		
Immunoglobulins, serum		
IgA	76–390 mg/dL	0.76–3.90 g/L
IgE	0–380 IU/mL	0–380 kIU/L
IgG	650–1500 mg/dL	6.5–15 g/L
IgM	40–345 mg/dL	0.4–3.45 g/L
Iron	50–170 µg/dL	9–30 µmol/L
Lactate dehydrogenase, serum	45–90 U/L	45–90 U/L
Luteinizing hormone, serum/ plasma (LH)	Male: 6–23 mIU/mL	6–23 U/L
	Female:	
	Follicular phase, 5–30 mIU/mL	5–30 U/L
	Midcycle, 75–150 mIU/mL	75–150 U/L
	Postmenopause, 30–200 mIU/mL	30–200 U/L
Osmolality, serum	275–295 mOsm/kg	275–295 mOsm/kg
Parathyroid hormone, serum, N-terminal	230–630 pg/mL	230–630 ng/L
Phosphatase (alkaline), serum (p-NPP at 30°C)	20–70 U/L	20–70 U/L
Phosphorus (inorganic), serum	3.0–4.5 mg/dL	1.0–1.5 mmol/L
Prolactin, serum (hPRL)	<20 ng/mL	<20 µg/L
Proteins, serum		
Total (recumbent)	6.0–8.0 g/dL	60–80 g/L
Albumin	3.5–5.5 g/dL	35–55 g/L
Globulin	2.3–3.5 g/dL	23–35 g/L
Thyroid-stimulating hormone, serum or plasma (TSH)	0.5–5.0 µU/mL	0.5–5.0 mU/L
Thyroidal iodine (^{123}I) uptake	8–30% of administered dose/24 hr	0.08–0.30/24 hr
Thyroxine (T_4), serum	4.5–12 µg/dL	58–154 nmol/L
Triglycerides, serum	35–160 mg/dL	0.4–1.81 mmol/L
Triiodothyronine (T_3), serum (RIA)	115–190 ng/dL	1.8–2.9 nmol/L
Triiodothyronine (T_3) resin uptake	25–38%	0.25–0.38
Urea nitrogen, serum (BUN)	7–18 mg/dL	1.2–3.0 mmol urea/L
Uric acid, serum	3.0–8.2 mg/dL	0.18–0.48 mmol/L
Cerebrospinal Fluid		
Cell count	0–5 cells/mm^3	0–5 × 10^6/L
Chloride	118–132 mEq/L	118–132 mmol/L
Gamma globulin	3–12% total proteins	0.03–0.12
Glucose	50–75 mg/dL	2.8–4.2 mmol/L
Pressure	70–180 mm H_2O	70–180 mm H_2O
Proteins, total	<40 mg/dL	<0.40 g/L
Hematology		
Bleeding time (template)	2–7 min	2–7 min
Erythrocyte count	Male: 4.3–5.9 million/mm^3	4.3–5.9 × 10^{12}/L
	Female: 3.5–5.5 million/mm^3	3.5–5.5 × 10^{12}/L
Erythrocyte sedimentation rate (Westergren)	Male: 0–15 mm/hr	0–15 mm/hr
	Female: 0–20 mm/hr	0–20 mm/hr
Hematocrit (Hct)	Male: 40–54%	0.40–0.54
	Female: 37–47%	0.37–0.47

continued

Test	Conventional Units	SI Units
Hematology—cont'd		
Hemoglobin A_{1C}	≤6%	≤ 0.06%
Hemoglobin, blood (Hb)	Male: 13.5–17.5 g/dL	2.09–2.71 mmol/L
	Female: 12.0–16.0 g/dL	1.86–2.48 mmol/L
Hemoglobin, plasma	1–4 mg/dL	0.16–0.62 mmol/L
Leukocyte count and differential		
Leukocyte count	4500–11,000/mm³	$4.5-11.0 \times 10^9$/L
Segmented neutrophils	54–62%	0.54–0.62
Bands	3–5%	0.03–0.05
Eosinophils	1–3%	0.01–0.03
Basophils	0–0.75%	0–0.0075
Lymphocytes	25–33%	0.25–0.33
Monocytes	3–7%	0.03–0.07
Mean corpuscular hemoglobin (MCH)	25.4–34.6 pg/cell	0.39–0.54 fmol/cell
Mean corpuscular hemoglobin concentration (MCHC)	31–37% Hb/cell	4.81–5.74 mmol Hb/L
Mean corpuscular volume (MCV)	80–100 µm³	80–100 fl
Partial thromboplastin time (activated) (aPTT)	25–40 sec	25–40 sec
Platelet count	150,000–400,000/mm³	$150-400 \times 10^9$/L
Prothrombin time (PT)	12–14 sec	12–14 sec
Reticulocyte count	0.5–1.5% of red cells	0.005–0.015
Thrombin time	<2 sec deviation from control	<2 sec deviation from control
Volume		
Plasma	Male: 25–43 mL/kg	0.025–0.043 L/kg
	Female: 28–45 mL/kg	0.028–0.045 L/kg
Red cell	Male: 20–36 mL/kg	0.020–0.036 L/kg
	Female: 19–31 mL/kg	0.019–0.031 L/kg
Sweat		
Chloride	0–35 mmol/L	0–35 mmol/L
Urine		
Calcium	100–300 mg/24 hr	2.5–7.5 mmol/24 hr
Creatinine clearance	Male: 97–137 mL/min	
	Female: 88–128 mL/min	
Estriol, total (in pregnancy)		
30 wk	6–18 mg/24 hr	21–62 µmol/24 hr
35 wk	9–28 mg/24 hr	31–97 µmol/24 hr
40 wk	13–42 mg/24 hr	45–146 µmol/24 hr
17-Hydroxycorticosteroids	Male: 3.0–9.0 mg/24 hr	8.2–25.0 µmol/24 hr
	Female: 2.0–8.0 mg/24 hr	5.5–22.0 µmol/24 hr
17-Ketosteroids, total	Male: 8–22 mg/24 hr	28–76 µmol/24 hr
	Female: 6–15 mg/24 hr	21–52 µmol/24 hr
Osmolality	50–1400 mOsm/kg	
Oxalate	8–40 µg/mL	90–445 µmol/L
Proteins, total	<150 mg/24 hr	<0.15 g/24 hr

questions

DIRECTIONS: Each numbered item or incomplete statement is followed by several options. Select the best answer to each question. Some options may be partially correct, but there is only **ONE BEST** answer.

1. A woman brings her 75-year-old mother to your office with complaints of memory problems. Her only other medical history is hypertension and a hip fracture. She relates that her mother has had progressive difficulty remembering for the past 2 years. She has problems with names, losing her keys, and forgetting appointments. She has written checks twice for the same bill and she is concerned about her independence. She has no urinary symptoms or other focal neurologic complaints. Her examination is normal except for a score of 20 (out of 30 points) on the Folstein mini-mental status examination. First-line evaluation should include all of the following *except:*
   A. Vitamin B_{12}
   B. TSH
   C. RPR
   D. Noncontrast head CT
   E. Lumbar puncture

2. You are called to see a 62-year-old man in the hospital who complains of a nosebleed that started 10 minutes ago. He is on a step-down unit for an evaluation of atypical chest pain. His past medical history is significant for hypertension and hyperlipidemia. His current medications include aspirin, a β-blocker, and a statin. His current nurse expresses concern about possible alcohol abuse. His most recent vital signs are pulse 70 bpm, blood pressure 140/80 mm Hg, respiratory rate 14, and oxygen

saturation 97% on room air. Upon entering the room, you observe a man in moderate distress due to a steady stream of blood coming from his right nares. Which of the following is the best initial step?
   A. Apply external pressure to the nares for 10 minutes.
   B. Place anterior nasal packing to prevent further bleeding.
   C. Place posterior nasal packing to prevent further bleeding and aspiration.
   D. Place both anterior and posterior nasal packing.
   E. Obtain ENT consult because of duration of bleeding.

3. A 60-year-old man with a previous history of myocardial infarction comes to your office because of progressive shortness of breath. He tells you he is unable to lie flat in bed because he gets breathless if he does so. Which of the following is *not* a sign of heart failure?
   A. Elevated jugular venous pressure
   B. Rales
   C. Hepatomegaly
   D. Edema
   E. Right parasternal lift

4. A 60-year-old woman presents to your office. Her past medical history is significant for stage 1 breast cancer diagnosed at age 45 and allergic rhinitis. Her medications include over-the-

counter loratadine. She is single, has one grown child, and is the CEO of a small local company. She is an ex-smoker with a 20 pack-year history. She relates progressive painless reduction of vision in both eyes over the previous 6 months. She reports that vision seems impaired in bright sunlight and while driving at night. She denies any medical problems. On examination, her visual acuity measures 20/50. Which of the following is the most likely diagnosis?

A. Corneal abrasion
B. Dermatochalasis
C. Cataract
D. Acute angle closure glaucoma
E. Central retinal artery occlusion

5. A 46-year-old woman presents with fatigue, generalized weakness, and lack of energy. She complains of morning stiffness lasting 2 to 3 hours. She also notes swelling in both hands with painful joints. Her symptoms have been present for 4 months. She is afebrile with stable vital signs. On physical examination, her MCPs and PIPs are tender and swollen on both hands. What is the next step to confirm the diagnosis?

A. Hand and wrist x-rays
B. Laboratory testing including rheumatoid factor, ESR, CBC, chemistry panel, and liver function tests
C. Lyme titer
D. Both A and B

6. A 26-year-old man presents to your clinic with a chief complaint of a "rash." He works as a cashier at a local restaurant. His past medical history is unremarkable. His only medication is as-needed acetaminophen. Examination reveals red plaques with silvery scale, mainly on the trunk, elbows, and knees. The following statements are true regarding this condition *except:*

A. A seronegative arthritis is associated with this disease.
B. Nail involvement is uncommon.
C. Auspitz sign can be elicited on scraping the lesions.

D. Topical corticosteroids are considered first line of treatment.
E. Severe cases may be associated with electrolyte imbalance.

7. A 79-year-old man comes to the emergency room with a myocardial infarction. He has had two previous myocardial infarctions and has made himself DNR (do not resuscitate) with the help of his long-time primary care physician. The cardiologist who admits him wants to take him for percutaneous transluminal coronary angioplasty (PTCA). There is a chance that the patient will arrest or have significant cardiac arrhythmias while undergoing the procedure. The cardiologist reverses the DNR order (i.e., he makes the patient a full code) for the procedure without talking to the patient. When asked about this by the patient's nurse, the cardiologist says that the PTCA is a temporary intervention and often resuscitation efforts are necessary even in younger, healthier patients. The nurse calls the ethics committee to inquire about this, as the patient has clearly stated to many people his wishes to be DNR. Which of the following statements is most accurate?

A. The cardiologist is correct; DNR orders can be reversed by physicians who "know better" than the patient.
B. The cardiologist is correct; the DNR order can be reversed without the patient's approval if it is only for one procedure.
C. The cardiologist is incorrect; a 79-year-old should not have a PTCA because he has outlived his life expectancy and should be DNR.
D. The cardiologist is incorrect; the patient's wishes must be respected at all times, providing that the patient has a clear understanding of the risks and benefits of treatment and DNR orders.
E. Further investigation to the cost-effectiveness of PTCA in elderly patients is needed.

8. A 19-year-old white man presents to the emergency department because of right-sided

abdominal pain, nausea, and vomiting for the past 2 days. He takes no medications and has previously been completely well. On physical examination he looks unwell, his temperature is 38°C, his pulse is 102/minute, and his blood pressure is 105/65 mm Hg. On abdominal examination there is right lower quadrant tenderness and guarding. The most likely diagnosis is acute appendicitis. Which of the following would provide the most certain confirmation of the diagnosis?

A. A positive Rovsing's sign
B. A positive psoas sign
C. A positive Murphy's sign
D. Tenderness to the right on rectal examination
E. Ultrasound examination showing a swollen appendix in the right lower quadrant

9. A 33-year-old woman without a significant past medical history reports to you for a routine annual gynecologic office visit. She complains of fatigue and generalized weakness, which is occasionally accompanied by nausea. Her vital signs reveal a supine blood pressure of 102/76 mm Hg and a standing blood pressure of 84/52 mm Hg. You notice that she has a bronze darkening of her skin. You order some laboratory studies. An electrolyte panel, including calcium and magnesium, is normal except for serum sodium of 126 mEq/L. Which of the following options is the most appropriate test to order next?

A. ACTH stimulation test
B. Serum aldosterone
C. 24-hour urine cortisol
D. Abdominal CT scan
E. Toxicology screen

10. A 34-year-old woman presents to your office with symptoms of amenorrhea and acne of 7 months' duration. Her past medical history is unremarkable and her only medication is a multivitamin. Her review of symptoms is negative for shortness of breath, chest pain, and abdominal pain. On physical examination, you

notice that she is obese and has facial hair and acne. Her pregnancy test is negative. Your most appropriate next step in the differential diagnosis of her hyperandrogenic state is to obtain which of the following?

A. CT scan of the adrenal glands and the ovaries
B. Measurements of circulating testosterone and dehydroepiandrosterone (DHEA) levels
C. Oral glucose tolerance test
D. Adrenal and ovarian vein catheterization studies
E. No further testing is needed. Start the patient on oral contraceptive pills and follow up in 12 months.

11. A 34-year-old man presents to the emergency department with a 2-day history of fever and headache. He reports no sick contacts and seems somewhat lethargic. On examination his temperature is 38.0°C with a pulse of 92 bpm and a BP of 110/64 mm Hg. Kernig's and Brudzinski's signs are negative, as is a funduscopic examination. A lumbar puncture is performed in the ED. It reveals a WBC count of 3000 with 85% neutrophils, a CSF glucose count of 40 mg/dL, and a CSF protein count of 70 mg/dL. What is the appropriate antimicrobial therapy at this time?

A. Vancomycin and ceftriaxone
B. Vancomycin, ceftriaxone, and dexamethasone
C. Vancomycin, ceftriaxone, and ampicillin
D. Vancomycin, ceftriaxone, ampicillin, and dexamethasone
E. Vancomycin, ceftriaxone, and acyclovir

12. A 17-year-old man is brought to the emergency department because of confusion. The patient is accompanied by his girlfriend. She reports that he has been previously healthy and is on no medications. She reports that the patient does not use any alcohol or other drugs. She believes that the confusion started after he returned from working on her car in a garage. What should be done next?

A. Measure oxygen saturation by pulse oximetry.

B. Place the patient on 2 L oxygen by nasal cannula and titrate up to maintain oxygen saturations above 98%.

C. Place the patient on 100% oxygen by face mask.

D. Recommend that the patient purchase a carbon monoxide detector and avoid working with cars in enclosed spaces.

E. Check an arterial blood gas.

13. A 10-day-old female infant is seen in the emergency department with a rectal temperature of 38.8°C and lethargy. There were no complications during the delivery, and the parents report no issues during the time their child spent at home. The couple has a 5-year-old son at home who had a "cold," but they reported that they had kept him away from the infant. An examination reveals no localizing signs of infection, but the infant is very lethargic. She is admitted to the pediatric ward and started on IV antibiotics after blood, urine, and CSF cultures are sent. What initial antibiotic regimen would be most appropriate?

A. Ampicillin and cefotaxime
B. Ampicillin and ceftriaxone
C. Gentamicin only
D. Ceftriaxone only

14. A 43-year-old white woman with a history of diabetes mellitus, hypertension, and trigeminal neuralgia presents with daily headaches of 6 months' duration. She has not seen a physician in 3 years. Her headaches have prevented her from completing normal daily tasks. You find that she has not had any age-appropriate cancer screening. She has a grandmother who developed invasive ductal carcinoma of the left breast at the age of 60. What is the current recommendation for breast cancer screening for this patient?

A. Screening mammogram 5 years earlier than her grandmother's diagnosis age
B. Screening mammogram every 4 years
C. Screening mammogram every 6 months
D. Screening mammogram every 1 to 2 years

E. There is no necessity for mammography at this time

The following background information applies to questions 15 and 16: A 65-year-old woman with a history of end-stage renal disease (ESRD), on hemodialysis three times per week, is admitted to the emergency department with a potassium level of 6.8 mEq/L. Her ECG shows peaked T waves. She receives 1 ampule of calcium gluconate, 10 units of regular insulin, and 1 ampule of 50% dextrose. Repeat serum potassium 20 minutes later is 6.9 mEq/L.

15. Which of the following would be the most appropriate therapy to correct this patient's hyperkalemia?

A. Administration of a kayexalate 30 g
B. Repeat insulin 10 units + 1 ampule of D_{50}
C. Repeat ECG
D. Administer 1 ampule of sodium bicarbonate
E. Hemodialysis

16. The patient may have which of the following complications as a result of her chronic renal failure?

A. Shortened bleeding time
B. Macrocytic anemia
C. Hypophosphatemia
D. Metabolic alkalosis
E. Hyperparathyroidism

17. A 25-year-old man presents with a 1-day history of watery diarrhea, four to five times in the last 24 hours, associated with mild abdominal discomfort. He is on no medications. Six months ago he had a physical examination, because his company required him to, and no abnormality was found. On examination he is afebrile, his blood pressure is 110/70 mm Hg and pulse is 64 bpm. Systemic examination was normal. What is the most appropriate course of action?

A. Admit this patient, because you cannot predict if his diarrhea will worsen.
B. Give him 1 L of 5% dextrose in saline and send him home with instructions to call you if the diarrhea worsens.

C. Prescribe an oral antimicrobial agent and loperamide and send the patient home.

D. Order stool cultures and serum electrolysis before deciding on further management.

E. Recommend an oral glucose-electrolyte solution and send the patient home.

18. A 68-year-old woman underwent a total right knee replacement 5 days ago. She is obese, and has a history of diabetes mellitus, hypertension, and coronary artery disease; 25 years ago, she was diagnosed with breast cancer, which was treated with lumpectomy, radiation, and chemotherapy. She quit smoking 5 years ago. She now presents with a sudden onset of shortness of breath. Examination reveals an anxious obese female with a respiratory rate of 28/minute, a well-healed surgical scar on the right knee, and scattered bilateral wheezes. What is the most likely diagnosis?

A. Exacerbation of chronic obstructive pulmonary disease

B. Congestive heart failure

C. Pulmonary embolism

D. Anxiety attack

E. Sepsis

The following background information applies to questions 19 and 20: A 32-year-old male lawyer comes to your office complaining of chest pain, palpitations, and shortness of breath associated with fear of losing control for the last month. The symptoms occur intermittently and last for about half an hour. The symptoms usually occur when he is meeting with clients and have caused significant impairment in his work.

19. What is the best next step in treatment?

A. A full cardiac workup

B. Reassurance and support

C. Check thyroid functioning

D. Complete blood counts

E. Plasma calcium level

20. The test comes back normal. Which of the following is the treatment of choice?

A. Cognitive behavioral therapy

B. Fluoxetine

C. Low-dose benzodiazepines

D. Cognitive behavioral therapy in combination with fluoxetine

E. Supportive therapy plus psycho-education

21. A 30-year-old woman complains of right knee pain. The knee is erythematous, tender, and swollen. She was recently diagnosed with an inflammatory arthritis characterized by swelling of bilateral MCP and PIP joints in her hands, as well as her knees and left shoulder. She denies fever, but has been complaining of fatigue. She denies alcohol, tobacco, and drug use. An arthrocentesis of the knee is performed. Which of the following is most likely to represent the synovial fluid from this patient?

A. Viscous, transparent, yellow, WBC 200/mm^3, PMN 20%,

B. Low viscosity, yellow, WBC 7000/mm^3, PMN 60%

C. Opaque, cloudy, WBC 100,000/mm^3, PMN 90%

D. Bloody, WBC 200/mm^3, PMN 50%

The following background information applies to questions 22 to 24: A 55-year-old, previously healthy man presents to your emergency room. He complains of a 2-month-long history of a progressive headache, tingling in his right arm, and blurry vision. The patient has a 25 pack-year history of smoking and drinks liquor occasionally. He works in a car factory and has a high school education. His vital signs are blood pressure 145/95 mm Hg, heart rate 78 bpm, and a temperature of 38°C. Physical examination is remarkable for mild obesity, wheezing bilaterally, and 1+ edema of the lower extremities. On funduscopic examination, you find papilledema. Neurologic examination is remarkable for right-sided hemisensory loss, right pronator drift, and problems with naming complex objects.

22. The patient's examination findings localize to which of the following areas?

A. Left pons

B. Right pons

C. Right cerebellum
D. Left cerebral cortex
E. Right cerebral cortex

23. After assuring that he is stable, what is your first step in evaluating the patient's symptoms?
A. Head CT
B. Lumbar puncture
C. Carotid ultrasound
D. Ophthalmology consult
E. Chest x-ray

24. The CT shows a large left temporal parietal mass with significant mass effect. CT of the chest shows a right upper lobe spiculated mass. Of the following brain tumors, which is the most likely in this 55-year-old man?
A. Metastatic lung cancer
B. Medulloblastoma
C. Glioblastoma multiforme
D. Schwannoma
E. Meningioma

25. A 65-year-old man with a past medical history significant for COPD is brought to the emergency department by his wife. She relates a history of a few days of malaise, myalgias, and a generalized headache recently followed by the onset of a watery diarrhea. Today he developed a high fever, shortness of breath, a nonproductive cough, and confusion. A chest x-ray in the ED reveals bilateral patchy areas of broncho-pneumonia. Which organism is most likely responsible for the pneumonia?
A. *Streptococcus pneumoniae*
B. *Chlamydophila pneumoniae*
C. *Mycoplasma pneumoniae*
D. *Pseudomonas*
E. *Legionella*

26. A young man is found lying on the ground next to a convenience store and is brought in to the hospital by the police. He is unresponsive and smells of alcohol. His past medical history, social list, and possible medications are not available. An examination reveals no signs of trauma.

Cardiopulmonary and abdominal examinations are within normal limits. Which of the following should be done next?
A. Send a blood toxicology screen.
B. Send a urine toxicology screen.
C. Administer oxygen, 0.4 mg IV naloxone, 50 mL intravenous 50% dextrose, and 100 mg intravenous thiamine.
D. Send the patient for an urgent CT scan of the brain.
E. Do nothing other than protect his airway; given enough time, the effect of alcohol will wear off and he should recover.

27. A 42-year-old woman presents to your outpatient clinic for an evaluation of 3 weeks of right wrist pain. The patient noted that the pain began suddenly after she fell in the parking lot after slipping on the ice. She notes that she used her hand to break her fall. The patient reports that she needed to go to the emergency department the next day because of severe wrist pain. X-rays were taken and were negative per the report she hands you. She describes her pain as a severe ache, which increases with flexion and extension of the wrist. Her physical examination is remarkable for limited flexion and extension of the wrist as well as increased pain with active wrist extension. She also has pain over the anatomic snuffbox and palmar side of her wrist. How would you advise the patient?
A. She most likely has a wrist sprain and should be treated in a brace for 2 weeks.
B. She most likely has a stress fracture of her distal radius from overusing her hand at work.
C. She most likely has continued pain from a bony contusion.
D. She most likely has continued pain from tendonitis of her wrist.
E. She most likely has a scaphoid fracture and should be referred to a specialist.

28. An 80-year-old man presents to your outpatient clinic with a chief complaint of fatigue over the last year. He has a history of type 2 diabetes,

congestive heart failure, and hypertension. His medication regimen includes aspirin 81 mg, lisinopril 40 mg, hydrochlorthiazide 25 mg, glipizide 10 mg, atorvastatin 20 mg, and amlodipine 10 mg. He has been cold all the time and has gained about 20 pounds. He denies orthopnea and chest pain but does note dyspnea on exertion. On examination you note a blood pressure of 144/89 mm Hg and a pulse of 68 bpm, and his face seems a little "puffy." His cardiopulmonary examination reveals no significant abnormalities. The neck examination reveals no jugular venous distention, but there is a mildly enlarged symmetrical goiter. He has 1+ bilateral lower extremity edema, and you note that he has slowed deep tendon reflexes. What is the treatment of choice for this disorder?

A. Radioactive iodine treatment
B. Methimazole
C. Subtotal thyroidectomy
D. Levothyroxine
E. β-Blocker

29. A 60-year-old man comes to you because of persistent fever of 10 days' duration and a newly diagnosed cardiac murmur. About 3 weeks ago he had a dental extraction. You suspect the patient has bacterial endocarditis. All of the following may be present in bacterial endocarditis *except:*

A. Congestive heart failure
B. Splinter hemorrhages
C. Osler's nodes
D. Heberden's nodes
E. Roth's spots

30. A 52-year-old man presents to your office for evaluation of right shoulder pain. The patient notes that pain has been present for 2 months. He has had trouble sleeping at night. The patient notes increased pain with brushing his teeth. He has difficulty putting his shirt on in the morning. Physical examination is remarkable for a painful arc of motion and impingement signs. The patient also has significant weakness with examination of his right arm compared to his

left. He is right-handed. Which of the following tests could be performed in your office today to help establish a diagnosis?

A. Perform an injection with cortisone and reexamine the patient.
B. Perform an injection with a local anesthetic and reexamine the patient.
C. Perform x-rays, then reexamine the patient.
D. Perform an injection with cortisone and a local anesthetic.
E. Perform an MRI.

31. A 30-year-old woman presents to the office with a 3-day history of a unilateral red eye. Her vision is decreased and she has significant light sensitivity (photophobia). There is a mucus-like discharge present. She reported having the "flu" with fever 2 weeks earlier. There is no history of exposure to an individual with a red eye, no history of contact lens wear, and no other associated nonocular findings. Past medical history is positive for a recent "cold sore" and a history of "hay fever." The patient is currently taking multivitamins and oral contraceptive pills. Based on the history presented, what is the best course of action?

A. Gentamicin ophthalmic solution four times a day for presumed bacterial conjunctivitis
B. Cool compresses and observation for presumed viral conjunctivitis
C. Ophthalmologic referral for presumed acute angle closure glaucoma
D. Ophthalmologic referral for presumed herpes simplex virus–related ocular disease
E. Observation and topical antihistamines for presumed allergic conjunctivitis

32. A 55-year-old man comes to you because he has been experiencing symptoms of heartburn for 15 years, for which he takes over-the-counter antacids. He has lost 5 pounds in the last 2 months after going on a diet and starting to exercise regularly. He has a 20 pack-year smoking history, but plans to quit sometime this year. His past medical history is only remarkable for laproscopic cholecystectomy. He

takes no regular medications. On questioning, he does complain of dysphagia, but only if he eats his food in a hurry. On examination, his weight is 95 kg, with a BP of 138/88 mm Hg and a pulse of 88 bpm. His abdominal examination is normal. What is the next step in the patient's management?

A. Recommend a proton pump inhibitor.
B. Order a barium swallow.
C. Order an upper gastrointestinal endoscopy.
D. Recommend he continue with over-the-counter antacids.
E. Refer the patient for pH studies.

33. An 8-year-old girl is brought to your clinic by her mother for an urgent visit. She presents with severely pruritic, thick, scaly plaques on both antecubital fossae. Her past medical history is significant for recurrent UTIs, for which she is currently undergoing an evaluation with a local urologist. She is currently not on any medications but did take a sulfa antibiotic 2 months ago. Examination also reveals prominent skin folds beneath both eyelids. What is the most likely diagnosis for her condition?

A. Pyoderma
B. Plaque psoriasis
C. Atopic dermatitis
D. Allergic contact dermatitis
E. Pityriasis lichenoides chronica

34. A 42-year-old woman, gravida 2, para 2, presents to your office for an annual physical examination. She attained menarche at age 13 and gave birth to her first child at age 25. She does not have a family history of breast cancer. She has never had a breast biopsy or an abnormal mammogram in the past. She is a smoker. On physical examination, you palpate a 1.5-cm, firm, mobile mass in her left breast. There are no axillary lymph nodes palpable and the rest of the physical examination is normal. You obtain a mammogram, which is interpreted as "normal." What is the most appropriate next step in the management of this patient?

A. Obtain a fine needle aspiration biopsy of the mass with or without an ultrasound.
B. Breast MRI

C. Repeat mammogram
D. Excisional biopsy of the mass
E. Reassure the woman; she probably has fibrocystic changes. She should take vitamin E and oral contraceptive pills and return in a year for her annual examination.

35. An 11-month-old male infant presents with his parents to the emergency department with a history of intermittent periods of crying and irritability for the past several hours, associated with emesis. Physical examination shows moderate abdominal tenderness and guaiac-positive stools. An acute abdominal series is performed and no free air or air-fluid levels are seen. An abdominal ultrasound demonstrates an intussusception. What should be done next?

A. CT scan of the abdomen
B. Upper gastrointestinal series
C. Barium contrast enema
D. Surgery to reduce the intussusception
E. Esophagogastroduodenoscopy

36. A 67-year-old white man with a past medical history of hypertension, hyperlipidemia, smoking, and a 4.0-cm abdominal aortic aneurysm (AAA) presents to your office complaining of vague lower abdominal and flank pain of 1 day's duration. His medications include hydrochlorothiazide, atenolol, lovastatin, and aspirin. His temperature is 37.3°C, his pulse is 88 bpm, and his blood pressure is 115/60 mm Hg. What is the appropriate management of this patient?

A. Outpatient workup of abdominal pain including imaging studies to evaluate for an increase in the size of the AAA
B. Transfer to the emergency department for CT scan with IV contrast of the abdomen
C. Elective repair of the AAA without further investigations
D. Admission to the hospital for aortography
E. Treat the patient empirically for possible pyelonephritis.

37. You recently read an article where the authors used a t-test to compare the incidence of pneumonia in smokers and nonsmokers; the *p*

value was <0.01. Which of the following is true regarding the data in this article?

A. There is no real difference between smokers and nonsmokers; the observed difference could have been due to chance alone.
B. There is a <1% probability that the difference observed between smokers and nonsmokers was due to chance alone.
C. There is a <0.01% probability that the difference observed between smokers and nonsmokers was due to chance alone.
D. The difference between the groups is likely to be accounted for by nonrandom sampling.
E. There is a 99% probability that the difference observed between smokers and nonsmokers was due to chance alone.

38. A 1-year-old boy comes to your office with a 1-day history of fever, poor oral intake, and irritability. His parents seem very concerned. This is only the second illness that their son has had and he is their first child. The father currently smokes cigarettes, but "never in the house." The child's height and weight are in the 60th and 40th percentiles, respectively. Which of the following best describes the American Academy of Pediatrics treatment guidelines for otitis media?

A. All children under 6 years old should receive antibiotics.
B. Children over 2 years old with known otitis media should be observed for at least 48 hours before receiving antibiotics.
C. Children over 2 years old should only receive antibiotics for recurrent otitis media.
D. Infants less than 6 months old should receive antibiotics.
E. In children greater than 16 months, observation for 48 hours is indicated prior to antibiotic therapy.

39. A 40-year-old female patient has episodic dry cough of several years' duration. She has no other symptoms. Examination reveals normal vital signs, an oxygen saturation of 98% on room air, a body mass index of 22 kg/m². Examination of the heart and lungs is normal. What is the most likely diagnosis?

A. Asthma
B. Gastroesophageal reflux (GERD)
C. Postnasal drip
D. Pulmonary tuberculosis
E. CHF

40. A 19-year-old woman is brought to the emergency department by her college roommate. The friend reports that the patient has been talking about suicide recently. Upon entering their room, the roommate found the patient leaning over the sink vomiting. She has brought a bottle of pills, which she suspects the patient ingested. The pharmacy is able to identify the pills as acetaminophen. Serum is sent for liver function tests, which come back normal. The patient is given activated charcoal and *N*-acetylcysteine. Which of the following is most appropriate at this time?

A. Ask the patient to sign a contract for her safety, and discharge her home with a referral for outpatient psychiatric evaluation.
B. Admit the patient; liver function tests should rise by day 2 or 3.
C. Consult the liver transplant team for transplant evaluation.
D. Give a prescription for *N*-acetylcysteine, instruct the patient and her roommate on its use, and send the patient home.
E. Prescribe an antidepressant and send the patient home.

41. A 58-year-old woman presents to your office with painless rectal bleeding, generally associated with bowel movements. Her past medical history includes hyperlipidemia. She underwent a total abdominal hysterectomy 5 years ago for uterine fibroids. Her current medications include atorvastatin and aspirin. Examination reveals a well-looking female in no distress with normal vital signs and external nonbleeding hemorrhoids. No other pathologic change is noted. What would you recommend?

A. Order an upper GI endoscopy to exclude aspirin-induced gastritis.
B. Ask that she stop taking aspirin and call you in 10 days if the bleeding persists.

C. Reassure her and tell her that the bleeding will resolve spontaneously.

D. Recommend immediate surgery.

E. Recommend a colonoscopy.

42. A 65-year-old man presents to the emergency department by ambulance. The neighbors had called 911 when they found the patient confused and sitting on the couch. He had not left his home in days, which was unusual for this patient. Upon arrival, the patient is moderately confused and unable to provide a good history. He has not seen a physician in 20 years and does not have any medical records at your institution. His neighbors report that he had been complaining of back pain for the last several weeks. They were unable to get the patient to stand because of weakness in his lower extremities. The patient also notes that he has some pain in his lower abdomen as well. Physical examination shows 2/5 strength in the lower extremities. Reflexes are depressed bilaterally as well. Rectal examination reveals decreased tone. Straight urinary catheterization produces 1500 mL of urine. Which of the following is your next step in management?

A. The patient requires a stat spine surgery consult.

B. The patient should be admitted to the medicine service for observation, rehydration, and serial examinations.

C. The patient should undergo a workup for malignancy.

D. The patient should undergo an MRI within 48 hours.

E. No further evaluation is required until the patients laboratory tests are reviewed, including muscle enzyme evaluation.

43. An 18-year-old woman is brought to the emergency room by her parents. She complains of seeing visions of herself dying for the last few hours. The patient is reported to have been more withdrawn in the last 2 weeks, spending most of her time in her room or out with her friends. She has no previous psychiatric history. On examination, she appears alert but confused. What is the next step?

A. Inpatient psychiatric hospitalization for suicidal ideation

B. Combination of antipsychotic and antidepressant medications

C. Urine toxicology screen

D. Obtain collateral history from her friends

E. None of the above

44. A 23-year-old woman comes to your office with a complaint of nasal congestion, facial pain, and purulent discharge. On examination, she has yellow-green rhinorrhea, congestion of bilateral nares, and pain to palpation of the sinuses. Which of the following would be most helpful for making a diagnosis of acute sinusitis?

A. Yellow-green rhinorrhea

B. Symptoms for longer than 5 days

C. Low-grade fever

D. An antecedent viral respiratory infection

E. The presence of an otitis media as well

45. A 56-year-old woman presents with a sudden onset of severe midsternal chest pain, which radiates to the back. This occurred while she was eating a large steak dinner. She is diaphoretic but has no shortness of breath or palpitations. She has a history of hypertension and diabetes, and a family history of coronary artery disease. She has no history of pulmonary disease. Examination reveals a blood pressure of 150/80 mm Hg in the right upper extremity and 120/70 mm Hg in the left upper extremity. Her heart rate is 110 bpm, and a soft early diastolic murmur in the aortic area is audible. The rest of the examination is normal. What is the diagnosis?

A. Acute coronary syndrome

B. Acute pulmonary embolus

C. Left-sided pneumothorax

D. Esophageal rupture

E. Acute aortic dissection

46. A 28-year-old nulliparous woman has been trying to conceive for more than a year without success. Her periods are regular, and she has no previous history of pelvic infections. Her physical and

pelvic examinations are normal and her vaginal and cervical cultures are negative. Her husband has a normal semen analysis. Her cycles are determined to be ovulatory and her laboratory workup is negative. Her hysterosalpingogram shows normal filling, but distal occlusion. Her laparoscopy confirms bilateral tubal occlusion with tubal distortion and adhesions distally. What is the most likely etiology for the adhesions?

A. *Trichomonas vaginalis*
B. *Gardnerella vaginalis*
C. *Chlamydia trachomatis*
D. *Neisseria gonorrhoeae*
E. *Treponema pallidum*

47. A 55-year-old man with a past medical history of hypertension and hyperlipidemia presents to your office with an acute onset of fevers, chills, dysuria, urinary frequency, and perineal/low back pain. On examination he appears to be moderately ill, with a temperature of 39.3°C, pulse of 105 bpm, and a blood pressure of 115/60 mm Hg. His cardiopulmonary and abdominal examinations are negative. He has no CVA tenderness. A urine dip in the office reveals trace blood, 2+ leukocytes, and negative nitrates. Of the following tests, which is most likely to lead to the correct diagnosis?

A. Urine culture
B. Renal ultrasound
C. Prostate examination
D. Blood cultures
E. CT scan of the abdomen

48. A 35-year-old Polish woman presents with fatigue, weakness, light-headedness, and mild exertional shortness of breath. She was found to have a hemoglobin of 9.2 g%, a hematocrit of 29%, and a total WBC count of 3100 with an absolute neutrophil count of 200 and a platelet count of 88,000. The peripheral smear showed 23% blasts of lymphoid origin. A bone marrow biopsy confirmed the presence of 90% lymphoid blasts of pre-B cell character. A diagnosis of pre-B cell acute lymphatic leukemia was made. Cytogenetic studies showed the presence of t(9,22). She immediately received induction

chemotherapy with vincristine, daunorubicin, and prednisone, which resulted in complete remission. What is the next best step in the management of this patient?

A. Start consolidation chemotherapy
B. No further treatment necessary until she relapses
C. Allogeneic bone marrow transplant
D. Radiation therapy
E. Start rituximab

49. A 20-year-old woman presents with red plaques with dusky centers and blisters on her palms and soles. She had a fever and cold sores 5 days ago, but a review of systems is otherwise unremarkable. Her past medical history is negative. She is on oral contraceptive pills, but denies any over-the-counter medications or supplements. She works as a waitress and is currently a one pack per day cigarette smoker. Which statement concerning the patient's condition is correct?

A. The condition is mostly elicited by an allergic reaction.
B. Oral corticosteroids are proved to improve the condition.
C. Mucosal lesions heal with scarring.
D. Among infections, EBV is the most common precipitating agent.
E. The lesions are nontender to palpation.

50. A 25-year-old female nurse presents to the emergency department with complaints of frequent episodes of symptomatic hypoglycemia with normal food intake. The recurrent symptoms are beginning to affect her work and she finds that she needs to take frequent breaks for snacks to prevent the hypoglycemic attacks. She denies any significant medical problems and states that her only medication is oral contraceptive pills. You check a C-peptide level, and it is low. What is the most likely diagnosis?

A. Insulinoma
B. Glucagonoma
C. A factitious disorder
D. New onset diabetes mellitus
E. MEN I

answers

1. **E** (lumbar puncture) is correct. First-line evaluation should include CMP, CBC, TSH, vitamin B_{12}, RPR, and HIV when appropriate. Head CT should be considered as part of this workup to rule out normal-pressure hydrocephalus. These are all treatable causes of dementia. LP is not part of the routine workup for classic Alzheimer's dementia. It should be considered when infection and carcinomatous meningitis are considerations.

   A (vitamin B_{12}), **B** (TSH), **C** (RPR), and **D** (noncontrast head CT) are incorrect. These are all included in the recommended first-line evaluation.

2. **A** (apply external pressure to the nares for 10 minutes) is correct. The initial step for this patient is conservative management by pressure applied to the external nares. This will stop most anterior epistaxis.

   B (place anterior nasal packing to prevent further bleeding) is incorrect. Anterior packing should be placed if compression is not effective.

   C (place posterior nasal packing to prevent further bleeding and aspiration) and **D** (place both anterior and posterior nasal packing) are incorrect. Posterior packing should be used if a posterior bleed has been identified or for brisk anterior bleeds that do not respond to conservative measures.

   E (obtain ENT consult because of duration of bleeding) is incorrect. If conservative measures fail, the patient should be seen by ENT.

3. **E** (right parasternal lift) is correct. The right parasternal lift is indicative of right ventricular hypertrophy. It is a sustained systolic lift at the lower left sternal border.

   A (elevated jugular venous pressure) is incorrect. It is a sign of congestive heart failure and is an important sign of right-sided heart failure.

   B (rales) is incorrect. It is a nonspecific sign but is often found in congestive heart failure.

   C (hepatomegaly) is incorrect. It is a finding in right-sided heart failure. If sustained pressure is applied over the liver there may be elevation of the jugular venous pressure. This is referred to as the hepatojugular reflux.

   D (edema) is incorrect. Dependent edema can be present in heart failure. It is important to remember that if the patient is bedridden, edema may be more easily detected over the sacrum rather than the lower extremities.

4. **C** (cataract) is correct. The patient's history suggests a cataract. A cataract is clinically important if it causes a significant decline in visual function. Patients often complain of decreased visual acuity but may also experience increased glare, double vision, and decreased contrast sensitivity. Symptoms may worsen in either especially bright or dim light. Often patients will complain of difficulty driving at night because of increased glare with oncoming headlights.

A (corneal abrasion) is incorrect. A corneal abrasion often presents with acute pain, usually with an associated history of eye trauma.

B (dermatochalasis) is incorrect. Dermatochalasis refers to the redundant, baggy eyelid skin that occurs with age.

D (acute angle closure glaucoma) is incorrect. Patients suffering an acute angle closure attack present with the sudden onset of pain, blurred vision, and photophobia. They may also complain of seeing halos around light sources that result from cornea swelling or edema.

E (central retinal artery occlusion) is incorrect. Occlusion of the central retinal artery (usually embolic) causes sudden, painless, unilateral blindness. This is a true ocular emergency in which every minute counts.

5. **D** (both A and B) is correct. The clinical presentation of symmetrical polyarticular arthritis mainly affecting the hands is consistent with rheumatoid arthritis. Her prolonged morning stiffness (>1 hour) also supports the diagnosis of RA. Hand and wrist x-rays are indicated to establish a baseline but may not show typical changes early in the disease. The laboratory testing should include a rheumatoid factor and ESR but the remaining studies are indicated because she will likely be started on DMARD therapy.

A (hand and wrist x-rays) and **B** (laboratory testing including rheumatoid factor, ESR, CBC, chemistry panel, and liver function tests) are incorrect. See the preceding explanation.

C (Lyme titer) is incorrect. Infectious serologic tests may be warranted in some cases but are not needed in an afebrile patient with symptoms of several months' duration. Her current symptoms are atypical for Lyme disease.

6. **B** (nail involvement is uncommon) is correct. This patient has psoriasis. Psoriasis is associated with nail involvement in up to 70% of patients. The nail involvement may be in the form of loss of transparency of the nail plate, pitting, crumbling of the nail plate, and debris underneath the nail plate. Such involvement can be an important clue to the diagnosis of psoriasis.

A (a seronegative arthritis is associated with this disease) is incorrect. Psoriasis is associated with arthritis in up to 30% of patients. The arthritis is most commonly an asymmetrical involvement of the joints. A rheumatoid arthritis–like involvement may also be seen; however, the rheumatoid factor is negative. Mutilating arthritis, as well as involvement of the axial skeleton, can also be seen.

C (Auspitz sign can be elicited on scraping the lesions) is incorrect. On scraping the plaques of psoriasis, the silvery scale can be easily removed. This leaves behind multiple bleeding spots on the skin. This finding is known as Auspitz sign and is diagnostic for psoriasis.

D (topical corticosteroids are considered first-line treatment) is incorrect. Topical corticosteroids and vitamin D analogs, such as calcipotriol, are first-line treatment for stable plaque psoriasis.

E (severe cases may be associated with electrolyte imbalance) is incorrect. Psoriasis can involve large areas of the body, leading to a condition called erythroderma. Another potentially serious presentation of psoriasis is pustular psoriasis. Both these conditions can be associated with electrolyte abnormalities and should be monitored.

7. **D** (the cardiologist is incorrect; the patient's wishes must be respected at all times, providing that the patient has a clear understanding of the risks and benefits of treatment and DNR orders) is correct. Patient autonomy is paramount in this situation. If the patient understands the risks, benefits, and alternatives to PTCA and still wants to be DNR, his wish should be honored. Physicians' judgments do not override a patient's autonomy in this setting.

A (the cardiologist is correct; that DNR orders can be reversed by physicians who "know better" than the patient), **B** (the cardiologist is correct; the DNR can be reversed without the patient's approval if it is only for one procedure), **C** (the cardiologist is incorrect; a 79-year-old should not have a PTCA because he has outlived his life expectancy and should be DNR), and **E** (further investigation to the cost-effectiveness of PTCA in elderly patients is needed) are incorrect. See the preceding explanation.

8. **E** (ultrasound examination showing a swollen appendix in the right lower quadrant) is correct. Ultrasound demonstration of a swollen appendix, often associated with focal tenderness, provides the most definitive confirmation of the clinical diagnosis of acute appendicitis.

A (a positive Rovsing's sign) is incorrect. A positive Rovsing's sign is a helpful physical sign of local peritoneal irritation, secondary to acute appendicitis and is elicited by palpating firmly in the left lower quadrant. The patient complains of pain in the right lower quadrant.

B (a positive psoas sign) is incorrect. A positive psoas sign is also a physical sign of local retroperitoneal irritation, secondary to acute appendicitis.

C (a positive Murphy's sign) is incorrect. Murphy's sign is the abrupt interruption in inspiration while palpating the right upper quadrant and is suggestive of acute cholecystitis, not appendicitis.

D (tenderness to the right on rectal examination) is incorrect. A rectal examination is mandatory and can often be the only positive physical finding in acute appendicitis, particularly when the appendix is retrocecal.

9. **A** (ACTH stimulation test) is correct. The patient's history and physical examination suggest adrenal insuffiency. A Cortrosyn or ACTH stimulation test is the best test to screen for glucocorticoid deficiency.

B (serum aldosterone) is incorrect. A serum aldosterone level is not needed to diagnose adrenal insufficiency.

C (24-hour urine cortisol) is incorrect. Random serum and urinary cortisol levels may be in the low normal range at baseline; thus, a stimulation test is a better way to test reserve. Remember, glucocorticoid deficiency occurs before mineralocorticoid deficiency.

D (abdominal CT scan) is incorrect. A CT scan would not be helpful at this point in time—the patient is not complaining of any abdominal pain.

E (toxicology screen) is incorrect. A toxicology screen may be warranted in a patient with unexplained symptoms, but this patient's history and physical examination are consistent with adrenal insufficiency.

10. **B** (measurements of circulating testosterone and DHEA levels) is correct. This patient has the clinical features of PCOS (polycystic ovary syndrome). The characteristic features of PCOS include obesity, hirsutism (hyperandrogenism), oligomenorrhea or secondary amenorrhea, insulin resistance, enlarged ovaries by ultrasound, and infertility. The diagnosis of PCOS is based upon clinical and biochemical criteria. Two out of three of the following are required to make the diagnosis of PCOS: oligomenorrhea, clinical or biochemical signs of hyperandrogenism, and polycystic ovaries (by ultrasound). In this patient, the next step in the diagnosis would be to obtain serum levels of androgens, namely, DHEA and testosterone.

A (CT scan of the adrenal glands and the ovaries) is incorrect. CT scan of the adrenals and ovaries to evaluate for the presence of an androgen-secreting ovarian tumor would be required only if the androgen levels were very elevated and other diagnostic features of PCOS were not found.

C (oral glucose tolerance test) is incorrect. Oral glucose tolerance test is required to assess for the presence of impaired glucose tolerance and diabetes mellitus but is not a diagnostic test for PCOS.

D (adrenal and ovarian vein catheterization studies) is incorrect. Adrenal and ovarian vein catheterization studies are not required.

E (start the patient on oral contraceptive pills and follow up in 12 months) is incorrect. Oral contraceptive pills with nonandrogenic progesterones can be used to treat hirsutism, regulate periods, and protect the endometrium if this patient does not desire a pregnancy. However, the diagnosis should be established first.

11. **B** (vancomycin, ceftriaxone, and dexamethasone) is correct. This patient's case is most consistent with bacterial meningitis. Infecting organisms vary with the age of the patient and the mode of entry. The most common agents are *Streptococcus pneumoniae* (pneumococcus), *Neisseria meningitidis*, and *Haemophilus influenzae*. Important other populations are neonates (group B streptococci, *E. coli*, *Listeria monocytogenes*), infants and young children (*H. influenzae* if unvaccinated), elderly and the

immunocompromised (*Listeria*), and postneurosurgical patients (*Staphylococcus epidermidis*)

If bacterial meningitis is suspected, immediately start empiric coverage with broad-spectrum antibiotics (i.e., vancomycin and ceftriaxone); vancomycin covers resistant pneumococccus. Ampicillin can be added if *Listeria* is suspected—in this case, it is not. Dexamethasone should be given in all cases of suspected bacterial meningitis because, with pneumococcal meningitis, it has been shown to reduce risk of death in adults and the risk of sensorineural hearing loss in children. Narrow antibiotic coverage as culture results become available.

A (vancomycin and ceftriaxone), **C** (vancomycin, ceftriaxone, and ampicillin), and **D** (vancomycin, ceftriaxone, ampicillin, and dexamethasone) are incorrect. See the preceding explanation.

E (vancomycin, ceftriaxone, and acyclovir) is incorrect. Viral meningitis is usually a self-limited process. If herpes simplex virus is suspected (many CSF RBCs), start acyclovir.

12. **C** (place the patient on 100% oxygen by face mask) is correct. This patient has carbon monoxide poisoning. Other manifestations of carbon monoxide poisoning include agitation, fecal and urinary incontinence, angina, nausea, vomiting, and hepatic necrosis. Physical examination is of little help in establishing the diagnosis. The patient should be given 100% oxygen to hasten the elimination of carbon monoxide. Oxygen should be continued until the patient is asymptomatic.

A (measure oxygen saturation by pulse oximetry) is incorrect. Most pulse oximeters measure carboxyhemoglobin as oxyhemoglobin, so pulse oximetry will give a falsely elevated reading.

B (place the patient on 2 L oxygen by nasal cannula and titrate up to maintain oxygen saturations above 98%) is incorrect. See the explanation for option C.

D (recommend that the patient purchase a carbon monoxide detector and avoid working with cars in enclosed spaces) is incorrect. Immediate medical intervention is necessary.

E (check an arterial blood gas) is incorrect. Blood gas analysis measures the oxygen dissolved in blood, which is unaffected by carbon monoxide, resulting in normal PaO_2 readings.

13. **A** (ampicillin and cefotaxime) is correct. Ampicillin is necessary to treat a possible *Listeria* infection. Ampicillin with cefotaxime would provide adequate coverage for the most common pathogens in this age group, i.e., group B streptococci, *E. coli,* and *Listeria.*

B (ampicillin and ceftriaxone) and **D** (ceftriaxone only) are incorrect. Ceftriaxone is contraindicated in neonates because of the risk of kernicterus secondary to the displacement of bilirubin from albumin.

C (gentamicin only) is incorrect. See explanation for option A.

14. **D** (screening mammogram every 1 to 2 years) is correct. Screening mammography, with or without clinical breast examination (CBE), is recommended every 1 to 2 years for women above the age of 40 years. Screening mammography is not recommended for women below the age of 40, both because the incidence of breast cancer is very low and also because the breasts have dense fibrous tissue, making interpretation difficult.

A (screening mammogram 5 years earlier than her grandmother's diagnosis age), **B** (screening mammogram every 4 years), **C** (screening mammogram every 6 months), and **E** (there is no necessity for mammography at this time) are incorrect. See the explanation for option D.

15. **E** (hemodialysis) is correct. This patient has a history of end-stage renal disease (ESRD) and, therefore, significantly impaired potassium excretion. Correction of hyperkalemia is best achieved in this population with dialysis. The indication for acute dialysis in this patient is hyperkalemia refractory to medical management. Her ECG has already shown the effects of elevated potassium, with rising levels despite medical therapy.

A (administration of a kayexalate 30 g) is incorrect. Kayexalate (sodium polystyrene sulfonate) will take at least 30 minutes to start acting and, with rising serum levels, will not be enough to lower serum levels effectively.

B (repeat insulin 10 units + 1 ampule of D_{50}) and **D** (administer 1 ampule of sodium bicarbonate) are incorrect. Insulin and sodium bicarbonate will transiently shift potassium intracellularly but will not effectively treat refractory hyperkalemia.

C (repeat ECG) is incorrect. Although a repeat ECG is helpful in monitoring the cardiac effects of hyperkalemia, treatment directed at lowering the serum potassium level is critical at this time.

16. **E** (hyperparathyroidism) is correct. An inability to excrete phosphorus on a chronic basis is the result of a reduced GFR. Hyperphosphatemia coupled with hypocalcemia leads to increased PTH secretion (secondary hyperparathyroidism), which has a phosphaturic effect and increases bone turnover. This disorder in calcium, phosphorus, and bone metabolism is typically referred to as renal osteodystrophy.

B (macrocytic anemia) is incorrect. Most patients with ESRD suffer from either a microcytic hypochromic anemia primarily as a result of iron deficiency anemia or a normochromic, normocytic anemia from erythropoietin deficiency.

A (shortened bleeding time) is incorrect. These patients are subject to prolonged bleeding time primarily as a function of platelet dysfunction in the uremic milieu. The etiology is multifactorial. It may be exacerbated as well because of chronic anemia.

C (hypophosphatemia) is incorrect. See explanation for option E.

D (metabolic alkalosis) is incorrect. Metabolic acidosis develops in renal failure because the kidney is unable to excrete H^+ ions, related to its inability to produce sufficient ammonia (NH_3) to buffer protons in the urine.

17. **E** (recommend oral glucose-electrolyte solution and send the patient home) is correct. The patient most likely has acute viral diarrhea, which is a self-limiting illness. An oral glucose-electrolyte solution (such as the WHO-oral rehydration solution), if taken appropriately, would prevent dehydration and electrolyte imbalance.

A (admit this patient, because you cannot predict if his diarrhea will worsen) is incorrect. The patient does not need to be admitted.

B (give him 1 L of 5% dextrose in saline and send him home with instructions to call you if the diarrhea worsens) is incorrect. The patient is not clinically dehydrated so he does not require a bolus of intravenous fluid.

C (prescribe an oral antimicrobial agent and loperamide and send the patient home) is incorrect. Antimicrobial agents are not indicated for acute watery diarrhea.

D (order stool cultures and serum electrolysis before deciding on further management) is incorrect. Stool cultures are usually of no value in acute watery diarrhea.

18. **C** (pulmonary embolism) is correct. This patient has several risk factors for developing deep vein thrombosis, especially of the lower extremities, and therefore pulmonary embolism. Risk factors for deep vein thrombosis and pulmonary embolism include immobility, lower extremity joint replacement, a prior history of deep vein thrombosis, malignancy, obesity, and the nephrotic syndrome.

A (exacerbation of chronic obstructive pulmonary disease) and **E** (sepsis) are incorrect. See explanation for option C.

B (congestive heart failure) is incorrect. Congestive heart failure is a possibility but is not the first diagnosis to consider in this patient.

D (anxiety attack) is incorrect. An anxiety attack should not be considered in this patient in the absence of any precipitating factor and prior history. A potentially life-threatening illness such as pulmonary embolism should always be excluded first.

19. **C** (check thyroid functioning) is correct. This patient most likely has episodes of severe anxiety. However, it is important to exclude organic disease, which may exaggerate his symptoms. Hyperthyroidism can present with episodes of anxiety and palpitations.

A (a full cardiac workup) is incorrect. It is unlikely that he has cardiac disease in view of his age and the fact that his symptoms only occur when he is in a stressful situation.

B (reassurance and support) is incorrect. See explanation for option C.

D (complete blood counts) is incorrect. See explanation for option C.

E (plasma calcium level) is incorrect. Hypercalcemia or hypocalcemia does not present with anxiety.

20. **D** (cognitive behavioral therapy in combination with fluoxetine) is correct. Behavioral therapy will help the patient to understand the reason for his symptoms when in a stressful environment through relaxation and imagery. Fluoxetine, an antidepressant, will also help with anxiety.

    A (cognitive behavioral therapy), **B** (fluoxetine), and **E** (supportive therapy plus psycho-education) are incorrect. See explanation for option D.

    C (low-dose benzodiazepines) is incorrect. Benzodiazepines, while useful in aborting an anxiety attack, have the potential for addiction.

21. **B** (low viscosity, yellow, WBC 7000/mm^3, PMN 60%) is correct. This patient with rheumatoid arthritis and active synovitis is most likely to have inflammatory synovial fluid. Infection may coexist and the fluid should always be sent for culture and sensitivity.

    A (viscous, transparent, yellow, WBC 200/mm^3, PMN 20%) is incorrect. This option represents a noninflammatory effusion.

    C (opaque, cloudy, WBC 100,000/mm^3, PMN 90%) is incorrect. This option represents an infectious effusion.

    D (bloody, WBC 200/mm^3, PMN 50%) is incorrect. This option is consistent with a hemorrhagic effusion.

22. **D** (left cerebral cortex) is correct. Right-sided sensorimotor symptoms and aphasia localize to the left cerebral hemisphere. The aphasia suggests this is a cortical lesion probably in or near the temporal lobe. Further language testing would be needed to more precisely localize the lesion.

    A (left pons), **B** (right pons), **C** (right cerebellum), and **E** (right cerebral cortex) are incorrect. See explanation for option D.

23. **A** (head CT) is correct. A head CT should be completed as the initial imaging modality in suspected space occupying lesion as the cause of symptoms.

    B (lumbar puncture) is incorrect. Because the patient has papilledema, a lumbar puncture is contraindicated without imaging.

    C (carotid ultrasound), **D** (ophthalmology consult), and **E** (chest x-ray) are incorrect. None of these options would provide the necessary diagnostic information in this patient.

24. **A** (metastatic lung cancer) is correct. Lung cancer is the most common *metastatic* tumor to the brain in adults. Overall, metastatic tumors to the brain are more common than primary brain tumors, making this the most likely diagnosis for this patient.

    C (glioblastoma multiforme) is incorrect. GBM is the most common *primary* brain tumor of adults.

    B (medulloblastoma), **D** (schwannoma), and **E** (meningioma) are incorrect. See explanation for option A.

25. **E** (*Legionella*) is correct. The patient's history indicates *Legionella*. The "atypical" pneumonia (*Legionella, Mycoplasma,* viruses) is insidious in onset. Lower fevers, nonproductive cough, headaches, myalgias, and the

absence of organisms on Gram stain of sputum characterize these infections. *Legionella* often has extrapulmonary symptoms (confusion and diarrhea). The presenting symptoms of pneumonia vary with the infecting agent. The "typical" pneumonia has an acute onset with fever, chills, productive cough, and pleuritic chest pain. The organisms involved are usually *S. pneumoniae*, *H. influenzae*, *Moraxella catarrhalis*, *S. aureus*, anaerobes, and gram-negative bacilli (i.e., *Klebsiella pneumoniae*). Some of the common organisms seen in the elderly with underlying lung disease are *S. pneumoniae*, *H. influenzae*, *Legionella pneumophila*, and *Moraxella catarrhalis*.

A (*Streptococcus pneumoniae*), **B** (*Chlamydophila pneumoniae*), **C** (*Mycoplasma pneumoniae*), and **D** (*Pseudomonas*) are incorrect. See explanation for option E.

26. **C** (administer oxygen, 0.4 mg IV naloxone, 50 mL intravenous 50% dextrose, and 100 mg intravenous thiamine) is correct. The very first thing that needs to be done in patients with suspected intoxications is to be certain that the vital signs are stable and the airway has been protected. Once this is ensured the patient should be given 50% dextrose solution to reverse any hypoglycemia that may have developed. Because other drugs such as opioids may be contributing to the unresponsive state, naloxone should be given, even if there is no history of opioid ingestion.

A (send a blood toxicology screen), **B** (send a urine toxicology screen), **D** (send the patient for an urgent CT scan of the brain), and **E** (do nothing other than protect his airway) are incorrect. Oxygen administration is easily done and prevents hypoxemia while the patient is being evaluated. Toxicology screens and a CT scan of the head are also important investigations which should be done later as part of the evaluation.

27. **E** (she most likely has a scaphoid fracture and should be referred to a specialist) is correct. Fractures of the scaphoid are one of the most commonly missed fractures. Fractures can be caused by a fall on an outstretched hand. Patients complain of central wrist pain. On examination they display pain over the anatomic snuffbox and decreased range of motion of the wrist. X-rays can be negative initially and may require further imaging for evaluation. A qualified specialist should treat these fractures.

A (she most likely has a wrist sprain and should be treated in a brace for 2 weeks), **B** (she most likely has a stress fracture of her distal radius from overusing her hand at work), **C** (she most likely has continued pain from a bony contusion), and **D** (she most likely has continued pain from tendonitis of her wrist) are incorrect. See the explanation for option E.

28. **D** (levothyroxine) is correct. Hypothyroidism may be insidious, especially in the elderly, and occasionally it may be hard to distinguish hypothyroidism from hyperthyroidism. However, this patient's cold intolerance, weight gain, and slowed deep tendon reflexes suggest the diagnosis of hypothyroidism. A TSH would help confirm the diagnosis. Replacement therapy with L-thyroxine is the treatment of choice. If the patient has symptomatic coronary disease, then starting a lower than projected maintenance dose is prudent.

A (radioactive iodine treatment), **B** (methimazole), and **E** (β-blocker) are incorrect. These are treatments for hyperthyroidism, not hypothyroidism.

C (subtotal thyroidectomy) is incorrect. Subtotal thyroidectomy is generally not performed except with a very large goiter that is causing local compressive symptoms.

29. **D** (Heberden's nodes) is correct. These are bony lesions seen arising from the base of the terminal phalanx of the fingers. They are typically seen in the chronic phase of osteoarthritis.

A (congestive heart failure) is incorrect. Congestive heart failure can occur if severe mitral or aortic regurgitation results secondary to bacterial endocarditis or if there is associated myocarditis. Congestive heart failure occurs in about 30% of patients with bacterial endocarditis.

B (splinter hemorrhages) is incorrect. See explanation for option D.

C (Osler's nodes) is incorrect. These painful tender swellings on the fingertips are believed to be due to a vasculitic process.

E (Roth's spots) is incorrect. These are hemorrhages in the retina with a central pale spot. They are the result of microemboli and can be seen in bacterial endocarditis.

30. **B** (perform an injection with a local anesthetic and reexamine the patient) is correct. The history and portions of the physical examination suggest an impingement-type syndrome (rotator cuff pathology). However, significant weakness is generally not present and suggests possible rotator cuff tear or other pathology. An injection followed by a reexamination would help sort out whether the weakness is secondary to pain or if another disorder is present (e.g., a rotator cuff tear).

A (perform an injection with cortisone and reexamine the patient), **C** (perform x-rays, then reexamine the patient), **D** (perform an injection with cortisone and a local anesthetic), and **E** (perform an MRI) are incorrect. See the preceding explanation.

31. **D** (ophthalmologic referral for presumed herpes simplex virus–related ocular disease) is correct. When dealing with an "acute red eye," it is imperative to establish a history of the present illness. One should explore the course of development, the presence of a discharge (bacterial infections produce more than viral), pain, recent upper respiratory infection (suggesting viral conjunctivitis), photophobia (suggesting iritis), foreign body sensation, itching (suggesting allergic conjunctivitis), burning, associated fever or rash, or decreased visual acuity. Elements of the past ocular history may be relevant, including glaucoma and contact lens wear. A history of atopic disease may be important in the diagnosis of allergic conjunctivitis. A history of herpes simplex virus labialis may be significant. In this patient, the history of herpes labialis and significant photophobia are related to herpes simplex virus–related ocular disease.

A (gentamicin ophthalmic solution four times a day for presumed bacterial conjunctivitis), **B** (cool compresses and observation for presumed viral conjunctivitis), **C** (ophthalmologic referral for presumed acute angle closure glaucoma), and **E** (observation and topical antihistamines for presumed allergic conjunctivitis) are incorrect. See the explanation for option D.

32. **C** (order an upper gastrointestinal endoscopy) is correct. The history of long-standing gastroesophageal reflux and smoking predisposes the patient to esophageal cancer. This is best detected by an upper gastrointestinal endoscopy, which also provides the opportunity to biopsy any abnormality. Smoking cessation should be recommended to all patients.

A (recommend a proton pump inhibitor), **B** (order a barium swallow), and **E** (refer the patient for pH studies) are incorrect. See the explanation for option C.

D (recommend he continue with over-the-counter antacids) is incorrect. Proton pump inhibitors are more effective than over-the-counter antacids in preventing the symptoms of gastroesophageal reflux disease.

33. **C** (atopic dermatitis) is correct. Involvement of the flexural area in a child with severely itchy and lichenified plaques is suggestive of atopic dermatitis. In addition, the presence of a prominent skin fold under both eyelids, which is known as the Dennie-Morgan fold, is seen in atopic individuals.

A (pyoderma) is incorrect. Pyoderma usually presents as red, crusted, or pustular lesions. They may look severely inflamed and may be weepy.

B (plaque psoriasis) is incorrect. Plaque psoriasis usually presents on the extensor surfaces, instead of flexor surfaces. The plaques are erythematous and covered with a silvery white scale. On scraping the lesions, the skin comes off easily, leaving bleeding pinpoints. This is known as the Auspitz sign.

D (allergic contact dermatitis) is incorrect. Chronic allergic contact dermatitis can present as thick, lichenified, scaly plaques. The flexor areas can be affected in airborne contact dermatitis. However, the clue in this question is the presence of the Dennie-Morgan fold, which is seen in atopic dermatitis.

E (pityriasis lichenoides chronica) is incorrect. Pityriasis lichenoid chronica is a skin condition characterized by small uniform papular lesions with mica-like scale. These are generalized lesions and do not localize to the flexor areas.

34. **A** (obtain a fine needle aspiration biopsy [FNAB] of the mass with or without an ultrasound) is correct. Mammography is recommended as part of the evaluation of any woman age 35 or older who has a breast mass. However, mammography usually cannot determine whether a lump is benign. In addition, mammography misses 10% to 20% of clinically palpable breast cancers. Thus, a negative mammogram should not stop further investigation. FNAB can be performed if the lump remains easily palpable and feels cystic (round, smooth, and not hard) and the patient wants quick resolution of the issue. If fluid is obtained and is not bloody and the mass disappears completely, the patient can be reassured and followed in 4 to 6 weeks to check for recurrence or re-accumulation. A recurrence suggests the need for surgical referral. Bloody fluid should be sent for cytologic testing. If the lump does not feel cystic, the patient may be referred for ultrasound. If ultrasound shows a solid mass, the patient should undergo FNAB, core needle biopsy, or excisional biopsy. If a solid lump is small (<1 cm) and is not clinically suspicious (e.g., is soft, not fixed, not new, and not changing), it is likely to be a fibroadenoma and the patient can be followed with physical examination every 3 to 6 months. Solid masses with malignant or suspicious cytologic features should receive definitive therapy or excisional biopsy. Masses that are not suspicious need careful follow-up.

B (breast MRI) is incorrect. Breast MRI is being evaluated for screening women at high risk for breast cancer, such as those with *BRCA1* and *BRCA2* mutations, a group for which the sensitivity of mammography is low. MRI should not be used for routine screening, diagnosis, or staging of the breast carcinoma outside a clinical trial.

C (repeat mammogram) is incorrect. Repeat mammogram will not add much diagnostic value and should not be done.

D (excisional biopsy of the mass) is incorrect. Excisional biopsy of the mass may be required if the cytologic appearance is suspicious after FNAB, but is not the initial test of choice.

E (reassure the woman; she probably has fibrocytic changes) is incorrect. Reassuring the woman that the mass is fibrocystic disease can only be done if the cytologic test comes back negative.

35. **C** (barium contrast enema) is correct. Barium contrast enema is both diagnostic and therapeutic in the management of most patients with an intussusception.

A (CT scan of the abdomen) is incorrect. CT scan will not provide any additional information and also exposes the young child or infant to unnecessary radiation.

D (surgery to reduce the intussusception) is incorrect. Surgery should be reserved for patients in whom gangrene or perforation of the bowel is suspected or in those patients in whom the intussusception is recurrent.

B (upper gastrointestinal series) and **E** (esophagogastroduodenoscopy) are incorrect. See the preceding explanations.

36. **B** (transfer to the emergency department for CT scan with IV contrast of the abdomen) is correct. The presence of vague abdominal pain in a patient with a known AAA constitutes an emergency because rupture, dissection, or leak of the abdominal aneurysm must be ruled out. Mesenteric ischemia and visceral perforation are other important diagnostic considerations. This patient should be immediately transferred to a setting where rapid evaluation and, if necessary, surgical or endovascular intervention can be undertaken. CT scan would be the diagnostic modality of choice, as it would best define the anatomy and the relationship of the AAA to adjacent structures.

A (outpatient workup of abdominal pain) is incorrect. A newly symptomatic aortic aneurysm demands urgent evaluation in a setting where surgery can be performed rapidly if needed.

C (elective repair of the AAA without further investigations) is incorrect. There are other diagnostic possibilities. Although leakage or impending rupture is the direst possibility, it is not the only one. Urgent evaluation in a center capable of intervening rapidly either surgically or via an endovascular approach is the best option.

D (admission to the hospital for aortography) is incorrect. CT scan provides more information and is noninvasive.

E (treat the patient empirically for possible pyelonephritis) is incorrect. Although pyelonephritis is in the differential diagnosis, the more dire diagnostic possibility is leak or impending rupture. It would be appropriate to test his urine, but urgent evaluation of the aneurysm should be undertaken simultaneously.

37. **B** (there is a <1% probability that the difference observed between smokers and nonsmokers was due to chance alone) is correct. A p value provides a numerical value of the probability that chance alone accounts for the difference observed. If expressed as a percentage, it gives the probability that the result occurred by chance alone. A p of <0.01 means that there is less than 1% probability that the observed difference occurred by chance alone.

A (there is no real difference between smokers and nonsmokers; the observed difference could have been due to chance alone), **C** (there is a <0.01% probability that the difference observed between smokers and nonsmokers was due to chance alone), **D** (the difference between the groups is likely to be accounted for by nonrandom sampling), and

E (there is a 99% probability that the difference observed between smokers and nonsmokers was due to chance alone) are incorrect. See the explanation for option B.

38. D (infants less than 6 months old should receive antibiotics) is correct. According to the most recent guidelines, all infants younger than 6 months and all children 6 months to 2 years with severe illness or definitive otitis media should receive antibiotics. Patients over 2 years old should be given antibiotics for known otitis media, but be observed if the diagnosis is not certain. Recurrence of otitis media is not an indication for treating with antibiotics.

A (all children under 6 years old should receive antibiotics), B (children over 2 years old with known otitis media should be observed for at least 48 hours before receiving antibiotics), C (children over 2 years old should only receive antibiotics for recurrent otitis media), and E (in children greater than 16 months, observation for 48 hours is indicated prior to antibiotic therapy) are incorrect. See the explanation for option D.

39. C (postnasal drip) is correct. Postnasal drip is the most common cause of an idiopathic cough. A trial of a first-generation antihistamine and decongestant is usually the first intervention tried.

A (asthma), B (GERD), D (pulmonary tuberculosis), and E (CHF) are incorrect. Asthma, GERD, and postnasal drip can all present with a chronic cough and no other symptom. Angiotensin-converting enzyme inhibitors are also a cause of chronic dry cough. A therapeutic trial with bronchodilators will help confirm or exclude the diagnosis of asthma. For GERD, which presents with cough, twice the usual dose of a proton pump inhibitor is necessary for 2 to 3 months before a response is apparent.

40. B (admit the patient) is correct. Because the patient is vomiting, it is likely that she ingested the acetaminophen tablets at least 4 hours ago. Evidence of liver damage is manifest about 24 to 48 hours later, and maximal hepatic abnormalities may not occur until 4 to 6 days following ingestion. The blood level of acetaminophen about 4 hours after ingestion correlates reasonably well with the degree of hepatic damage. Activated charcoal and gastric lavage are generally not useful if done more than 4 hours after ingestion. The concern with acetaminophen is fulminant hepatic failure, and this requires prompt treatment with *N*-acetylcysteine. Laboratory monitoring should include electrolytes, LFTs, and PT/INR. The patient's mental status should be closely followed, as well.

A (ask the patient to sign a contract for her safety, and discharge her home with a referral for outpatient psychiatric evaluation), C (consult the liver transplant team for transplant evaluation), D (give a prescription for *N*-acetylcysteine, instruct the patient and her roommate on its use, and send the patient home), and E (prescribe an antidepressant and send the patient home) are incorrect.

41. E (recommend a colonoscopy) is correct. This patient is at risk of a colon malignancy because she is over the age of 50. This condition must be ruled out by colonoscopy, even if the patient has hemorrhoids that could explain the bleeding.

A (order an upper GI endoscopy to exclude aspirin-induced gastritis), B (ask that she stop taking aspirin and call you in 10 days if the bleeding persists), C (reassure her and tell her that the bleeding will resolve spontaneously), and D (recommend immediate surgery) are incorrect. Brisk bleeding from the upper gastrointestinal tract can result in fresh blood per rectum, and the patient usually has signs of shock. Emergency surgery is generally not indicated for hemorrhoidal bleed.

42. **A** (the patient requires a stat spine surgery consult) is correct. This patient's history and physical indicate possible cauda equina syndrome, which is a surgical emergency. Fracture, disk herniation, infection, and tumor can cause sudden compression of nerve roots, causing significant neurologic compromise. Patients can have decreased anal sphincter tone, urinary retention, erectile dysfunction, and saddle anesthesia. Neurologic symptoms can be rapidly progressive. Patients often complain of paresthesia and inability to ambulate because of weakness. Patients should be immediately referred to a spine specialist for an emergency evaluation as prolonged nerve compression can lead to permanent deficits. An emergent MRI is the imaging modality of choice. Treatment often requires surgical decompression.

  B (the patient should be admitted to the medicine service for observation, rehydration, and serial examinations), **C** (the patient should undergo a workup for malignancy), **D** (the patient should undergo an MRI within 48 hours), and **E** (no further evaluation is required until the patient's laboratory tests are reviewed, including muscle enzyme evaluation) are incorrect. See the explanation for option A.

43. **C** (urine toxicology screen) is correct. This is a common presentation of recreational drug abuse. The prevalence of drug abuse is increasing in metropolitan areas in men and women alike. Mood changes, including bouts of anger, being withdrawn and uncommunicative, decreased motivation,

deterioration in the quality of work, a change in friends, becoming deceitful, and having problems with cash flow are some telltale signs.

  A (inpatient psychiatric hospitalization for suicidal ideation), **B** (combination of antipsychotic and antidepressant medications), **D** (obtain collateral history from her friends), and **E** (none of the above) are incorrect. This patient gives no history of depression, so medications for depression are not indicated. Speaking with her friends will be unhelpful because they themselves are likely to be using recreational drugs and will therefore not betray their friend.

44. **D** (an antecedent viral respiratory infection) is correct. Most sinusitis and rhinitis is viral, with a small percentage of patients developing a secondary bacterial infection. A history of viral upper respiratory infection would be most useful.

  A (yellow-green rhinorrhea) is incorrect. Purulent rhinorrhea is the result of breakdown of the nasal mucosa by either viral or bacterial infections and is a poor indicator of bacterial etiology.

  B (symptoms for greater than 5 days) is incorrect. A typical viral rhinitis may last for 7 to 10 days, so symptoms beyond 5 days would not necessarily indicate acute bacterial sinusitis.

  C (low-grade fever) is incorrect. Low-grade fever is not specific for acute bacterial sinusitis.

  E (the presence of an otitis media as well) is incorrect. See the explanation for option D.

45. **E** (acute aortic dissection) is correct. The chest pain radiating to the back, the difference in blood pressure readings in the upper extremities, and the diastolic murmur in the aortic area indicative of aortic regurgitation are highly suggestive of an aortic dissection.

A (an acute coronary syndrome) is incorrect. Although central chest pain occurs with ACS, radiation to the back is uncommon. Also, blood pressure difference in the upper extremities is not present. If a new murmur in ACS is heard, it is likely due to mitral regurgitation secondary to papillary muscle rupture or ischemia.

B (acute pulmonary embolus) is incorrect. Pulmonary embolus may cause chest tightness but not severe chest pain. When present, chest pain is pleuritic and indicates peripheral pulmonary infarction resulting in a pleuritic reaction. The patient is also usually short of breath.

C (left-sided pneumothorax) is incorrect. Spontaneous pneumothorax typically occurs in young (20- to 30-year-old) men who are tall and smokers with subpleural blebs. All individuals who develop a pneumothorax usually have an underlying lung disease.

D (esophageal rupture) is incorrect. The pain is severe and constant but upper extremity differences in blood pressure are not a feature. Forceful vomiting or retching often precedes chest pain.

46. **C** (*Chlamydia trachomatis*) is correct. Women with tubal factor infertility apparently induced by past episodes of PID often give no history of PID. In addition, up to one third of women without a history of PID harbor persistent *Chlamydia trachomatis* in the upper genital tract, despite the absence of clinical findings except infertility. Most cases of PID are secondary to *C. trachomatis* or *N. gonorrhoeae*. PID is frequently a result of mixed infection with facultative, anaerobic, and sexually transmitted pathogens, including group B streptococci, *H. influenzae, G. vaginalis,* anaerobes, and genital mycoplasmas (*M. hominis, U. urealyticum*). Upper genital tract infections can also be caused by hematogenous dissemination of

Mycobacterium tuberculosis, contiguous spread from intra-abdominal sepsis, and ascending infection from IUDs or postsurgical instrumentation. Approximately 30% of women with chlamydial infection will develop PID if left untreated.

A (*Trichomonas vaginalis*) is incorrect. *Trichomonas vaginalis* is a flagellated protozoan that causes the sexually transmitted infection trichomoniasis. Classic signs and symptoms include a purulent, malodorous discharge with associated burning, pruritus, dysuria, frequency, and dyspareunia. Physical examination often reveals erythema of the vulva and vaginal mucosa; the classic green-yellow frothy discharge is observed in 10% to 30% of affected women. Punctate hemorrhages may be visible on the vagina and cervix. Treatment is by oral or intravaginal metronidazole. The partner should also be treated. The woman should be screened for HIV, hepatitis B and C, and syphilis.

B (*Gardnerella vaginalis*) is incorrect. Bacterial vaginosis is more common among women with pelvic inflammatory disease, but has not shown to be independently responsible for this disease. Three of the four criteria (Amstel criteria) are necessary for diagnosis. They include: grayish white discharge; vaginal pH greater than 4.5; positive whiff-amine test, defined as the presence of a fishy odor when 10% KOH is added to vaginal discharge samples and the presence of clue cells on saline wet mount. Bacterial vaginosis infection during pregnancy can increase the risk of preterm labor. However, routine screening in all pregnant women is not recommended. Treatment is by oral metronidazole (oral or intravaginal clindamycin can be used in pregnancy).

D (*Neisseria gonorrhoeae*) is incorrect. Although PID due to *N. gonorrhoeae* infection may be more acutely symptomatic, PID due to *C.*

trachomatis tends to be associated with higher rates of subsequent infertility.

E (*Treponema pallidum*) is incorrect. Treponema pallidum is the spirochete that causes syphilis. It is not a causative organism implicated in PID.

47. **A** (urine culture) is correct. Acute bacterial prostatitis is uncommon but characterized by the rapid onset of high fever, chills, dysuria, frequency, hesitancy, low back pain, and perineal discomfort. Fever is common and the patient may appear septic. A rectal examination shows a swollen, tender prostate; epididymitis may also be present. A UA and a urine culture should be collected. Because cystitis often accompanies prostatitis, a urine culture and sensitivity will usually reveal the offending organism. Oral TMP-SMZ or fluoroquinolone (FQ) should be started empirically. If the patient appears septic, IV FQ and gentamicin should be started. Antibiotic therapy should be tailored to the sensitivities from the culture and continued for 4 weeks.

C (prostate examination) is incorrect. Prostatic massage is contraindicated with acute bacterial prostatitis, due to the risk of bacteremia.

B (renal ultrasound), **D** (blood cultures), and **E** (CT scan of the abdomen) are incorrect. See explanation for option A.

48. **C** (allogeneic bone marrow transplant) is correct. As with acute myeloid leukemia, patients with acute lymphatic leukemia require induction chemotherapy, which usually includes vincristine, daunorubicin, and prednisone. The presence of the chromosomal marker t(9,22) in a patient with acute lymphatic leukemia carries a poor prognosis. The only potential for cure in these patients is allogeneic bone marrow transplant.

A (start consolidation chemotherapy) and **B** (no further treatment necessary until she relapses) are incorrect. See explanation for option C.

D (radiation therapy) is incorrect. Radiation therapy has a role in preventing CNS relapse in acute lymphatic leukemia.

E (start rituximab) is incorrect. Rituximab is a monoclonal antibody against CD-20 that is used in the treatment of non-Hodgkin's lymphoma.

49. **E** (the lesions are nontender to palpation) is correct. This clinical scenario indicates the patient has erythema multiforme. The prodrome of fever and cold sores indicates that she had a preceding HSV infection, which is a common cause of erythema multiforme. The skin rash appears as crops of erythematous lesions with acral distribution. Lesions can have dusky centers and appear targetoid. The centers may show blistering. The eruption is usually asymptomatic, although some patients may report mild itching.

A (the condition is mostly elicited by an allergic reaction) is incorrect. As discussed in option E, the condition is a self-limited mild reaction to a preceding infection. Unlike erythema multiforme, Stevens-Johnson syndrome and toxic epidermal necrolysis are reactions of the skin, which involve the mucous membranes, as well as the skin in a more severe form. These are seen as a reaction to medications in 80% to 95% of the patients.

B (oral corticosteroids are proved to improve the condition) is incorrect. There are no trials to support the use of oral corticosteroids in erythema multiforme.

C (mucosal lesions heal with scarring) is incorrect. In mild erythema multiforme, the mucosal lesions heal without scarring, unlike severe forms such as toxic epidermal necrolysis, which heals with scarring.

D (among infections, EBV is the most common precipitating agent) is incorrect. See preceding discussion. Among infections, herpes simplex virus is the most common preceding infection.

50. **C** (a factitious disorder) is correct. Hypoglycemia associated with elevated insulin and a low C-peptide is associated with exogenous insulin (often surreptitious) use.

A (insulinoma), **B** (glucagonoma), and **E** (MEN I) are incorrect. Hypoglycemia associated with elevated insulin and C-peptide levels may be caused by an insulinoma (alone or with MEN I) or insulin secretagogues such as the sulfonylureas. In the latter case drug substitution is always a consideration.

D (new onset diabetes mellitus) is incorrect. New onset diabetes generally does not present with hypoglycemia.

questions

DIRECTIONS: Each numbered item or incomplete statement is followed by several options. Select the best answer to each question. Some options may be partially correct, but there is only **ONE BEST** answer.

1. Atrial fibrillation is the most common atrial arrhythmia. It is associated with all of the following *except:*
   A. A pulse deficit
   B. Thyrotoxicosis
   C. Pulmonary embolus
   D. Atrial septal defects
   E. Calcium channel blocker use

2. An 18-year-old man presents to your office for an urgent visit with complaints of a 20-pound weight loss over several months, shortness of breath, paroxysmal nocturnal dyspnea, orthopnea, and palpitations. On examination you note an irregular heart rhythm, as well as lid lag and retraction. ECG confirms your suspicion of atrial fibrillation with a rate of 112 bpm. What is the drug of choice in this situation?
   A. Amiodarone
   B. Methimazole
   C. Furosemide
   D. Warfarin
   E. Levothyroxine

3. A 32-year-old male respiratory therapist comes for a physical examination prior to starting a new job at a nursing home in October. He has never had chickenpox but has received all his routine childhood immunizations. His last tetanus booster was 12 years ago. A screening test for varicella and hepatitis B reveals no antibodies. Which vaccinations should he receive?

   A. Tetanus, hepatitis B, influenza
   B. Tetanus, hepatitis B, influenza, *S. pneumoniae*
   C. Tetanus, hepatitis B, *S. pneumoniae,* varicella
   D. Hepatitis B, varicella, influenza
   E. Tetanus, hepatitis B, influenza, varicella

4. A 50-year-old obese man without a significant past medical history presents to the emergency room with severe pain in his right great toe, which began yesterday and rapidly worsened overnight. He has just returned from a business trip, and admits to drinking several beers per day while on his trip. The right great toe is warm, erythematous, swollen, and tender to palpation. A basic chemistry panel and complete blood count are normal. The synovial fluid shows negatively birefringent needle-shaped crystals under polarized light microscopy. Cultures are pending. What is the most appropriate initial therapy?
   A. Oral corticosteroids
   B. Probenecid
   C. Allopurinol
   D. Indomethacin

5. A 54-year-old postmenopausal woman who has never been on hormone therapy comes to you complaining of vaginal dryness and painful intercourse. She has a past medical history significant for a deep vein thrombosis of her right lower extremity after cholecystectomy 10

years ago. She has also been told that her HDL cholesterol is low and her triglycerides are elevated; she is adopting diet and exercise changes for these. Her father died of coronary artery disease at the age of 44; he was a smoker. She also gets hot flashes, especially at night, but she manages to cope with this by wearing light clothing and lowering the ambient temperature in the room. She has occasional episodes of urinary incontinence when she coughs or sneezes. Physical examination reveals atrophic vaginal changes. Urinary dipstick is negative for infection. What is her best management option for the vaginal atrophy?

A. Vaginal cream containing estrogen
B. Oral cyclic estrogen-progesterone therapy
C. Transdermal estrogens
D. Selective serotonin reuptake inhibitors
E. Estrogen-containing vaginal cream with oral progestins for 12 days of the month

6. A 14-year-old girl presents to the emergency department after being bitten by an animal, probably a raccoon by report, while camping out in her backyard. Her father is very concerned about rabies. Which of the following statements concerning rabies is correct?

A. Rabies represents a meningitis that is caused by a rhabdovirus following a bite from an infected animal.
B. Dogs are a common vector in the United States.
C. Once the diagnosis is considered, rabies is fairly easy to diagnose.
D. The incubation period is generally 1 to 3 months.
E. Once a clinical diagnosis of rabies is made, the prognosis is favorable.

7. A 7-year-old boy presents to his pediatrician's office with a 1-week history of low-grade fever, sore throat, and cough. Physical examination demonstrates faint bibasilar crackles. Chest x-ray demonstrates bilateral interstitial infiltrates. Which is the most likely causative organism?

A. *Streptococcus pneumoniae*
B. *Mycoplasma pneumoniae*

C. *Staphylococcus aureus*
D. *Haemophilus influenzae*
E. *Escherichia coli*

8. A 25-year-old man presents with low back pain, which has gradually progressed over the past 6 months. He initially attributed the pain to a prior football injury. He notes stiffness in the morning lasting for over an hour, but feels better after exercise or with ibuprofen. He takes no other medications. Regarding his social history, he is currently looking for work. He never finished college, but is thinking of going back "at the right time." He is living with his girlfriend and denies tobacco or drug use, but does admit to drinking 8 to 10 beers over the weekends. Physical examination shows moderately decreased range of motion in the lumbar spine. What is likely to be most helpful in confirming the diagnosis?

A. Sacroiliac x-rays
B. MRI of the lumbar spine
C. Trial of oral corticosteroids
D. Trial of intra-articular corticosteroids
E. No further workup is necessary.

9. You are currently rotating on the neurology consult service. You are called to see a patient following a cardiopulmonary arrest. Circulation was restored after 30 minutes of resuscitory efforts. The patient is now in the intensive care unit and intubated. He is a 65-year-old man and has an extensive history of coronary heart disease with coronary stenting. His pre-arrest ejection fraction was 35%. His pulse is 65 bpm and his blood pressure is 135/84 mm Hg. He does not require any blood pressure support. You are asked to evaluate the patient for hypoxic ischemic coma and brain death. Which of the following examination findings can persist despite brain death?

A. Corneal reflexes
B. Respiratory effort on cessation of mechanical ventilation
C. Withdrawal from noxious stimuli
D. Oculocephalic reflexes
E. Deep tendon or stretch reflexes

10. A 25-year-old 8th grade schoolteacher and mother of a child in daycare presents to your office with a unilateral red eye, 5 days after her son began topical ocular antibiotics for a bilateral red eye. She has a 10-year history of migraine headaches, for which she needs to take a triptan medication about once a month. Her husband is a construction worker with a history of alcohol abuse. Although her vision is not decreased, there is significant mucopurulent discharge. Her son had resolution of symptoms in 2 days. What is the most likely diagnosis?
A. Bacterial conjunctivitis
B. Viral epidemic conjunctivitis
C. Herpes simplex virus conjunctivitis
D. Fungal conjunctivitis
E. Allergic conjunctivitis

11. A 21-year-old man comes to the office with complaint of constant worrying about germs and fear of getting contaminated for the last year. He reports that his symptoms have progressively worsened to the point where he bathes seven or eight times a day and is afraid of going out of the house. His past medical history is significant for allergic rhinitis, but he is not taking any medications, because he "doesn't like medicine." He is a junior in a local community college studying finance. He reports that his grades are good. He is currently living at home with his parents, and he denies any tobacco, alcohol, or drug use. What is the most likely diagnosis?
A. Major depression
B. Schizophrenia
C. Social phobia
D. Antisocial personality disorder
E. Obsessive compulsive personality disorder

12. A 12-year-old boy presents to your clinic for evaluation of low back pain. The patient has noted pain for the past several months. He denies any acute injury, but does note increasing pain when he participates in gymnastics practice. The patient did take a few weeks off from practice, but the pain returned shortly after resumption. Physical examination is remarkable

for decreased flexibility of his hamstrings bilaterally. His back pain is exacerbated with extension but not flexion. Minimal muscle spasm is present. Straight leg raise is negative. His neurologic examination is normal. What is the most likely cause of this patient's back pain?
A. Osteoarthritis of the facet joints
B. Cauda equina syndrome
C. Spinal stenosis
D. Spondylolysis
E. Mechanical low back pain

13. A 35-year-old woman is evaluated 3 days after she passed a kidney stone following 2 days of right-sided renal colic. She has a 12-year history of recurrent episodes of calcium oxalate kidney stones. At age 15, she developed Crohn's disease. Current laboratory studies show a creatinine 1.1 mg/dL, sodium 141 mEq/L, potassium 2.8 mEq/L, chloride 112 mEq/L, bicarbonate 19 mEq/L. A urinalysis was remarkable for a specific gravity of 1.015, pH 6.5, 2+ heme, no protein, 5 to 10 RBC/hpf.

A plain x-ray of the abdomen and pelvis shows multiple 1-mm calcifications overlying both renal shadows. Which of the following is the most likely cause of the renal stone disease in this patient?
A. Idiopathic hypercalciuria
B. Cystinuria
C. Renal tubular acidosis
D. Struvite (infection) stone disease
E. Medullary sponge kidney

14. A 72-year-old man with a 75 pack-year smoking history has recurrent episodes of hemoptysis, cough productive of whitish sputum, and a 20-pound weight loss of 10 months' duration. He was recently diagnosed with small cell lung cancer and was started on cisplatin and VP-16. At his most recent office visit he was found to be febrile and was admitted to the hospital. Empiric antibiotic therapy is begun. Which drug interaction should you be concerned about?

A. Augmentin and VP-16
B. Amphotericin B and cisplatin
C. Piperacillin-tazobactam and cisplatin
D. Imipenem and cisplatin
E. Amphotericin B and VP-16

15. A 58-year-old woman is brought to the emergency department by the EMS. She was found to be confused and drowsy. She has been to your emergency department once before, and records indicate that she has hypertension, gastroesophageal reflux disorder, and major depressive disorder. There was no documentation of her medications during that visit. On examination her temperature is 37.5°C, heart rate is 104 bpm, BP 100/70 mm Hg, and respiratory rate 18. An ECG shows QT prolongation. You suspect that her presentation is the result of one of her medications. Which of the following medications is most likely responsible?
A. Lisinopril
B. Hydrochlorothiazide
C. Omeprazole
D. Amitriptyline
E. Paroxetine

16. A 46-year-old man presents with colicky abdominal pain of 2 days' duration. He also complains of nausea, and has noted some vomiting over the last 14 hours. His past medical history is unremarkable except for an appendectomy done at age 14 years. He appears in mild distress. His vital signs reveal a temperature of 37.3°C, pulse of 92 bpm, and BP of 130/84 mm Hg. Examination confirms the presence of abdominal distention and reveals hyperperistaltic bowel sounds. You recommend that he receive intravenous fluids and that any electrolyte abnormalities be corrected. What else would you recommend?
A. Saline enemas until clear
B. Placement of a nasogastric tube
C. Placing a rectal tube
D. A mesenteric angiogram to exclude mesenteric ischemia
E. Treatment with an oral rehydration solution

17. A 30-year-old woman presents with sudden onset of painful red nodules on both anterior shins. She is otherwise in good health, and her only medication is oral contraceptive pills. She denies any headaches, chest pain, shortness of breath, and abdominal pain. She works in the editorial department of a local paper. Which is the correct statement concerning her condition?
A. This condition is not associated with inflammatory bowel disease.
B. A sinus CT is an important part of the workup.
C. Males are up to six times more commonly affected than females.
D. These lesions do not ulcerate and scar.
E. Staphylococcal infections are the leading cause in children.

18. A patient who was previously diagnosed with bacterial sinusitis returns to your clinic in 4 months and is frustrated that she continues to have frequent purulent discharge, nasal congestion, postnasal drip, and cough. Which of the following best describes the etiology of acute and chronic sinusitis?
A. Most chronic sinusitis is due to penicillin-resistant *Haemophilus influenzae*.
B. Most acute sinusitis in adults is due to *Moraxella catarrhalis*.
C. Anaerobic gram-positive organisms cause most acute sinusitis.
D. Most chronic sinusitis is polymicrobial.
E. Most chronic sinusitis is viral in origin.

19. A 54-year-old woman is found to have a left-sided pleural effusion when she presents to her doctor's office because of shortness of breath. Pleural fluid analysis is as follows: pleural/serum LDH ratio is 0.8, pleural/serum protein ratio is 0.7, pH is 7.4. What kind of pleural effusion does this patient have?
A. Transudate
B. Exudate
C. Mixed transudate and exudates
D. Not enough information to comment on the type of effusion
E. Empyema

20. A 45-year-old man is seen the emergency room because of hematemesis. He has not vomited blood in the last 2 hours. He has a history of hypertension for which he takes HCTZ. He is an ex-smoker (10 pack-year history) and drinks one beer per day. He reports he has been having nausea, vomiting, and some diarrhea for the past 48 hours. This morning, he noticed some hematemesis. He didn't want to come to the ER, but he started to feel dizzy, and his wife brought him in. His blood pressure is 100/70 mm Hg and pulse is 110 bpm when lying flat and 80/60 mm Hg and 126 bpm when standing. What is the next step in this patient's management?
   A. Send blood for CBC and wait for the hemoglobin result before transfusing packed red blood cells.
   B. The patient has stopped bleeding so he can be observed.
   C. Place one large-bore intravenous catheter in each upper extremity, and start intravenous fluids.
   D. Send the patient for an urgent esophagogastroduodenoscopy (EGD).
   E. Pass a Sengstaken-Blakemore tube.

21. A 74-year-old man presents to the emergency department for evaluation of chest pain. He was previously healthy and has not seen a physician in 5 years. He relates that his chest pain started 30 minutes ago and is related to exertion but improves with rest. His pain was relieved after sublingual nitroglycerin was given by a paramedic. On physical examination, his blood pressure is 148/89 mm Hg and heart rate is 82 bpm. Cardiopulmonary examination is normal. Lower extremity edema is absent. Electrocardiogram is normal. Complete blood counts are within normal limits. His complete chemistry panel is remarkable only for a creatinine of 2.6 mg/dL. A review of previous laboratory workup reveals an old creatinine of 0.5 mg/dL. What is the most important next step in evaluating this patient's decreased renal function?

A. Obtain a renal ultrasound.
B. Calculate the fractional excretion of sodium.
C. Obtain urine microscopy.
D. Obtain x-rays of both hands.
E. Obtain a kidney biopsy.

22. A 14-year-old girl presents to the emergency department after a hot iron fell onto her leg. She denies other injuries, and a quick, focused physical examination confirms this. Her right leg has a well demarcated burn with an erythematous base and blistering. The area is tender to touch, and there are copious clear secretions. What degree burn is this?
A. First-degree burn
B. Second-degree, superficial burn
C. Second-degree, deep partial-thickness burn
D. Third-degree burn
E. Fourth-degree burn

23. A 2-month-old male infant was just diagnosed with a urinary tract infection after presenting with fever and irritability. The infant was admitted to the pediatric ward for IV antibiotics and subsequently improved (fevers resolved, repeat urine culture normal, and oral intake greatly improved). Prior to discharging the patient, the pediatrician wants to order diagnostic imaging. What specific imaging studies should the pediatrician order?
A. Imaging studies are not recommended.
B. Abdominal CT scan
C. Renal ultrasound and a voiding cystourethrogram (VCUG)
D. Plain films of the abdomen
E. Abdominal MRI

24. A 24-year-old primigravid woman at 30 weeks' gestation is admitted with abdominal pain for the last 4 hours. She has noticed a pinkish vaginal discharge. She is afebrile. A physical examination reveals uterine contractions occurring every 10 minutes. Fetal heart tracing is reactive without any decelerations. A pelvic examination reveals pooling of amniotic fluid in the posterior fornix and a positive Nitrazine test. A urinalysis and vaginal and cervical swab is

obtained. All of the following are appropriate measures in the management of this case *except:*
A. Administering antibiotics
B. Intramuscular betamethasone injections
C. Administering ritodrine
D. Abdominal ultrasound
E. Immediate delivery by intravaginal prostaglandin induction and intravenous oxytocin augmentation or cesarean section if this fails

25. A 45-year-old woman is in your office for follow-up. She was diagnosed with CREST syndrome (limited cutaneous scleroderma) 3 years ago. Recently she was found to have hypertension. You started her on an ACE inhibitor. She does not smoke or drink. Which of the following patterns of autoantibodies is the patient most likely to have?
A. ANA, dsDNA, anti-Smith
B. ANA, anti-Jo-1
C. ANA, anticentromere
D. ANA, anti-scl-70

26. A 38-year-old man presents to your office with an acute severe headache behind his right eye. It has recurred five times within the last 2 days and lasts 45 minutes each time. He has ipsilateral tearing and rhinorrhea. He is pacing around your office and hits his head against the door to alleviate the pain. He works as an accountant and is married with two young children. He takes no medication, and his past medical history is significant for a cervical "whiplash" injury 10 years ago due to a motor vehicle accident. He reports a history of intermittent headaches. What is the most appropriate first-line therapy?
A. Narcotics
B. 8 to 10 L of oxygen by nonrebreather face mask
C. Acetaminophen
D. Lorazepam

27. A 5-year-old boy comes to the emergency department after developing acute shortness of breath and stridor while at preschool. On

examination, the patient is in moderate respiratory distress, has stridor, and is noted to have swelling of the tongue and lips. The patient's vital signs include a temperature of 37.2°C, a heart rate of 120 bpm, and a respiratory rate of 26. What is the first step in this patient's management?
A. An immediate ABG to assess the degree of airway compromise
B. AP and lateral x-rays of the neck to identify a foreign body
C. Elective intubation for airway protection while assessing the cause of the patient's stridor
D. Subcutaneous epinephrine followed by intravenous steroids
E. Aggressive IV fluid resuscitation

28. A 50-year-old woman who grew up in South Asia comes to you for a physical examination. She is asymptomatic and felt she should see a physician because she is now 50 years of age. On cardiac examination, you hear a loud first sound, a loud P_2, and a mid-diastolic rumble. What condition does this patient likely have?
A. Aortic regurgitation
B. Aortic stenosis
C. Mitral stenosis
D. Mitral regurgitation
E. A small atrial septal defect

29. A 12-year-old girl presents to the emergency department with a few days' history of severe itching, mainly on her hands, feet, and axillae. Her past medical history is unremarkable, and she takes no medications. She has linear and papular lesions on examination of the affected areas. Her mother and younger brother also complain of itching. Which of the following statements regarding this condition is true?
A. Application of 5% permethrin cream is effective in this condition and safe in pregnancy.
B. Household contacts rarely need to be treated.
C. Oral ivermectin is considered to be nonefficacious against the organism.

D. A simple scraping of the lesions, when examined under the microscope, is rarely diagnostic.

E. Scalp and face are uncommon sites of involvement.

30. A 54-year-old female secretary who works in a hospital is currently receiving chemotherapy for her recently diagnosed metastatic breast cancer. Over the last 2 weeks she has developed pain, swelling, and mild erythema over her right thigh. A duplex ultrasound of the right lower extremity demonstrated venous thrombosis involving the right femoral vein and the right popliteal vein. What is the best management strategy for this patient?

A. Start heparin 5000 units subcutaneously twice daily.

B. Start heparin IV and bridge to oral warfarin; continue warfarin for 3 months only.

C. Start oral warfarin without bridging with IV heparin; continue warfarin for 6 months.

D. Start heparin IV and bridge to oral warfarin; continue warfarin indefinitely.

E. Give heparin IV for 3 months only.

31. A 65-year-old man presents to the emergency department in August. He explains that he worked on his car all day long, and probably did not drink enough fluids. He complains of feeling very hot. Vital signs show temperature 39.5°C, heart rate 98 bpm, BP 130/90 mm Hg, and respiratory rate 22. On examination, his skin is clammy. What condition is this patient experiencing?

A. Heat edema

B. Heat cramps

C. Heat syncope

D. Heat exhaustion

E. Heatstroke

32. A 55-year-old woman is brought to the emergency room by her husband. He reports a 5-day history of nausea, vomiting, and diarrhea. She has become increasing lethargic over the past day. Her past medical history includes type II diabetes (diet controlled), hypertension that is controlled by HCTZ, and osteoarthritis for which she takes naproxen as needed (at least a couple of times a week). Her blood pressure on initial evaluation is 102/65 mm Hg with a pulse of 98 bpm. She is very lethargic but answers questions appropriately in short sentences. A screening examination is nonfocal. Her laboratory results reveal a BUN of 100 mg/dL and a creatinine of 4.3 mg/dL. Which of the following statements concerning her acute renal failure (ARF) is correct?

A. A potassium level of 6.5 mEq/L would be an indication for emergent dialysis.

B. NSAIDs can cause acute interstitial nephritis (AIN) and her urine would reveal hematuria.

C. Her BUN/creatinine ratio is not consistent with a prerenal cause of her ARF.

D. A fractional excretion of sodium (FeNa) over 1% rules out a prerenal cause of ARF.

E. A heme-positive dipstick without microscopic RBCs in the urine is generally indicative of rhabdomyolysis.

33. A 75-year-old woman undergoes coronary artery bypass graft. On postoperation day 4, nurses note that the patient is not sleeping and appears to be talking to unseen people in the room. She does not know where she is or the time or date. She recognizes her daughter, but not the hospital staff. What is the most likely diagnosis?

A. Alzheimer's dementia

B. Delirium

C. Multi-infarct dementia

D. Stroke

E. None of the above

34. A 55-year-old man presents to you because he has gained 15 pounds. His wife complains that he has begun to snore excessively, and he episodically stops breathing when he sleeps. You confirm your clinical suspicion of sleep apnea by a nocturnal polysomnogram. The patient and his wife are now in your office to review the results of the testing. Which of the following statements is correct?

A. The prevalence of sleep apnea increases with age.

B. Morning headaches are not associated with sleep apnea.

C. A neck circumference greater than 15 inches in males is a clue that the individual could have sleep apnea.

D. All patients who snore have sleep apnea.

E. Sleep apnea does not cause pulmonary hypertension.

35. A 75-year-old man with a history of hypertension, diabetes, and osteoporosis presents for a 4-month follow-up appointment. His medications include metformin, ACE inhibitor, β-blocker, calcium, vitamin D, and alendronate. He is a retired medical worker. His wife of 45 years is present. She is concerned about a hand tremor the patient has developed, and is worried about Parkinson's disease. Which of the following statements regarding Parkinson's disease patients is correct?

A. Head titubation is an uncommon feature.

B. Micrographia is an uncommon feature.

C. Bradykinetic movements are not characteristic.

D. Postural tremor is more common than a rest tremor.

E. Most patients do not have a good response to carbidopa/levodopa initially.

36. A 58-year-old female presents to your office because of mild rectal bleeding and a burning sensation in the rectal region, associated with severe pain while defecating and immediately after defecating. This severe pain lasts about 30 to 40 minutes and is followed by a dull ache in the rectal region. Which condition does this patient most likely have?

A. Thrombosed external hemorrhoid

B. Anal cancer

C. Anal fissure

D. Internal hemorrhoids

E. Adenocarcinoma of the rectum

37. A 24-year-old gravida 3 para 0 woman with a history of a previous induced abortion and an ectopic pregnancy presents to the emergency room at 5 weeks' gestation with a history of left lower quadrant abdominal pain. Her vital signs are stable and pelvic examination reveals a closed cervix and no evidence of vaginal bleeding. She has tenderness corresponding to the pain but no guarding or rigidity. Transvaginal ultrasound (TVUS) does not reveal any intrauterine gestation. Her serum quantitative β-hCG is 1400 IU/L. What is the next step in the evaluation of this patient?

A. Culdocentesis

B. Transabdominal ultrasound

C. Dilatation and curettage

D. Laparoscopy

E. Repeat serum β-hCG and transvaginal ultrasound in 48 hours

38. An 8-month-old infant is brought to the emergency department with a 4-day history of fever, diarrhea, and vomiting. Initially, the infant was started on Pedialyte, but the mother became concerned that he was not getting enough nutrition and began giving the baby boiled skim milk for the next 48 hours. On physical examination, the baby appears irritable with a high-pitched cry. His skin has a "doughy" feel to it. The fontanel is flat, and his eyes do not appear sunken. He weighs 10 kg, and has a pulse of 130 bpm, blood pressure of 80/45 mm Hg, and temperature of 38°C. A serum sodium is found to be 155 mEq/L. Over what period of time should the fluid deficit be corrected?

A. 8 hours

B. 6 hours

C. 24 hours

D. 48 hours

39. A 69-year-old man presents to your office with complaints of fatigue. He has a history of smoking for 45 years, chronic obstructive pulmonary disease (COPD), and hypertension for 8 years treated with hydrochlorothiazide. His blood pressure is 105/68 mm Hg. His laboratory studies show the following:

Serum sodium   129 mEq/L
Serum potassium   3.2 mEq/L
Serum chloride   85 mEq/L
Serum bicarbonate   38 mEq/L
Arterial blood gas (on room air): pH 7.50, P_{CO_2} 50 mm Hg, P_{O_2} 70 mm Hg

Which of the following options best describes this patient's acid-base disturbance?
A. Respiratory acidosis secondary to COPD
B. Metabolic alkalosis induced by diuretic use
C. Primary hyperaldosteronism
D. Hyperventilation and respiratory alkalosis
E. Respiratory alkalosis secondary to COPD

40. A 24-year-homeless woman presents to a local medical shelter for a "check-up." She is currently an active IV drug abuser (IVDA) and works as a prostitute as a means to obtain her drugs. She is coming in today to make sure she is "clean." A screening physical examination reveals no abnormalities except for bilateral "track" marks related to her IVDA. Results of testing include: negative HIV testing, negative remote hepatitis panel, positive RPR (rapid plasma reagin), negative gonococcus and chlamydia, and a Pap smear that revealed ASCUS (atypical squamous cells of undetermined significance). What would the next step be?
A. Order an FTAB (fluorescent treponemal antibody-absorption test)
B. Order a VDRL (Veneral Disease Research Laboratory test)
C. Recheck her HIV test
D. Begin a course of oral penicillin therapy
E. Begin a course of IM penicillin therapy

41. When monitoring a patient on an HMG CoA reductase inhibitor, what should be checked periodically?
A. An electrocardiogram to detect coronary artery disease
B. Serum creatinine
C. Blood glucose
D. Creatinine kinase
E. Hemoglobin levels

42. A 26-year-old man presents to your clinic complaining of abdominal pain. The pain began today and is periumbilical in location. He feels very nauseated. He takes no medications but is a pack a day smoker. You are concerned about possible acute appendicitis. What are the classic symptoms of acute appendicitis?
A. Right lower quadrant pain
B. Nausea and vomiting
C. Fever
D. All of the above
E. Both A and B

The following applies to questions 43 and 44: A healthy 65-year-old white man presents to your office with complaints of bilateral red eye with associated foreign body sensation, burning, and a "heavy feeling" about the eye. The symptoms have been present for approximately 2 months without significant change. The patient notes a small "bump" is present in the lower left lid which was initially painful to touch but which is now smaller, firm, and nontender. The swellings have been recurrent. The patient denies any current exudative-type drainage but does have significant tearing in both eyes.

43. What is the most likely diagnosis?
A. Bacterial or viral conjunctivitis
B. Recurrent attacks of acute angle closure glaucoma
C. Herpes simplex keratitis
D. Blepharitis with internal hordeolum
E. Corneal abrasion

44. What would the best management for this patient be?
A. Routine bacterial culture of the eyelids followed by a 7- to 10-day course of oral antibiotics
B. Hot soaks to the eyelids twice a day with a topical gram-positive antibiotic ointment applied to both lids once a day
C. Viral culture of the eyelids
D. Herpes simplex virus culture of the eyelids

E. Send the patient home with a topical anesthetic four times a day with scheduled ophthalmology follow-up in 1 week

45. A 14-year-old high school girl presents to your clinic with complaints of bilateral knee pain. The patient reports pain for approximately 2 months. Pain is worse with squatting, going down stairs, and after playing soccer. She denies any injury. The patient is poorly able to localize the exact location of her pain. Physical examination is remarkable for bilateral crepitus with knee flexion. She has no effusion or instability of her ligaments. She has increased pain at extremes of flexion but none with compression of her meniscus. What would be the most appropriate next step in the treatment of this patient?
A. Reassurance
B. Immediate referral to a specialist
C. Bilateral MRIs of her knees
D. Long-leg cast of her more symptomatic knee
E. Tell her she has to quit the soccer team.

46. A researcher is investigating the use of a new serum marker, enzyme X, as a screening tool for patients at risk for lung cancer. A group of 2000 patients are enrolled and 1000 are found to have cancer. The presence of enzyme X is confirmed in 75 of the 1000 patients found to have cancer, but is absent in the remaining 925 with cancer. In the 1000 patients without cancer, enzyme X is positive in 100 patients, but not in 900 patients. What is the sensitivity and positive predictive value of enzyme X?
A. Sensitivity = 7.5% and positive predictive value = 43%
B. Sensitivity = 90% and positive predictive value = 43%
C. Sensitivity = 7.5% and positive predictive value = 49%
D. Sensitivity = 43% and positive predictive value = 88%
E. Sensitivity = 7.5% and positive predictive value = 90%

47. A 52-year-old man presents with left lower quadrant pain. You have been seeing him for the past 2 years for type II diabetes, which is diet controlled. His last HBA1C was 6.8%, and he has recently lost 15 pounds to decrease his weight to 225 pounds. His only medication is aspirin. He has never smoked, and only drinks alcohol once or twice a year. The pain has been present for 6 days. He rates it as a 6 out of 10, and it has increased over the last 24 to 48 hours. He also thinks he had a fever last night, and "just doesn't feel well." He reports some constipation, but denies any nausea/vomiting or urinary symptoms. You suspect he has diverticulitis. What is the procedure of choice to help confirm your impression?
A. Plain film of the abdomen taken with the patient lying flat
B. CT scan of the abdomen
C. Ultrasound of the left lower quadrant
D. Colonoscopy
E. MRI of the abdomen

48. A 46-year-old woman presents with proximal muscle weakness over the past 2 months. She was originally thought to have a viral infection, but her symptoms did not improve and she returned to her primary care physician. Initial workup included a CBC, BMP, TSH, and CXR, all of which were unremarkable. She is now seeing you for a second opinion. She denies any recent travel and has no pets. She reports no medication use. She does have Raynaud's phenomenon and describes a photosensitive rash on her chest and neck. Physical examination reveals a violet eruption on her upper eyelids and an erythematous papular rash over the anterior chest and neck. What laboratory tests are most appropriate to help support the diagnosis?
A. ESR
B. Creatine kinase (CK)
C. Antinuclear antibody (ANA)
D. Rheumatoid factor

49. A 28-year-old man walks into the emergency department complaining of chest pain. He refuses to speak to the triage nurse and demands that a doctor see him immediately. Vital signs are temperature 37.9°C, heart rate 98 bpm, respirations 16, BP 198/96 mm Hg. Physical examination reveals dilated pupils, epistaxis, and mild confusion. ECG shows sinus tachycardia. Which of the following agents should not be used in this case?

A. Metoprolol
B. Nitroprusside
C. Phentolamine
D. Diltiazem
E. Lorazepam

50. A 65-year-old previously healthy Irish gentleman has noticed a 15-pound weight loss in the past 4 months. He had visited Egypt 5 months ago, where he noticed occasional episodes of dysuria and episodic gross hematuria, which would resolve spontaneously. Three months ago he developed a dull persistent ache in his abdomen. A CT scan of his abdomen showed a complex right renal mass, which was interpreted as a possible clear cell adenocarcinoma. Staging revealed no invasion of the renal capsule or Gerota's fascia. There was no evidence of metastasis. What is the next best step in managing this patient?

A. Right radical nephrectomy alone
B. Bilateral radical nephrectomy followed by hemodialysis and renal transplantation
C. Right nephrectomy and systemic chemotherapy
D. Chemotherapy alone
E. Chemotherapy and radiation therapy

answers

1. **E** (calcium channel blocker use) is correct. Calcium channel blockers are used to control ventricular rate in patients with atrial fibrillation. They are, however, not the drugs of choice.

   A (a pulse deficit) is incorrect. Pulse deficit refers to difference between the rate as counted by auscultation of the heart and by palpating the pulse. The ventricular rate, as measured by auscultation, is always higher.

   B (thyrotoxicosis), **C** (pulmonary embolus), and **D** (atrial septal defects) are incorrect. Thyrotoxicosis, pulmonary embolus, and atrial septal defect are all associated with atrial fibrillation.

2. **B** (methimazole) is correct. This patient's history and physical findings are consistent with hyperthyroidism. In patients who have hyperthyroidism from either Graves' disease or a multinodular goiter, methimazole is an oral medication that is used. A β-blocker would also be appropriate to help slow the heart rate and treat other hyperadrenergic symptoms.

   A (amiodarone) and **D** (warfarin) are incorrect. Amiodarone and warfarin are generally not needed because treatment of the underlying hyperthyroidism helps resolve the atrial fibrillation.

   C (furosemide) is incorrect. Furosemide may be needed if the physical examination or chest

x-ray demonstrates evidence of congestive heart failure.

   E (levothyroxine) is incorrect. The addition of levothyroxine would only worsen the situation.

3. **E** (tetanus, hepatitis B, influenza, varicella) is correct. Health care workers should be vaccinated against varicella if they never had the disease nor antibodies, as well as hepatitis B and annually for influenza. All patients should receive a tetanus booster every 10 years. Although high-risk patients should be vaccinated for pneumococcus, it is not routinely indicated for health care workers unless they have risk factors which include diabetes, alcoholism, cardiovascular disease, chronic pulmonary disease, and those who are immunosuppressed.

   A (tetanus, hepatitis B, influenza), **B** (tetanus, hepatitis B, influenza, *S. pneumoniae*), **C** (tetanus, hepatitis B, *S. pneumoniae*, varicella), and **D** (hepatitis B, varicella, influenza) are incorrect. See the explanation for option E.

4. **D** (indomethacin) is correct. The patient has gout, based on the clinical history and presence of crystals. The drug of choice is indomethacin, although any other NSAID or colchicine is also appropriate.

   B (probenecid) and **C** (allopurinol) are incorrect. Antihyperuricemic therapy (allopurinol or probenecid) should not be initiated during an acute attack.

A (oral corticosteroids) is incorrect. Oral corticosteroids are generally not first-line therapy.

5. **A** (vaginal cream containing estrogen) is correct. This patient has atrophic vaginitis and the best benefit is provided by estrogen therapy. However, she has significant risk factors for oral estrogen therapy including a history of venous thromboembolism, elevated triglycerides, and a family history of coronary artery disease. Therefore, vaginal creams containing estrogen are her best option. Vaginal estrogen therapy will provide relief for her vaginal atrophy and urinary symptoms but will not help with her vasomotor symptoms.

B (oral cyclic estrogen-progesterone therapy) is incorrect. Oral cyclic estrogen-progesterone therapy contains higher doses of estrogen and progesterone and is not required. Also, they will induce cyclic bleeding, which may not be desired by most women.

C (transdermal estrogen) is incorrect. Transdermal estrogen has similar risks and benefits as compared to oral estrogen therapy. However, the risk for hypertriglyceridemia is lower with transdermal estrogen therapy, due to bypassing of the first pass hepatic metabolism.

D (selective serotonin reuptake inhibitors) is incorrect. Selective serotonin receptor antagonists are being used to symptomatically relieve hot flashes; they do not treat vaginal atrophy and urinary symptoms.

E (estrogen-containing vaginal cream with oral progestins for 12 days of the month) is incorrect. Progestin therapy for 12 days of the month is required with oral estrogen and transdermal estrogen therapy for endometrial protection in all women with an intact uterus. They are not required for most forms

of vaginal estrogen therapy because the systemic absorption and subsequent endometrial thickening are low. However, any woman who presents with postmenopausal bleeding while on vaginal estrogen-containing cream should always have an endometrial biopsy to evaluate endometrial disease.

6. **D** (the incubation period is generally 1 to 3 months) is correct. Rabies is an encephalitis caused by a rhabdovirus following a bite from an infected animal. Animal vectors vary geographically in the United States and include bats, skunks, raccoons, coyotes, and foxes. After inoculation, the virus travels retrograde along the nerves toward the central nervous system, where it replicates and disseminates. The incubation period is dependent in part on the distance the virus must travel to reach the brain, but averages 1 to 3 months.

A (rabies represents a meningitis that is caused by a rhabdovirus following a bite from an infected animal) is incorrect. See explanation for option D.

B (dogs are a common vector in the United States) is incorrect. Dogs are uncommon vector in the United States since animal vaccination was introduced, but remain a common vector in developing countries.

C (once the diagnosis is considered, rabies is fairly easy to diagnosis) is incorrect. No single simple diagnostic test is available. Saliva, serum, CSF, and neck biopsy (cutaneous nerve) tissue should be sent for testing after consultation with the state laboratory. Brain tissue from the animal should be tested, if available.

E (once a clinical diagnosis of rabies is made, the prognosis is favorable) is incorrect. Untreated rabies infection invariably results in death within a week after onset of clinical symptoms, usually from respiratory failure.

Bites from a potentially infected animal must be assessed for the need for prophylaxis.

7. **B** (*Mycoplasma pneumoniae*) is correct. This is the typical presentation for pneumonia caused by *Mycoplasma pneumoniae* or *Chlamydia pneumoniae* infection. In pneumonia caused by these organisms, the physical findings are less impressive than the chest x-ray findings, which often shows extensive infiltrates. A macrolide is the antibiotic of choice.

    A (*Streptococcus pneumoniae*) and **C** (*Staphylococcus aureus*) are incorrect. *Staphylococcus* generally causes pneumonia in a child who is recovering from a viral pneumonia.

    D (*Haemophilus influenzae*) is incorrect. Most pneumonias in children of all ages are caused by viruses such as the respiratory syncytial virus, influenza viruses, parainfluenza viruses, and adenoviruses.

    E (*Escherichia coli*) is incorrect. *E. coli* is not a common cause of pneumonia.

8. **A** (sacroiliac x-rays) is correct. The patient is a young man with some elements on history and physical examination that could be consistent with an inflammatory back pain, such as ankylosing spondylitis. A sacroiliac x-ray revealing sacroiliitis would help confirm the diagnosis. A positive HLA-B27 serologic test would also support the diagnosis.

    B (MRI of the lumbar spine) is incorrect. MRI may be helpful but is not the accepted standard for diagnosis.

    C (trial of oral corticosteroids) and **D** (trial of intra-articular corticosteroids) are incorrect. Trials of corticosteroids are not appropriate prior to establishing the diagnosis.

    E (no further workup is necessary) is incorrect. See explanation for option A.

9. **E** (deep tendon or stretch reflexes) is correct. DTRs persist despite brain death. These reflexes are part of the spinal circuit and do not require transmission to the brain.

    A (corneal reflexes), **B** (respiratory effort on cessation of mechanical ventilation), **C** (withdrawal from noxious stimuli), and **D** (occulocephalic reflexes) are incorrect. The remainder of the examination findings must be absent to declare a patient brain dead.

10. **A** (bacterial conjunctivitis) is correct. The significant mucopurulent discharge would favor a bacterial conjunctivitis, but it is certainly not diagnostic. If bacterial conjunctivitis is highly suspected, topical antibiotics can be started. Seven to ten days of treatment is usually sufficient. Never use an antibiotic-steroid combination, or steroids alone, as this may lead to significant complications, including the potentiation of herpes simplex virus as well as worsened bacterial and viral infections.

    B (viral epidemic conjunctivitis) is incorrect. Viral conjunctivitis usually runs its course, but may lead to serious sequelae. Treatment usually consists of keeping the eye clear of accumulating discharge, cool compresses, and contagious precautions. Topical antibiotics may be added for possible bacterial infection if the diagnosis is in doubt. Viral conjunctivitis can be contagious for approximately 2 weeks from the onset of symptoms. Patients should be advised to use prudent hand washing and to avoid sharing of towels or pillows.

    C (herpes simplex virus conjunctivitis), **D** (fungal conjunctivitis), and **E** (allergic conjunctivitis) are incorrect. See the explanations for options A and B.

11. E (obsessive compulsive personality disorder) is correct. This disorder is characterized by preoccupation with rules, cleanliness, and perfection in whatever the patient does, to the point that these concerns interfere with efficiency, personal relationships, and the ability to complete tasks.

A (major depression) is incorrect. In major depression, a depressed mood; crying; loss of pleasure in activites that previously were pleasurable; changes in appetite, weight, and sleep; lack of energy; feeling of worthlessness; and in severe cases suicidal thoughts are present.

B (schizophrenia) is incorrect. Schizophrenia is characterized by deterioration in the ability to function in society, delusions, hallucinations, abnormal psychomotor behavior, and disturbances in the form and content of thought.

C (social phobia) and D (antisocial personality disorder) are incorrect. See the preceding explanations.

12. D (spondylolysis) is correct. Spondylolysis is more common in children and adolescents than in adults. Males tend to be more affected than females. Spondylolysis is a fracture through the pars interarticularis of the vertebral body. It is most common in the fourth and fifth lumbar vertebrae. The defect is caused by repetitive trauma to the spine, and is considered more of a stress fracture than a direct traumatic injury. Patients who undergo activities that place them in extension or hyperextension are at risk. Symptoms are variable; ranging from completely asymptomatic to constant pain even at rest. Pain is localized to the lower back but can radiate to the buttock and posterior thigh bilaterally. Physical examination may reveal muscle spasm (especially the hamstrings) and point tenderness along the vertebral body. Pain is often exacerbated by lumbar extension and single leg stand. Muscle strength and neurologic findings are otherwise unremarkable.

A (osteoarthritis of the facet joints), B (cauda equina syndrome), C (spinal stenosis), and E (mechanical low back pain) are incorrect. See the explanation for option D.

13. C (renal tubular acidosis) is correct. This patient's history and current diagnostic studies are consistent with type 1 renal tubular acidosis (RTA) as the cause of her nephrolithiasis. Typically, the serum bicarbonate concentration is low and the serum chloride concentration is elevated, reflecting a nonanion gap metabolic acidosis. The urine pH is inappropriately alkaline (>5.5) in view of the metabolic acidosis, and hypokalemia is frequently seen. Type 1 RTA is associated with several systemic disorders, including IBD and Sjögren's syndrome.

A (idiopathic hypercalciuria) is incorrect. See explanation for option C.

B (cystinuria) is incorrect. Cystinuria is not associated with systemic acidosis, hypokalemia, or nephrocalcinosis.

D (struvite [infection] stone disease) is incorrect. Struvite stones are always associated with infected alkaline urine.

E (medullary sponge kidney) is incorrect. Medullary sponge kidney may be associated with nephrocalcinosis but does not usually cause metabolic acidosis or hypokalemia.

14. B (amphotericin B and cisplatin) is correct. Cisplatin is a nephrotoxic drug and causes damage to the proximal tubules. The renal manifestation of cisplatin toxicity includes oliguria, rising BUN, creatinine, proteinuria, hypokalemia, and hypocalcemia.

Amphotericin B is also nephrotoxic and therefore should be used with care in patients receiving cisplatin.

A (augmentin and VP-16), **C** (piperacillin-tazobactam and cisplatin), **D** (imipenem and cisplatin), and **E** (amphotericin B and VP-16) are incorrect. VP-16 toxicity is related to its myelosuppressive effects. Renal failure is not a common side effect of augmentin, piperacillin, tazobactam, or imipenem.

15. **D** (amitriptyline) is correct. Amitriptyline is a tricyclic antidepressant. It has marked anticholinergic effects. Adverse reactions include confusion, drowsiness, dry mouth, constipation, hypotension, arrhythmias, blurred vision, and urinary retention.

A (lisinopril) is incorrect. The side effects of lisinopril include hypotension, dizziness, cough, diarrhea, elevation in the serum creatinine and potassium levels, and angioedema. With an overdose, hypotension is the usual finding.

B (hydrochlorothiazide) is incorrect. Side effects due to hydrochlorothiazide are generally metabolic and include hypokalemia, hyponatremia, hyperglycemia, and hypercalcemia.

C (omeprazole) is incorrect. Omeprazole can cause headache, abdominal pain, nausea, vomiting, and in toxic doses hypothermia, sedation, and convulsions.

E (paroxetine) is incorrect. Paroxetine overdose can cause nausea, vomiting, drowsiness, and dilated pupils.

16. **B** (placement of a nasogastric tube) is correct. This patient probably has bowel obstruction. The most likely cause would be adhesions that most likely developed after the appendectomy. Besides adhesions, irreducible hernias such as inguinal or femoral hernias are

the two main causes of small bowel obstruction and should be sought on physical examination. The diagnosis is made clinically and can be confirmed by erect plain films of the abdomen or CT scan of the abdomen which will show air-fluid levels and distended bowel loops.

A (saline enemas until clear) is incorrect because there is no evidence that this problem is due to constipation or fecal impaction.

C (placing a rectal tube) is incorrect because there is no evidence that this problem is due to constipation or to fecal impaction.

D (a mesenteric angiogram to exclude mesenteric ischemia) is incorrect because the patient's age and the absence of risk factors of vascular disease render it unlikely that this patient has mesenteric vascular disease.

E (treatment with an oral rehydration solution) is incorrect because the symptoms are most suggestive of bowel obstruction, not gastroenteritis. Administration of anything by mouth is likely to provoke vomiting.

17. **D** (these lesions do not ulcerate and scar) is correct. Painful red nodules on the shins of a female on oral contraceptives indicate that she has erythema nodosum. This is a reactive condition that occurs in response to infections, drugs, inflammatory bowel diseases, and other conditions. The lesions heal with a bruise-like pigmentation. These lesions resolve without any scarring or ulceration. Other causes should be looked at if the lesions ulcerate or scar.

A (this condition is not associated with inflammatory bowel disease) is incorrect. Erythema nodosum can be associated with inflammatory bowel disease such as ulcerative colitis and Crohn's disease.

B (a sinus CT is an important part of the workup) is incorrect. A chest x-ray is an important part of the workup. Tuberculosis, as well as sarcoidosis, has been known to be associated with erythema nodosum. This may be a primary presentation of these conditions, which can be diagnosed on a chest x-ray.

C (males are up to six times more commonly affected than females) is incorrect. Females are three to six times more commonly affected than males. The average age at presentation is 20 to 30 years.

E (staphylococcal infections are the leading cause in children) is incorrect. In young children, streptococcal infections are a common preceding cause of the development of tender erythema nodosum nodules on the legs.

18. **D** (most chronic sinusitis is polymicrobial) is correct. Most chronic sinusitis is polymicrobial, so treatment should be directed toward broader coverage, including coverage for penicillin-resistant *Streptococcus pneumoniae.*

A (most chronic sinusitis is due to penicillin-resistant *Haemophilus influenzae*) is incorrect. *Haemophilus influenzae* is a frequent cause of acute sinusitis, but penicillin-resistant *H. influenzae* is not a frequent cause of chronic sinusitis.

B (most acute sinusitis in adults is due to *Moraxella catarrhalis*) is incorrect. *Moraxella catarrhalis* is a frequent cause of acute sinusitis in children, but is not a common cause in adults.

C (anaerobic gram-positive organisms cause most acute sinusitis) is incorrect. Most acute sinusitis is caused by *S. pneumoniae,* not anaerobes.

E (most chronic sinusitis is viral in origin) is incorrect. See explanation for option D.

19. **B** (exudate) is correct. If any of the following criteria are met, the patient has an exudative effusion: pleural fluid protein/serum protein ratio greater than 0.5, pleural fluid LDH/serum LDH ratio greater than 0.6, or pleural fluid LDH greater than two thirds the upper limits of normal of the serum LDH. All exudative pleural effusions should be investigated. Some causes of an exudative effusion are malignancy, tuberculosis, pulmonary embolism, trauma, and collagen vascular disease.

A (transudate), **C** (mixed transudate and exudates), **D** (not enough information to comment on the type of effusion), and **E** (empyema) are incorrect. See the explanation for option D.

20. **C** (place one large-bore intravenous catheter in each upper extremity, and start intravenous fluids) is correct. This patient has suffered a major upper gastrointestinal bleed. He needs to be rapidly stabilized. Giving intravenous fluids through large-bore catheters is appropriate until packed red blood cells are available for transfusion.

D (send the patient for an urgent EGD) is incorrect. An EGD should not be performed on an unstable patient.

E (pass a Sengstaken-Blakemore tube) is incorrect. A Sengstaken-Blakemore tube can be placed if the patient is actively bleeding. The tube placement requires a physician skilled in its placement. Intravenous somatostatin and vasopressin (now less often used) are more widely available and easier to use.

A (send blood for CBC and wait for the hemoglobin result before transfusing packed red blood cells) and **B** (the patient has stopped bleeding so he can be observed) are incorrect. See explanation for option C.

21. **C** (obtain urine microscopy) is correct. The first step in the workup of a patient with decreased renal function (decreased GFR) is determining if the renal failure is acute or chronic. For this purpose, it is essential to obtain prior levels of serum creatinine and results of urinalyses to assess proteinuria. Prior evidence of elevated creatinine and proteinuria will not be diagnostic of any specific condition but will point toward the presence of established chronic kidney disease rather than an acute process. If old laboratory values are not available, always assume the renal failure is acute. A urinalysis and urine microscopy can be vital in helping determine the underlying cause of the renal failure.

A (obtain a renal ultrasound) is incorrect. Renal ultrasound is a valuable tool to assess kidney size and exclude hydronephrosis; however, it would not be the next step is evaluating this patient's renal dysfunction.

B (calculate the fractional excretion of sodium) is incorrect. Calculation of the fractional excretion of sodium is a useful tool in the evaluation of acute renal failure (prerenal versus renal), but before proceeding with additional workup an attempt to distinguish acute from chronic kidney disease needs to be made.

D (obtain x-rays of both hands) is incorrect. Abnormal hand x-rays showing signs of renal osteodystrophy would be consistent with a history of chronic kidney disease, but a normal radiograph in this setting would be of little help.

E (obtain a kidney biopsy) is incorrect. Obtaining a kidney biopsy in this case would be quite premature, as less invasive testing has not yet been done.

22. **B** (second-degree, superficial burn) is correct. Second-degree superficial burns are characterized by pink to bright red discoloration, associated blistering and often plentiful exudates. They are painful and often associated with edema. These burns heal in 2 to 3 weeks without scarring

A (first-degree burn) is incorrect. First-degree burns are usually caused by the sun or a minor injury caused by a flame. The burn site is generally light pink, the surface is without any exudates with minimal edema. It is painful. These burns heal in a few days.

C (second-degree, deep burn) is incorrect. This type of burn has a pale or mottled pale appearance, the bullae tend to be small, the site is moist but less so then the second-degree, superficial burn with moderate edema. Pinprick sensation is diminished. These burns are difficult to distinguish from third-degree burns. The surrounding skin is very painful.

D (third-degree burn) is incorrect. The burn site is pale or charred and parchment-like, there is anesthesia, and the area is inelastic and leathery.

E (fourth-degree burn) is incorrect. The burn site is charred and often extends to the underlying bone or the muscles. It can be difficult to distinguish this from a third-degree burn.

23. **C** (renal ultrasound and a voiding cystourethrogram) is correct. A renal ultrasound should be ordered to ensure that the infant does not have any anatomic abnormality of the kidney. A vesicoureteral reflux is excluded by a VCUG. Infants with vesicoureteral reflux are prone to repeated episodes of urinary tract infections. These, in turn, can lead to renal scarring and ultimately to renal failure if the infections are not diagnosed early and treated appropriately.

A (imaging studies are not recommended), **B** (abdominal CT scan), **D** (plain films of the abdomen), and **E** (abdominal MRI) are incorrect. Plain films would not be helpful, and neither CT or MRI would give information about vesicoureteral reflux.

24. E (immediate delivery by intravaginal prostaglandin induction and intravenous oxytocin augmentation or cesarean section if this fails) is correct. This woman has preterm prelabor rupture of membranes (PPROM) and is most likely in preterm labor. In general, preterm delivery is the greatest risk to the fetus with PPROM at less than 32 weeks of gestation. This diagnosis of preterm labor is based upon clinical criteria of regular painful uterine contractions (four every 20 minutes or eight every 60 minutes) accompanied by cervical dilation and effacement documented cervical change (cervical dilatation more than 1 cm or cervical effacement of at least 80%). Antenatal corticosteroids and prophylactic antibiotics should be given. Antenatal corticosteroids promote pulmonary maturation in the preterm fetus and reduce the risk of respiratory distress syndrome of the newborn and intraventricular hemorrhage. Prophylactic antibiotics prolong the latent period between the time of membrane rupture and the onset of labor and significantly reduce the frequency of maternal and neonatal infection. Tocolytics are used to attempt to delay delivery 48 hours in women with preterm labor who are receiving steroids for fetal lung maturation. Abdominal ultrasound can be used either alone or as part of the biophysical profile to assess fetal well-being.

    When the pregnancy reaches 32 to 34 weeks, amniotic fluid is tested for fetal lung maturity. If mature, induction may be performed depending on the obstetrician. However, if testing suggests immature lungs, then manage expectantly until pulmonary maturation occurs. Earlier delivery would be indicated if the patient developed clinical evidence of infection or went into labor or the FHR testing was nonreassuring.

Antibiotic prophylaxis for possible GBS colonization should be given during labor in the absence of a documented, recent negative GBS culture.

    A (administering antibiotics), B (intramuscular betamethasone injections), C (administering ritodrine), and D (abdominal ultrasound) are incorrect. See explanation for option E.

25. C (ANA, anticentromere) is correct. This is the profile for limited cutaneous scleroderma.

    A (ANA, dsDNA, anti-Smith) is incorrect. This profile represents SLE.

    B (ANA, anti-Jo-1) is incorrect. This profile represents polymyositis/dermacomyositis.

    D (ANA, anti-scl-70) is incorrect. This profile represents diffuse cutaneous scleroderma.

26. B (8 to 10 L of oxygen by nonrebreather face mask) is correct. This is an example of cluster headache. These headaches typically respond to high-flow oxygen. Other first-line agents could include the triptan class of medications.

    A (narcotics), C (acetaminophen), and D (lorazepam) are incorrect. See the explanation for option B.

27. D (subcutaneous epinephrine followed by intravenous steroids) is correct. This patient is presenting with upper airway obstruction due to an allergic reaction. Patients with allergic reactions presenting with edema of the lips, tongue, and uvula are at risk for progressive airway compromise. These patients should immediately be given subcutaneous epinephrine followed by nebulized epinephrine, intravenous antihistamines, and intravenous steroids, as necessary.

    A (an immediate ABG to assess the degree of airway compromise) is incorrect. An ABG in this patient will not indicate the degree of airway obstruction, may be relatively normal until respiratory failure, and may delay appropriate treatment while you are awaiting the results.

B (AP and lateral x-rays of the neck to identify a foreign body) is incorrect. The patient's symptoms are not consistent with foreign body obstruction, so x-rays of the neck should be delayed.

C (elective intubation for airway protection while assessing the cause of the patient's stridor) is incorrect. The underlying cause of the upper airway obstruction is easily treatable, so intubation should be delayed if possible.

E (aggressive IV fluid resuscitation) is incorrect. See explanation for option D.

28. **C** (mitral stenosis) is correct. Rheumatic fever is endemic in parts of Asia, Africa, and South America. The pulmonary and tricuspid valves are rarely involved. The loud P_2 is indicative of associated pulmonary hypertension.

A (aortic regurgitation) is incorrect. The murmur of aortic regurgitation is typically early diastolic and best heard in the aortic area in expiration with the patient leaning forward.

B (aortic stenosis) is incorrect. The murmur is an ejection systolic murmur. When aortic stenosis is severe, the pulse is slow rising, the pulse pressure narrow, and the apical impulse is thrusting and displaced laterally.

D (mitral regurgitation) is incorrect. The murmur is a pansystolic apical murmur and may be associated with a thrill.

E (a small atrial septal defect) is incorrect. The second heart sound is fixed and widely split. The murmur is a systolic flow murmur across the pulmonary valve secondary to right ventricular volume overload.

29. **E** (scalp and face are uncommon sites of involvement) is correct. Severe itching mainly on the extremities and flexural areas, along with linear lesions, is suggestive of scabies. Another important clue is the involvement of other family members with similar symptoms. Scalp and face are uncommon areas of involvement in older children and adults. Involvement of the scalp and face can be seen in infants and immunocompromised individuals. A condition in which there is generalized involvement in the form of crusted lesions and infestation with numerous mites is termed Norwegian scabies. This is highly contagious, and in this case, there may be involvement of the face and scalp.

A (application of 5% permethrin cream is effective in this condition and safe in pregnancy) is incorrect. Permethrin cream 5% is an effective treatment for scabies and it has a low incidence of toxicity. It is preferred that a second application is done 7 days later to ensure complete clearance. Permethrin should not be used in infants younger than 2 months or in pregnant or nursing women.

B (household contacts rarely need to be treated) is incorrect. Household contacts need to be examined and treated. This ensures that there is no reinfection, because this condition is spread through close contacts and fomites.

C (oral ivermectin is considered to be nonefficacious against the organism) is incorrect. Ivermectin is an antiparasitic agent, which is effective against scabies mite. One or two oral doses are required.

D (a simple scraping of the lesions, when examined under the microscope, is rarely diagnostic) is incorrect. A simple scraping or shaving of the top of the linear burrows or papules, when examined microscopically, can demonstrate the mites, eggs, or fecal pellets and can aid in diagnosis.

30. **D** (start heparin IV and bridge to oral warfarin; continue warfarin indefinitely) is correct. The patient has deep vein thrombosis (DVT). She requires anticoagulation with heparin (given as an initial IV bolus followed by a continuous infusion) to maintain the partial thromboplastin time between two and three times the control value, and continued until 24 hours after the INR is elevated to two to three times normal as a result of warfarin.

A (start heparin 5000 units subcutaneously twice daily) is incorrect. This is only prophylactic anticoagulation and is inadequate in the treatment of DVT.

B (start heparin IV and bridge to oral warfarin; continue warfarin for 3 months only) is incorrect. Because the patient developed a DVT and has underlying malignancy (which results in a hypercoagulable state), lifelong anticoagulation is indicated. Low-molecular-weight heparin can also be used until the INR is in the therapeutic range.

C (start oral warfarin without bridging with IV heparin; continue warfarin for 6 months) and **E** (give heparin IV for 3 months only) are incorrect. See explanation for option D.

31. **D** (heat exhaustion) is the correct answer. Heat exhaustion is considered to be a precursor of a heatstroke and therefore should be treated aggressively. Dehydration is believed to be the underlying cause for many of the symptoms. In addition to the symptoms mentioned, the patient may complain of nausea, vomiting, and marked fatigue. Hyperventilation is common.

A (heat edema) is incorrect. This condition is characterized by swelling of the lower extremities when an individual travels to a hot environment. It is attributed to vasodilatation in the skin and muscles with associated venous stasis. These in turn lead to interstitial fluid accumulation in the lower extremities.

B (heat cramps) is incorrect. Heat cramps are involuntary spasms of major muscles, are very painful, and occur in individuals who are not used to intense activity. Dehydration and electrolyte imbalance may play a role. Body temperature is usually normal.

C (heat syncope) is incorrect. Heat syncope occurs in a hot environment. Dehydration is coupled with vasodilatation, which in turn potentiates loss of vasomotor tone and results in the syncopal episode.

E (heatstroke) is incorrect. In heatstroke the patient is usually comatose or delirious with an elevated body temperature (usually above 41°C) and hot, dry skin.

32. **E** (a heme-positive dipstick without microscopic RBCs in the urine is generally indicative of rhabdomyolysis) is correct. The dipstick is reacting to myoglobin in the urine that is seen in rhabdomyolysis.

A (a potassium level of 6.5 mEq/L would be an indication for emergent dialysis) is incorrect. Initial serum potassium of 6.5 mEq/L is very serious and would require aggressive workup and treatment. If initial treatment was not successful, or if the patient is anuric, dialysis would generally be indicated.

B (NSAIDs can cause acute interstitial nephritis and her urine would reveal hematuria) is incorrect. NSAIDs can be responsible for AIN, but the UA in such cases generally reveals WBCs, WBC casts, and less often eosinophils.

C (her BUN/creatinine ratio is not consistent with a prerenal cause of her ARF) is incorrect. This patient's BUN/creatinine ratio is >20:1 and consistent with a prerenal cause of ARF.

D (a fractional excretion of sodium (FeNa) >1% rules out a prerenal cause of ARF) is incorrect. An FeNa may not be accurate in patients who recently received diuretics.

33. B (delirium) is correct. Delirium is a confusional state with associated agitation, hallucinations, tremors, and misperception of sounds, sight, or touch. Not all of these components are necessary to make a diagnosis of delirium. It is important to determine the cause of the delirium, which may be neurologic, metabolic, or secondary to medications or infections. Delirium is common in the hospitalized elderly patient and is usually mutifactorial.

A (Alzheimer's dementia) and **C** (multi-infarct dementia) are incorrect. With Alzheimer's dementia the disease is generally slowly progressive and usually manifests itself initially as memory loss, without the episodic sudden deterioration characteristic of multi-infarct dementia.

D (stroke) and **E** (none of the above) are incorrect. See the explanation for option B.

34. A (the prevalence of sleep apnea increases with age) is correct.

B (morning headaches are not associated with sleep apnea) is incorrect. Morning headaches occur in about 15% of all patients with sleep apnea. The headache is attributed to hypercapnia.

C (a neck circumference greater than 15 inches in males is a clue that the individual could have sleep apnea) is incorrect. A neck size greater than 17 inches correlates better than the body mass index with the likelihood of sleep apnea, possibly because of the greater amount of soft tissue that can compromise the airway.

D (all patients who snore have sleep apnea) is incorrect.

E (sleep apnea does not cause pulmonary hypertension) is incorrect. Sleep apnea is a

well-recognized cause of secondary pulmonary hypertension. Also, there is increasing evidence that sleep apnea is associated with cardiovascular disease and low HDL.

35. A (head titubation is an uncommon feature) is correct. Head titubation is a common feature of essential tremor, not Parkinson's disease.

B (micrographia is an uncommon feature), **C** (bradykinetic movements are not characteristic), **D** (postural tremor is more common than a rest tremor), and **E** (most patients do not have a good response to carbidopa/levodopa initially) are incorrect. Micrographia, bradykinesia, rest tremor, and a good initial response to carbidopa/levodopa are all seen in Parkinson's disease.

36. C (anal fissure) is correct. Anal fissures are a common cause of minor degrees of rectal bleeding associated with severe pain. The fissure is a result of the passage of hard stools. Bleeding usually occurs after the act of defecation. Examination reveals a semielliptical defect in the anal skin extending radially. Most fissures respond to conservative treatment.

A (thrombosed external hemorrhoid), **B** (anal cancer), **D** (internal hemorrhoids), and **E** (adenocarcinoma of the rectum) are incorrect. See explanation for option C.

37. E (repeat serum β-hCG and transvaginal ultrasound in 48 hours) is correct. There is a high suspicion of ectopic pregnancy in this patient because of the historical features and the ultrasound findings. However, the serum β-hCG levels fall in the discriminatory hCG zone. The discriminatory hCG zone refers to the hCG level that distinguishes patients with intrauterine pregnancies in whom a gestational sac can be seen from those in whom it cannot be seen by transvaginal ultrasonography. The gestational sac may be observed by TVUS in patients with β-hCG concentrations above 1500 to 2000 IU/L. The absence of an intrauterine gestational sac at β-hCG concentrations above 2000 IU/L strongly suggests an ectopic pregnancy. However, the absence of an intrauterine sac is nondiagnostic when associated with hCG values below the discriminatory zone. These findings are consistent with an early viable intrauterine pregnancy or an ectopic pregnancy or a nonviable intrauterine pregnancy. A serum β-hCG concentration less than 1500 IU/L with a TVUS examination that is negative should be followed by repetition of both of these tests in 2 days to follow the rate of rise of the hCG. β-hCG concentrations usually double every 1.5 to 2 days until 6 to 7 weeks of gestation in viable intrauterine pregnancies. If the β-hCG concentration does not double over 48 to 72 hours and a repeat TVUS examination does not show an intrauterine gestation, then the pregnancy is nonviable, such as an ectopic gestation or intrauterine pregnancy is destined to abort. A normally rising β-hCG concentration should be evaluated with TVUS until an intrauterine pregnancy or an ectopic pregnancy can be demonstrated. A falling β-hCG concentration is most consistent with a failed pregnancy (e.g., arrested pregnancy, blighted ovum, tubal abortion, spontaneously resolving ectopic pregnancy). The rate of fall is slower with an ectopic pregnancy than with a completed abortion. Weekly β-hCG concentrations should be monitored until the result is negative for pregnancy.

A (culdocentesis) is incorrect. Culdocentesis is employed to detect blood in the cul-de-sac, a finding that can be easily demonstrated by transvaginal ultrasound. Blood often escapes from the fimbriated end of the tube with tubal pregnancy or may be the result of a ruptured hemorrhagic ovarian cyst. Therefore, a culdocentesis positive for blood does not confirm either tubal rupture or the presence of an extrauterine gestation.

B (transabdominal ultrasound) is incorrect. Transabdominal ultrasound is less sensitive than transvaginal ultrasound in early pregnancies and is unlikely to add much in this patient.

C (dilatation and curettage) is incorrect. Dilatation and curettage is not required until the diagnosis has been made.

D (laparoscopy) is incorrect. The patient is hemodynamically stable and a laparoscopy is not required in the current situation.

38. **D** (48 hours) is correct. The signs of irritability, tachycardia, doughy skin, and flat fontanel indicate moderate dehydration (10%) in the setting of hypernatremic dehydration. The classic history for infants presenting with hypernatremic dehydration usually includes a history of the infant's being given boiled skim milk or concentrated formula. These children will often appear clinically less dehydrated than children with hyponatremic dehydration. Hypernatremic dehydration is due to loss of free water. In such cases, the fluid deficit should be corrected over 48 hours so as not to lower the serum sodium too quickly in order to avoid cerebral edema.

A (8 hours), **B** (6 hours), and **C** (24 hours) are incorrect. See explanation for option D.

39. **B** (metabolic alkalosis induced by diuretic use) is correct. This patient's presentation is suggestive of volume-sensitive (contraction) alkalosis—relative hypotension and hypochloremia—most likely due to diuretic therapy. The primary acid-base disorder is metabolic alkalosis indicated by a pH >7.4 and an elevated serum bicarbonate.

A (respiratory acidosis secondary to COPD) and **D** (hyperventilation and respiratory alkalosis) are incorrect. See explanation for option B.

C (primary hyperaldosteronism) is incorrect. Primary hyperaldosteronism may also cause a metabolic alkalosis. However, one would expect a greater degree of hypokalemia (<3.0 mg/dL) in a patient with primary hyperaldosteronism who is also on a diuretic.

E (respiratory alkalosis secondary to COPD) is incorrect. The level of P_{CO_2} is appropriate compensation for the increased bicarbonate (not a primary disorder as seen in COPD).

40. **A** (order an FTAB) is correct. This patient's positive RPR without any physical signs or symptoms suggest latent syphilis. For secondary, latent, and tertiary syphilis, a rapid plasma reagin (RPR) or Venereal Disease Research Laboratory test (VDRL) should be performed; a positive result indicates that the patient has or has had syphilis. False positive results may occur in many disease states, so a confirmatory test (FTAB, the fluorescent treponemal antibody-absorption test) must be performed.

D (begin a course of oral penicillin therapy) and **E** (begin a course of IM penicillin therapy) are incorrect. The treatment for all stages of syphilis is penicillin. The recommended regimen for primary or secondary syphilis is IM penicillin (i.e., one dose of benzathine penicillin G); an alternative is doxycycline for 2 weeks. For latent syphilis, three weekly doses of IM penicillin or 4 weeks of doxycycline is sufficient. For tertiary syphilis, IV penicillin must be given for 2 weeks.

B (order a VDRL) and **C** (recheck her HIV test) are incorrect. See explanation for option A.

41. **D** (creatinine kinase) is correct. Statins can cause myopathy and affect liver function; therefore, it is recommended that creatinine kinase and transaminase levels be checked before initiating treatment and periodically thereafter.

A (an electrocardiogram to detect coronary artery disease), **B** (serum creatinine), **C** (blood glucose), and **E** (hemoglobin levels) are incorrect. Statins have no effect on the electrocardiogram, serum creatinine, blood glucose, or hemoglobin levels.

42. **D** (all of the above) is correct. Acute appendicitis results from obstruction of the appendiceal lumen, usually from fecaliths, fibrous bands, foreign bodies, parasites, or lymphoid hyperplasia. Appendiceal inflammation and edema cause increased wall tension, eventually disrupting blood flow leading to ischemia and ultimately to appendiceal perforation. The time from obstruction to perforation may be as little as 24 hours. The four classic symptoms of appendicitis are: right lower quadrant (RLQ) abdominal pain, anorexia, nausea and vomiting, and fever. However, less than one half of patients have typical signs and symptoms of appendicitis. Appendicitis usually begins as periumbilical abdominal discomfort, followed by anorexia, nausea, and often vomiting. After several hours, the pain usually moves to the RLQ due to regional peritoneal irritation.

A (right lower quadrant pain), **B** (nausea and vomiting), **C** (fever), and **E** (both A and B) are incorrect. See explanation for option D.

43. **D** (blepharitis with internal hordeolum) is correct. In blepharitis, the lipid glands within the lid may become plugged. This results in a deficiency of lipid in the tear film that normally lubricates and protects the ocular surface. Patients may complain of eye and lid discomfort including burning and itching, as well as a "gritty" sensation. Signs include eyelid erythema and edema, crusting or scaling of the eyelid margins, and a red eye. The glands may become secondarily infected, usually with staphylococci, leading to bacterial toxin production with associated ocular inflammation. Hordeola are acute bacterial infections involving the lid sebaceous glands or the lash (cilia) follicle. The onset can be rapid, and an inflammatory mass forms. Staphylococci are the usual offending bacteria.

A (bacterial or viral conjunctivitis), **B** (recurrent attacks of acute angle closure glaucoma), **C** (herpes simplex keratitis), and **E** (corneal abrasion) are incorrect. See explanation for option D.

44. **B** (hot soaks to the eyelids twice a day with a topical gram-positive antibiotic ointment applied to both lids once a day) is correct. Treatment of blepharitis requires patient education as to the chronicity of the problem and eyelid hygiene (warm washcloth compresses followed by gentle scrubbing). An application of an antibiotic-corticosteroid ointment may reduce the infectious and inflammatory components of the disorder, but this requires closer monitoring. If these measures are unsuccessful, oral doxycycline may be useful. A hordeolum points toward the lid margin and usually drains spontaneously, although its resolution can be hastened by the application of warm compresses, antibiotic ointment, and occasionally oral antibiotics.

A (routine bacterial culture of the eyelids followed by a 7- to 10-day course of oral antibiotics), **C** (viral culture of the eyelids), **D** (herpes simplex virus culture of the eyelids), and **E** (send the patient home with a topical anesthetic four times a day with scheduled ophthalmology follow up in 1 week) are incorrect. See explanation for option B.

45. **A** (reassurance) is correct. Patellofemoral pain is one of the most common types of knee pain in adolescents. Pain is localized to the anterior knee and is caused by overuse and irritation of the patellar facets (femoral condyles) and posterior surface of the patella. Patients report pain that increases with increased activity, stair climbing, squatting, and moving from the sitting to standing position. Females are more often affected than males. Treatment is aimed at reassuring the patient, anti-inflammatory medication, and physical therapy to strengthen the muscles surrounding the knee.

B (immediate referral to a specialist), **C** (bilateral MRIs of her knees), **D** (long-leg cast of her more symptomatic knee), and **E** (tell her she has to quit the soccer team) are incorrect. See explanation for option A.

46. **A** (Sensitivity = 7.5% and positive predictive value = 43%) is correct. Create a 2 × 2 table based on test results and absence or presence of disease:

	Disease Present	Disease Absent
Test positive	TP	FP
Test negative	FN	TN

Filling in the blanks, the test is positive in 75 with cancer (TP = 75) and negative in 925 with cancer (FN = 925); the test is positive in 100 without cancer (FP = 100) and is negative in 900 patients without cancer (TN = 900).

	Cancer	No Cancer
Test positive	75	100
Test negative	925	900

Sensitivity = patients with a positive test with disease/all patients with disease
= TP/(FN + TP) = 75/(925 + 75) = 0.075
= 7.5%

Specificity = patients with a negative test without disease/all patients without disease
= TN/(FP + TN) = 900/(900 + 100) = 0.90
= 90%

PPV = value of a positive test in predicting disease
= TP/(TP + FP) = 75/(75 + 100) = 0.428
= 42.8%

NPV = value of a negative test in predicting disease
= TN/(TN + FN) = 900/(900 + 925)
= 0.493 = 49.3%

B (sensitivity = 90% and positive predictive value = 43%), **C** (sensitivity = 7.5% and positive predictive value = 49%), **D** (sensitivity = 43% and positive predictive value = 88%), and **E** (sensitivity = 7.5% and positive predictive value = 90%) are incorrect. See explanation for option A.

47. **B** (CT scan of the abdomen) is correct. A CT of the abdomen will show evidence of diverticulitis and an associated abscess.

A (plain film of the abdomen taken with the patient lying flat) is incorrect. An erect film of the abdomen may identify air under the diaphragm if there is a perforation.

C (ultrasound of the left lower quadrant), **D** (colonoscopy), and **E** (MRI of the abdomen) are incorrect. MRI and ultrasound are not indicated.

48. **B** (CK) is correct. The clinical history of symmetrical proximal muscle weakness and the described rash is consistent with polymyositis/dermatomyositis. A markedly elevated CK (or other muscle enzymes) is a very helpful laboratory finding in diagnosing this condition. EMG and a muscle biopsy consistent with PM/DM would confirm the diagnosis.

A (ESR), **C** (ANA), and **D** (rheumatoid factor) are incorrect. Although both ANA and rheumatoid factor may be positive in PM/DM, they are not specific for PM/DM.

49. **A** (metoprolol) is correct. This patient likely has acute cocaine intoxication. Additional features of cocaine intoxication (which is a hyperadrenergic state) include seizures, dyspnea, and ventricular arrhythmias. The chest pain (which may not always predict an acute coronary syndrome), tachycardia, and elevated blood pressure are all suggestive. Using a β-blocker will allow unopposed alpha activity and can cause a hypertensive crisis or induce ventricular arrhythmias.

B (nitroprusside), **C** (phentolamine), **D** (diltiazem), and **E** (lorazepam) are incorrect. Lorazepam can be used to calm a patient and nitroprusside, phentolamine, and diltiazem can all be used to control the blood pressure. Phentolamine is the antihypertensive agent of choice.

50. **A** (right radical nephrectomy alone) is correct. The patient has stage I renal cell cancer for which a radical nephrectomy is indicated. Absence of tumor invasion of the renal capsule of Gerota's fascia is consistent with stage I renal cell cancer (RCC).

B (bilateral radical nephrectomy followed by hemodialysis and renal transplantation), **C** (right nephrectomy and systemic chemotherapy), **D** (chemotherapy alone), and **E** (chemotherapy and radiation therapy) are incorrect. There is no proven role for bilateral nephrectomy, adjuvant chemotherapy, or radiation therapy in stage I RCC.

Index

Note: Page numbers followed by f indicate figures; those followed by t indicate tables; and those followed by b indicate boxed material.